Attention mediates the way in which we experience the world around us. In this comprehensive and insightful text, the authors provide clear and concise explanations of the phenomenon, accessible to both the motivated student and the informed expert alike. If you want to understand the nature of reality, the insights in this book will enable you to do so.

—**Peter Hancock, PhD,** Provost & Distinguished Research Professor, University of Central Florida, Orlando, FL; Fellow, American Association for the Advancement of Science; Author, *Hoax Springs Eternal: The Psychology of Cognitive Deception*

With their broad experience and many contributions, Proctor and Vu have produced a lucid, comprehensible text that provides an excellent summary of attention writ large. This is a challenge because, from its simple, intuitive origins, attention has become an overarching concept reflecting the operation of several distinct mechanisms. This text succeeds by emphasizing their family resemblance and by detailing studies that illustrate how attention research is conducted and how the research methods and theory have co-evolved.

—**Charles E. (Ted) Wright, PhD,** Professor of Cognitive Sciences, University of California, Irvine, Irvine, CA

Proctor and Vu bring their encyclopedic knowledge of attention to bear in this comprehensive review of the subject. Any student of attention must keep this book by their side at all times. The work is invaluable.

—**David A. Rosenbaum, PhD,** University of California, Riverside, Riverside, CA

The book provides an insightful and comprehensive review and appraisal of the science of attention and its relationship to advanced information technologies. It is a must-have volume for all individuals interested in the subject matter of attention.

—**Gavriel Salvendy, PhD,** University Distinguished Professor, University of Central Florida, Orlando, FL; Member, National Academy of Engineering (NAE); APA Fellow

D0911902

ATTENTION

ATTENTION
Selection and Control
in Human Information Processing

Robert W. Proctor
Kim-Phuong L. Vu

 AMERICAN PSYCHOLOGICAL ASSOCIATION

Published by
American Psychological Association
750 First Street, NE
Washington, DC 20002
https://www.apa.org

Order Department
https://www.apa.org/pubs/books
order@apa.org

In the U.K., Europe, Africa, and the Middle East, copies may be ordered from Eurospan
https://www.eurospanbookstore.com/apa
info@eurospangroup.com

Typeset in Meridien and Ortodoxa by Circle Graphics, Inc., Reisterstown, MD

Printer: Gasch Printing, Odenton, MD
Cover Designer: Anthony Paular Design, Newbury Park, CA

Library of Congress Cataloging-in-Publication Data

Names: Proctor, Robert W., author. | Vu, Kim-Phuong L., author.
Title: Attention : selection and control in human information processing /
  by Robert W. Proctor and Kim-Phuong L. Vu.
Description: Washington, DC : American Psychological Association, [2023] |
  Includes bibliographical references and index.
Identifiers: LCCN 2022006531 (print) | LCCN 2022006532 (ebook) |
  ISBN 9781433833861 (paperback) | ISBN 9781433840456 (ebook)
Subjects: LCSH: Attention. | Human information processing.
Classification: LCC BF321 .P746 2023 (print) | LCC BF321 (ebook) |
  DDC 153.7/33--dc23/eng/20220614
LC record available at https://lccn.loc.gov/2022006531
LC ebook record available at https://lccn.loc.gov/2022006

https://doi.org/10.1037/0000317-000

Printed in the United States of America

10 9 8 7 6 5 4 3 2 1

CONTENTS

PREFACE

We all know that our ability to attend to events and thoughts and to act on them is limited. If you are reading this preface and attending closely to the content, you cannot attend simultaneously to other events that are happening in your immediate environment. When focused on a task, you tend to block out stimulation that is not relevant to your task goals, although you cannot do so entirely, and a sudden sound or other event may interrupt you. You can focus attention internally or externally and toward specific locations and objects. You can also attend to action goals or the movements of the body needed to accomplish those goals. If you initiate an action that you no longer want to complete, you can countermand it before execution is completed. These are all things that people can do by directing their attention, but exactly how these are done has been the subject of speculation and research from antiquity to the present.

Within psychology, attention was a foundational topic in the establishment of the field as a science. Wilhelm Wundt, who is credited with starting the first laboratory devoted to psychological research in 1879, studied attention, and William James provided tour de force coverage of attention in his 1890 book, *The Principles of Psychology*. Research on attention prospered through the early 20th century and then resumed a prominent role in the "cognitive" or "information processing" revolution in the 1950s. The initial research in the contemporary era was based on applications to military technology. However, it also provided the earliest theories of human information processing in adults. Moreover, attention has been studied across the life span with healthy individuals and in individuals with attentional disorders. Beginning in the 1980s, research on attention has been in the frontline of advances in cognitive neuroscience and human interactions with technology.

Earlier in this century, we noted a lack of accessible texts on the topic and tried to remedy that situation by writing *Attention: Theory and Practice* (2004), for which Addie Johnson and Robert Proctor were the coauthors, with guest chapter coauthors (Edward H. F. de Haan, Roy P. C. Kessels, Robert D. Melara, Mark R. Nieuwenstein, and Kim-Phuong L. Vu). Since then, more attention research has been conducted than in the entire history of research on the topic. Although many of the classic studies and basic principles of attention covered in that book are still relevant, it became clear to us that an expanded, augmented, and updated treatment was needed. Our goal for this book is to present a coherent, accessible view of research that falls broadly under the heading of *attention*, conveying the essential issues and major findings and relating them to interests of the readers. We provide sufficient details regarding experiments and theories so that the reader can follow and evaluate the results and conclusions. In each chapter, we cover the theories of attention and the behavioral research conducted to support or argue against them. Some of this research focuses on determining the underlying mechanisms of attention through performance, whereas other studies emphasize neural underpinnings. We provide a balanced view of current debates to encourage readers to think critically about the issues rather than strongly stating our own positions. Finally, the research is related to applications throughout the book.

The book is intended to be used as a text for upper-level undergraduate courses in attention and graduate-level courses or seminars on attention in particular or cognition in general. In addition, it should serve as a resource for basic and applied researchers in a variety of areas who want thorough coverage of what is known about this core aspect of psychology. Pedagogical features of the book include key points of facts, phenomena, and theories in the chapter summaries and boxes highlighting specific applications and implications of the research on attention described in the chapters.

We thank Addie Johnson for encouraging this updating of the prior book and the coauthors of chapters in the Johnson and Proctor book. We also thank Darryl Schneider for sharing some of his course materials with one of us (RWP). In addition, we thank Christopher Kelaher for encouraging us to propose and develop the book, Judy Barnes for her editorial development of the book, Erin O'Brien for her careful copyediting, and Ann Butler for her detailed work during the production process. Finally, we would like to acknowledge the two reviewers of our initial manuscript who provided detailed, constructive comments that improved the final manuscript.

ATTENTION

1

Historical Overview of Research on Attention

The topic of *attention*—how people select information for perception, cognition, and action—is arguably the core of cognitive psychology. Interest in attention predates the founding of psychology as a discipline in 1879 and was prominent in the work of the earliest psychologists. Many of the most well-known and widely studied phenomena relate to attention, and attention was at the center of the "cognitive" revolution in the 1950s, which led to its current prominence. The topic of attention is embedded within all areas of psychology. Moreover, given the ever-increasing information demands on individuals in contemporary society, due to the expansion of media and technology, the subject of attention is more relevant now than ever.

In today's physical, cyber, and social worlds, people are increasingly bombarded with various stimuli, only some of which are relevant to current goals. Just a few will affect our behavior, and even fewer will reach our consciousness. The information conveyed by the stimuli may not be consistent, and the multiple stimuli may each require a different action—actions that often are incompatible with each other. Think of driving in heavy traffic while operating the automobile's entertainment system, following driving directions from a navigation system, and engaging in a conversation with one or more passengers. Alternatively, consider the task of flying an aircraft. The pilot must process information from numerous visual displays and the outside world while listening to and talking with air traffic controllers and other members of the flight crew, selecting and operating appropriate controls, and being prepared to detect

https://doi.org/10.1037/0000317-001
Attention: Selection and Control in Human Information Processing, by R. W. Proctor and K.-P. L. Vu

and identify emergency warning signals. Driving and flying thus require selection among competing stimuli, the concurrent performance of several subtasks, and the monitoring of the environment for changes. How people select among competing external and internal stimuli and control their thoughts and actions in a manner to achieve goals is of central concern in the study of attention.

The topic of attention is a major part of contemporary cognitive psychology and cognitive neuroscience, as well as of a variety of other areas in psychology and the interdisciplinary field of human factors engineering. Processes encompassed within the category of attention play critical roles in essentially all aspects of perception, cognition, and action, influencing the choices you make. For example, when performing a task such as remembering the name of someone you have met only once before, you must process the retrieval cue (the person's face or who they are with) and then shift to evaluating the possible alternative names for retrieval. In a more complex task, such as deciding which car to buy, attention must be directed to the different properties that the new car should have, and the most important goals (e.g., staying within budget) must be kept in mind. As these examples illustrate, the study of attention should be of interest to anyone who wants to learn more about human behavior and cognition and gain insight into how selective processes guide their thought and behavior.

As noted, because of its relevance to much of human experience, attention has been of importance to the field of psychology since its earliest days. This research was first summarized in the book *The Psychology of Attention* by Théodule Ribot (1890), in which he distinguished a spontaneous (i.e., automatic) mode of attention from a voluntary one. Spontaneous attention is most fundamental and is caused by emotional states, whereas voluntary attention is built on spontaneous attention through education and training. Voluntary attention was presumed to be accompanied by a feeling of effort because of the need to inhibit and direct attention.

Eighteen years later, two landmark texts devoted to the topic of attention were published: Edward B. Titchener's (1908/1973) *Lectures on the Elementary Psychology of Feeling and Attention* and Walter B. Pillsbury's (1908/1973) *Attention*. These texts put the study of attention in psychology on a firm footing. Titchener included several laws of psychology, among which the *law of prior entry* is the most well known. According to this law, "the stimulus for which we are predisposed requires less time than a like stimulus, for which we are unprepared, to produce its full conscious effect" (Titchener, 1908/1973, p. 251). In the book, Titchener described the discovery of attention as one of three major achievements of experimental psychology to that point, stating, "the doctrine of attention is the nerve of the whole psychological system" (p. 173).

Pillsbury (1908/1973) provided a similarly strong assessment of the importance of attention, asserting that effects of attention "extend to every part of the physical organism, and are among the most profound facts of mind" (p. 1). The quotes of Titchener and Pillsbury make apparent the central weight placed on attention in the early days of psychological science and also, in part, why the topic of attention has continued to receive considerable research in this era: It relates to selection and control of perception, cognition, and action.

The history of research on attention can be broken up into six periods:

1. philosophic work preceding the founding of the field of psychology in the last half of the 1800s;

2. the period from the founding of psychology until 1909;

3. the period from 1910 until 1949, during which behaviorism flourished, and interest in attention waned to some extent;

4. the resurgence of widespread interest in attention during the period of the cognitive and engineering psychology revolutions from 1950 to 1974;

5. the experimental research on attention from 1974 to 1999; and

6. contemporary research with emphasis on cognitive control, multitasking, training, cognitive neuroscience, and applications dating from 2000 to the present.

In the sections that follow, we summarize the major research and theories of attention during each period. This historical context is essential to provide a foundation for the more detailed treatments of specific topics in subsequent chapters.

THE PHILOSOPHICAL PERIOD

Interest in attention began in the field of philosophy before the founding of psychology as a scientific discipline. Because the topic of attention was originally discussed by philosophers, many ideas about the nature of attention held today can be traced back to the views held by them (Posner, 2017). Among the issues they considered was the role of attention in conscious awareness and thought and whether attention was directed voluntarily or involuntarily toward objects and events. The characterization of attention provided by each philosopher reflected that individual's larger metaphysical view of the nature of things and how we come to know the world. We briefly describe the treatments of attention provided by a few eminent philosophers.

The importance of empirical investigation was emphasized by Juan Luis Vives (1492–1540) in his book, *De Anima et Vita*, in 1538. He is most well known for his views on memory (Murray & Ross, 1982), in which attention played a significant role. According to Vives, the more closely one attends to stimuli, the better they will be retained. Learning consists of the formation of associations, and retrieval from memory occurs through automatic activation of associated ideas or intentional, effortful search.

The first extended treatment of attention was that of Nicolas Malebranche (1638–1715) in his book *The Search After Truth* (1674/1980; see Berlyne, 1974). Malebranche held that we have access to ideas, or mental representations of the external world, but not direct access to the world itself. He considered attention to be necessary to prevent perception and ideas from becoming confused and to make some clearer by drawing attention to them.

The concept of *apperception*, introduced by Gottfried Leibniz (1765), refers to an act that is necessary for an individual to become conscious of a perceptual event. Events can be perceived unconsciously but will not enter conscious awareness without apperception. Leibniz emphasized a reflexive view of attention, in which attention is directed automatically to events and ideas that demand it (McRae, 1976). However, attention also has a voluntary and directed aspect (Leibniz, 1948/1985). Leibniz was a mathematician who discovered the differential calculus. Not surprisingly, he had the ambition of basing psychology and other sciences in mathematics (Klempe, 2021), a goal also of current quantitative modelers of attention.

From 1704 until his death in 1716, Leibniz corresponded with Christian Wolff (1679–1754) and had considerable influence on his thinking (Richards, 1980). Wolff published two books on psychology, *Psychologia Empirica* in 1738 and *Psychologia Rationalis* in 1740 (see English translations in Richards, 1980). He distinguished an empirical approach (introspection), which he argued would benefit from mathematical analyses, from a deductive, theoretical approach. Each book included a chapter with *attention* in the title (Richards, 1980). With regard to attention, Wolff (1740) also described several general properties that have been emphasized in subsequent textbooks (Hatfield, 1998, p. 5):

- The greater the attention, the smaller the part of the visual field to which it extends;

- with equally distributed attention, that part of a whole which otherwise is cognized most clearly will come to the fore; and

- conscious attention acts to combine spatial representations and temporal processes into ordered whole events in the part of the visual field to which it is directed.

Johann Herbart (1776–1841) agreed with Leibniz and Wolff that an event had to be apperceived to enter conscious awareness. However, he stressed that apperception involved relating newly perceived ideas to ones already contained in the mind (Herbart, 1824–1825). All new perceptual experience occurs in relation to prior perceptions. This apperceptive process occurs through associations among mental contents. Herbart also was the first person to apply mathematical modeling systematically to the study of psychology. The conceptual structure of his mathematical psychology was supplied by Immanuel Kant (1724–1804), specifically, Kant's view that knowledge of the observable world is a constructed mental representation (Leary, 1980). This view led Herbart to stress the study of the self as a dynamically changing representation composed of mental entities, mainly through introspections about experience. Whereas Kant was skeptical about the use of mathematics for understanding and predicting mental events, Herbart argued that a mathematical account could be used to predict the existence, magnitude, and duration of mental events (Boudewijnse et al., 1999).

A popular view in the first part of the 19th century was that people are incapable of attending to more than one thing at once. However, William S. Hamilton (1788–1856) argued that the span of attention is more than one object. He proposed measuring its size by throwing marbles on the floor and determining how many of them could be apprehended at once: "If you throw a handful of marbles on the floor, you will find it difficult to view at once more than six, or seven at most, without confusion" (Hamilton, 1859, p. 254). Jevons (1871) followed up Hamilton's idea for testing the span of apprehension and estimated it to be four items.

In summary, many philosophers and early psychologists gave attention a central role in perception and thinking. They introduced several issues that continue to be examined in contemporary research, such as the extent to which attention is directed automatically or intentionally. Although they conducted little experimental research themselves, their conceptual analyses of attention laid the foundation for the scientific study of attention in following years.

THE PERIOD FROM 1860 TO 1909

The philosophical analyses of attention led to some predictions that could be tested experimentally, as in Hamilton's work. Also, in the mid-1800s, psychophysical methods were being developed that allowed measurement of the relation between physical stimulus properties and the psychological perceptions of them (Fechner, 1966; Weber, 1846/1978). Thus, it was a small step to infer that attention can be investigated using an experimental approach.

Speed of Mental Processes

The first laboratory devoted to psychological research was founded in 1879 by Wilhelm Wundt (1832–1920), who was responsible for introducing the study of attention to the field. As a laboratory assistant in physiology at Heidelberg, Germany, Wundt became interested in the issue of the astronomers' *personal equation* (see Woodworth, 1938). This refers to systematic, individual differences between astronomers in their measures of the time for the transit of stars. Astronomers in the late 18th and early 19th centuries measured time by determining when the stars and planets crossed the meridian, using an "eye-and-ear" method (Sheehan, 2013). This measurement was made with a telescope that had an eyepiece equipped with a number of equidistant vertical wires (see Figure 1.1). The astronomer recorded the times at which a particular star crossed each of the wires by noting the distance of a star from one of the wires coinciding with two beats of a clock, heard immediately before and after the star crossed the wire. These times were averaged to find the time at which the star crossed the meridian. This method was generally accepted because it allowed comparison across different observatories.

FIGURE 1.1. Depiction of a Star Crossing the Wires in the Field of View of a Meridian or Transit Telescope

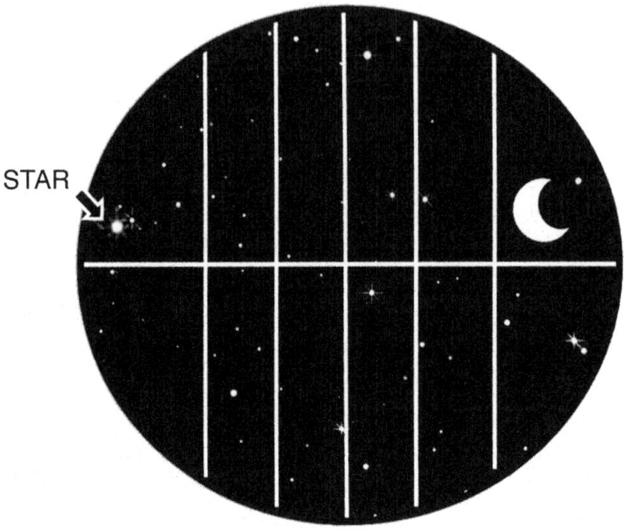

Nevil Maskelyne, then royal astronomer at the Royal Observatory Greenwich in England, noticed in 1795 that his assistant, David Kinnebrook, made measurements that were as much as 800 milliseconds (ms) longer than his own. Because this disparity continued into 1796, Maskelyne fired Kinnebrook for being incapable of making accurate observations. More than 20 years later, Friedrich Wilhelm Bessel (1784–1846), director of Prussian King Friedrich Wilhelm III's observatory at Königsberg, noted this incident. He then conducted a relatively controlled experiment in which he and a well-trained assistant made transit measurements on alternate nights for several nights using the eye-and-ear method for two sets of five stars. Their measurements showed an even greater difference between observers. This difference between observers is what became known as the personal equation, which Bessel indicated was "involuntary" because it could not be overcome by practice and training (Hoffmann, 2007). Since then, it has been noted that the eye-and-ear method involves several aspects of attention, the most obvious being switching attention between visual and auditory modalities.

Wundt was among those who became interested in the possible role of attention. Around 1860, he set up an apparatus to simulate this situation. As described by Blumenthal (1980),

> Wundt suddenly realized that he was measuring the speed of a mental process, that for the first time, he thought, a self-conscious experimental psychology was taking place. *The time it takes to switch attention* [emphasis added] voluntarily from one stimulus to another had been measured—it varied around a tenth of a second. (p. 121)

This insight led Wundt to emphasize the voluntary control of attention.

The first demonstration that the speed of neural processing could be measured came from Herman von Helmholtz (1821–1894). By positioning an electrode at different places on a frog nerve-muscle preparation, Helmholtz was able to calculate the speed at which the nerve impulse was propagated as approximately 30 meters per second (Schmidgen, 2002). He applied the method similarly to humans by stimulating sensory areas on the skin at different distances from the brain and measuring the time to respond. The difference in times between the long and short distances was used to estimate the speed of neural processing, which was approximately 60 meters per second.

These findings led to more formal studies measuring the speed of mental processes in humans conducted by Franciscus C. Donders (1818–1889). De Jagger's (1865/1970) dissertation, conducted under Donders's supervision, provided the initial account of the experiments conducted in Donders's lab. The experiments focused on measuring the time required to identify a stimulus and select a motor response. In one set of experiments, participants were required to respond to a red light with the right hand and a white light with the left hand. The mean reaction time was 356 ms, which was 172 ms longer than a simple reaction (executing a single response when a stimulus is presented) to the same stimuli. De Jagger interpreted this time as the duration of the central processes involving stimulus discrimination and response initiation.

Donders (1868/1969) formalized the method used by De Jagger, known as the *subtractive method,* emphasizing specifically that the time for a particular process could be estimated by adding that process to a task and taking the difference in reaction time between the two tasks. He distinguished three types of reactions: *a* (simple reaction), *b* (choice reaction), and *c* (go or no-go reaction; responding to one stimulus but not another). These types of reactions allowed separate measures of the stimulus identification and decision processes that were assessed together by De Jagger. The difference between the c and a reactions was presumed to reflect the time for stimulus identification, and the difference between the b and c reactions was considered as the time for "expression of the will" (p. 424). Donders's assertion that the time for distinct mental processes can be measured and his method for modeling human information processing are precursors to contemporary methods that are described in Chapter 2 of this volume.

Reaction-time research, in general, and the study of action selection, in particular, flourished throughout the remainder of the 19th century (see Jastrow, 1890; D. K. Robinson, 2001). Other classic reaction-time experiments include those of Exner (1882), who noted that performance of simple reaction tasks was characterized by voluntary preparation that occurs before presentation of the stimulus, with the reaction being a reflexive response to the stimulus. L. Lange (1888) extended this work further by distinguishing between preparatory sets that focused on the sensory and motor stages of the task (D. K. Robinson, 2001). A motor set, which involved focusing attention on the response, produced fast, reflexive responses of the type described by Exner. In contrast, a perceptual set, which involved focusing attention on the stimulus, required apperception and an intentional act of will to initiate the response, resulting in slower responses.

An initial demonstration that choice-reaction time increases as a function of the number of possible stimulus–response alternatives—that is, as a function of uncertainty regarding which response will be required—was provided by Merkel (1885, described in Woodworth, 1938). In Merkel's experiment, the Arabic numerals 1 through 5 were assigned to the left hand and the Roman numerals I through V to the right hand, in left-to-right order. Results showed that when the number of alternatives increased from two to 10 choices, mean reaction time increased from approximately 300 ms to a little over 600 ms. This relation, which indicates that the probabilities of occurrence of stimuli influence the time to respond to whichever one occurs, was rediscovered in the early 1950s by Hick (1952) and Hyman (1953). Their work resulted in the formulation of what is known as Hick's law, or the Hick-Hyman law, which is described in detail in Chapter 2.

Effects of Attention

The relation between attention and perception was one of the first topics to be studied in experimental psychology. At the end of the 19th century, Helmholtz (1894/1968) provided evidence suggesting that attention is essential for visual perception. Using himself as subject and pages of briefly visible printed letters as stimuli, he obtained evidence that attention could be directed in advance of the stimulus presentation to a particular region of the page, even though his eyes were kept fixed at a central point. As depicted in Figure 1.2, Helmholtz focused on an illuminated pinhole in the dark display (labeled *central fixation*) of a type of tachistoscope (a box used to briefly illuminate the display) and directed his attention to a particular peripheral location (labeled *attention shift*), after which the display was briefly illuminated by discharge of a spark (labeled

FIGURE 1.2. Depiction of the Stimulus Display Helmholtz Used to Study Attention Shifts

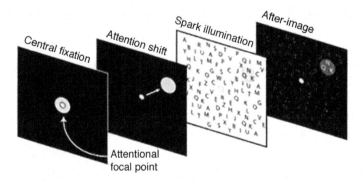

Note. From *Orienting of Attention* (p. 5), by R. D. Wright and J. M. Ward, 2008, Oxford University Press. Copyright 2008 by Oxford University Press. Reprinted with permission.

spark illumination), from which he could report the letters at the attended location. In his words, "With a subsequent discharge I could direct my perception to another section of the field, while always fixating on the pinhole, and then read a group of letters there" (p. 259).

Helmholtz also found that attention was limited: The letters in the largest part of the visual field, even in the vicinity of the fixation point, were not automatically perceived. Based on these observations, Helmholtz (1894/1968) concluded that attention can be covert and concentrated on a part of the visual field on which the eyes are not fixated.

The idea that attention was an inner activity that caused ideas to be present to differing degrees in consciousness was emphasized by Wundt (1880, 1907b). He distinguished between perception, which was the entry into what he called "the field of attention," and apperception, which was responsible for entry into the inner focus. He assumed that the focus of attention could be narrow or wide, a view that has enjoyed popularity in contemporary research on attention (C. W. Eriksen & St. James, 1986). Cowan and Rachev (2018) noted similarities between Wundt's "embedded system's" view of attention and the contemporary working memory models of Cowan and others, described in Chapter 7. Wundt (1907a) identified three components of attention: increased clearness of ideas, muscle sensations in the same modality as the ideas, and emotions related to the ideas on which attention is focused. Wundt used the word *voluntarism* to describe his school of psychology, which emphasized volition, or the study of conscious decision and choice. He held that psychological processes could be understood only in terms of their goals or consequences and that apperception and attention are processes of active synthesis.

The conditions of an act of attention are found not only in the environment but also in the individual, as shown by demonstrations of the role of task set on performance. *Task set* refers to the readiness to carry out an instructed action in response to a given stimulus. One of the earliest investigations of task set was conducted by Oswald Külpe (1904), who used briefly displayed nonsense syllables of different colors as stimuli. The instructions were to determine the number of letters displayed, the colors and their positions, or the letters and their positions. Performance was best when the judgments that had to be made coincided with the task for which the observer had been set (Wilcocks, 1925). The attributes included different letters or colors of syllables in the display and their locations. Külpe's results showed that the participants were able to report the chosen attribute more accurately when it was instructed in advance than when it was not.

A student of Külpe's, Watt (1904/1906), related a similar effect, which he explained as an *Einstellung* ("task set") that people create in constituting the instructed *Aufgabe* ("task") before stimulus presentation. Ach (1905/1964) provided one of the best demonstrations of task set, presenting the numbers 6 and 2 as stimuli to participants. They yielded a response of 8, 4, or 12, depending on whether the instructed task was to add, subtract, or multiply the numbers.

Ach's results indicated that the same stimuli can yield different responses based on the task set.

The views of William James (1890/1950) on attention are probably the most well known of the early psychologists. His definition of attention is widely quoted:

> It is the taking possession by the mind, in clear and vivid form, of one of what seem several simultaneously possible objects or trains of thought. Focalization, concentration, of consciousness are of its essence. It implies withdrawal from some things in order to deal effectively with others. (pp. 403–404)

The emphasis on clearness is similar to that of Wundt, Titchener, and Pillsbury.

Researchers at the beginning of the 20th century debated how this increased clearness was obtained. Ernst Mach, Carl Stumpf, and others favored the view that this increase was direct, whereas Wundt, Külpe, and others held the view that the increase was accomplished indirectly by inhibiting the sensations that were not attended to (Pillsbury, 1908/1973). One difficulty with resolving the issue of how attention influences clearness is illustrated by an experiment conducted by Mach and Stumpf. They agreed that attention to a stimulus increases its perceived intensity, but whereas Mach thought that this effect of attention occurs for all stimuli, Stumpf thought that attention benefits only weak sensations. As described by Titchener (1908/1973), Mach and Stumpf listened to a harmonium together to determine whether attention to one of the clearly audible component tones in a chord increases its strength. Regrettably, Mach concluded that it did, but Stumpf concluded that it did not. Thus, their introspections did not allow them to agree on an answer to this question. The debate about whether attention increases the clearness of attended events or decreases the clearness of unattended events presaged the ongoing argument in psychology regarding whether, and how, attending is accomplished through excitatory and inhibitory mechanisms (e.g., Slagter et al., 2016; see also Chapter 5, this volume).

Although James considered clarity to be a central feature of attention, he is known for taking a functionalist view that emphasized the selective aspect of attention, as illustrated in the last sentence of the earlier quote from James. This functional, selective aspect of attention has been stressed in most research of the past 70 years (Pashler, 1998). Still, the issue of conscious awareness remains vital and is attracting increased interest (e.g., Simione et al., 2019).

James (1890/1950) suggested three categories for characterizing attention. The first is that attention can be directed to actual objects or mental representations of them. Also, attention can be linked to the present event or removed from it. Finally, attention can be automatically attracted to objects or spaces or voluntarily directed to them. James also indicated that attention makes people perceive, think, and remember better than they would without it. Although most studies of attention historically have been on perceiving and identifying stimuli, its influence on memory also was considered. Pillsbury (1908/1973) was explicit about the role of attention in memory, saying, "Retention is dependent on the degree of attention that was given at the moment of learning"

(p. 148). Note the similarity of this quote to Vives's view, cited earlier. Pillsbury also stressed the role of attention in retrieving information from memory.

Also, psychologists have been interested in the role of attention in selection and control of action. In his textbook on attention, Pillsbury (1908/1973) noted that all acts of attention are accompanied by some motor activation. Motor responses include both voluntary and involuntary orienting toward a source of stimulation, as well as other more overt actions. In agreement with Pillsbury, James (1890/1950) said, "Organic adjustment, then, and ideational preparation or preperception are concerned in all attentive acts" (p. 444). A similar view was advocated recently by Hommel et al. (2019), who promoted what they call a synthetic approach to attention that considers perceptual-motor interactions across the information-processing system.

Lotze (1852) and Harleß (1861) introduced the idea that the links between movements and their mental representations are bidirectional, thus allowing the representations to directly produce the movements. This idea came to be called *ideomotor action*, a term first coined by Carpenter (1852) to explain the effect of suggestion on muscular movement independent from conscious intent. Carpenter was interested mainly in explaining phenomena such as dowsing, in which a divining rod might be "pulled" to the earth by the presence of water under the ground, that were attributed to supernatural forces. His idea was that the individual's expectancies and thoughts affected the motor system and thus unintentionally caused the movements. James (1890/1950) agreed with Carpenter's views and was a strong advocate of the ideomotor theory of action. Margaret Washburn (1871–1930) also emphasized the motoric nature of attention, theorizing that associations between stimuli and motor responses become linked in mental images through attention to stimuli (Washburn, 1914). In more recent research, Greenwald (1970), Hommel (2019), Pfister (2019), and others have advocated ideomotor theories of action.

A common idea with respect to attention is that if a task requires attention, it will interfere with simultaneous performance of another task that also requires attention (Keele, 1973). Binet (1890) was one of the first individuals to suggest that attention could be understood in terms of interference. He found that mental addition interfered with a task of rhythmically squeezing a rubber ball a specified number of times. However, this interference did not occur when the timing and number of squeezes did not have to be monitored. In another demonstration of the link between action and attention, Welch (1898) found that a strong grip could not be maintained while performing demanding mental tasks.

In sum, around 1860, the philosophical approach dominated the study of psychology in general and attention in particular. During the period from 1860 to 1909, the study of attention was transformed, as was the field of psychology as a whole, to one of scientific inquiry with emphasis on experimental investigations. By 1909, many phenomena of concern to contemporary attention researchers had been discovered and investigated, and the study of attention was central to the field of psychology. However, the situation was one captured by Ribot (1890) in the first sentence of his book: "Psychologists have given much study to the effects of attention, but very little to its mechanism" (p. 7). Unfortunately, emphasis on the study of attentional mechanisms was largely delayed until the middle of the 20th century.

THE PERIOD FROM 1910 TO 1949

Lovie (1983) conducted a search of *Psychological Index* and *Psychological Abstracts* from 1911 to 1960 and found that the number of articles on the topic of attention exceeded 100 in all but the 1911–1920 decade. Figure 1.3 depicts results of a search of the PsycInfo database we conducted for the word *attention* in the title and subject categories. It illustrates the rise of interest in the topic of attention in contemporary psychology.

One often reads that research on attention essentially ceased between 1910 and 1949 (Keele, 1973; Moray, 1969; Neisser, 1976). However, although not evident from Figure 1.3 due to its scale, attention research never disappeared, as indicated by Lovie's (1983) tallies of more than 100 articles on the topic being published in all but 1 decade before 1960. Not only was research on attention conducted continuously throughout the first half of the 20th century, but this research also provided a close link both to the work before 1910 and contemporary work. Lovie (1983) noted that research during this period pursued the ideas expressed in the work of Broadbent and others following the increased interest in attention in the 1950s.

Among the essential works on attention was that of Jersild (1927), who published a classic monograph, "Mental Set and Shift." In it, he reported a

FIGURE 1.3. Research on Attention: Number of Publications as Indicated by a PsycInfo Search Conducted on December 15, 2021

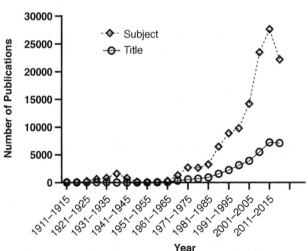

series of experiments in which participants had to make judgments regarding each stimulus in a list as a function of whether a single task was to be performed or two tasks in alternating order. The major finding was that in many situations, the time to complete the list was longer for mixed lists than for pure lists of a single task. Although Jersild's study did not generate much interest for many years, since the mid-1990s, there has been a resurgence of interest in task-switching costs, making it one of the hottest areas of research on attention (e.g., Koch et al., 2018; see also Chapter 6, this volume).

Another significant contribution during this era is the discovery of the *psychological refractory period effect* by Telford (1931). He noted that numerous studies showed that stimulation of neurons was followed by a refractory phase during which the neurons were less sensitive to stimulation. Telford conducted an experiment to answer the question "Do voluntary responses, judgments and simple associative processes produce effects in the organism which serve as a barrier against immediate repetition, that can be identified with a refractory phase?" (p. 7). One of Telford's tasks required participants to make a simple reaction by pressing a key whenever a tone occurred. The interval between successive tones varied between 0.5, 1, 2, and 4 seconds. Responses were considerably slower when the stimulus followed the preceding one by a short interval than when the interval was longer. This finding, that reaction time to the second of two stimuli or tasks is increased when the interval between their onsets is short, was shown subsequently to be a pervasive phenomenon that occurred for choice reaction tasks as well. This psychological refractory period effect has been a constant source of research and theoretical speculation for the past 90 years (e.g., Klapp et al., 2019; Welford, 1952).

The same year as Telford, Bills (1931) reported a study on what would now be called *mind wandering*, or lapses of attention, but that he called "blocks." In a series of experiments, he had participants perform various tasks (e.g., color naming) as fast as possible for 7 to 10 minutes and, in a final experiment, an hour. Performance of all tasks showed blocks or pauses of varying durations in which no response occurred. The blocks tended to bunch together, suggesting a relatively rhythmic fluctuation of attention. The frequency of the blocks was about three per minute, but the frequency and length of the blocks were reduced by practice and increased by fatigue. Errors tended to coincide with the blocks, suggesting that their cause was linked to the low level of task engagement implied by the blocks.

One of the most well-known studies in the field of psychology was conducted by Stroop (1935/1992), who demonstrated that stimulus information that is irrelevant to the task can have a major impact on performance (the *Stroop effect*). He had participants name the ink colors for a list of 100 stimuli. In the crucial list, the stimuli spelled incongruent color words, and the participants were instructed to name the ink color while ignoring the color word (see Figure 1.4). Participants took an average of 110 seconds to name a list of this type, compared with 63 seconds to name the colors when presented in the form of solid squares. Thus, the naming time nearly doubled in the presence of conflicting

FIGURE 1.4. A Monochrome Version of the Stroop Task

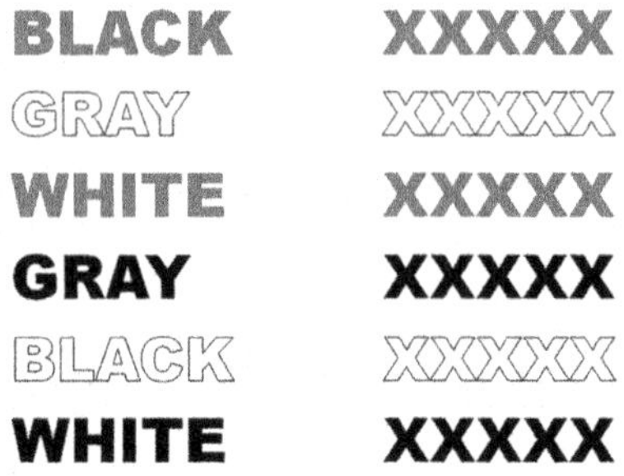

BLACK	**XXXXX**
GRAY	XXXXX
WHITE	**XXXXX**
GRAY	**XXXXX**
BLACK	XXXXX
WHITE	**XXXXX**

color words. Another finding of Stroop's was that the time to name the color words was unaffected by incongruent ink colors. The time to read 100 words for that list was 43 seconds, compared with 41 seconds for those words presented in black ink. Thus, the interference with color naming was asymmetric: Irrelevant words interfered with naming ink colors, but irrelevant ink colors did not interfere with naming color words.

The Stroop task provides one of the best methods for examining a variety of issues relevant to attention in young adults and more specialized populations of people. When the article was reprinted in 1992, MacLeod (1992) referred to the Stroop task as the "gold standard" of attentional measures and noted that citations of the article increased over the period of 1974 to 1990, from a low of 25 in 1974 to 80 in 1990. MacLeod's words, "The Stroop effect . . . continues to play a key role in the understanding of attention" (p. 12), are still true today.

Among the research conducted in the 1930s and 40s, that on preparatory set or mental set was among the most important (Gibson, 1941). Mowrer et al. (1940) established that preparatory set does not necessarily involve motor adjustments such as body posture and muscle tension. They reached this conclusion based on the finding that expectancy for one of two possible stimulus events was a critical factor influencing reaction time. They pointed out the consistency of their findings with those of Wundt (1880), who found that reaction time was longer when the participant did not know whether the stimulus would be visual, auditory, or tactual than when the sensory modality was known. Gibson (1941) provided a thorough, highly critical, review of the literature on set, noting, "The concept of set or attitude is a nearly universal one in psychological thinking despite the fact that the underlying meaning is indefinite, the terminology chaotic, and the usage by psychologists highly individualistic" (p. 781).

In the late 1940s, two influential works in cognitive neuroscience appeared. One was Hebb's (1949) book, *The Organization of Behavior: A Neuropsychological Theory*. In that book, Hebb pulled together research in neuroscience and psychology to provide a theory based on both. His theory was built around the concept of a *cell assembly*, a neural response in the brain corresponding to sensory information that activates specific motor responses. According to

Hebb, "Each assembly action may be aroused by a preceding assembly, by a sensory event, or—normally—by both. The central facilitation from one of these activities on the next is the prototype of 'attention'" (p. xix). In other words, each assembly action can be primed by others. Hebb's theory was one of the earliest connectionist models to try to relate brain and behavior. Even more pointedly, in criticizing much theorizing that did not include attention as a component, Hebb stated, "Since everyone knows that attention and set exist, we had better get the skeleton out of the closet and see what can be done with it" (p. 5). In essence, that is what the research described in this book is all about.

Moruzzi and Magoun (1949) conducted studies on cats that similarly showed the contribution of a brain region, the reticular formation, to arousal and alertness. The reticular formation is composed of many brain nuclei and projects into the forebrain, brain stem, and cerebellum. Moruzzi and Magoun stimulated various components of the reticular formation in sedated cats and found that electroencephalogram measures showed changes like those when the cat entered a waking state. Their study provided strong evidence that the reticular activating system mediates arousal by way of afferent pathways from the system to cortical and other brain areas.

In sum, although the proportion of psychological research devoted to the topic of attention was less during this period than in prior decades, many significant discoveries were made. Much of the recent research on attention has focused on developing theoretical accounts of the phenomenon of task-switching costs, the effects of irrelevant information in the Stroop and related tasks, and the psychological refractory period effect in dual-task performance, all of which were discovered during this time. Moreover, the insights of Hebb (1949), Moruzzi and Magoun (1949), and others spurred the analysis of brain networks underlying attention.

THE PERIOD FROM 1950 TO 1974

The period from 1950 to 1974 saw a revival of interest in the characterization of human information processing. This revival is sometimes called the "cognitive revolution," but we think that it is more accurately characterized as the information-processing revolution (Xiong & Proctor, 2018). The revolution was stimulated by developments in communication theory and by renewed interest in measuring and characterizing stages of information processing. Research on attention in this period is characterized by an interplay between application and theory. One of its founders, George A. Miller (2003), gives 1956, the year in which he published his classic article "The Magic Number Seven Plus or Minus Two," as the inaugural year. However, he also specified that major advances had occurred in the prior years of the decade. This is true both for the view of the human as an information-processing system and the study of attention, for which seminal research in the modern era dates to the late 1940s (e.g., K. J. W. Craik, 1948, and Saltzman & Garner, 1948).

Although many areas of investigation contributed to the rise of the information-processing approach, research on attention and performance was at the forefront of advances, providing, among other things, the first formal processing model (Broadbent, 1958). It is customary to read that the approach relies on an analogy of humans to computers, but the fundamental idea is that humans are complex systems that can be analyzed in the same way as nonhuman systems (Posner, 1986; Proctor & Vu, 2006b).

The information-processing revolution was based on three pillars (Xiong & Proctor, 2018). The first of these, the systems concept, comes mainly from cybernetics (Wiener, 1950). Cybernetics provided the idea that everything ranging from neurophysiological mechanisms to societal activities can be modeled as structured control systems with feedforward and feedback loops. A second and closely related significant contributor was information theory (Shannon & Weaver, 1949), which provided a way to quantify entropy (uncertainty) and information and promoted theorizing in terms of information flow. The final pillar was statistical theory and the concept of null hypothesis testing, coupled with advances in experimental design, which afforded the means for making scientific inferences from the results of controlled experiments using small group designs (Fisher, 1937). Statistical theory also provided the basis for conceptualizing human decision making in other situations (Peterson et al., 1954). An additional influence was the advent of artificial intelligence and the possibility of simulating human cognition (Hovland, 1960). All these contributions came together in the early 1950s to provide the basis for most research on cognition in general and attention in particular since that time.

Experiments on the maintenance of vigilance, or sustained attention, that exemplified the interplay between theory and application were reported by Mackworth (1950/1961). This research originated in concerns about the performance of World War II radar operators in detecting infrequently occurring signals. It has continued to generate interest because of its relevance to industrial monitoring tasks and theoretical issues in attention. Mackworth introduced a "clock" test in which a pointer moved in steps of 12 minutes of arc per second, but 12 times in 20 seconds, it made a double jump of 24 minutes. The participant was to report the double jumps by pressing a key whenever one occurred. The proportion of double jumps detected decreased across the first half hour or so of the vigil. Research on the nature of this *vigilance decrement* and the factors that affect its magnitude has been conducted continuously since Mackworth's influential study (e.g., Neigel et al., 2020).

Cherry (1953) produced one of the groundbreaking works on attention. He studied the problem of auditory selective attention or, as he called it, the *cocktail-party phenomenon*. He was concerned with the issues of how we can select one voice to attend to among several and what information is remembered from the unattended messages. Cherry used a procedure called dichotic listening in which he presented different messages to each ear through headphones. Participants were to repeat aloud, or shadow, one of the two messages while ignoring the other. This was a relatively easy task for them to do. Moreover, when subsequently asked questions about the unattended message, participants were unable to describe anything about it except physical characteristics, such as the gender of the speaker.

Broadbent (1958) conducted an experiment that produced converging results with those of Cherry (1953). He presented participants with a set of three digits one after the other to one ear and another set at the same time to the other ear, with instructions to recall as many digits as possible. Participants tended to recall all the digits presented to one ear before trying to recall the digits presented to the other ear. To account for findings such as his and Cherry's, Broadbent developed the first complete model of attention, called filter theory (see Chapter 3, this volume). He proposed that the nervous system acts as a single-communication channel of limited capacity. According to filter theory, information is held in a preattentive temporary store, and only sensory events that have some physical feature in common (e.g., spatial location) are selected to pass into the limited capacity processing system. Broadbent's filter theory implies that the meaning of unattended messages is not identified. He also proposed that an amount of time that is not negligible is required to shift the filter from one channel of events to another.

Later studies showed that the unattended message could be processed beyond the physical level, in at least some cases (Treisman, 1960). To explain the finding that the meaning of an unattended message can influence performance, Treisman (1960) reformulated filter theory into filter-attenuation theory. According to this theory, early selection by filtering still precedes stimulus identification, but attenuated signals may be sufficient to allow identification if the stimulus has a low identification threshold, such as a person's name or an expected event. Deutsch and Deutsch (1963) took an alternative approach, proposing that unattended stimuli are always identified and that the bottleneck occurs in later processing. This view is called late-selection theory, in contrast to the filter and filter-attenuation theories, which are called early-selection theories. The issue posed by the distinction between the early- and late-selection theories is whether meaning is fully analyzed. This issue continues to be debated; for example, Weissman et al. (2018) evaluated conditions under which selection seems to be early versus late.

In the early 1970s, there was a shift from studying attention with auditory tasks to visual tasks. A view that regards attention as a limited-capacity resource that can be directed toward various processes became popular. Kahneman's (1973) model is the most well known of these unitary-capacity, or resource, theories. According to the theory, attention is a resource that can be divided up among distinct tasks in different amounts. The available supply of this resource varies as a function of arousal and task demands, and allocation strategies determine the tasks and processes to which the resource is devoted when the demand exceeds the supply. Posner and Boies (1971) distinguished two attentional components in addition to processing capacity, alertness and selectivity, and demonstrated how the separate effects of these components could be isolated in behavioral experiments.

In the early 1970s, the first controlled experiments that used psychophysio-logical techniques to study attention were conducted on humans (e.g., Hillyard et al., 1973). These experiments used methods that allow brain activity relating to the processing of a stimulus, called *event-related potentials*, to be measured from electrodes placed on the scalp. The difference between event-related potential patterns obtained under different conditions, such as when a person is attending to a stimulus versus when the person is not, can provide evidence about the nature of the neural mechanisms underlying the processing of specific stimuli.

Techniques were also developed to perform single-cell recordings in alert monkeys. Wurtz and Goldberg (1972) provided evidence that neurons in the superior colliculus (a midbrain area involved in sensory integration) are involved in a shift of visual attention to the location of a critical region of the visual field before the onset of eye movements. Tanji and Evarts (1976) offered similar evidence that an instruction signal as to whether a forthcoming movement would be a push or pull of a lever led to anticipatory activity in the motor cortex while the monkey was waiting for a signal to trigger the movement.

The research during this period yielded considerable information about the mechanisms of attention, specifically those involved in auditory attention. The most notable development was the introduction of detailed information-processing models of attention and performance, beginning with Broadbent's (1958) filter theory. The realization that such models can be developed and tested paved the way for many advances in our understanding of attention.

THE PERIOD FROM 1975 TO 1999

Research on attention flourished during the last quarter of the 20th century. This is evident in Figure 1.3, which shows that the number of articles with *attention* in the title increased from approximately 700 in the period ending in 1980 to more than 3,000 for the period ending in 2000. Researchers continued to conduct behavioral (and psychophysiological) research directed toward many of the tasks, issues, and phenomena of the previous period, but the range of research expanded.

Many studies showed that it is easier to perform two tasks together when they use different stimulus or response modalities than when they use the same modalities. Performance is also better when one task is verbal and the other is visuospatial than when they are the same type. On the basis of these find-ings, Navon and Gopher (1979) proposed that attention is better viewed as multiple resources. Wickens (1980) extended the multiple-resource view by proposing that different attentional resources exist for distinct sensory modali-ties, coding modes, and response modalities. Multiple-resource theory captures the fact that multiple-task performance typically is better when the tasks use different input–output modes than when they use the same modes. Although useful for application guidelines, the concept of multiple resources is limited as a theory of attention because its flexibility allows new resources to be added to fit any finding showing the specificity of interference (Navon, 1984).

Another distinction that became prominent is between space-based and object-based approaches to attention. In the *space-based* approach, a widely used metaphor for visual attention is a spotlight that is presumed to direct attention to everything in its field (e.g., Posner, 1980). The attentional spotlight can presumably be dissociated from the direction of gaze (a view for which Helmholtz, 1894/1968, provided evidence many years earlier). Studies showed that when a location is cued as likely to contain a target stimulus but then a probe stimulus is presented at another location, a spatial gradient surrounds the attended location such that items nearer to the focus of attention are processed more efficiently than those farther away from it (LaBerge, 1983). Evidence suggested that the attentional spotlight can be moved to a location either voluntarily or involuntarily (attention is captured by an abrupt stimulus onset).

Treisman and Gelade (1980) developed a highly influential variant of spotlight theory called feature integration theory to explain the results from visual search studies, in which participants detect whether a target is present among distractors. Feature integration theory assumes that basic features of stimuli are encoded into feature maps in parallel across the visual field at a preattentive stage. Search for a target distinguished from distractors by a single feature can be based on processing occurring during this preattentive stage. The second stage involves focusing attention on a specific location and combining the features at that location into an object. Searching for a target distinguished from distractors by a conjunction of features requires attention, and search performance decreases as the number of distractors increases.

Object-based models of attention view objects as the primary units on which attention operates. The primary reason for proposing such models is that numerous findings suggest a processing cost when attention must be directed toward two different objects, even when spatial factors are controlled (Duncan, 1984).

Priming studies were also popular during this period. In such studies, a prime stimulus precedes a target stimulus to which the participant is to respond; the prime can be the same as or different from some aspect of the target. When it is the same as or a close associate of the target stimulus, the prime facilitates responding to the target. For example, Meyer et al. (1975) found that the time to say the name of a visual word (e.g., BUTTER) or classify it as a word (vs. nonword) was less when it was preceded by an associated word (e.g., BREAD). Posner and Snyder (1975) and Neely (1977) varied the onsets between a prime stimulus and the target stimulus and provided evidence for two types of priming effects, one that is rapid and automatic and the other that is slower and intentional. Neely found that a category prime (e.g., Bird) facilitated processing of a word from that category at short intervals, without a cost for processing words not from the category. At longer intervals, though, the category benefit was accompanied by a cost for stimuli from a nonprimed category.

A phenomenon called *negative priming* was introduced, for which responding to a stimulus is slower when that stimulus had to be ignored on the prior trial (e.g., it was the word of Stroop color stimulus). This phenomenon was originally attributed to inhibitory processes from the prime trial affecting the probe trial, but the specific cause of negative priming remains unresolved (Labossière & Leboe-McGowan, 2018).

Another view that gained some adherents is that of *selection-for-action*. According to this view, first advocated by Neumann (1987) and Allport (1987), attentional limitations should not be attributed to a limited capacity resource or mechanism. Instead, the limitations are byproducts of the need to coordinate action and ensure that the correct stimulus information is controlling the intended responses. An application of this approach is the executive-process interactive control model presented by Meyer and Kieras (1997a, 1997b), which attempts to account for limitations in multiple-task performance in terms of strategic factors rather than structural capacity limitations. The view is represented more recently in Hommel et al.'s (2019) synthetic approach, which suggests that the emphasis should be on selection processes relevant to behavior and the systems that implement them.

During this period of research, a focus was on gathering neuropsychological evidence pertaining to the brain mechanisms that underlie attention. Cognitive neuroscience, of which studies of attention are a major part, made great strides due to the continued development of neuroimaging technologies. These include the measurement of event-related brain potentials with scalp electrodes, positron emission tomography, and functional magnetic resonance imaging. These techniques, described in Chapter 2, allow the activity of different brain regions during the performance of a variety of tasks to be examined (e.g., Leonards et al., 2000). Likewise, *spatial neglect*—a reduced ability to attend to and respond to stimuli on the side opposite a cerebral lesion (typically right hemisphere lesion and left visual field neglect)—provided evidence regarding the brain mechanisms underlying visual attention (Heilman & Valenstein, 1979; Heilman, Watson, & Valenstein, 1985). Among the most influential articles in the area of attention was Posner and Petersen's (1990) "Attentional Systems of the Brain," which distinguished three separate but interrelated subsystems of the attentional system. One subsystem is concerned with orienting to sensory events, another to detecting events to which conscious processing may be directed, and the third to maintaining an alert state. Posner and Petersen's depictions of each subsystem were based on a variety of neuroscience data from animals and humans.

Significant advances were also made toward expanding the theories and methods of attention to address a range of applied problems. Applications of research on attention are many, but two major areas can be identified. The first concerns ergonomics in its broadest sense, ranging from human–machine interactions to improvement of work environments. Examples of this work include *mental workload* (the measurement of the mental demands placed on a person; Gopher, 1994) and *situation awareness* (a person's understanding of the situation in which they are involved; Endsley, 1995b), for both of which measurement became increasingly sophisticated during the period (see Chapter 9). The second major area of application is clinical neuropsychology, which benefited substantially from adopting cognitive models and methods to describe and investigate damaged systems in neurological patients (see Chapter 3).

THE PERIOD FROM 2000 TO 2020

Research on attention continued to grow during the first 2 decades of the 21st century. One need only note from Figure 1.3 that the number of articles with *attention* in the title from 2000 to 2020 approximately equals the total number of articles before that time. We will not describe the research from this era in much detail because it will be covered throughout the remainder of the book. However, the following are some highlights.

A popular view is that attention has three distinct functions—alerting, orienting, and executive control—that are implemented in distinct neural systems (Fan & Posner, 2004). Work on executive control based on sequential effects in tasks for which some irrelevant aspect of stimulation can correspond or not with relevant information became a central focus of investigation. Botvinick et al.'s (2001) conflict resolution model initiated much of this interest. Bidirectional relations between perception and action came to the forefront, as in the theory of event coding (Hommel et al., 2001). Another widely investigated topic is the influence of action video game play on attention and performance; a meta-analysis concluded that playing action video games enhances top-down attention and spatial cognition (Bediou et al., 2018). Research on the neural bases of attention has continued to grow, as has research on the role of attention in social interactions. Findings of attention research have been applied to online education, social media, driving, and other human interactions with technology (see Box 1.1).

BOOK COVERAGE

In this chapter, we touched on many of the topics that subsequent chapters cover in detail. By necessity, we cannot address all topics on attention. For this book, we selected topics and studies that illustrate how research on attention is conducted and advances. Part of what we want students and researchers to learn is how research and theory coevolve. Consequently, we present evidence to support alternative views and only state definitive conclusions where they seem warranted. As you will see, the data show a lot of agreement about the fundamental phenomena and the factors that influence them, and the issues

BOX 1.1 | **HUMAN FACTORS AND ERGONOMICS**

Human factors and ergonomics (HFE) is a "scientific discipline concerned with the understanding of interactions among humans and other elements of a system, and the profession that applies theory, principles, data, and other methods to design in order to optimize human well-being and overall system performance" (International Ergonomics Association, n.d., para. 1). HFE grew out of World War II, when human error was a leading cause of aviation and naval accidents (Proctor & Van Zandt, 2018). Many researchers studied factors that impacted human performance, including attentional factors in perception, cognition, and action. By understanding human information processing, researchers were able to design products and systems to increase performance and safety. Chapter 1 provides an overview of the history of research on attention, and this box is intended to highlight how "old issues" relating to attention are directly applicable to "new issues" associated with the design of modern products and systems. Thus, history repeats. Table B1.1 highlights historical trends in attention research and shows how similar issues resurface years later.

TABLE B1.1. Applications of Attentional Theories and Phenomena

Theory	Phenomena	Applications
Philosophical Work		
Vives: Notion that the more closely one attends to stimuli, the better they will be retained.	Depth of processing: The deeper you process information at encoding, the better retention.	Study strategies that relate new information to prior knowledge and other contexts result in better learning and retention of that material.
Hamilton: Notion that more than one object or event can be attended at the same time, but with less efficiency.	Cost of concurrence: Just having to keep track of two tasks, even though 100% of attention is devoted to one of the tasks results in poorer performance than performing that same task alone.	Driving modes on smartphones: Driving modes prevent distraction during driving (e.g., alerts from text messages, emails, apps). Even if one is not actively responding to the alerts generated from the phone, the possibility of getting an alert can influence driving performance.
Founding of Psychology (1860 to 1909)		
Wundt: Notion that it takes time to switch attention.	Task-switching cost: It takes longer to respond to stimuli on task-switch than task-repeat trials.	Multitasking: Multitasking performance is poorer than single task performance in most situations.
Pillsbury: Retention is dependent on the degree of attention given to the material at the moment of learning.	Encoding specificity: Retention is better when the recall environment matches the learning environment.	Transfer appropriate training: Training should focus on directing learners to code information in a manner consistent with how they will retrieve it.

BOX 1.1 | **HUMAN FACTORS AND ERGONOMICS *(Continued)***

**TABLE B1.1. Applications of Attentional Theories and Phenomena
*(Continued)***

Theory	Phenomena	Applications
Period of 1910 to 1949		
Jersild: The time to switch between tasks is typically longer than the time to repeat the same task.	Task switching effect: Slowing of response to a second task if it follows performance of another task rather than the same task.	Multitasking: There is a cost of multitasking, even though performance can become more efficient with practice.
Stroop: Stimulus information that is related but irrelevant to the defined task can have a major impact on performance.	Stroop effect: Irrelevant color words interfere with relevant task of naming ink colors.	Brain training: Practice at the Stroop task is used in a variety of games intended to promote attentional and cognitive control.
Information-Processing Revolution (1950–1974)		
Mackworth: It is difficult to sustain attention.	Vigilance decrement: Decreased ability to detect infrequent events over time.	Automation monitoring: Automation monitoring is similar to performing a vigilance task, making the human a bad "back up" for detecting automation failures.
Broadbent: The nervous system acts as a single-communication channel of limited capacity.	Cocktail-party effect: Attended conversation is processed and understood; unattended conversation cannot be recalled. But attention can be given to unattended conversation if it is highly salient.	Online learning: Students who multitask during class show poorer performance on retention tests. Moreover, students who sit in view of other students multitasking with other media also show poorer performance.

are about the best ways to explain the underlying mechanisms of these phenomena. As researchers learn more about a topic and have additional data to inform their theories, the issues become more refined, and debates arise. Ongoing debates do not mean a lack of progress; they are part of the scientific process. Although the resolution of issues may sometimes occur relatively quickly, more often, many decades are required to arrive at a consensus.

One point on which researchers agree is that "attention" is an overarching concept for which there are subcategories based on distinct mechanisms. Some have called for the abandonment of the term "attention" because of the broad range of topics it encompasses (Hommel et al., 2019). However, there is considerable family resemblance (Medin et al., 1987; Wittgenstein, 1953) among the subcategories of attention, relating to selection and control at all stages of information processing, which we argue warrants viewing attention as an encompassing category. The widespread research conducted under the umbrella of attention suggests that most researchers agree with us. In terms of practical implications of the research on attention, we show how this work is relevant to multitasking in everyday environments such as driving and remote learning, monitoring automation, cognitive "brain" training, and behavioral interventions for developmental disorders of attention. In the remainder of the book, you will see that much has been learned about the topics considered under "attention" and how they apply to everyday life, although, as noted earlier, there is still more to learn.

CHAPTER SUMMARY

In this text, we take a scientific approach to the study of attention. That means that the emphasis is on empirical testing, most often in controlled laboratory environments (Proctor & Capaldi, 2006). This testing allows claims to be evaluated in terms of what Strevens (2020) called the *iron rule of explanation*, to which he attributes scientific progress:

1. Strive to settle all arguments by empirical testing.

2. To conduct an empirical test to decide between a pair of hypotheses, perform an experiment or measurement, one of whose possible outcomes can be explained by one hypothesis (and accompanying cohort) but not the other. (p. 96)

Implications of this approach are that details of research are crucial and that alternative theories have to be taken into consideration.

In this context, it is essential to distinguish facts, phenomena, and theories—which we emphasize in the Chapter Summary section of each chapter. Because the concept of attention is multifaceted, the distinctions between these classifications in some cases are somewhat fuzzy. In this chapter, we have introduced facts, phenomena, and theories regarding attention, into which we will delve in more detail in the remaining chapters. This chapter thus provides a base on which understanding of the science of attention and its applications can build in the subsequent chapters. Several facts, phenomena, and theories are summarized here, and many more will be explained and highlighted throughout the book in the Key Points sections at the end of each chapter. There is typically agreement on the facts and phenomena but less agreement on theories because they involve interpretation of the facts and phenomena.

We have tried to make it apparent in this chapter that contemporary research on attention owes a considerable debt to the work on attention conducted since the earliest days of the field of psychology. Forty years ago, Posner (1982) made this point eloquently, stating the following:

> One can see emerging from psychological research in the area of attention a cumulative development of theoretical concepts that rely on principles, some over 100 years old, that are now elaborated in ways that were essentially unavailable to earlier researchers. (p. 168)

He also noted,

> The cumulative nature of work on attention is not widely appreciated, in part because of a failure to recognize that the methods used in current studies arose in empirical findings of the past and also because attention is a concept that can be studied at many levels. (p. 168)

Among the findings Posner referred to are that each mental operation requires a measurable period (Donders, 1868/1969), two events occurring close together in time are processed sequentially (Wundt, 1912), internal events can have facilitatory or inhibitory properties (Pavlov, 1960), and reflexive orienting to stimuli may occur (Sokolov, 1963).

In the Introduction to his collection of readings, *The Psychology of Attention*, Posner (2017) again posed the question of progress and once more answered it affirmatively:

> Is there a cumulative development of work on attention? Can we argue that recent work answers issues raised earlier, even in the distant past? Based on my reading I think the answer is yes, despite many changes in language and method. (p. 2)

We hope that this chapter will help you appreciate the history of research on attention in its own right, as well as for the foundation it provides for ongoing investigations into this central aspect of human perception, cognition, and action that we describe in the remainder of this book.

KEY POINTS

- **Fact:** Attention is a topic that has attracted considerable interest over many centuries.

- **Fact:** Empirical investigations of attention began in the last half of the 19th century and introduced reaction-time procedures to study attention that are still used today.

- **Fact:** Attention was a focus of experimental psychology through the first part of the 20th century.

- **Fact:** Much research shifted to a behavioral emphasis in the first half of the 20th century, with the study of attention continuing but in a secondary role.

- **Fact:** Attention research has flourished since the middle of the 20th century due to the development of theories and models that characterize human information processing in detail and the progress of technologies that allow examination of neural correlates of attention.

- **Fact:** Perhaps more than any other aspect of cognitive psychology, attention research has benefited from an interplay between basic and applied studies.

- **Fact:** Selection and control are key factors in all aspects of human information processing—perception, cognition, and action, and their interactions— at the individual and social levels.

- **Phenomenon:** Many phenomena introduced here, such as the Stroop effect, the psychological refractory period effect, and the cocktail-party effect, will resurface throughout the book.

- **Theory:** Many theories of attention have been proposed and tested over the years, resulting in a refinement in the understanding of attention.

- **Fact:** The interplay between theory and data from controlled experiments is essential to the progress that has been made in the way that attention is understood.

2

Information Processing and the Study of Attention

It is apparent that attention takes many forms and has many roles. Specifying the functions of attention in detail requires an understanding of the stages involved in performing an act. That is, to specify the role of attention in performance, it is necessary to describe the course of human information processing, including expectancies and preparation. For example, attending to a region of space may affect perception by making stimulus processing more efficient for certain locations or objects in that region. Attending to information can also affect later stages of processing. For instance, paying attention to certain aspects of a scene might lead to better memory of other information associated with the perceived objects or events. It is also the case that a certain level of arousal or alertness is necessary to perform any task. Finally, preparation for a specific action may alter other processes of perception and cognition.

HUMAN INFORMATION PROCESSING

The *information-processing approach* focuses on the processes by which information in a stimulus at the receptors is translated into thought and action. Because these processes themselves are unobservable, an assortment of techniques has been developed to gain insight into their nature. This chapter describes the techniques and paradigms that can be used to determine the processes involved in perceiving, classifying, and acting on stimuli. Traditionally,

https://doi.org/10.1037/0000317-002
Attention: Selection and Control in Human Information Processing, by R. W. Proctor and K.-P. L. Vu

behavioral measures of speed and accuracy of task performance have been the most widely used ones. However, electrophysiological measures are taking an increasingly key role in making the unobservable observable. For example, by measuring the electrical activity produced in the brain during the performance of a task, it is often possible to obtain otherwise unobservable evidence as to the stage of processing influenced by an experimental manipulation. Also, neuroimaging and brain stimulation techniques implemented over the past few decades allow us to determine not just the processes of cognition but how these processes may be realized in the brain.

A basic model of human information processing distinguishes processes of perception, cognition, and action (Proctor & Vu, 2021; Wickens & Carswell, 2021). As shown in Figure 2.1, these processes can be decomposed further and are influenced by attention and memory. It is often assumed that, from the onset of a stimulus event, the processes occur sequentially and the results of one processing stage form the input to the next. An attentional system selects some sources of information for processing over others, and a memory system maintains the information of immediate relevance to the current task and brings prior knowledge to bear on the task. Intention and task goals guide information processing for the task, and feedback enables adjustments and corrections. This model does not depict all aspects of human information processing, but it is useful for organizing the effects of several factors on performance.

Specific models differ in the proposed properties of the stages of information processing, including whether attention is required, whether particular processes can be executed simultaneously or must be performed sequentially, and the extent to which one process affects another (Proctor & Vu, 2021; Wickens & Carswell, 2021). Among the variants are ones that emphasize influences of the body and motoric processes on perception and cognition (e.g., embodied cognition; M. R. Robinson & Thomas, 2021). However, all variations rely on the basic idea that processing can be usefully described in terms of more-or-less distinct cognitive activities. This idea is also central to many advances in cognitive neuroscience and applied human factors. In this section, we describe information theory, which had a large impact on the contemporary study of attention, and the more general idea of information-processing stages.

Information Theory

An essential idea in the human information-processing approach is that the human is not just a receiver of information but a transmitter of information, as well. In this sense, the human can be described as a communication channel (Shannon & Weaver, 1949). As with any other communication channel (e.g., a phone line), it is possible to talk about the rate of information transfer and the efficiency of transmission. For example, a dispatcher might have the task of relaying information from different sources to workers in the field. The dispatcher's performance depends on the quality of the information from different sources and the speed and reliability of their equipment. It also depends

FIGURE 2.1. The Three-Stage Information-Processing Framework

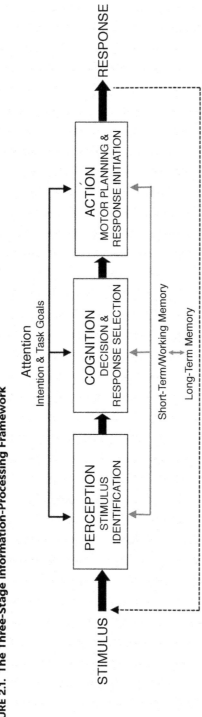

on how quickly and accurately the information is relayed. To describe the rate of information transmission, we need to quantify the information, and then we can examine the time it takes to receive and transmit a given amount of information.

Technically, information is available whenever there is some uncertainty about what will occur. If the switchboard operator makes a mistake and gives a message received from one source back to that same source, the original source is none the wiser, and we can say that no information has been transmitted. In other words, if reduction of uncertainty does not take place, no information is transmitted. The amount of information in a stimulus depends in part on the number of possible stimuli that could occur in a given context. For example, if the same stimulus occurs repeatedly, there is no room for reduction in uncertainty about what stimulus will occur. In contrast, if different stimuli are possible, there will be uncertainty about what will happen next, and the stimulus will, by definition, convey information. The amount of information in a stimulus is expressed in bits (*bi*nary un*its*). When stimuli are equally likely, the number of bits in a stimulus is computed as $\log_2(N)$, where N is the number of alternatives.

In the 1950s and 1960s, many experiments were conducted concerning the information-processing efficiency of the human operator (Fitts & Posner, 1967), with efficiency described as the rate of information transmission in bits per second. This measure was used to compare the effectiveness of different coding schemes or the efficiency of one operator compared with another. In Chapter 1, we mentioned *Hick's law*, which relates task performance to information transmitted. According to Hick's law, reaction time in a task is linearly related to the amount of information transmitted. With equally likely stimuli and perfect performance, reaction time increases by a constant amount each time the number of possible stimuli is doubled (see Figure 2.2). The slope of the function relating information transmitted and reaction time is a measure of processing efficiency. This law continues to inspire research on the mechanisms of information processing to this day (see Proctor & Schneider, 2018, for a review). Because information-processing models typically do not focus exclusively on uncertainty, information theory is not now widely used in psychology. However, its use is advocated in neuroscience (Timme & Lapish, 2018) and applied areas such as human–computer interaction (Liu et al., 2019).

Information and Stages

A common approach to human information processing is to suppose that information is processed in a series of discrete stages (see Figure 2.1). In this approach, a stage can be viewed as a processing component in which the output of one component serves as the input for the next. A stage does not necessarily correspond to a particular circuit or structure in the brain but indicates a function (or process) carried out during a period. How the stages are structured and the way they interact is the subject of much research. Methods used to study these stages and the role of attention are the subject of the next section.

FIGURE 2.2. The Relation Between Reaction Time and Information Transmitted According to Hick's Law

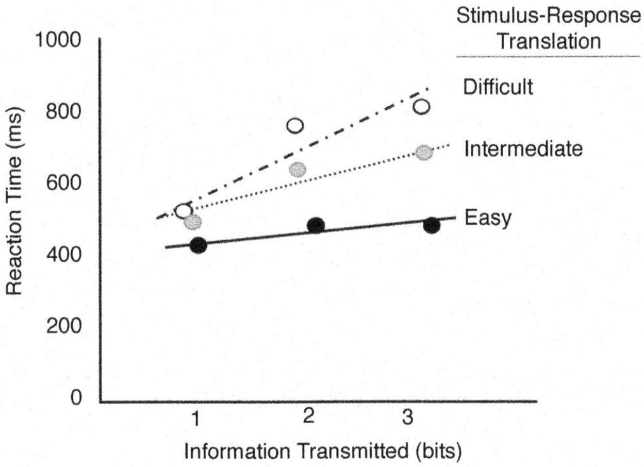

Note. The slope of the line reflects the efficiency with which information can be processed.

BEHAVIORAL METHODS USED TO STUDY ATTENTION

Whether someone is attending to a stimulus, an event, or an action seems simple. We can ask a person about content that was presented in a message or see whether they looked at some component of a display. However, as will be evident, matters are not so simple. Early research on attention in psychology concentrated heavily, though not exclusively, on introspections (self-observations) about awareness under controlled experimental conditions (e.g., Külpe, 1922/1964; Titchener, 1910). Since the information-processing revolution, the emphasis has been on behavioral and, increasingly, neuro-physiological measures. Behavioral methods include metrics of reaction time, accuracy of decisions, and trade-offs between speed and accuracy.

Reaction Time

Many methods used to study attention are based on reaction time. Typically, a participant is given a task to perform in which a particular response is to be made when a stimulus event, called the target stimulus, occurs. Instructions are to respond as fast as possible without making many errors, and reaction time is measured from the onset of the stimulus to the registration of the response. The required response is often a key press because the time for motor execution is minimal. Reaction time is usually measured in milliseconds (ms) for correct responses, averaged across several trials in the various conditions to provide the data from individual participants that make up the group analysis. Error rates are typically low, given the instructions to respond accurately, and are analyzed secondarily. By examining various details of mean reaction times and the distributions of reaction times in various conditions, it is possible to obtain evidence relevant to many issues about attention and human performance.

Subtractive Method

One topic of interest is the time needed to complete various processes. One of the most important events in experimental psychology was the realization that the time to complete mental processes could be measured. The development of this idea since the establishment of psychology as a science was discussed in Chapter 1, beginning with Wundt's observations of the time to switch attention from one stimulus to another (Blumenthal, 1980) and Helmholtz's measurement of neural transmission time (Schmidgen, 2002). The measurement of information-processing time was set on a firm footing with Donders's (1868/1969) use of the *subtractive method* for measuring the duration of processes. Recall that this method consists of comparing tasks that differ only in the processing stage of interest and taking the difference in completion times for the two tasks as a measure of the time needed to complete the process of interest.

In an application of this technique, Posner and Mitchell (1967) estimated the time to name letters. They did this by comparing the time to make a same or different classification of two letters that were identical in form (e.g., *RR*) with the time needed to make the classification when the letters were only identical in name (e.g., *Rr*). Posner and Mitchell found that judgments were 75 ms faster in the former case than in the latter. Reasoning that the letters with the same form could be judged as being the same or different based on visual information alone, whereas the letters presented in different cases required in addition that the name of each form be determined, Posner and Mitchell concluded that the naming process takes approximately 75 ms.

It should be noted that application of the subtractive logic, as in this example, depends on assumptions that the processing stages (e.g., perceive letters, name letters, select response "same" or "different," make response) are serial and independent and that the insertion of the additional process does not alter the basic task structure. The latter assumption is called *pure insertion*. Posner and Mitchell's (1967) application of the subtractive method in determining the time to name letters could be questioned because the time to process the letters might be affected by the forms of the letters, with processing proceeding more efficiently when the same stimulus occurs twice rather than when there are two different stimuli (Harding & Cousineau, 2022; Proctor, 1981).

Conditions that might lead to the violation of the assumption of pure insertion were observed soon after Donders (1868/1969) published his landmark paper. For example, L. Lange (1888) noted that emphasizing the response to be made—rather than the stimulus to be processed—led to shorter reaction times. Thus, the addition of instructions that change the focus of the participant (or task set) from the stimuli to the responses might lead to changes in one or more other stages of processing. Other studies have shown that although responses to simple and choice reaction tasks have similar characteristics, as Donders claimed, more physical force is exerted in responding in the Go/No-go task than in simple or choice reaction tasks (Ulrich et al., 1999). Further, Q. Zhang et al. (2018) found that electrical brain activity showed evidence of violation of pure insertion under conditions that reaction time did not. Participants were to enter two numbers or their two-digit product, which was one independent variable. In one condition, the digits were presented directly, whereas, in another condition, one was represented by a letter, for which the digit had to be substituted (e.g., $c = 3$). The variables had separate effects, which were assumed to reflect multiplication and substitution stages, respectively. However, electrical brain activity provided evidence that adding the substitution process also increased the duration of the response-selection stage, and adding the multiplication process decreased the duration of the motor stage.

Additive Factors Method

The subtractive method is used to compute the time needed to complete a known process. That is, the researcher makes assumptions about what the processes are and then compares tasks to measure the duration of the process of interest. A more basic question concerns the number and nature of the information-processing stages themselves. The *additive factors method*, developed by Sternberg (1969), is a method for determining which stages are involved in a particular task. That is, it can be used to infer the presence of specific stages.

In the additive factors method, several factors (i.e., independent variables) are manipulated, and the effects of these manipulations on time to perform the task are examined. Essentially all tasks involve the three information-processing stages. For example, driving requires monitoring displays in the vehicle and events outside of the vehicle (perception), decision making when changing lanes or routes (response selection), and steering the vehicle (motor). Similarly, having a phone conversation involves hearing the other person (perception), understanding what was said and deciding how to respond (response selection), and talking (motor). Some factors, though, influence one processing stage more than others, and additive factors analysis can help determine which stage is most impacted.

Which stage is most impacted by traffic levels in a driving task? An experiment can be designed to answer that question in which response time to an unexpected event is measured under low or high traffic levels and whether the driver is talking with a hands-free or hand-held phone. If the factors have additive effects (i.e., if the effect of traffic level does not depend on the use-of-phone factor), they are assumed to affect different stages (see Figure 2.3, left panel). If the factors interact, such that the effect of one depends on the level of the other, they are assumed to affect the same processing stage (see Figure 2.3, right panel). When it is known which stage is affected by one of the factors (e.g., use of a hand-held or hands-free phone most likely affects motor processing time), the underlying processing stages can be inferred. This is achieved by examining the patterns of interactions (e.g., if the use of the

FIGURE 2.3. **Hypothetical Example of Additive and Interactive Effects**

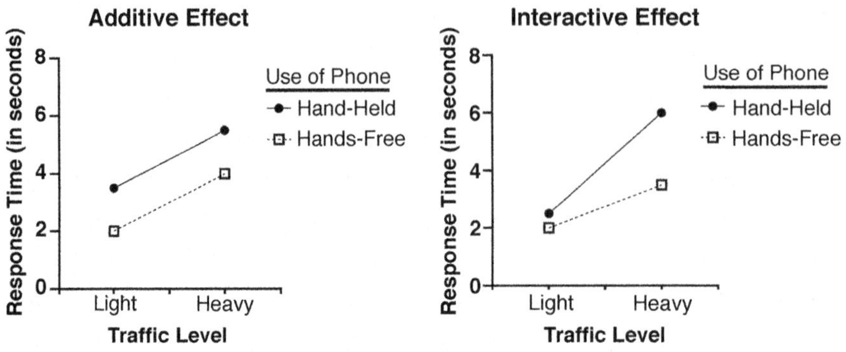

phone interacts with traffic level, both variables affect the motor stage; if the effects of the two factors are additive, the effect of traffic level is primarily affecting another stage, e.g., perception or response selection).

The additive factors method and subtractive logic can also be applied in an everyday task of buying an item on an e-commerce website to determine stages of the task and the time involved in those stages. The time it takes to acquire a product is the sum of all the sub-steps: (a) ordering the product (includes searching and checking out with the product) + (b) processing time (i.e., time for the company to receive your order and prepare your product for shipping) + (c) shipping time (time for the product to get from distribution to your destination). Assuming that these three stages are independent, the total time (T_{total}) from ordering to receiving your product is the sum of the time it takes for ordering, processing, and shipping your product ($T_{total} = T_{ordering} + T_{processing} + T_{shipping}$). For example, if it takes 30 minutes (.02 day) to order the product, 1 day to process it, and 3.5 days to ship it, the total time for you to receive the product is 4.52 days. If weather delayed the shipping by 2 days, the total time to receive the product is also extended by 2 days, to 6.52 days. That is, additional time added to any of the three steps increases the total time by the same amount. Subtractive logic can also be used to determine how long a specific step takes. For example, if it took 8 days for you to receive your product and the ordering and processing time remains .02 and 1 day, respectively, you can calculate the shipping time to be 6.98 days ($T_{shipping} = T_{total} - T_{ordering} - T_{processing}$).

The e-commerce example illustrates that effects are additive when factors affect different stages. That is, bad weather affecting the shipping route only extends the shipping time. When the factors influence a common stage, the effect of one factor can depend on the levels of the other. That is, bad weather can cause delays and extend shipping time (e.g., 2 days). Also, the COVID-19 pandemic might reduce the number of drivers available, which can delay delivery times (e.g., 1 day). Combined, the smaller number of drivers, along with the bad weather, can cause a temporary backlog of items, resulting in additional delays (e.g., 1 day). Thus, the delay time of 4 days is longer than that of 3 days (2 for shipping + 1 for reduced workforce) when the two factors are measured in isolation. Despite the possibility that the assumptions underlying additive factors analysis do not always hold (e.g., processes may operate concurrently, or a given process may output partial rather than complete information; McClelland, 1979; Roberts & Sternberg, 1993), a fairly consistent picture of the stages of information processing has emerged from applications of the additive factors logic in research studies (Sanders, 1990).

Response Accuracy

Accuracy of performance is analyzed as a dependent variable, often with methods in which response speed is not emphasized, but errors will be likely. In such studies, the proportion of correct responses or errors may be reported. A key consideration when interpreting accuracy is that the probability of an error depends on the number and probability of the response alternatives: The more alternatives, the lower the percentage correct expected by chance alone. Moreover, accuracy can be affected not only by a person's sensitivity to the critical information but also by their bias to give one response or another. These can be distinguished using signal detection methods and theory.

Signal Detection Methods and Theory

In this section, we describe a method for separating effects on response accuracy due to the sensitivity of the observer (i.e., the ability to perceptually process information) from effects due to the setting of a response criterion. This method, based on signal detection theory (e.g., D. M. Green & Swets, 1966; Kellen & Klauer, 2018), has been used with a wide variety of tasks, ranging from perceptual discrimination to recognition memory, to determine whether differences in performance between participants or tasks can be attributed to differences in the ability to discriminate among stimuli or a change in response bias or both.

Signal detection methods are applied to situations in which a participant must indicate whether a stimulus (signal) was present. For example, in a perceptual discrimination experiment, the signal might be a flash of light or a tone of a specific frequency, and in a memory experiment, the "signal" might be a word that was presented earlier in the experiment. An assumption is that signals are not equally clear on all trials but contain a random amount of noise that can detract from their discriminability. Noise might be due to external sources, such as the visual or auditory background, or internal sources, such as physiological variations in blood pressure. It is assumed that the quality of the signal varies along a single continuum of sensory evidence, ranging from relatively little evidence that a stimulus was present on a given trial to relatively convincing evidence. "Noise" trials, in which no stimulus was present, are also assumed to contain some evidence that a signal is present. Thus, the signal and noise trials can be depicted by distributions along a continuum of sensory evidence (see Figure 2.4, right half). Signal detection methods can only be applied when the distributions overlap, such that uncertainty about whether the signal was present exists in some trials. If the signal and noise distributions

FIGURE 2.4. Combinations of State of the World and Responses, and Distributions of Noise (Signal Absent) and Signal + Noise (Signal Present) Trials as a Function of Sensory Evidence

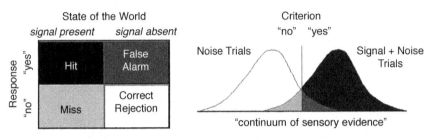

Note. "State of the world" refers to whether the signal was actually present or absent, and "response" refers to whether the operator said the target was present (yes) or absent (no). When the evidence exceeds the response criterion (the vertical line in the right panel), the "yes" response is made.

overlap completely, it is impossible to know whether a signal was present, and performance will be at chance.

In a typical signal detection experiment, the stimulus is presented on some proportion of the trials, and observers indicate on each trial whether they think the target stimulus was present. The experiment can be described as shown in Figure 2.4. On each trial, the signal was either present or absent, and the observer responded "yes" (the signal was present) or "no" (the signal was not present). Thus, there are four possible outcomes on a given trial: a "hit," a false alarm, a correct rejection, or a miss (see Figure 2.4, left half). Because the miss rate and the correct rejection rate can be derived from the hit rate and false alarm rates, respectively, performance can be completely described by just focusing on the hit rate and false alarm rate.

Although it might seem that a high hit rate indicates good performance, this is not always the case. To measure the sensitivity of the observer, it is also necessary to consider the false alarm rate. The sensitivity of the observer is high when the hit rate is high relative to the false alarm rate—that is, when the observer is accurate at discriminating signal and noise trials. High sensitivity can be conceptualized as indicating that there is little overlap between the signal and noise distributions. The most common measure used to describe sensitivity is d', which is equal to z(false-alarm rate) $- z$(hit rate). The z scores are obtained from normal distribution z tables and reflect the distance between the mean and criterion of each distribution (see Figure 2.5).

A key assumption of signal detection methods is that the results of a given experiment do not depend on the sensitivity of the observer alone but also on the decision criterion the observer uses. The decision criterion is defined as the point along the continuum of sensory evidence at which the person perceives enough information to make a "yes" response (see Figure 2.5). A conservative observer requires more information than a liberal observer. The more conservative the criterion setting, the less often the observer will say "yes," and

FIGURE 2.5. Neutral and Conservative Response Criteria for the Same *d'* Value

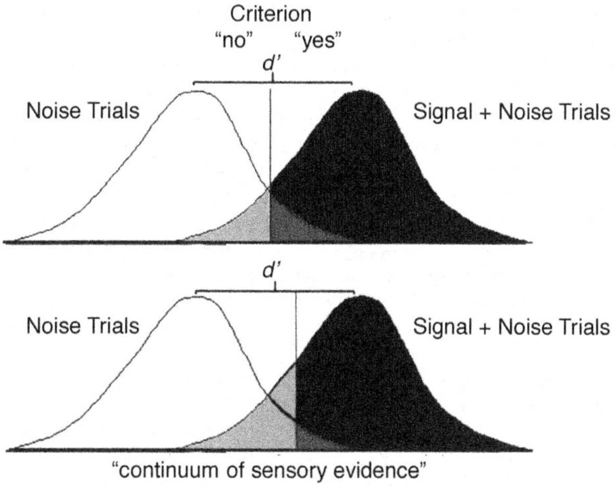

Note. The upper panel illustrates a neutral criterion and the lower panel a more conservative criterion. Both the hit and false alarm rates will be lower with the conservative criterion.

the lower the hit and false alarm rates (see Figure 2.5, bottom row). There are different ways to characterize the response criterion, with one measure being β (beta), the ratio of the height of the signal distribution to that of the noise distribution at the location of the decision criterion. Response bias has been assumed to be influenced by a number of factors, including payoffs that encourage observers to be more liberal (e.g., pay 20¢ for a hit and penalize 1¢ for a false alarm) or more conservative (e.g., pay 10¢ for a hit and penalize 10¢ for a false alarm) or the use of different probabilities for signal and noise. Both the degree of overlap of the distributions and the location of the response criterion can be computed from the observed hit and false alarm rates.

Signal detection methods have been widely used to study the effects of variables such as drugs, alcohol, and sleep loss on performance. The major question is whether such variables affect the sensitivity of the observer or the response criterion. An example related to attention is a study by Rosenstreich and Ruderman (2016) that examined the relation between self-reported mindfulness (awareness of the present moment) and performance on a recognition memory test. Participants initially filled out a questionnaire that measured five facets of mindfulness. They then studied two lists of words, one under full attention and another while performing an additional task of classifying the pitch of rapidly presented tones. Signal detection analyses were conducted of "old" (previously presented) and "new" responses on the recognition tests performed after each list. The analyses showed that memory sensitivity was less when attention was divided during the study phase than when it was not, but this effect was not moderated by any mindfulness facet. Responses were biased more toward "no" for the list studied under divided attention than for the list studied with full attention, and this difference was moderated by the mindfulness facet of "being nonjudgmental" about the self and others. The difference in response bias was evident for the participants classified as low on this facet but not those classified as high. The authors interpreted their results as suggesting that mindfulness did not allow participants to focus attention better on the words being studied during the study phase but may have indirectly affected decision processes on the recognition test.

Rather than analyzing a single yes–no point for each condition, as in Rosenstreich and Ruderman's (2016) study, a more complete analysis of sensitivity, bias, and the underlying distributions can be achieved through varying response bias and obtaining a *receiver-operating characteristic* (ROC) curve. Each ROC curve represents a single value of *d'*, as depicted in Figure 2.6. The curves show the possible combinations of hit and false-alarm rates that can be achieved solely by varying the response criterion through payoffs or probabilities that would maximize the value of the outcome (Lynn & Barrett, 2014). For example, Donkin et al. (2014) had participants view a memory set of displays of one to eight colored squares. Each display was followed by a colored square in one location to which a response of "change" or "no change" of color was to be made. The probability of change was varied between trial blocks to induce different criterion settings. Distinct ROC curves of decreasing sensitivity as memory set size increased were obtained, and probability biased the response criterion toward change or no change, as expected. Donkin et al. then conducted a more detailed analysis, which we will not describe here, to evaluate alternative models of the nature of the memory representation. Signal detection theory and ROC analysis have had considerable influence not only on basic research but also on applications (Wixted, 2020), examples of which are provided in Box 2.1.

FIGURE 2.6. Receiver Operating Characteristic (ROC) Curves for Two Sensitivity Levels (*d'* Values)

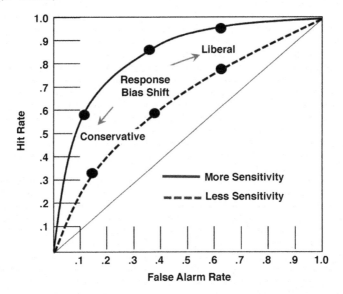

BOX 2.1 | SIGNAL DETECTION IN APPLIED SETTINGS

Signal detection methods provide a robust measurement of an operator's sensitivity (or accuracy) in a detection task. In many applied settings, human operators must detect a critical stimulus or event that is presented within background noise. Figure B2.1 shows some examples of different applied situations where signal detection methods have been used.

FIGURE B2.1. Example Applications of Signal Detection Theory

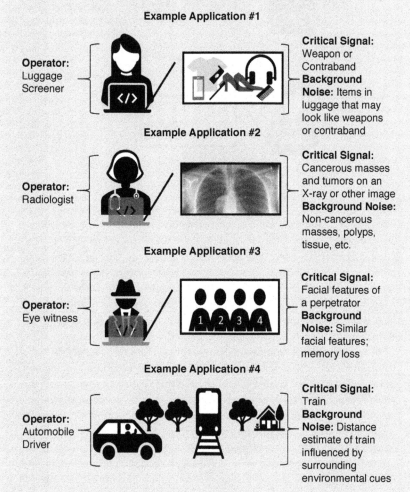

Example Application #1

Operator: Luggage Screener

Critical Signal: Weapon or Contraband
Background Noise: Items in luggage that may look like weapons or contraband

Example Application #2

Operator: Radiologist

Critical Signal: Cancerous masses and tumors on an X-ray or other image
Background Noise: Non-cancerous masses, polyps, tissue, etc.

Example Application #3

Operator: Eye witness

Critical Signal: Facial features of a perpetrator
Background Noise: Similar facial features; memory loss

Example Application #4

Operator: Automobile Driver

Critical Signal: Train
Background Noise: Distance estimate of train influenced by surrounding environmental cues

(continues)

BOX 2.1 | **SIGNAL DETECTION IN APPLIED SETTINGS** *(Continued)*

FIGURE B2.1. Example Applications of Signal Detection Theory *(Continued)*

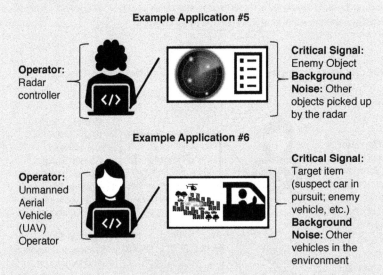

Example Application #5

Operator: Radar controller

Critical Signal: Enemy Object
Background Noise: Other objects picked up by the radar

Example Application #6

Operator: Unmanned Aerial Vehicle (UAV) Operator

Critical Signal: Target item (suspect car in pursuit; enemy vehicle, etc.)
Background Noise: Other vehicles in the environment

In all these cases, the goal is to have operators maximize the hit rate (HR), or the number of correct detections, and minimize the false alarm rate (FAR), or the number of incorrect detections. Signal detection methods provide a measure of d' for sensitivity (i.e., accuracy), and operators with higher d' values have higher sensitivity. It should be noted that sensitivity is based in part on the operator's natural ability, but it can also be increased through training or providing operators with tools that make it easier for the operator to discriminate targets from distractors.

In applied settings, another useful measure is that of a diagnosticity ratio (DR), where DR = HR divided by FAR. The DR can be based on a single pair of HR and FAR values. Wixted (2020) showed that DR can be used to test the effectiveness of two types of lineup procedures used by police for eyewitness identification of suspects. The first lineup procedure had a photo of six individuals presented simultaneously, and the second one had the individuals presented one at a time, serially. When comparing the HRs and FARs, the serial photo lineup yielded lower HRs and FARs, which could be interpreted as the procedure only making the eyewitnesses more conservative in their judgments (i.e., making fewer positive identifications). However, when the DR metric was used, the DR values were higher for the serial than simultaneous photo lineup procedures in most cases. This finding indicates that using the serial photo lineup procedure led to more accurate identification of the perpetrator in eyewitness identification. This higher accuracy may be result from being able to attend to the features of the suspect rather than trying to compare them across suspects.

Reaction Time and Accuracy

As should be apparent, in any situation for which responses are to be made quickly, a person will make errors. As noted, errors are often analyzed in reaction-time experiments but typically play a secondary role because the error rate is low. Thus, even when reaction time is the primary dependent measure in an experiment, accuracy is also measured. Having measures of both reaction time and accuracy is important to determine whether a *speed–accuracy trade-off* has occurred. In general, reaction time and accuracy are inversely related, such that, in a given task, increases in response speed are accompanied by reduced accuracy of performance (Heitz, 2014).

Figure 2.7 shows a typical speed–accuracy trade-off operating characteristic. The S-shaped form of the function reflects that when responses are relatively fast, any decreases in reaction time are accompanied by large costs in accuracy. Similarly, when accuracy is already high, it can only be increased at large costs in time to respond. Asking participants in an experiment to "respond as quickly as possible without making too many errors" is essentially asking them to find an optimal point on the speed–accuracy trade-off function. Speed–accuracy trade-off is said to occur when fast responses are accompanied by high error rates and vice versa. When this occurs, it is impossible to know whether differences between conditions are inherent in the task or simply due to the adoption of a different setting on the speed–accuracy trade-off function.

A distinction has been made between two types of speed–accuracy trade-off: macro and micro (Pachella, 1974). *Macro trade-off* is the most commonly studied type and refers to the setting on the speed–accuracy trade-off function within a particular condition or experiment. For example, some participants might adopt a risky strategy, resulting in fast reactions and many errors, whereas others may be more conservative, making few errors but taking a longer time to respond. Thus, macro trade-off reflects the strategy adopted by the participant and corresponds to adopting a setting on the speed–accuracy trade-off function. The influence of macro trade-off has been examined by using instructions that emphasize speed or accuracy or by using deadlines to induce different levels of time pressure (e.g., Wickelgren, 1977). *Micro trade-off* refers to the

FIGURE 2.7. A Speed–Accuracy Trade-Off Operating Characteristic

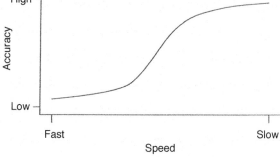

relation between speed and accuracy for trials within a single speed–accuracy emphasis condition. Micro trade-offs can be obtained by rank ordering reaction times and grouping them into bins from shortest to longest (e.g., quantiles). Plotting mean reaction time and accuracy for the respective bins yields a function showing the relation between speed and accuracy across the reaction-time distribution. Panis et al. (2020) applied such an analysis to several visual search tasks to examine the temporal dynamics of processing in them.

Modeling Speed and Accuracy

Sequential Sampling Models

A customary way to model relations between speed and accuracy is to use sequential sampling models (Donkin & Brown, 2018). Such models include thresholds, or criteria, for each response and a noisy evidence accumulation process. At the onset of a stimulus, evidence builds up over time, generally toward the response alternative assigned to the stimulus, and a response is executed when a threshold is reached. If presentation conditions are such that the stimulus is perceptible, it will be identified correctly if a sufficiently long time is allowed before responding. However, in a study for which response speed is emphasized, participants need to respond quickly. Due to noise in the accumulation process, if the response thresholds are set low, the threshold for an incorrect response may be the one that is exceeded first, resulting in an error.

Sequential sampling models distinguish three factors (Wagenmakers et al., 2007). *Drift rate* is the speed at which evidence builds up toward the correct response, and it will be larger the more discriminable the stimulus alternatives are. The second factor is the *response threshold settings*, which reflect speed–accuracy bias. Under constant stimulus and response conditions, reaction times will be shorter and incorrect responses more frequent when the threshold settings are more liberal than when they are more conservative. Models often include a third factor, a constant for all other processes that do not influence the response-decision time.

Some models—called race models—incorporate multiple accumulators that "race" to the thresholds, whereas others have a single accumulator that is between two thresholds and moves toward one or the other at any moment in time (Van Zandt, 2000). We cover only the most widely used of the latter models, the diffusion model (Ratcliff, 1978), to convey how data can be modeled with sequential sampling. This model is depicted in Figure 2.8 for a lexical decision task in which a person must respond as to whether a letter string is a word or nonword by making a key press. After stimulus onset, there is a brief period of nondecision time in which initial processing is done without any buildup toward a threshold. At the end of this period, the information accumulation process starts. This process is a continuous random walk (Wiener diffusion) in which the information accumulates over time toward one threshold or the other. (Note that Wiener, cited in Chapter 1 with regard to cybernetics, developed this process to model Brownian motion of particles suspended in liquid or gas.)

FIGURE 2.8. Depiction of a Diffusion Model for Lexical Decisions

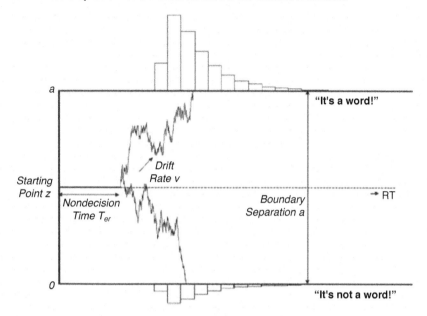

Note. Evidence builds up from starting point z toward one response boundary by a random walk. The drift rate v determines the speed at which the evidence builds up. When the evidence reaches a response boundary (*a* for "word" and *o* for "not a word"), a response is made. The bars represent the reaction-time distributions for correct "word" and incorrect "nonword" responses. From "Response Times and Decision-Making," by C. Donkin and S. D. Brown, in E.-J. Wagenmakers and J. T. Wixted (Eds.), *Stevens' Handbook of Experimental Psychology and Cognitive Neuroscience: Vol. 5. Methodology* (4th ed., p. 372), 2018, John Wiley & Sons (https://doi.org/10.1002/9781119170174.epcn509). Copyright 2018 by John Wiley & Sons. Reprinted with permission.

The drift rate is a function of the discriminability of the stimuli. For example, if the nonwords are the string XXXXX, the evidence will move quickly toward the appropriate threshold on a given trial, whereas if the nonwords differ from the words in only a single letter, the drift rate will be much less due to the greater similarity to a word. In the latter case, to respond accurately, the response boundaries will need to be set much wider. So, speed–accuracy trade-off can be modeled by the separation between the boundaries, whereas bias toward one response or the other (e.g., through instructions) can be modeled by moving the location of one boundary relative to the starting point to be less than the location of the other.

Connectionist and Neural Network Models

A second approach to modeling attention and other cognitive processes goes under the names of connectionist models, parallel distributed processing models, and neural networks. These models are constructed with modules that consist of elements and links between them. Presentation of a stimulus produces activation at the lowest levels of the system, which then propagates through the rest of the system, producing activation in subsequent units according to the link strengths. Sets of modules may be organized into distinct pathways, which may interact at any level of the system. A well-known application to attention is a model developed by J. D. Cohen et al. (1990) to explain performance in the Stroop task (see Figure 2.9). As described in Chapter 1, the Stroop effect is that reaction time to name a stimulus color is longer when the stimulus spells a color name that conflicts with the font color. The effect is asymmetric: When the task is word reading, performance is unaffected by whether the color conflicts with the color word.

The architecture depicts a situation in which two possible ink colors (red or green) and two possible color words (RED and GREEN) occur equally often in a series of trials. The color and color word each produces activation in distinct pathways. The input layer has an excitatory connection to the corresponding unit at the intermediate level and an inhibitory connection to the alternative unit. The task demand units modulate the activation in the pathways according to whether the task is to name the color or read the word. The remaining links are between the intermediate units and the response units. The asymmetry in the Stroop effect—that color words interfere with color naming but not vice versa—can be modeled by having stronger links to the responses from

FIGURE 2.9. J. D. Cohen et al.'s (1990) Connectionist Model for the Stroop Task

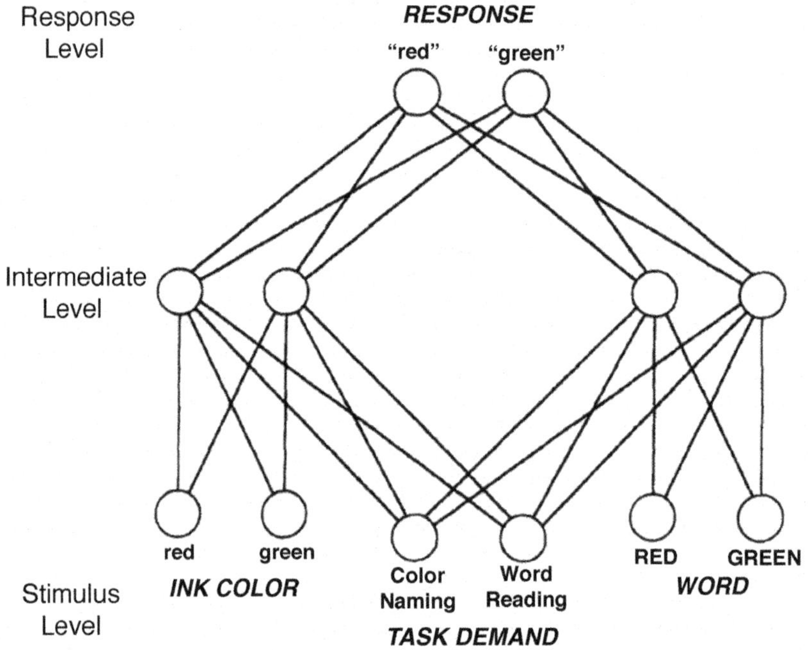

Note. Adapted from "On the Control of Automatic Processes: A Parallel Distributed Processing Account of the Stroop Effect," by J. D. Cohen, K. Dunbar, and J. L. McClelland, 1990, *Psychological Review*, 97(3), p. 336 (https://doi.org/10.1037/0033-295X.97.3.332). Copyright 1990 by the American Psychological Association.

the color word pathway than from the ink color pathway. J. D. Cohen et al.'s (1990) model is based on individual, discrete units for the stimuli and responses, but other models may distribute the inputs and outputs across many units (Mesulam, 1990).

Production System Models

Production system models originated in artificial intelligence as computer programs that were intended to emulate an expert's problem-solving and decision-making processes (H. A. Simon, 1979). A *production system* consists of a set of productions, each comprising a condition (IF) and an action (THEN). Whenever the condition is satisfied, the action will be produced. An early artificial intelligence program of this type was MYCIN, which diagnosed bacterial diseases in the manner of a trained physician (Shortliffe, 1976).

Production system models were then adopted to simulate human cognition. Newell and Simon (1972) were among the first to apply such models to human problem solving. Later, production systems provided the basis for architectures of human information processing intended to represent perceptual, cognitive, and motoric processes. These architectures offer computational frameworks in which simulations of alternative models for the performance of specific tasks can be developed. Among the most well known are SOAR (Laird, 2012), EPIC (Kieras, 2017), and ACT-R (adaptive control of thought—rational; J. R. Anderson et al., 2004). We describe ACT-R as an exemplar because of its widespread use.

The ACT-R architecture consists of several modules that carry out different aspects of information processing. Each module has a buffer that enables communication within and between modules. Modeling in ACT-R requires specifying declarative knowledge (a network of interrelated facts) for the domain or task being modeled and procedural knowledge in the form of production rules for execution of actions (Salvucci, 2017). The declarative knowledge is represented in the form of chunks, which vary in base-level activation and associative activation attributable to the current task goals. A highly activated chunk can be retrieved easily and fast. The IF part of the production rules consists of the chunk patterns that need to be matched by the current contents of the modules. When those patterns are activated, the production rule executes its actions transforming the set of patterns active in the buffers. From stimulus onset to response, computational models can be developed to simulate task performance under various conditions.

The emphasis on cognitive control in the name for the architecture should make clear that there is a close relationship to attention, and this is particularly evident in applications of ACT-R to control information processing in complex cognitive tasks (J. R. Anderson et al., 2004) and multitasking (Salvucci & Taatgen, 2011). J. R. Anderson et al. (1997) illustrated how ACT-R can be applied to tasks like visual search, in which visual attention needs to move across a display screen. They emphasized that ACT-R's focus of attention can be guided by looking in particular locations and directions, looking for specific features, and requesting to scan for objects that have yet to be attended to.

Eye Tracking and Related Measures

When someone talks about visually attending to a stimulus, they often mean that they are looking directly at it. Although attention can be decoupled from visual fixation, knowing where a person is looking in a display or scene can be informative about where their attention is directed. Studies conducted in the first half of the 20th century by Huey (1908) and others using rudimentary recording techniques established many of the fundamental facts about eye tracking (Rayner, 1978). Studies of military aircraft pilots' fixations and eye-movement patterns were conducted in the later 1940s by Fitts et al. (1950). Their measurements of the frequency of fixations on the various instruments of an aircraft instrument panel and the successive eye movements between the instruments led to a revision of the layout of the panel. The most widely cited research related to attention for many years was that of Yarbus (1967), who conducted studies of eye movements when looking at complex scenes. Yarbus showed that fixation patterns are determined by both the image properties and the task that a person intends to perform.

Research on eye tracking exploded in the 1970s due to the development of devices that could be interfaced with a computer to provide continuous online recording of eye movements (Rayner, 1978). Rayner (1998) summarized many of the advances made during the prior 20 years of research. He emphasized the development of innovative techniques allowing the visual display to change contingent on the eye position and the development of cognitive theories that made it possible to use eye-movement records to test implications in a variety of information-processing tasks, particularly in reading. Within the past 10 to 15 years, eye-tracking technology has improved in many ways, including affordability, miniaturization, and mobility, enabling widespread access for researchers to eye-tracking systems that allow detailed measurements of where one is looking and how the eyes move when one is performing a task.

The eyes move regularly from one stationary position to another. The periods in which the eyes are relatively stationary are *fixations*. It is during fixations that visual sensory information is processed. Because the eye and visual system are designed to process detailed information only from a small region of the retina in which acuity is highest (the fovea), during a fixation, the region in central vision will be processed in detail. However, some information relevant to perception and eye movements can be processed from the visual periphery. Fixation duration can vary, being as short as 50 ms and as long as several hundred ms when examining complex images (Salthouse & Ellis, 1980). Commonly reported measures include number of fixations on various areas of interest, mean fixation duration, and so on.

The eye movements between successive fixations are called *saccades*. They are fast and accurate, and processing of visual sensory input is suppressed during the saccades, which is called *saccadic suppression*. A consequence of this suppression and the fact that visual acuity decreases the further from the periphery a stimulus is located is that attending to a central point when two stimuli are relevant may lead to better performance. Hüttermann et al. (2014) obtained results consistent with this hypothesis for soccer players' detection of a goalie's direction of movement when making a penalty kick, which requires attention to both the ball and the goalie.

Two to three saccades per second typically occur (Pierce et al., 2019). A distinction can be made between involuntary visually guided saccades and volitional saccades that are voluntarily generated and more reliant on cognitive processes. The direction and distance of the saccades of both types can provide information about where a person is attending, whereas volitional saccades can also provide evidence about the person's goals and knowledge. For instance, regressive saccades when reading text, for which the reader returns to earlier phrases, provide indications that the person lacks understanding and has decided to recheck information. Also, gaze paths integrate fixations and saccades across time, which can provide evidence of the strategy a person is using to acquire information (Mäkisalo et al., 2013).

Attention plays a role in the control of eye movements (Greenlee & Kimmig, 2019). For example, B. Fischer (1986; B. Fischer et al., 1997) compared saccadic reaction times for two tasks. In one, called a *gap task*, the fixation point was switched off, and after a delay (the gap), a target stimulus appeared in the visual periphery to which the participant was to execute a saccade. In the other, called the overlap task, the central fixation point stayed on so that it overlapped temporally with the peripheral target stimulus. Reaction times were longer in the overlap task (240 ms on average) than in the gap task, which showed a bimodal distribution with peaks in the range of 100 to 120 ms and slightly less than 200 ms. B. Fischer interpreted these results as showing that attention must be disengaged from the fixation point in the overlap task, whereas in the gap task, attention can be disengaged during the blank period after fixation point offset, allowing an automatic "express" saccade to be triggered at target stimulus onset.

Most eye trackers also measure pupil diameter. Although people are aware that pupil size increases when lighting levels are low and decreases when lighting levels are high, they are unaware that pupil size is also affected by cognitive factors (see Chapter 11). Specifically, the pupils dilate when attentional demands, emotional arousal, and cognitive load are high. Because these measures are consistent and reliable, changes in pupil diameter provide real-time measures of attentional demands and emotional reactions. Kahneman (1973) defined attention as mental effort and advocated pupil dilation as a physiological measure of mental effort because it is sensitive to levels of difficulty within tasks. Pupil dilation is also capable of distinguishing processing requirements between task domains and is sensitive to individual differences in processing capacity (Laeng & Alnaes, 2019). Van den Brink et al. (2016) measured changes in pupil diameter when participants performed a sustained attention task. Pupil size correlated with behavioral indicators of attention, with pupil diameter being smaller during lapses of attention.

Blinking can also be an indicator of attentional demands because people blink less when they are paying attention than when they are not. Paprocki and Lenskiy (2017) analyzed participants' eye-blink rate variability during a 5-minute resting period and 10-minute IQ test. Blink rate variability during rest was positively correlated with performance on the IQ test, suggesting that blink rate variability dynamics at rest may carry information about cognitive ability.

COGNITIVE NEUROSCIENCE

Cognitive neuroscience analyzes neurophysiological processes, primarily in the brain, to elucidate the neural mechanisms that underlie cognition. Our concern specifically is with the neural basis of attention. We provide a brief description of several key regions of the brain here; a more thorough description can be found in Gage and Baars (2018). The *frontal lobe* is, as its name implies, at the front of the brain and is involved in higher level cognitive functions, including attentional control. It includes a region called *Broca's area* that is associated with speech production, as well as the primary motor area and three other regions involved in motor control: the premotor, supplementary motor, and cingulate motor areas. The *parietal lobe* is located behind the frontal lobe and is divided into two regions with different functions, one that subserves the skin senses and the other of which is involved in sensorimotor spatial processing and motor planning. The *temporal lobe*, located below the parietal lobe, contains the primary auditory cortex, a region involved in phonological representation, and structures that are involved in pattern recognition and memory. The *occipital lobe* is at the back of the brain and includes the primary visual cortex and other sections devoted to vision. A further terminological distinction in reference to the lobe is that "anterior" describes front or forward and "posterior" back or backward. "Superior" and "inferior" are adjectives used to describe top or bottom locations, respectively.

Other points to note are the following. Representation is lateralized such that the left cortical hemisphere receives sensory input from the right side and controls motor output from that side of the body, with the opposite for the right hemisphere. Also, two visual pathways, ventral and dorsal, carry out relatively distinct functions for visual perception. The *ventral pathway* goes from the occipital lobe to regions in the temporal lobe that are involved in detailed form perception. The *dorsal pathway* extends from the visual cortex to the parietal lobe and is involved in global aspects of vision. The former is sometimes said to process "what" and the latter "where." The "where" pathway has also been characterized as the "how" pathway due to the parietal lobe's role in action selection and control. As noted initially, we emphasize that this description is an extreme oversimplification; systems involving many cortical and subcortical brain areas are involved in all fundamental operations of attention. This simplified description should be sufficient, though, for understanding the results of cognitive neuroscience studies that are presented later in the book.

Electrophysiological Measures

Behavioral measures of human information processing can be supplemented by correlates of the physiological processes that underlie such processing. The most widely used of these are electrophysiological measures based on the voltage fluctuations within the brain that can be measured by electrodes placed on the scalp (i.e., the electroencephalogram [EEG]).

EEG Waves

The *EEG* measures ongoing brain waves that emanate from the brain's neural activity. The brain waves fall into four primary bands that range in wave frequency and are associated with high arousal down to the lowest level of arousal (see Figure 2.10). Evidence suggests that oscillations in all these frequency bands are related to many perceptual, cognitive, and action control processes (Harmony, 2013). The highest frequency brain waves are *beta waves*, for which the frequency is approximately 13 to 30 Hz. They are found when

FIGURE 2.10. EEG Waves, Frequency Ranges, Characteristics, and Key Properties

Wave (frequency)	Characteristics	Key properties

Beta (13–30 Hz) 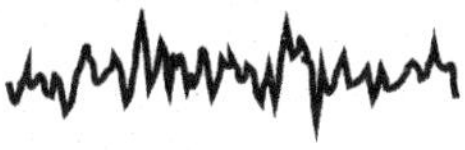	Awake, normal alertness, engaged in cognitive activity	• Increased activity:
		  o when movements are inhibited
		  o precedes correct responding
		  o faster responses are made to target stimuli
		• Decreased activity:
		  o when preparing movement execution
		  o slower responses are made to target stimuli

Alpha (8–12 Hz) 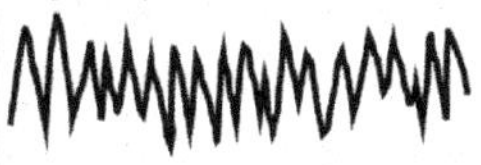	Calm, relaxed	• Inhibit task-irrelevant input • Facilitate processing of task-relevant input

Theta (4–7 Hz) 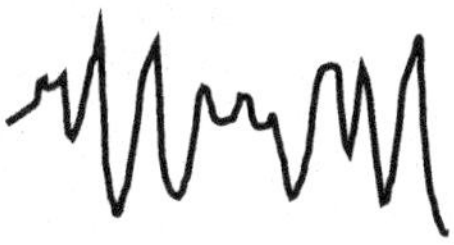	Day dreaming, mind wandering, deep relaxation, meditation	• Adjusting behavior to uncertainty
		• Burst activity:
		  o prior to quick responses
		  o involved in disinhibiting motor responses to achieve goals

Delta (1–3 Hz) 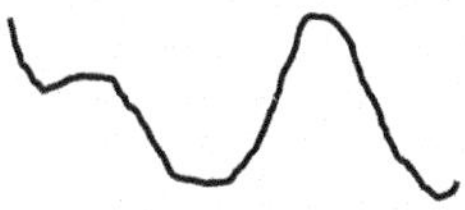	Sleep, dreaming	• Inhibition of:
		  o advanced cortical brain systems
		  o prepared responses
		• Increased activity for tasks that require focusing on internal representations (e.g., mentally doing math problems)

a person is in a normal, awake state and indicate that the brain is aroused and engaged in cognitive activity. Beta wave activity decreases when movements are prepared for execution (Pfurtscheller & Berghold, 1989) and increases when movements must be inhibited (Y. Zhang et al., 2008). Kamiński et al. (2012) found that beta-band activation was related to fast versus slow responding to target stimuli. Faster responses were preceded by higher EEG activation in the beta band over parieto-occipital regions, which they attributed to increased alertness. Gola et al. (2013) compared older and younger adults when performing a visual attention task. For both age groups, beta power showed increases in activity preceding correct responses but not incorrect responses. High-performing older adults did not differ from young adults in terms of beta-band power increases, but low-performing older adults showed less beta power. Consequently, Gola et al. concluded that low-performing older adults have deficits in activation and sustaining attentional processes.

Alpha waves are in the range of 8 to 12 Hz and occur when a person is in a calm state. Some evidence suggests that a person can control alpha activity to inhibit irrelevant stimuli and facilitate the processing of relevant information (Van Diepen et al., 2019). Speculative results have suggested that high-power alpha activity does not inhibit neural activity throughout the alpha cycle but mainly in specific segments of it (Mathewson et al., 2011). Findings of this type led Van Diepen et al. (2019) to speculate that alpha activity involves phasic bursts of inhibition that decrease activity in parts of the cortex, allowing for selective information processing and reallocation of resources.

The next frequency band is *theta waves*, for which the frequency is 4 to 7 Hz. Waves in the theta band are prominent when a person is daydreaming or, in current vernacular, mind wandering. However, they have also been implicated as playing a role in cognitive control and memory (Cavanagh & Frank, 2014). Cavanagh and Shackman (2015) went further in arguing that theta activity in the midline of the frontal lobes is correlated with adjusting behavior and response to uncertainty. Similarly, Delorme et al. (2007) found bursts in medial prefrontal theta waves preceding quick responses and suggested that the bursts indexed cortical activity involved in disinhibiting motor responses to rewarding or goal-fulfilling events.

The final level is *delta waves*, in the region of 1 to 3 Hz. These are associated with sleep and dreaming and have been attributed to inhibition of advanced cortical brain systems. However, evidence has indicated that delta waves are also involved in the performance of laboratory tasks. Increases in power in the delta wave region are often reported for tasks that require focusing on an internal representation, like those that require mental arithmetic. For example, Harmony (2013) reported that in a go/no-go task, power increased at 1 Hz on both go and no-go trials during a period 100 to 300 ms after stimulus onset in central, parietal, and temporal regions. However, in the no-go condition, power also increased in frontal regions, suggesting that the delta waves in that region reflect processes involved in inhibiting the prepared response. On the basis of these findings, Harmony concluded that the delta waves reflect inhibitory oscillations that reduce the activity of brain networks that would interfere with accomplishing the intended task.

In summary, task-related EEG changes are associated with decision making and cognitive control processes. Although different bands are associated with specific attentional functions, they are often used in conjunction with behavioral analyses to establish correlations. For example, Karamacoska et al. (2018) analyzed amplitude in the delta and theta bands for states progressing from relaxation (resting state with eyes closed) to eyes open and from eyes open to performance of a go/no-go task. Delta power increased from eyes open to the go/no-go task, and larger increases were associated with longer go reaction time and lower accuracy.

Event-Related Potentials

The EEG reflects all neural processing occurring within a given time interval and, as such, is not informative about the specific processes occurring at different points in time after an event onset. *Event-related potentials* (ERPs) are usually computed to narrow down the range of activity examined at a given moment (Luck, 2014). The ERP is calculated by averaging together many single-trial EEGs, starting from (i.e., time-locked to) a particular external event, usually the onset of a stimulus. As shown in Figure 2.11, electrical activity is generally recorded at several scalp sites. This is done for many trials, which are then averaged together to eliminate random noise and any electrical activity that is not temporally related to the processing of the stimulus. The resulting average waveform is the ERP, and it reflects only the neural activity associated with the information processing performed in response to the stimulus.

An advantage of ERP relative to behavioral measures is that it is measured throughout the intervening time between the presentation of the stimulus and the response, allowing precise measurement of the time course of attentional and other cognitive processes. Typical ERPs in reaction to a visual stimulus are

FIGURE 2.11. Schematic Depicting ERP Components to a Visual Signal

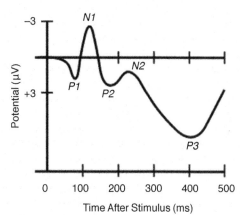

Note. ERP = event-related potential.

shown in Figure 2.11. The waveforms have components that can vary in latency and amplitude, as well as across electrode locations. The ERP components can be associated with specific cognitive activities. Spatial localization of processes in the brain from the electrode locations is imprecise due to what is called the "inverse problem" of working backward from the electrodes to the source of the neural generation (Slotnick, 2005). Despite this limitation, ERPs with a scalp distribution over the posterior areas of the brain are likely to reflect an influence of attention on sensory processes, whereas those with a frontal scalp distribution are likely to reflect an influence of attention on a higher level of cognition.

The components of the ERP are designated by the letters *N* or *P* to indicate whether the component is negative going or positive going, and a number to indicate the serial order in the event sequence (e.g., N1 is the first negative-going component). Because different research groups follow different conventions, attention should be paid to the *y*-axis of an ERP plot to determine whether the ERP has been plotted with positive going downward and negative going upward (as in Figure 2.11) or vice versa. Stimulus-locked ERPs in visual tasks show several positive and negative components, which are denoted as NP80 (a small negative/positive complex peaking at 80 ms after stimulus onset; also denoted as C1), P1, N1, P2, N2, and P3, in their temporal order of appearance. The earliest components (C1, P1, and N1) are assumed to reflect mainly bottom-up (i.e., stimulus-driven) processing. For visual stimuli, the polarity of C1, which appears to be generated in the early visual processing cortical areas (the primary visual cortex), depends on the position of a stimulus (V. P. Clark & Hillyard, 1996): C1 is positive for a stimulus that onsets in the lower part of the visual field and negative for one that onsets in the upper part. Its magnitude is affected by contrast and other stimulus features (Luck, 2014).

The P1 component is sensitive to the side of stimulus presentation: It is larger when measured at the brain hemisphere contralateral to the side of presentation (Heinze et al., 1990). Although, like C1, it reflects stimulus parameters, P1 is also modulated by selective attention to the left or right visual field (Luck et al., 2000) and attentional load (Fu et al., 2010). The N1 component comprises three subcomponents (V. P. Clark & Hillyard, 1996; Wijers et al., 1997) and could reflect a process that discriminates relevant from irrelevant stimuli (Vogel & Luck, 2000). N1 is also greater for stimuli at attended spatial locations than at unattended locations, suggesting that attention enhances early perceptual processing (Luck & Girelli, 1998).

The P2 wave occurs at central (denoted, e.g., Cz) and frontal (e.g., Fz) sites after the N1 component. Enlargement of the P2 wave is found in an oddball task when the oddball differs in a simple feature but not a complex feature combination (Luck, 2014). In an *oddball paradigm*, a standard stimulus is repeated in a series. Occasionally, a distinct "oddball" occurs, and the participant is asked to respond to it or mentally count the occurrences of the oddball stimulus. Thus, the enhancement of the P2 wave is interpreted as an indicator of change detection.

For the N2 wave that follows the P2 wave, it is useful to distinguish frontal and posterior locations. The frontal N2 is affected mainly by factors relating to response inhibition and response competition, topics we cover later in the book. The posterior N2, which can be decomposed into two components, is likely involved in categorization and focusing of attention (Luck, 2014). Specifically, N2pc (N2–posterior–contralateral) is thought to measure the covert orientation of attention. A target stimulus that is visible among a set of distractors produces an N2 component that is more negative at contralateral scalp sites than at ipsilateral scalp sites, and this difference defines the N2pc component (Woodman & Luck, 2003).

One of the most widely studied ERP components is the P3 (also denoted as P300 or P3b), which reaches its largest amplitude at centrally placed electrode sites and usually peaks between 330 to 600 ms after stimulus onset. The peak latency of the P3 component is assumed to reflect the end point of stimulus evaluation (Donchin et al., 1978; Kutas et al., 1977), although some studies have shown this component to be sensitive to variables that affect response-related processing (Nieuwenhuis et al., 2011; Verleger, 1997). Stimuli falling within the focus of attention only elicit a P3 component when the stimulus is relevant for performance—that is, when it is a target rather than a distractor (Hillyard & Kutas, 1983).

The dependency of the P3 component on target relevance is evident in the oddball paradigm. For trials in which an oddball stimulus occurs, a strong P3 component is evoked. The amplitude of this P3 component has been interpreted as reflecting processes involved in *memory updating* (Donchin & Coles, 1988) because only when the oddball stimulus appears does memory for the target need to be updated. It should be noted, though, that P3 amplitude may be affected by many variables, including task complexity and response-related factors (e.g., R. Johnson, 1993).

The oddball paradigm has also been used to examine the influence of changes in unattended auditory stimuli. In this case, a series of tones of short duration (e.g., 60 ms) is presented while participants perform a relatively passive task such as reading a book or even while they sleep (e.g., Atienza et al., 2001). Most of the time, a standard tone of a given frequency (e.g., 1,000 Hz) and duration is presented, but occasionally a deviant (oddball) tone of a slightly different frequency (e.g., 1,032 Hz), intensity, or length is presented. The difference between the ERPs elicited by the standard and deviant tones is largest over the frontal-central brain areas and has been denoted as the *mismatch negativity* (MMN). The MMN has been interpreted as the outcome of a preattentive process that registers the "mismatch" between new sensory input and the representation of the standard stimulus, which is stored in auditory sensory memory (Näätänen, 1992). The MMN arises from the auditory cortex, and it has been argued that the mismatch negativity can be modulated by attention (Woldorff et al., 1998).

Another frequently used measure derived from the EEG is the *lateralized readiness potential* (LRP). The LRP seems to be a pure measure of motor preparation (e.g., J. Miller & Hackley, 1992; Smulders et al., 2012). The LRP is measured above the primary motor areas and is obtained using a double subtraction procedure to remove activity that is not related to the side of the required response. Relatively high contralateral activity to the side of the required response hand indicates that motor activation is larger for the required response, whereas higher ipsilateral activity indicates that motor activation is larger for the incorrect response. The LRP can be computed time-locked to the onset of the stimulus or the response, yielding measures of the duration of the processes that occur before the start of the LRP (and thus before readiness to respond) and after the start of the LRP (Osman & Moore, 1993). When a manipulation (e.g., varying signal quality) affects the start of the stimulus-locked LRP but not the start of the response-locked LRP, it can be concluded that a process before the moment of correct motor activation is affected. An influence of a manipulation on the start time of the response-locked LRP but not on that of the stimulus-locked LRP indicates that a process after motor activation is affected. Varying speed–accuracy instructions have such a response-locked effect (Osman et al., 2000; van der Lubbe et al., 2001).

Neuroimaging and Neurostimulation Techniques

Although ERPs provide precise data about the time course of information processing, they do not provide much information about which brain areas are involved in specific activities. Methodologies for human brain imaging allow the determination of areas of brain activity. The most well-known techniques used to provide information about the localization of processes are *positron emission tomography* (PET) and *functional magnetic resonance imaging* (fMRI). In both, people perform a cognitive task (e.g., a task requiring selective attention) while in a scanner. Blood flow rates in different regions are measured, which are assumed to vary as a function of neural activity. The blood flow during the task is compared with that during baseline testing (i.e., without the specific cognitive aspect of interest) to isolate the brain region that is unique to the process of interest. In this way, cerebral regions associated with specific task components can be visualized (see the images in Figure 2.12 for people trained to direct attention externally vs. internally).

In PET research, a radioactive marker is inhaled by or injected into the participant. These marker molecules can then be used to measure brain metabolism as the markers move with the regional cerebral blood flow (rCBF). Images of the locations of the markers thus reveal where blood flow was necessary to provide oxygen. Areas that show an increase in rCBF during a cognitive task are presumed to be actively involved in the underlying process (Narayana et al., 2017). PET can be sensitive to methodological differences between tasks and, because of the nature of the vascular response, is limited in spatial resolution (Corbetta, 1998). A classic study in cognitive neuroscience and attention was conducted by Posner et al. (1988), in which they concluded that the PET data provided evidence that different regions of the brain are involved in processing visual, phonological, and semantic codes.

FIGURE 2.12. fMRI Images for Groups Trained With an External and Internal Focus of Attention

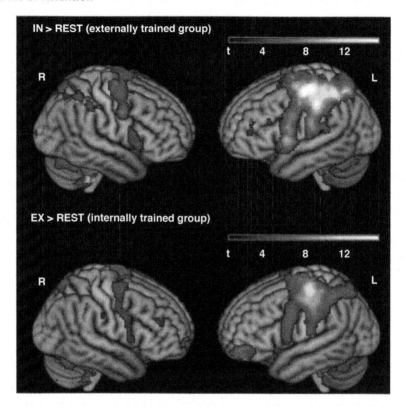

Note. From "Neural Correlates of Switching Attentional Focus During Finger Movements: An fMRI Study," by K. M. Zimmermann, M. Bischoff, B. Lorey, R. Stark, J. Munzert, and K. Zentgraf, 2012, *Frontiers in Psychology, 3*, p. 8 (https://doi.org/10.3389/fpsyg.2012. 00555). CC BY 3.0.

fMRI is more widely used than PET, in part because the magnets for measuring it are better in quality and cheaper in price, making it more accessible (Stamatakis et al., 2017). Moreover, it does not require participants to ingest radioactive materials. fMRI is based on the magnetic characteristics of the blood oxygen level–dependent (BOLD) response. Brain regions that are active during a given task or process require more oxygen, supplied through the blood. This increase in blood oxygen is measured using the specific magnetic properties of blood and the surrounding tissue (see Haxby et al., 1998, for a detailed overview of the use of fMRI as a research method to study attention). fMRI has a fairly high spatial resolution of about 1 centimeter and is becoming more and more accurate in the temporal domain. It has also become possible to study the BOLD response to a single event (e.g., with different stimulus types within a task), using a technique known as event-related fMRI (D'Esposito et al., 1999).

An approach to obtaining both temporal and spatial resolution is to measure ERPs and fMRI for the same tasks. Bayer et al. (2018) recorded both types of measures simultaneously for tasks requiring face processing and concluded that this joint analysis revealed attention-dependent coupling of early face processing with a cortical network distributed across several brain regions. Salmela et al. (2018) had participants perform identical experiments using visual and auditory attention tasks. In one experiment, they recorded ERPs, and in another, they recorded fMRI images. An ERP-based analysis was used to decompose the time-averaged fMRI pattern activity into distinct spatial maps, each of which corresponded to a short temporal ERP segment. Their analysis revealed eight cortical networks, three of which involved attention.

Another technology that uses blood oxygen levels to infer brain activity is functional near-infrared spectroscopy (fNIRS; Ferrari & Quaresima, 2012; Xu et al., 2019). Among the benefits of fNIRS is that it is not affected much by body movements and can be used in both laboratory and more naturalistic environments with a variety of participant populations (Pinti et al., 2020). In the lab, increases in workload demands of working memory and mathematical tasks have been found to be associated with increases in oxygenated hemoglobin and decreases in deoxygenated hemoglobin in the prefrontal cortex (Herff et al., 2014; Mandrick et al., 2013). Outside of the lab, fNIRS has been shown to be sensitive to the cognitive demands of tasks, including air traffic control (Harrison et al., 2014) and the operation of remotely piloted vehicles (Afergan et al., 2014). Perhaps most important, hyperscanning techniques with fNIRS allow measurement of the brain activity of two or more persons at the same time (Scholkmann et al., 2013). Studies have shown neural synchrony of the participants in tasks requiring cooperation (Yang et al., 2021) or synchronized performance (Babiloni & Astolfi, 2014). For example, in one study, pairs of singers showed more fNIRS neural synchrony in a condition that required singing together than in one that involved singing alone (Osaka et al., 2015).

An additional technique to map neural activity is *magnetoencephalography*, which is based on the electromagnetic characteristics of the electric field produced by firing nerve cells (P. Downing et al., 2001). Although the temporal characteristics of the activity of the brain revealed by these methods are detailed and accurate, their spatial resolution is not. In other words, it is difficult to link the electrical signal to a specific structure in the human brain other than in general terms such as "left posterior" or "right posterior" activity.

The final technique for localizing brain function is *transcranial magnetic stimulation* (TMS). Here, brief electromagnetic pulses are applied over a given area of the skull before or during a cognitive task using a current-producing coil that interferes with the underlying neural tissue (Stewart et al., 2001). Low-frequency TMS (< 1 Hz) is thought to produce a "virtual lesion"—that is, a transient dysfunction in the affected brain area. High-frequency TMS (> 5 Hz) might enhance neural activity, thus improving performance on a specific function (Wassermann & Lisanby, 2001). Because TMS can be manipulated as an independent variable, it can provide causal evidence rather than being restricted to correlational relations with performance and experience (Fernández & Carrasco, 2020).

In short, imaging and related techniques can be used to study in detail the functional characteristics of the human brain with relatively high resolution.

Although the temporal resolution is not as high, it is becoming progressively more precise as the imaging techniques increase in sophistication. With the help of such techniques, our knowledge of the neural basis of attention has greatly improved over the past decades. But, as pointed out by Uttal (2001) and reiterated by Pereira (2017), it is still an open question as to how much detail about localization of function the imaging techniques can ultimately provide. As Umiltà (2022) emphasized,

> Even if it were possible . . . to map specific mental processes into well-localized brain areas, the explanatory value of brain localization would be doubtful. Localizing a mental process in the brain would not explain that process. That is because any true explanation must be concerned with the *mechanisms* that instantiate a given mental process, not with where in the brain it is instantiated. Knowing the answer to the "where" question is no doubt helpful. However, the important question is the "how" question. (p. 572)

CHAPTER SUMMARY

This chapter provides a primer of the techniques used to conduct research on attention and performance. The concept of the human as an information processor plays an important role in empirical research and theory development. A simple three-stage model of information processing provides an adequate framework for organizing discussion and debate of issues such as the purpose and effects of attention. The three-stage framework will recur throughout the book as we address topics such as the locus of attentional selection, the location of processing bottlenecks, and the performance of multiple tasks. As new topics are addressed, details about the sort of processing that occurs—and the role of attention in that processing—will be discussed.

A range of techniques is available for delineating the processes involved in the selection and processing of information and the factors that influence them. Behavioral techniques focus on the outcome of information processing by measuring overt performance, such as the speed and accuracy with which a task is performed. Electrophysiological and neuroimaging techniques can be used to examine intermediate steps of processing, providing a picture of brain activity during task performance. These techniques can also be used, along with computational models and analytical methods, to explore and confirm hypotheses about attentional systems and their neural basis. The techniques introduced in this chapter recur throughout the book as we describe the nature of attention and its role in human performance.

KEY POINTS

- **Fact:** The cognitive, or information-processing, revolution in the 1950s introduced a variety of theories, conceptual tools, and methodologies to study human attention and performance.

- **Fact:** Objective measures of human performance—reaction time, response accuracy, and their relation—can be used to provide attentional data and evaluate attentional theories.

- **Fact:** Sophisticated methods and models can be used to test detailed predictions of theories.

- **Fact:** Signal detection methods have been widely used to distinguish effects of sensitivity from those of bias in response accuracy measures.

- **Phenomenon:** For any task, basic or applied, for which speed of responding is critical, speed can be traded off for accuracy, which is known as the speed–accuracy trade-off.

- **Theory:** Many theories of attention and performance treat information from the onset of a stimulus as building up over time by a noisy process toward one of two or more alternative responses.

- **Fact:** Eye trackers can be used to record both intentional and unintentional overt orienting of attention by measuring the properties of fixations and the saccades between them.

- **Fact:** EEG and neuroimaging methods can measure brain activity associated with attention and other cognitive processes, and other neurophysiological techniques are also available.

3

Selective Attention in Audition and Vision

For an individual to produce coherent behavior in the face of competing and distracting sources of stimulation, that person must select some things and ignore others. If unable to do so, the person would constantly be distracted by the stimuli with which they are bombarded. This would render them unable to carry out any controlled perception, cognition, or action. Thus, it is essential that people are aware of only a small portion of their surroundings at any moment, and only a limited range of objects can be attended to and acted on at any one time.

As William James (1890/1950) pointed out, concentration and focus are attention's essence. That seems to be even more so in the 21st century, when technological advances have increased the sources of stimulation, viewpoints, and possible actions with which people are continually bombarded. Although it is apparent that selective attention is necessary, its locus in the human information-processing system and the objects of selection remain controversial. For example, some evidence suggests that selection occurs at early, perceptual levels of processing, such that some stimuli are identified and others are not. Other evidence implies that selection does not occur until later levels after perceived information has achieved some semantic processing, thus allowing the meaning conveyed by unattended stimuli to influence performance.

The emphasis of this chapter is on fundamental aspects of selective attention in the auditory and visual sensory modalities, but much of the remainder of

https://doi.org/10.1037/0000317-003
Attention: Selection and Control in Human Information Processing, by R. W. Proctor and K.-P. L. Vu

the book delves into topics that also involve selective attention. In this chapter, we consider the following questions: At what stage of information processing is attention required or engaged to select information? On what is attention focused—locations in space or the objects in them? What makes selection easy or difficult? We begin by discussing the purpose of selective attention.

THE FUNCTION OF SELECTIVE ATTENTION

Attention for Perception

Some psychologists have proposed that attention is necessary for perception. For example, Carrasco (2018) wrote, "Visual attention is essential for visual perception" (p. 577). That is, the perceptual system is assumed to have limited processing capacity, an assumption made earlier by Broadbent (1958) for auditory perception. This limited capacity, which may have its basis in limitations of neural processing (Lennie, 2003), makes it necessary to select a subset of items to receive perceptual processing. In this view, called *early selection*, attention is needed to restrict sensory input to the perceptual system to prevent overload. Another hypothesis is that the task of combining all the separate features of an object, such as the contours, colors, and locations of a visual stimulus, if undertaken for all objects at the same moment, would result in a combinatorial explosion of the number of different possible reconstructions (e.g., Treisman et al., 1983). The proposed solution for this problem, called the *binding problem*, is to focus on a limited area for processing so that only the features within that area will be combined to reconstruct the objects present there.

Attention for Conscious Awareness and Clearness

As discussed in Chapter 1, an initial view regarding the function of attention was that it is needed to bring perceptual information to conscious awareness. James (1890/1950) described this role of attention as "anticipatory preparation" for the stimuli to come. This preparation is critical in determining what people become aware of (see also Wundt, 1907b). In this view, images of unattended visual objects are registered on the retina and may even be processed to the level of identification (e.g., to a semantic level), but attention is required to be aware of the objects.

Although this relation between attention and awareness seems straightforward, it is still a matter of debate. For example, Baier et al. (2020) proposed that the two processes are independent. Without going into details, they based this proposal on findings that attention capture by a color singleton (i.e., a stimulus that stands out because of its unique color) influenced performance separately from the effect of a visual mask on subjective awareness and accuracy of discriminating the target stimulus. There was no relation between the attention-grabbing property of the stimulus and measures relating to conscious awareness. Studies using various neurophysiological measures, such as electroencephalogram and functional magnetic resonance imaging (fMRI), also provide evidence that neural mechanisms of attention and consciousness can be dissociated (Maier & Tsuchiya, 2021).

A closely related proposal is that attention increases the perceived intensity of a stimulus and possibly other spatial and temporal dimensions as well (Carrasco & Barbot, 2019). This was the conclusion reached by Mach in his dispute with Stumpf in the early 20th century over whether attending to an audible component tone of a harmonium increased its perceived intensity (Titchener, 1908/1973; see also Chapter 1, this volume). Prinzmetal and colleagues (1997, 1998) conducted experiments examining the effect of attention on the appearance of stimulus brightness, contrast, color, location, orientation, and spatial frequency. The amount of attention available for observers to indicate the appearance of the objects was varied in several ways. One way was to present stimuli for a second task simultaneously, rather than successively, with those stimuli for the appearance task, based on evidence that the simultaneous task would require more attention. Results showed that the effect of attention was not to change the appearance of the stimuli, as Mach would have expected, but to decrease the variance of the observers' ratings. This decreased variability was proposed to be a consequence of a reduction of uncertainty about the exact stimulus value.

Attention for Action Selection and Control

Some researchers argue that rather than being linked to the limited capacity of the perceptual systems, attentional selection is needed to constrain and control possible actions. The basis for this view is that although the senses can register many different objects together, movement systems are limited to carrying out just one action at a time. Thus, Allport (1987) and Neumann (1987) advocated what Allport called *selection-for-action* processes, which selectively couple perception to action. Neumann similarly argued that the limits of attention are not due to processing capacity but rather to the necessity of mechanisms to coordinate and control action. In most tasks, just one category or mode of action is given priority to prevent conflicts. Attention is needed to constrain the selection of the appropriate action based on the incoming information.

Hommel (2010) elaborated this view, arguing, "Attention is a direct derivative of mechanisms subserving the control of basic motor actions" (p. 123) and proposing that attentional functions may be a by-product of action control. He based this argument in part on findings that stimulus and response representations can interact when they share features. For example, in a study by Müsseler and Hommel (1997), participants prepared a left or right key press, after which they pressed a key to indicate being ready. This press resulted in the onset of a masked visual arrowhead pointing to the left or right. Accuracy of report at the end of the trial of the direction in which the arrow pointed was lower when it pointed in the same direction as the response compared with when it pointed in the opposite direction. This outcome suggests that binding a left or right feature to the response reduced its availability for perception. Olivers and Roelfsema (2020) are among those who have advocated the view that action is essential to attention, stating, "Attention emerges from coupling relevant sensory and action representations within working memory. Importantly, this coupling is bidirectional" (p. 179). The emphasis on a bidirectional relation between perception and action has been prominent in psychological research during the first decades of the 21st century (Camus et al., 2018; Pfister, 2019).

Much of the early information-processing research on attention used auditory stimuli to address critical issues such as the nature of selective and divided attention and whether selection occurred early or late in processing. For that reason, we next review research on auditory selective attention using the *dichotic listening task*, in which separate messages are presented at the same time, each to a different ear. We summarize the major findings and phenomena for auditory selective attention, in which listeners attend to one message, ignoring the other. In the rest of the chapter, we describe phenomena and theories for visual selective attention.

AUDITORY SELECTIVE ATTENTION

Dichotic Listening Task

Everyone has had the experience of trying to follow two conversations at the same time, such as when you hear your name spoken at a party and try to hear what is being said while carrying on the current conversation. More often, we try to ignore one conversation to focus on another, such as when trying to follow the dialog of a film in a noisy theater. In these examples, two sources of auditory information are presented to both ears simultaneously. We try to follow one of the conversations while filtering out the other, relying only on our attentional capacities.

To control the presentation of the stimuli used to study the ability to select information, researchers in the 1950s developed the dichotic listening task in which separate sources of auditory information are presented to the two ears of the listener. For example, one might hear a list of spoken digits in one ear and a list of spoken letters in the other. Selecting one message is easier in dichotic listening than in monaural or binaural listening, in which the two messages are presented together to one ear or both ears (Egan et al., 1954). In dichotic listening, each message is presented with a large intensity difference (in each case, zero for one ear and easily audible for the other), but even more moderate differences comparable to those of spatial distinctions in everyday life improve selective listening considerably (Treisman, 1964a). Dichotic presentation gives the impression of separate streams of sound, each localized at the input ear. The localization is stronger than in monaural listening and of a different nature. Normally, localization rests on several cues, the most important being the differences in time (and phase of the sound waves) and intensity at which the information reaches each of the respective ears. These cues are absent in the dichotic listening task because each ear only receives one message. Even so, the task has often been used to study the limits of attention in selecting information.

Cherry (1953) was the first to use the dichotic listening technique to study attention, motivated by the question of how someone recognizes what one person is saying when others are talking at the same time, which is known as the *cocktail-party problem*. In his experiments, participants were required to shadow (repeat back immediately) one of the messages. People could do this remarkably well. When asked about the information presented to the unattended ear, however, they were able to report nothing more than that speech sounds had been present.

Cherry (1953) manipulated the message on the unattended ear to determine how much of the information was processed despite the instruction to attend to the opposite ear. He found that almost no one noticed when the unattended message changed languages from English to German. When it changed to backward speech, some participants showed no awareness of the change, whereas a few listeners identified the speech as having something odd about it. A subsequent study showed that all participants who reported detecting something unusual in the unattended message showed disrupted shadowing during the backward speech (Wood & Cowan, 1995). This result suggests a shift of attention to the message that was supposedly unattended. Participants who showed no disruption of shadowing did not report detecting the unusual nature of the speech, implying that attention is required to detect and report the unusual nature. In contrast to the changes that were not routinely noticed, listeners usually noticed a change in the gender of the speaker (and, thus, the pitch of the voice) or presentation of a 400-Hz tone. Cherry concluded that changes in perceptual features are typically identified, whereas changes in semantic content are not.

Bottleneck Models of Selective Attention

Filter Theory

Broadbent (1958) proposed an early selection bottleneck model of attention, called *filter theory*, which was based on this key property of auditory selection noted by Cherry (1953). The model characterized human processing as an information channel with limited capacity. Broadbent's views about the human as a limited capacity information channel were inspired by the then-recent developments in communications engineering. Information theory (see Chapter 2, this volume) provided an elegant way to model the transfer of information, and Broadbent saw the possibility of using this theory to quantify human information processing precisely. His first concern was specifying the point at which information processing is limited. He relied primarily on the experiments of Cherry (1953) and others (e.g., Webster & Thompson, 1954), in which it was found that participants could select information presented to one "information channel" (in this case, an ear) and ignore information presented to the other. Consequently, Broadbent hypothesized that attention operates to select information at an early stage, before the stimuli are identified, based on attributes, such as their locations, or features, such as pitch or loudness. According to his filter theory (see Figure 3.1), a selective filter protects the information-processing channel from being overloaded by too much information. This filter, which is "set" for basic stimulus characteristics such as location, pitch, or loudness, allows only some information to enter the system and excludes the rest.

As applied to dichotic listening, filter theory assumes that information from each ear first enters a buffer in which it can be held for a short time (the input tubes in Figure 3.1a; the short-term sensory store in Figure 3.1b). The filter is set to block entry into the limited capacity channel (the single tube in Figure 3.1a) of the input from one ear and allow that from the other ear to enter the channel, where it can be identified. The results of this analysis are then sent to a response system (motor buffer and effectors in Figure 3.1b) and may also be used to update expectations about what is likely to occur in the given situation. Filter theory is classified as an early-selection theory because information is assumed to be selected by the attention mechanism before stimulus identification. Broadbent's model captures the most obvious effects of attending to one message but not the other: People show little awareness soon thereafter of anything about the unattended message other than sensory features.

To test whether people are as insensitive to the unattended channel as it seemed in Cherry's (1953) study and as exemplified in Broadbent's (1958)

FIGURE 3.1. Simple and More Complete Depictions of Broadbent's (1957, 1958) Filter Theory

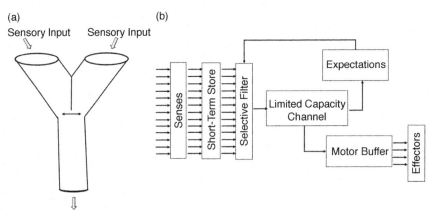

Note. (a) A simplified depiction in which the filter is shown as a solid vertical line, which can be set to block one side of the funnel, and (b) a detailed depiction where the selective filter is labeled as the mechanism that limits access to the limited capacity channel. Adapted from "A Mechanical Model for Human Attention and Immediate Memory," by D. E. Broadbent, 1957, *Psychological Review, 64*(3), p. 206 (https://doi.org/10.1037/h0047313). Copyright 1957 by the American Psychological Association.

model, Moray (1959) played the same word list to the unattended ear 35 times. He found that listeners were no more likely to report having heard the repeated words than words that were never presented. However, when the message played to the unattended ear is the same as that played to the attended ear, listeners notice the repetition when the lag between the repeated words is only a few seconds (Cherry, 1953; Treisman, 1964b). This result poses a problem for theories of attention that propose early selection of information based on a filter that monitors sounds fitting a certain sensory criterion, be that location, pitch, or intensity (e.g., filter theory; Broadbent, 1958). It also shows that more information may be processed than that of which people are normally aware.

More informative, Moray (1959) found that when a person's name was presented in the unattended message, followed by the message "You may stop now" or "Change to your other ear," 33% of the participants detected the occurrence of their name even though they had not received instruction indicating that it would occur. This phenomenon is replicable, as are most phenomena in basic research on attention. For example, Röer and Cowan (2021) found that 29% of their participants detected their own names but not other unexpected words, indicating that lack of expectancy was not the critical factor. This intrusion of one's name into conscious awareness should ring true to almost everyone because all of us have experienced times when we were in a crowd and detected our name being said, often not with respect to ourselves.

Treisman (1960) also provided evidence that the meaning of the unattended message was processed, at least to some extent. Participants shadowed a prose passage in one ear and ignored a different passage in the other ear. In the middle of the sequence, the passages switched ears so that the previously shadowed message was now in the to-be-ignored ear. Yet, participants often continued shadowing the original passage for a word or two before switching back to the message in the to-be-attended-to ear. One example provided by Treisman is

Shadowed Message: . . . SITTING AT A MAHOGANY/three POSSIBILITIES

Ignored Message: . . . . let us look at these/TABLE with her head
(p. 246),

with capital letters indicating what the participant was saying up to the switch (shown by the slashes) and then after the switch. The participant mistakenly said the word "TABLE," which fit the context of the message they were shadowing, before changing back for the next word.

Filter-Attenuation and Late-Selection Theories

On the basis of her results and Moray's (1959), Treisman (1960) proposed a modified version of Broadbent's (1958) filter theory, called *filter-attenuation theory*, according to which the unattended message is not blocked out entirely but only has its "volume" decreased, or attenuated. When the threshold for identifying a stimulus is low, either through prior experience (as with one's name) or the immediate context (as in the prose passages), the word is identified. In Figure 3.2b, the words B and C are shown as darker circles because they have had their thresholds lowered due to their relation to the prior word, A. Consequently, Word C may be identified even though it was presented in the unshadowed ear.

Deutsch and Deutsch (1963) and Norman (1968) went further than Treisman (1960) and argued that there is no significant processing limitation up to a categorical level of processing. In other words, they suggested that selection does not occur on the basis of an early selection filter (which sometimes allows specific stimuli to be identified) but after all stimuli have already been identified. According to this *late-selection* view, attention is not needed to perceptually process and identify items but to create a more durable representation of the information. That is, information that is not explicitly attended to will be seen or heard, but it will decay rapidly in the absence of attention and will not usually reach the level of conscious awareness. The basic contribution of late-selection theories is that the assumption that all information is processed to a semantic level can explain why relevant, though initially unattended to, information is identified.

Norman's (1968) late-selection theory is depicted in Figure 3.3 for the shadowing task. Words in both the attended and unattended ear receive full activation from sensory input. In addition, they receive activation based on

FIGURE 3.2. Treisman's (1960) Filter-Attenuation Theory

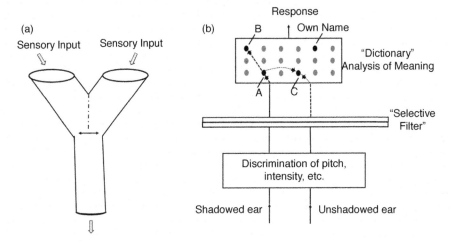

Note. (a) A depiction in which the filter is shown as a dashed vertical line, which can be set to attenuate the input from one side of the funnel, and (b) a depiction where the dashed line indicates the attenuated unattended message, and the filled circles indicate identification of the words. From "Contextual Cues in Selective Listening," by A. Treisman, 1960, *Quarterly Journal of Experimental Psychology, 12*(4), p. 247 (https://doi.org/10.1080/17470216008416732). Copyright 1960 by SAGE. Adapted with permission.

FIGURE 3.3. Depiction of Norman's (1968) Late-Selection Model

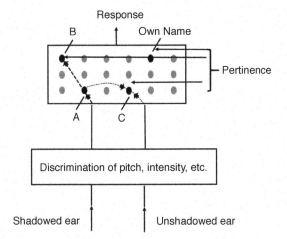

Note. Unshadowed input is analyzed fully and combines with pertinence for activation.

pertinence, which for Word B is its being in the shadowed ear and for Word C is its being based on any semantic relation to the prior word, A, in the attended message. The word that is attended to is the one with the greatest combined sensory and pertinence activation. Note that the activation of the words occurs before the limited-capacity processing stage (not depicted), thus placing the model within the category of late selection.

Factors Affecting the Ease of Selection

Early work with the dichotic listening paradigm led researchers to conclude that ears were like information channels and information could be more or less independently presented to each of these channels. As mentioned previously, localization of the message in dichotic listening is more extreme than in normal listening conditions. In the everyday world, location can be an effective cue for auditory selection, but there are limits on the resolution of auditory localization (van Opstal, 2016). For example, when several distinct stimuli are presented simultaneously and to both ears, it is difficult to tell more than a few apart (Scharf & Buus, 1986). Even under dichotic listening conditions, the number of messages that can be effectively isolated (and ignored) is limited. Treisman (1964a) showed this by creating a third "channel" as a result of presenting a message with equal intensity to both ears. This procedure creates the impression of a voice in the middle of one's head. Treisman found that shadowing one of the three channels was possible when a message was presented in only one of the other channels, but performance was impaired when messages were presented in all three channels.

Even when just two messages are played separately to the two ears, selection is not always efficient. In fact, sometimes, shadowing by ear is nearly impossible. For example, Treisman and Riley (1969) showed that it is also necessary to be able to separate the two streams of information based on temporal cues. In the relevant experiment, they synchronized lists of digits presented to each ear by first digitally processing each word so that it lasted precisely 250 milliseconds (ms). Two digits were presented simultaneously, one to each ear. Listeners made shadowing errors on about 25% of the digit pairs, with more than 10% including digits that should have been unattended to intruding into the listener's report. Apparently, it is not just the physical localization of the voices that makes selection easy in dichotic listening. The differences in onset times of the words in the messages also play a critical role in enabling efficient selection.

We mentioned earlier that the participants in Cherry's (1953) study noticed when the gender of the speaker on the unattended channel was changed. This suggests that people can detect the pitch of a message without actively attending to a channel. According to Broadbent (1958), this implies that pitch can be used to filter information. Because pitch is used as a filter, people notice when the pitch is changed, and the filter is no longer effective. This fact is illustrated in Treisman and Riley's (1969) experiment just described. When participants were instructed to stop shadowing if a letter occurred among the shadowed and to-be-ignored digit streams, both spoken by the same male, only 39% of the digits in the ignored stream were detected (compared with 70% in the shadowed stream). However, when the letter was spoken by a person of a different gender (female) than the digits (male), participants stopped shadowing on essentially all trials, even if the letter was in the to-be-ignored message. This result implies that the pitch difference was automatically detected in the message that was not being shadowed. In general, it is easier to tell simultaneously presented auditory messages apart if the different messages are presented in distinct pitches (Treisman, 1964c). For example, it is much easier to attend to one voice in the presence of another if the two voices are of different gender (and hence of different pitch) than if a member of the same gender as the speaker of the first speaks the second.

Processing of Unselected Information

In an attempt to distinguish early and late selection, J. L. Lewis (1970) conducted a study that yielded results consistent with the late selection view, using a reaction-time measure. His reasoning was that if an unattended word is identified, its meaning should affect the time to say the word presented simultaneously in the attended message. Participants performed a dichotic shadowing task in which a list of unattended words was paired with a list of attended, shadowed words, presented at a rapid rate of 66 ms per word. When the unattended word for a critical pair was a synonym of the word in the list being shadowed, reaction time to say the shadowed word was increased compared with when the words were unrelated.

Although J. L. Lewis (1970) interpreted these results as support for late-selection attention models, Treisman et al. (1974) questioned J. L. Lewis's premise that unattended words receive full semantic analysis before being filtered. They replicated his experiment with modifications to test the effect of position in the list, with the idea that it may take time for capacity to become fully saturated and attention to become focused on the attended message. Reaction time was longer when the paired word was a synonym than when it was not but only at the third position in lists and not the seventh position. On the basis of this and other results, Treisman et al. concluded that once attention has been focused on the attended channel, the meanings of unattended words are not processed and have no effect on performance.

However, other studies have typically found evidence for processing meaning. In one example, Rivenez et al. (2006) measured priming in a dichotic listening task. The task required participants to detect a target word from a specific category presented in a list of words in the attended ear. Sentences were presented in a chain in the unattended ear, some of which included a repetition prime (i.e., the same word) just before a target word in the attended ear. A high presentation rate of two words per second was used to prevent attention switches to the unattended ear, and a secondary task was performed at the same time. The results showed a priming effect similar to J. L. Lewis's (1970) result: Reaction times to the target word were reduced when it was preceded by the same word in the unattended message.

Corteen and Wood (1972) conducted a study in which the results also suggested that unattended words are processed to a semantic level. They first conditioned people to expect a mild but unpleasant shock after hearing the names of certain cities. The participants then performed a dichotic listening task in which the unattended message contained the conditioned city names, other city names, and unrelated nouns. The participants did not report hearing any city names, but they showed a change in galvanic skin response (GSR), a measure of the conductivity of the skin associated with stress. This change occurred with 38% of the conditioned names compared with 23% of other city names and 10% of unrelated nouns. Thus, although the conditioned names did not reach conscious awareness, they did seem to reach semantic analysis.

Although Corteen and Wood's (1972) results are consistent with the idea of semantic analysis of words on the unattended channel, they do not imply that all information on the unattended channel is fully processed. As is also suggested by the fact that one's own name is only recognized about a third of the time in a dichotic listening task, Corteen and Wood's result could be at least partly due to occasional lapses in selective attention wherein the to-be-ignored channel is monitored. That this may have been the case is suggested by a replication of the Corteen and Wood study conducted by Dawson and Schell (1982). Dawson and Schell replicated the main finding of Corteen and Wood but also found that the GSR to conditioned words on the unattended channel was often accompanied by evidence of attention lapses (shadowing errors or reports of having heard items on the unattended channel).

Other Neuropsychological Evidence of Speech Properties Being Processed Preattentively

Among the best evidence that higher level properties of speech can be processed before attentional selection comes from studies using an event-related potential (ERP) measure called the *mismatch negativity* (MMN; see Chapter 2). This component occurs in response to a deviant, or oddball, stimulus within a series of repeated standard stimuli (Näätänen et al., 2019). One of the essential features of the MMN is that it is relatively unaffected by attention and seems to reflect a preattentive process that detects the deviation from the other stimuli. All bottleneck models assume that physical features such as location and frequency can be processed preattentively. It is not surprising, then, that a physical deviation generates an MMN (Bissonnette et al., 2020; Tsogli et al., 2019). The question is whether higher level deviants, including lexical, semantic, and syntactical ones, do as well.

Pulvermüller and Shtyrov (2006) summarized evidence suggesting that the answer is positive in each case. It is essential that physical differences are controlled in the experimental design to assess the automaticity of processing of these deviants. In a study satisfying this criterion, Shtyrov and Pulvermüller (2002) used a pseudoword as a standard and a word as the deviant in one condition, with the roles reversed in another. In a third condition, both the standard and deviant were different words. The main finding was that the word deviant produced an MMN regardless of the lexicality of the standard, and the pseudoword deviant among words did not produce an MMN. This result pattern suggests that the word deviant retrieved a long-term memory trace. The MMN also shows sensitivity to semantic differences. Pulvermüller et al. (2004) found that the source of the MMN relative to a pseudoword was primarily over the left hemisphere for an abstract word but bilateral with more right-lateralized activation for a concrete, imageable word. This difference is expected because the right hemisphere is more specialized for visual imagery.

A final study we mention here, which is particularly well controlled (Bronkhorst, 2015), indicates an MMN for a syntactic distinction. Pulvermüller et al. (2008) recorded ERPs of syntactic processing to spoken sentences while participants engaged in other tasks that would demand attention to different extents. They watched a silent video film (weak distraction) or also performed a difficult acoustic signal detection task (strong distraction). The early MMN (< 150 ms) at left lateral sites distinguished grammatical from ungrammatical speech in both distraction conditions, and its magnitude was unaffected by whether the distraction task imposed weak or strong demands on attention. This study thus provides evidence that speech signals are processed to a syntactical level before attentional selection.

A question that could be asked is whether processing other than physical characteristics extends to the cochlear nerve, which is the pathway that conveys the sensory signal from the receptors in the cochlea of the inner ear to the brain. Picton et al. (1971) investigated this question by recording ERPs from the cochlear nerve and cortex while participants discriminated clicks in an attended ear and ignored clicks in the other ear. The cochlear nerve response showed no difference during attention to clicks compared with a control condition, but changes occurred in the amplitude of the cortical ERP as well as in a cortical component called the contingent negative variation, which is known to increase during attention to significant events. These results are consistent with the view that auditory stimuli are not filtered peripherally but at a higher level in the sensory system.

Most studies using methods like those of Picton et al. (1971) that examine transient effects of single stimuli have likewise reported no effects of attention before cortical responses (Price & Moncrieff, 2021). Relatedly, Varghese et al. (2015) measured subcortical steady-state responses (SSSR, obtained from the brain stem) under various conditions: listening to a monaural stimulus, attending to a specific ear during dichotic listening, and ignoring dichotic auditory stimuli while attending to visual stimuli. These manipulations had no effect on the SSSR, but they did affect alpha-wave cortical activity. The lack of effect on the cochlear nerve and brain stem measures implies that attention has little influence on auditory sensory processing.

Final Thoughts on Early and Late Auditory Selection

Research on auditory selection has shown from the earliest days that people exhibit little awareness when asked shortly thereafter about the information presented to an unattended channel. This robust finding was the basis for Broadbent's (1958) filter theory. Subsequent studies showed more subtle effects of information in the unattended channel, and much of the theoretical debate has hinged on the degree to which the unattended information is processed. It should be apparent from the discussions in this section that distinguishing empirically whether selection is early, as assumed by the filter-attenuation model, or late, as assumed by the late-selection models, is difficult. Both views allow that the meaning of items in an unattended message can be identified in at least some circumstances. The difference is mainly whether identification occurs only for specific items and contexts or routinely. Accounts like the filter-attenuation model allow meaning to be a factor in many situations because of top-down influences. Consequently, most evidence does not unambiguously distinguish between these views.

One attempt to reconcile the early and late selection views is perceptual load theory, developed by Lavie (1995; Lavie & Tsal, 1994), primarily for visual attention research. As evidence, Lavie (1995) reported experiments for which a distractor letter located above fixation produced interference with identifying a target letter aligned at fixation. In one experiment, the task was to identify whether a lowercase *z* or *x* was presented, and the distractor was an uppercase *Z* or *X*. When only a single letter was shown at fixation (low-load condition), the distractor interfered with responding when it was incompatible with the target (e.g., *z* accompanied by *X*). But when the target letter was one in a string of six letters, the distractor had no effect on performance. According to perceptual load theory, the perceptual system has limited processing capacity, but all stimuli are processed automatically if that capacity is not exceeded. Thus, under low perceptual load, irrelevant stimuli should affect performance. When the capacity is exceeded, attentional control processes determine what gets processed beyond preattentive feature analysis, excluding stimuli that are not relevant. This exclusion reduces or eliminates the influence of irrelevant stimuli. Thus, according to perceptual load theory, selection is late under conditions of low perceptual load and early under conditions of high perceptual load.

Although most relevant research on perceptual load theory has involved visual attention, S. Murphy et al. (2017) noted its potential applicability to auditory perception. They pointed out that for auditory stimuli, the evidence as to whether an increase in perceptual load for the relevant message reduces the effects of irrelevant stimuli is ambiguous. S. Murphy et al. noted that although reduced congruency effects have been obtained under conditions of high perceptual load based on a search for features versus conjunctions of features, the results of those studies could be attributed to cognitive load (executive control demand) rather than perceptual load. Results have been inconsistent for studies that used manipulations that more clearly affect perceptual load, such as similarity of targets and nontargets. The varied results led S. Murphy et al. to conclude that the evidence is mixed. Thus, it is not clear whether the results of auditory studies conform to perceptual load theory.

Despite the remaining issues regarding the conditions under which higher level properties of stimuli are processed, there is agreement that speech and other sounds can be selected based on elemental features, including spatial location and frequency. Selection is more difficult and processing more complex when it must be based on lexical, semantic, or syntactic distinctions. After reviewing the literature related to the cocktail-party phenomenon, Bronkhorst (2015) concluded that the processing depth of auditory stimuli depends on how relevant they are to the instructed task and what is currently being processed. This conclusion fits with an increasing emphasis on task set and processing dynamics in the 21st century.

VISUAL SELECTIVE ATTENTION

As with auditory attention, issues in visual selective attention have also focused on the long-standing controversy concerning the level of processing at which attention comes into play or, in other words, the extent to which visual stimuli can be processed without the application of attention. It is customarily assumed that visual information processing starts with basic feature information, such as the orientation, form, and color of items in a visual display. As with audition, at this level, information is precategorical in the sense that the meaning of the stimuli has not yet been processed. At a later time and a higher level of processing, stimuli are processed categorically or semantically.

Although the abilities of visual selection are impressive, selection is not perfect. For example, when driving your car along the highway, a particularly flashy or interesting billboard may distract you. Such distraction is most likely to occur when something relevant to you is present. That is, potentially relevant information sometimes gets past the selective mechanism, which would be consistent with the filter-attenuation and late-selection theories discussed for auditory information processing. Information that is familiar or fits the context of attended information may influence performance and break through to the level of conscious awareness.

Neisser extended the auditory research to visual selection in studies of selective reading (Neisser, 1969) and selective looking (Neisser & Becklen, 1975). The selective reading procedure was similar to the shadowing studies. Participants were to read a passage typed in red, and the red lines of the passage alternated on the page with strings of random words typed in black, which were to be ignored. The participants were able to perform the task with no increase in reading time relative to control pages without the black lines. If unwarned that they might be asked questions about the material in the black lines, almost all participants did not notice the word "Friday" being repeated in all black lines of three pages in a row. Sixty-five percent of unwarned participants did detect their name as occurring in the black lines. Neisser (1969) pointed out that these results were comparable to those obtained by Moray (1959) and others with the auditory shadowing task, implying similar selective processes for visual information processing.

Neisser and Becklen (1975) went a step further and presented participants with video scenes of two people playing a hand game, in which one person tried to slap a hand of the other, and a ball game, in which three people passed a basketball to each other while moving around (see Figure 3.4). Participants were to press a switch with the right index finger for each hand slap in the hand game and another switch with the left hand for each pass in the ball game. They performed in sessions with only one of the videos and with the videos superimposed. For the latter, in some sessions, participants were to respond only to events in one game; in others, they were to respond to events in both

FIGURE 3.4. Outlines of Video Images for Neisser and Becklen (1975)

A. Handgame Alone	B. Ballgame Alone	C. Handgame and Ballgame Superimposed
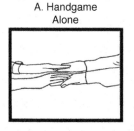	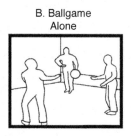	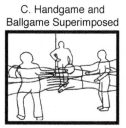

Note. From "Selective Looking: Attending to Visually Specified Events," by U. Neisser and R. Becklen, 1975, *Cognitive Psychology, 7*(4), p. 485 (https://doi.org/10.1016/0010-0285(75)90019-5). Copyright 1975 by Elsevier. Reprinted with permission.

games. Results showed nearly perfect performance when the instructions were to attend to one game and ignore the other but poor performance when the instructions were to attend to both games simultaneously. In other words, participants could selectively attend to a specific game but not divide attention across the games. In sessions that included unusual events in the unattended game (e.g., a handshake in the hand game), few participants reported noticing the events.

The Spotlight of Attention

The *spotlight metaphor* is a popular metaphor of attention, according to which, like a spotlight, selected information is highlighted and information outside the spotlight is not (Posner et al., 1980). Like a spotlight, attention can be moved to different regions of space to "illuminate" anything that might be present there, facilitating processing. When attention is cued to a location, simple detection reactions to stimulus onsets are faster (Posner, 1980; Posner et al., 1980), and identification of a target letter or word is enhanced (C. W. Eriksen & Hoffman, 1973; Folk et al., 1992). Locations of stimuli at nearby positions are displaced away from the spotlight as if they were repulsed (Suzuki & Cavanagh, 1997). Less obvious is whether the movements of attention are continuous, of constant speed, or whether attention is "turned off" at one location before being applied at another (Gabbay et al., 2019). A closely related metaphor is a *zoom lens*, which suggests that attention is more diffuse when it encompasses a larger area than a smaller one (C. W. Eriksen & St. James, 1986).

Focusing the Attentional Spotlight

Many studies have shown that the spotlight of attention can be adjusted to focus on a relatively small region or a larger region of space (e.g., C. W. Eriksen & Yeh, 1985). For example, LaBerge (1983) had people perform a task that required them to focus on just one letter (i.e., indicate whether the middle letter in a word was from a certain range of the alphabet) or on a whole word (i.e., indicate whether a word was a proper noun). On some trials, in place of a word, a row of four #s with a probe letter or digit in one of the five letter positions was presented (e.g., ###7#), and the person was to respond to the probe as quickly as possible. LaBerge found that response time depended on the focus of attention: If attention was focused on the middle letter, response times were fastest to the middle letter on the probe trials, intermediate to the letters adjacent to the middle letter, and slowest to the letters farthest away from the center (see Figure 3.5, solid line). However, if attention was devoted to the whole word, response time to the probe letter did not depend on its position (see Figure 3.5, dashed line).

Goodhew et al. (2016) used a similar method of having participants judge whether a centrally presented stimulus was a circle or ellipse for an inducer

FIGURE 3.5. Results of LaBerge's (1983) Experiment on the Focus of the Attentional Spotlight

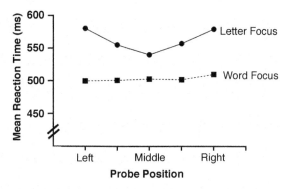

Note. Data from LaBerge (1983).

task on 80% of the trials. In some trial blocks, the stimuli were small (creating images about the size of the fovea), whereas, in others, they were much larger. For the probe trials, which occurred 20% of the time, an outline circular stimulus with a small spatial gap in it or a filled circular stimulus with a temporal gap (of 13 ms) was presented (see Figure 3.6b). For both tasks, the participant had to indicate whether a gap was present. Spatial gap detection was more accurate in the context of the smaller inducing stimuli than in that of the larger inducing stimuli, consistent with the hypothesis of attention being more tightly

FIGURE 3.6. Depiction of the Possible Stimuli for the Spatial and Temporal Gap Detection Tasks

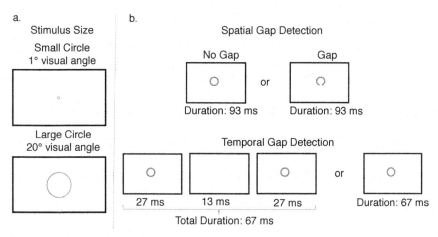

Note. From "Selective Spatial Enhancement: Attentional Spotlight Size Impacts Spatial but not Temporal Perception," by S. C. Goodhew, E. Shen, and M. Edwards, 2016, *Psychonomic Bulletin & Review, 23*(4), p. 1145 (https://doi.org/10.3758/s13423-015-0904-6). Copyright 2016 by Springer Nature. Adapted with permission.

focused in the former case. Temporal gap detection did not show a similar effect of the inducing stimuli, suggesting that the temporal judgments were independent of the distribution of visual attention.

However, the stimuli used in the prior studies were unfilled circles of different sizes (see Figure 3.6a). Consequently, participants may not have spread their attention across the entire inner region but instead only around the perimeter of the shape. When Lawrence et al. (2020) tested the influence of attention scaling using a method that required attending to information across the entire stimulus, they found that a narrow attention scale improved both spatial and temporal acuity. They noted that these findings are inconsistent with the view that attention has differential impacts on spatial and temporal processing and instead support the zoom lens model of C. W. Eriksen and St. James (1986).

The size of the attentional focus can also be manipulated by cuing different numbers of locations in a circular display. Using this method, C. W. Eriksen and St. James (1986; see Figure 3.7) found that response times to a target letter increased when the number of adjacent cued positions was larger. Moreover, the costs associated with incompatible items (noncued items that, if cued, would require a different response) depended on the size of the attentional focus: When the focus was larger, items in positions farther away from the target showed more interference than when the focus was smaller. The benefit in reaction time for cuing a smaller number of positions increased as the cue-display onset interval (cue-onset asynchrony) increased (see Figure 3.8), indicating that it takes time to focus attention. This result was one of the main findings that led C. W. Eriksen and St. James to propose that attention is like a zoom lens, for which there is an inverse relation between the illuminated area and the concentration of attentional resources.

Although a concentrated focus of attention on a region may facilitate selective attention to it, certain types of information may benefit from a broad, more diffuse attentional setting. Chong and Treisman (2005) found that participants

FIGURE 3.7. Displays Like Those Used by C. W. Eriksen and St. James (1986)

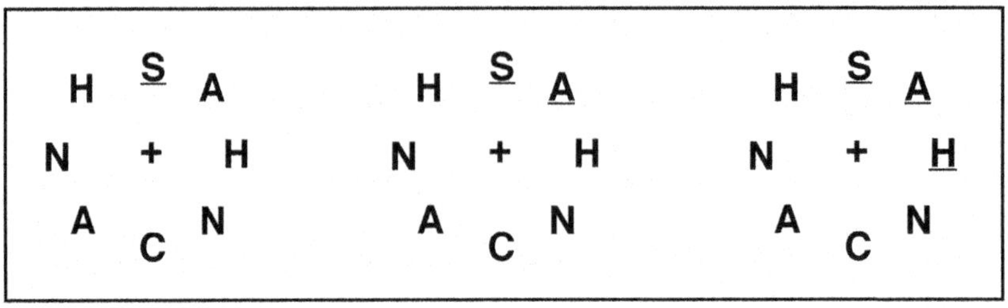

Note. Displays similar to those used by Eriksen and St. James (1986). One, two, or three adjacent positions were cued to vary the size of the attentional focus. From *Attention: Theory and Practice* (p. 68), by A. Johnson and R. W. Proctor, 2004, SAGE (https://doi.org/10.4135/9781483328768). Copyright 2004 by A. W. Johnson and R. W. Proctor. Reprinted with permission.

FIGURE 3.8. Time to Focus Attention

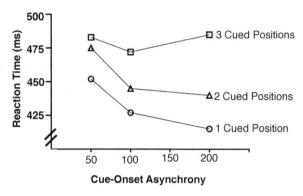

Note. Data from C. W. Eriksen and St. James (1986).

were able to identify the average size of sets of circles better when that task was combined with another task that required diffuse attention compared with one that required focused attention. Moreover, performance was just as good in the diffuse-attention dual-task condition as when the average-size task was performed alone. Finally, fMRI analyses show that the regions of neurons activated in the visual cortex are larger, with lower activation levels, for tasks in which attention is spread diffusely than for those in which it is focused (N. G. Müller et al., 2003).

Moving the Attentional Spotlight

If attention is like a spotlight (or zoom lens), it should be possible to move it across regions of space. Moreover, the spotlight should illuminate the area over which it passes. These assumptions of the spotlight metaphor have been tested by examining movements of attention. For example, using location cues (i.e., signaling the location to which attention should be directed) and targets at three distances from fixation, Tsal (1983) found that the time needed to focus attention at a location increased as the distance of the target increased. This finding led him to propose that attention travels through space at a constant velocity. However, this assumption has been criticized because the results can also be attributed to the time needed to identify targets in peripheral vision: More time is needed to identify targets that are more distant (and their cues) because of poorer visual processing in the periphery of the visual field (C. W. Eriksen & Murphy, 1987). Using a central cue to direct participants where to look, Remington and Pierce (1984) showed that attention could be moved just as quickly to a distant position as to a near position. In general, attention shifts can be well described by models that assume that the time taken to move attention is independent of the distance to be moved (e.g., Yantis, 1988). Rather than moving around the display in an analog fashion, it appears that attention jumps from one position to another such that resources are allocated to a new location as they are released at the old location (see also C. W. Eriksen & Webb, 1989).

Gabbay et al. (2019) reported evidence suggesting that some of the attentional spotlight can be directed to a new location while part of it is still focused on an initially cued location. In their study, participants searched arrays of four items (in left, right, up, or down locations) for a target defined by its red color. Each trial included a red-circle cue that appeared briefly and was followed after a short interval by a second red-circle cue in a different location or by no second cue. Not too surprisingly, there was a benefit on target identification when the target was in the single cued location. The crucial finding is that there was also a spatial benefit at the location of the first cue even when attention had been shifted to the location of the second cue, although that benefit was smaller than when the second cue was absent. The authors interpreted these and other results as suggesting that attention can be directed to a new cued location before it is completely disengaged from the first cued location. Furthermore, they used an electrophysiological measure called the steady-state visual evoked potential to provide evidence that the attentional spotlight can be divided across noncontiguous locations when the participant is sustaining attention to rapidly presented stimuli over several seconds (see also M. M. Müller et al., 2003).

Another study concentrated on rhythmic sampling of attention, which refers to visual attention operating periodically, regardless of whether it is focused on a single location or multiple locations. A. Chen et al. (2017) found that task difficulty is a factor influencing these periodic patterns of attention. Their experimental procedure is shown in Figure 3.9. Participants monitored two grating stimuli displayed on opposite sides of a fixation point that drifted left or right. The task was to detect a contrast reduction of 30-ms duration between the light and dark regions that occurred for one of the gratings. A cue event (four white disks presented around one of the gratings) occurred 1 to 1.2 seconds after fixation onset, but the cue was uninformative as to which grating would have the critical target event. The participant responded to the target event by pressing the corresponding left or right arrow key on a keyboard. The time course of performance was obtained by having the target appear at one of 50 temporal intervals, in steps of 20 ms, 0.1 to 1.08 seconds after cue onset. A difficult target discrimination version was set at a 65% threshold, whereas an easy version was set at a 75% threshold.

The main finding was that the dynamics of response accuracy showed a theta rhythm in the difficult discrimination version but oscillations at higher frequencies in the easy version. The authors interpreted this difference in frequency of the brain waves as suggesting that the attention spotlight switched faster between the two gratings when the task was easy than when the task was difficult, possibly to obtain more information per sample in the latter task. Regardless of whether these findings are attributed specifically to switching the attention spotlight, they indicate that sampling at the two locations occurs periodically.

FIGURE 3.9. Experimental Procedure of A. Chen et al. (2017)

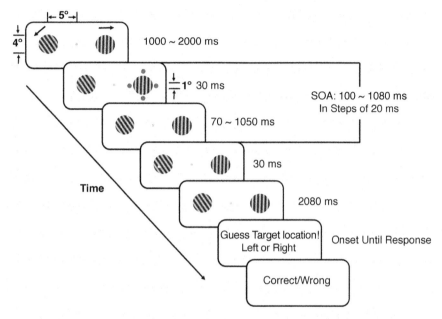

Note. Adapted from "Behavioral Oscillations in Visual Attention Modulated by Task Difficulty," by A. Chen, A. Wang, T. Wang, X. Tang, and M. Zhang, 2017, *Frontiers in Psychology, 8*, Article 1630, p. 3 (https://doi.org/10.3389/fpsyg.2017.01630). CC BY.

Resolution of the Attentional Spotlight

Several studies have shown that there is a gradient of attention about an attended location. For example, C. J. Downing and Pinker (1985) had participants maintain fixation on a central location and respond to a light onset at any of four locations aligned with the fixation location. On trials with a cue, a digit from 1 to 4 appeared at the central location to specify the likely location at which the light would appear. Participants were to direct attention to that location and respond as quickly as possible when any of the lights came on. The cost in reaction time when the light occurred at an uncued location, relative to a condition with no cue, was an increasing function of the visual angle between the cued location and the one in which the light occurred. Because these angles were 1°, 5°, 10.5°, and 15.5°, this result implies a gradient of attention that extends well beyond 1° of visual angle.

The implication of the spotlight metaphor that the gradient of attention should be space based may not be correct. For instance, regions of space that contain objects may be processed differently from empty regions of space. Cepeda et al. (1998) used a probe dot procedure in which a small dot, which only appeared on some trials, had to be responded to as quickly as possible to test whether attention is allocated differently to objects than to empty space. The probe response time indicates where attention is currently allocated. The main experimental task of Cepeda et al. was to select and identify one digit of a four-digit circular display based on its color while keeping the eyes fixated at the display center. Rather than responding to the digit right away, participants were to respond after an interval of 1,400 ms.

On 50% of the trials, the dot probe was presented in the interval between the primary-task stimulus and response. It could occur with equal probability at any of the digit positions or in one of the blank positions between the digits (for eight possible locations). Response times to the probes were fastest when the probe occurred at the position of the to-be-reported digit and slowest at the position of any other digit. An additional finding—that responses were faster when the probe occurred on blank positions far from the target than when the probe occurred on the position of a distractor digit—was interpreted as showing that the nonselected digits were inhibited. Responses to probes at blank positions near the target were faster than to probes at blank positions farther away, as in C. J. Downing and Pinker's (1985) study, consistent with the spotlight metaphor. However, this experiment suggests that rather than illuminating all areas within its focus, attention operates differently on objects than on empty space.

Is Selection Early or Late?

Many studies show evidence for visual early selection—and perhaps as many show evidence for late selection. An example of a study showing that processing does not proceed effortlessly to the point of stimulus identification (and thus depends on attention at an earlier stage) is that of Pashler (1984). In his experiment, participants were required to identify a letter at one of eight locations of a circular visual array as quickly as possible. The letters in the array were high or low contrast (white or gray on a black background), and a location cue indicating which letter should be identified was present for 150 ms during the display presentation. The cue was onset 200 ms before or after the array onset or simultaneous with it. The results showed a typical effect of stimulus contrast, with low contrast letters taking about 40 ms longer to identify than high contrast letters. Most important, this contrast effect was of similar size for all the cue conditions, including when the cue array was previewed for 300 ms before the cue. The independence of the contrast effect from the time of the cue onset suggests that the observers did not identify the letters until after the cue arrived, even when they had the opportunity to process letters before the cue (see also Pashler, 1998). This result is inconsistent with late selection and implies that identification was delayed until the cued letter was signaled.

Other studies using a cue procedure have also obtained results implying early selection. For example, Yantis and Johnston (1990) presented participants with a circular array of eight letters and asked participants to attend to one of the eight positions of the display, as indicated by a location cue. Participants indicated whether that position contained a specific target (e.g., the letter T).

On some trials, an extra target was present elsewhere in the display. If this redundant target was in a position adjacent to the cued location, responses to the target were faster than when no redundant target was present. However, if a redundant target was anywhere else in the display, it had no effect on performance. Yantis and Johnston thus concluded that attention was effectively allocated to a small region of space and that only stimuli present in that region were processed.

Although Yantis and Johnston's (1990) results are consistent with the hypothesis that attention is needed to perceive stimuli, Shiffrin et al. (1996) argued that basic visual information is processed in parallel across the visual field and that attention is only applied to a location when a response must be selected. Shiffrin et al. used a procedure like that of Yantis and Johnston, but instead of sometimes presenting a second target in the same display as the relevant target, they presented it first in a separate prime display (see Figure 3.10). As in prior studies, they found that the benefit of a redundant target and the cost associated with having a conflicting target (i.e., a target assigned to a different response) in the display were limited to locations adjacent to (or the same as) the target. However, these costs and benefits were essentially the same when the location cue appeared after the prime display as when it appeared before the prime display.

Shiffrin et al.'s (1996) findings suggest that all items in the prime display were processed to some extent, even though the observer had not yet been

FIGURE 3.10. Displays Similar to Those Used in the Compatible Cue Conditions of Shiffrin et al. (1996)

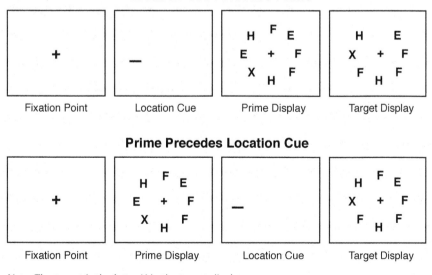

Note. The target is the letter X in the target display.

cued as to where to direct attention. Thus, Shiffrin et al. proposed a model of attention in which perceptual processing proceeds without attention to specific locations, but attention to locations is needed to select the appropriate response. They argued that the results using Yantis and Johnston's (1990) cuing paradigm can be attributed to response competition (i.e., stimuli associated with the same response benefit performance, and those associated with a different response hinder it) rather than perceptual interference. That response competition is the basis for the influence of flanking stimuli on performance is widely accepted for reasons described in Chapter 4.

The study by Shiffrin et al. (1996), as well as many other studies, have found that unattended stimuli are processed up to a semantic level. Such results favor the view that selection occurs after information has been categorized. A partial explanation for the conflicting results regarding whether selection is early or late may be that the level of selection depends on perceptual load (e.g., Lavie & Tsal, 1994; Treisman, 1969). According to Treisman (1969), early selection is necessary whenever perceptual load is high to prevent interference within the various perceptual analyzers. As noted earlier, Lavie (1995) and Lavie and Tsal (1994) have argued that when perceptual load is high, selection occurs early, and only selected items are fully identified. But when perceptual load is low, processing proceeds unhindered to the point of identification for all display elements.

Perceptual load can be manipulated in at least three different ways (G. Murphy et al., 2016). The first way is to vary the number of items in the relevant display, assuming that the difficulty of visual processing is an increasing function of array size. A second way is to vary the visual similarity between target stimuli and nontarget distractors, presuming that perceptual difficulty increases as the similarity increases. Finally, a third way is to manipulate the complexity of perceptual operations performed on the same stimuli. Performance measures have generally shown results consistent with perceptual load theory, with effects of irrelevant distractor stimuli being reduced under high-load conditions (G. Murphy et al., 2016). The main limitation is that there are alternative explanations for the findings, discussed later in this section.

Likewise, electrophysiological and neuroimaging studies have provided results consistent with a role of perceptual load in determining the level of selection. In ERP studies, components associated with early perceptual processing, the P1 and N1 components, are larger when perceptual load is high than when it is low. Handy and Mangun (2000) had people identify whether a letter to the left or right of fixation was an A or H. A left- or right-pointing arrow presented in the center of the screen 600 to 800 ms before the onset of the letter cued its location. The cue was valid on 73% of the trials and invalid on 27%. On low-load trials, the letter A or H was intact, making the two highly discriminable; on high-load trials, the arms of the A were pulled apart slightly and the arms of the H were tilted inward slightly, increasing the difficulty of the discrimination. The crucial finding was that in the high-load condition, P1 and N1 were larger when the letter occurred in the cued location than when it did not, but in the low-load condition, the two components were unaffected by expectancy. These findings are consistent with the view that increasing perceptual load induces early selection in visual processing.

Similar results have been obtained in neuroimaging studies. For example, Xu et al. (2011) implemented fMRI while participants performed a visual target-identification task with low and high perceptual loads. The stimuli were schematic faces, presented in a stream at fixation, to which a button was to be pressed whenever a target face was detected. For a low-load condition, the targets had a single distinctive feature (an elongated nose), whereas, for high load, targets could vary in face color, face shape, shape of the eyes, or shape of the mouth. In distractor conditions, the stream of stimulus faces was presented against a background of picture scenes, whereas in no-distractor conditions, the background was blank.

Results showed that distractor-related activation in the visual cortices for low perceptual load was greater than for high perceptual load. Low perceptual load was also associated with (a) increased activation in the midbrain reticular formation and medial prefrontal cortex, possibly reflecting increased arousal; (b) decreased activation in the temporoparietal junction, reflecting filtering of distractors; and (c) increased activation in frontostriatal circuits (which connect the frontal lobe to the basal ganglia) to reject distractors or select appropriate responses. At high perceptual load, increased top-down attentional control appears to contribute to the inhibition of distractor interference, as suggested by distractor-related concurrent deactivation in the frontostriatal circuits, midbrain area, part of the basal ganglia, and visual sensory cortices. These activation patterns may reflect different roles of the respective areas when selection is early (high load) versus late (low load).

Perceptual load theory has been subject to numerous criticisms, including evidence that several other factors are involved. One possibility is that the reduction of distractor interference under high load produced by varying set size may be due to dilution of the distractor effect by the presence of neutral items rather than the need to attend selectively (Tsal & Benoni, 2010). In a review of the extant literature using visual tasks, G. Murphy et al. (2016) concluded that perceptual and cognitive load are not the only factors influencing selective attention, although they may be major factors in some circumstances. But, as Benoni (2018), a critic of the theory, said, "In application, the theory can provide good predictions concerning the outcomes of selectivity, even without specifying the fundamental theoretical roles that determine these predicted outcomes" (p. 2044). In agreement with this opinion, G. Murphy and Greene (2016, 2017) showed the value of applying the theory to an analysis of driving and eyewitness testimony.

Final Thoughts on Early and Late Visual Selection

Benoni (2018) also gave perceptual load theory credit for initiating the focus on efficiency of perceptual selectivity rather than on locus of selective attention.

This change is reflected in contemporary models of visual search, described in Chapter 4, with increasing emphasis on task set and goals, and models of auditory selection that emphasize task relevance (Bronkhorst, 2015). Similar sentiments are expressed in the area of visual perception and working memory, with an emphasis on a close relation between perception and action. Most notable in this regard is the theory of event coding developed by Hommel et al. (2001), in which perception and action interact through networks of codes of perceptual-motor episodes called *event files*. This theory provided a framework for many advances in understanding all aspects of human information processing during the initial decades of the 21st century, with one of the advancements being the role of task goals in the retrieval and integration of event files (Hommel, 2019). Olivers and Roelfsema (2020) described the shift in emphasis as follows:

> Where previously attention has been regarded as the mental spotlight that serves to keep items alive on the mental canvas, according to the current view attention emerges from bridging perception and action, as sensory representations are made available for overt or covert operations. (p. 189)

HEMISPHERIC DIFFERENCES

Until now, we have treated selective attention to the left or right ear and left or right visual field as equivalent, but studies show that hemispheric differences can affect performance. Such differences can be shown for individuals with and without attentional deficits. In this section, we describe two differences: the right-ear advantage as an example of left-hemisphere dominance and spatial neglect as an example of right-hemisphere dominance.

Right-Ear Advantage

For auditory selective attention, beginning with research by Kimura (1961), evidence has accrued for a right-ear advantage in a variety of dichotic listening tasks that is attributed to the dominance of the left cortical hemisphere for speech processing (Westerhausen, 2019). The possible role of attention in producing this advantage is of interest, and researchers have examined how it changes across development and in aging and in adults with and without attention deficits. Moncrieff (2011) found that 80% of children ages 5 to 12 showed a right-ear advantage, in which they correctly identified more words presented in their right than left ear. Moreover, the right-ear advantage was larger for younger than older children.

Takio et al. (2009) found that the right-ear advantage could be modified by attentional control that develops across the life span. They tested participants ranging from 5 to 79 years of age (divided into five age groups: 5–7; 8–9, 10–11, 19–32, and 59–79 years old) in a dichotic recognition task in which they had to report the consonant–vowel syllable (e.g., /ma/) that was presented. Three conditions varied in terms of the attentional instructions. In the nonforced attention condition, participants were instructed to report the syllable that they heard most clearly (from either ear). In the forced-right attention condition, participants were instructed to attend to the right ear only and only report the consonant–vowel syllables presented in the right ear. Similarly, in the forced-left attention condition, participants were instructed to attend to the left ear only and report the consonant–vowel syllables presented in the left ear.

Takio et al. (2009) found an overall right-ear advantage that was larger for females than males and with the nonforced and forced-right instructions compared with the forced-left instructions. The participants in the 5-to-7, 8-to-9, and 59-to-79 age groups all showed a right-ear advantage, regardless of the attentional instructions. Children in the 10-to-11 age group were able to follow instructions to focus their attention to the left ear to reduce the right-ear advantage in the forced-left attention condition. But it was not until adulthood (i.e., 19–32 years) that participants were able to eliminate the right-ear advantage or even obtain a left ear advantage when following the instructions to direct their focus to the left ear. Note that the oldest adult group was not able to do this either, indicating a decline in attentional control with old age.

When free report of words at either ear is allowed, the right-ear advantage could reflect a bias to report that ear first rather than hemispheric specialization. It would seem that any such bias could be controlled by comparing performance when participants are instructed to attend to the left versus right ear. In that case, an overall right-ear advantage is typically obtained, as in the studies described previously (see also Foundas et al., 2006; Moncrieff & Dubyne, 2017). This result suggests that an instructed direction of attention to the left ear must overcome the bias to attend to the right ear. In agreement with this interpretation, Westerhausen (2019) concluded that selectively attending to the left ear is more cognitively demanding than attending to the right ear. This account is consistent with the findings that people with lower cognitive abilities have more difficulty attending to the left than right ear compared with people with higher cognitive abilities. Moreover, an fMRI study found more activation of the left-side prefrontal cortex and caudate nucleus (located near the thalamus) with attend-left instructions than attend-right instructions (Kompus et al., 2012); these areas are thought to play a role in cognitive control (Casey, 2005).

Øie et al. (2021) conducted a longitudinal study to examine the cognitive performance of individuals with early-onset schizophrenia (mean age of 16.2 years at the start of the study), attention-deficit/hyperactivity disorder (ADHD; mean age of 14.1 years), and healthy controls (mean age of 15.7 years). Participants were recruited in adolescence (Time 1), tested again 13 years later (Time 2), and tested once again 23 to 25 years later (Time 3). They were given a battery of cognitive tests, but only the results of the dichotic listening task for selective attention are described here. Overall, the schizophrenia group performed worse on the dichotic listening task than the other two groups. As shown in Figure 3.11, the schizophrenia group showed no right-ear advantage, whereas both the ADHD and healthy control groups did. Moreover, the

FIGURE 3.11. Right-Ear Advantage for Individuals With Clinical Diagnoses and Healthy Controls

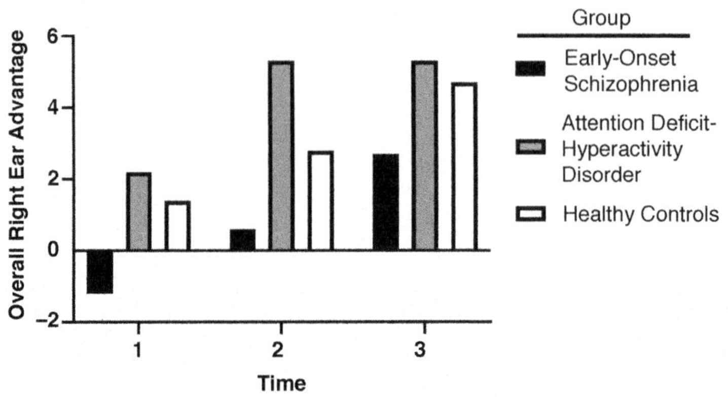

Note. Data reflect accuracy (correct answers in the dichotic listening task). The overall right-ear advantage is the difference between the right-ear advantage with forced right attention instructions and the left-ear advantage with forced left attention instructions.

group with ADHD showed a larger right-ear advantage than the healthy controls. These data suggest that adolescents and adults with ADHD have poorer attentional control than healthy adults.

The right-ear advantage is associated with auditory pathways from the right ear connecting more directly to the speech-dominant left cerebral hemisphere. When information is presented to the left ear, it is first relayed to the right hemisphere and then transmitted to the left one via the corpus callosum. Thus, individuals experiencing damage to the corpus callosum or having neurodegeneration in its regions should show a larger right-ear advantage than individuals with an intact corpus callosum. Utoomprurkporn et al.'s (2020) review and meta-analysis of many studies showed that patients with lesions to their corpus callosum have a larger right-ear advantage. Healthy adults showed no significant right-ear advantage (mean difference = 0.93%), but individuals with mild cognitive impairment and dementia (e.g., Alzheimer's disease) showed right-ear advantages of 5.7% and 24.4%, respectively. Individuals with dementia showed the largest right-ear advantage, resulting from the low recognition performance of information presented to the left ear. Again, this decrement in left-ear performance may result from corpus callosum changes known to occur in individuals with dementia. The findings of Utoomprurkporn et al. suggest that magnitude of right-ear advantage can be used as an early indicator of cognitive impairment and neural damage. But Øie et al. (2021) found no advantage or a smaller right-ear advantage among individuals with early onset of schizophrenia compared with healthy controls. These findings, taken together, suggest that a deficit in left-ear processing may be a side effect of long-term illness or even drug treatment.

Spatial Neglect

Hemispheric differences have also been studied in patients with spatial neglect. Attentional deficits frequently occur following brain damage, such as that caused by a stroke or accident. When damage occurs to both hemispheres, severe attentional deficits can occur (see Box 3.1 for a rare disorder called Bálint's syndrome). More common is damage to a single hemisphere. Left hemisphere damage may cause spatial neglect for the right side, and right hemisphere damage may cause neglect for the left side. In its most complete form, the patient does not acknowledge any type of stimulation from the side contralateral to the damaged hemisphere and attends to items toward the same side of the damaged hemisphere (i.e., the ipsilateral side; Parton et al., 2004). Neglect is not caused by primary sensory or motor deficits because patients can report seeing, hearing, and feeling stimuli and perform the appropriate actions on objects they perceive. Neglect can also be restricted to a single modality (e.g., visual or auditory; see Soroker et al.,1997) or a certain type of stimulus (e.g., pictures vs. text; see Robertson & Marshall, 1993).

Chakrabarty et al. (2017) indicated that some researchers (e.g., Kinsbourne, 1993) argued that rightward orientation by the left hemisphere is stronger than leftward orientation by the right hemisphere. Thus, when the left hemisphere is damaged, the resulting right neglect is not severe because the dominant rightward orientation can compensate. However, when the right hemisphere is damaged, the resulting left neglect tends to be more severe and enduring. Neglect following right hemisphere damage is also more common (Parton et al., 2004).

Attention theories of neglect indicate that it occurs because of the patient's inability to orient, select, and direct attention across spatial boundaries (Chakrabarty et al., 2017). Because neglect can vary in severity, several simple paper and pencil tests have been developed for diagnosing neglect (see Figure 3.12 for examples of results typically obtained from patients with right hemisphere damage or left neglect; also see Parton et al., 2004). In cancellation tasks, all stimuli or stimuli of a given category are to be crossed out. Left-neglect patients tend to fail to cross out stimuli on the left side of the paper. For copying tasks that require the individual to copy a model stimulus, left neglect is shown by patients who do not copy details present on the left side of the model stimulus. In a line-bisection task, where participants are asked to draw a vertical line in the middle of a horizontal line, left-neglect patients draw their line to the right of the middle. The patients performing these tasks can usually perform the task without any restriction of eye, head, or body movements. This indicates that the problem is not perceptual but reflects a failure to attend to the left.

Ferber and Karnath (2001) found that the line-bisection task was less effective in identifying individuals with spatial neglect than a letter cancellation task. Specifically, individuals tend to make fewer errors of omission in the line-bisection task, which could lead to missing neglect patients with mild

BOX 3.1 | **BÁLINT'S SYNDROME**

Bálint's syndrome (Bálint, 1909) is a rare neurological disorder that affects visuospatial attention and is characterized by difficulty in fixating the eyes in a position in space, executing goal-directed movements, and processing objects in visual scenes. Bilateral damage to the parietal lobes or parieto-occipital areas can lead to Bálint's syndrome (D'Imperio et al., 2017) and results in narrowed attentional focus and problems shifting attention between objects (Chakrabarty et al., 2017). Thus, unlike visual neglect patients who are unable to identify objects in a hemifield, patients with Bálint's syndrome have trouble identifying objects regardless of where they are located. Moreover, patients with Bálint's syndrome often show three distinct behavior patterns: ocular apraxia, optic ataxia, and simultanagnosia.

Ocular apraxia is a problem of visuomotor integration, in which the patient finds it difficult to fixate on a certain position in space. *Optic ataxia* refers to impaired oculomotor coordination. The patient is not able to execute goal-directed movements to visual targets, such as being able to point accurately at a location or grasp an object, but is able to execute controlled movements with their eyes closed (i.e., able to move their finger to touch their nose). *Simultanagnosia* refers to an inability to simultaneously perceive the different aspects of an object or a visual scene. In this case, the patient is unable to change their attentional focus of interest from one location to another, resulting in visual recognition impairments by not being able to see different aspects of an object or combine the aspects to recognize the object.

Researchers have studied patients with Bálint syndrome to determine neural underpinnings of attention and find ways for improving the performance of patients with the disorder. For example, D'Imperio et al. (2017) examined whether cues from different modalities about an object's identity can be used to facilitate visual object recognition in a patient with Bálint's syndrome by activating top-down processes (i.e., knowledge of objects). Patient M. R. was diagnosed with Bálint's syndrome after damage to the frontal areas of the brain. M. R.'s optic ataxia was shown by his inability to point at or grab static objects. Ocular apraxia was demonstrated by his inability to read, write, and voluntarily move his gaze to specified locations. Simultanagnosia was evident in M. R.'s inability to explore complex, multipart objects.

D'Imperio et al. (2017) used an experimental procedure in which a visual, auditory, tactile, or olfactory cue was paired with a visual stimulus illustrating overlapping objects (see Figure B3.1). The visual cue was an outline drawing of an object. The auditory cue was a natural sound made by the object, presented through headphones. The tactile cue was a real object that participants were able to touch. Finally, the olfactory cue was a real odor that the object would emit. Each cue was followed by a test stimulus, which had two overlapping images, rotated 45° from each other (see Figure B3.1), and M.R. was to identify both objects.

BOX 3.1 | **BÁLINT'S SYNDROME** *(Continued)*

FIGURE B3.1. Experimental Task Used by D'Imperio et al. (2017)

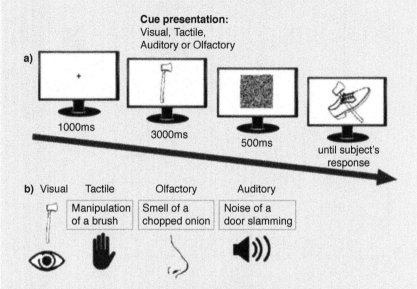

Note. a) Illustration of the sequence of events on each experimental trial and b) description of the different types of sensory cues. From "Visual and Cross-Modal Cues Increase the Identification of Overlapping Visual Stimuli in Balint's Syndrome," by D. D'Imperio, M. Scandola, V. Gobbetto, C. Bulgarelli, M. Salgarello, R. Avesani, and V. Moro, 2017, *Journal of Clinical and Experimental Neuropsychology*, *39*(8), p. 795 (https://doi.org/10.1080/13803395.2016.1266 307). Copyright 2017 by Taylor & Francis. Reprinted with permission.

On valid trials, one of the objects in the test stimulus was the cued object. On invalid trials, neither of the objects in the test stimulus was cued. M. R. was tasked with indicating whether the cued image was present in the test stimulus (a yes/no identification task) and then to discriminate both of the objects in the test stimulus. Results showed that the visual, tactile, and olfactory sensory cues were effective in reducing simultanagnosia by improving object identification and discrimination in overlapping figures. Thus, D'Imperio et al. (2017) concluded that using cues about an object in the same and different modalities activate the visual system to disambiguate the two overlapping images. Doing so allowed patient M. R. to identify objects he could not have identified otherwise. A case study of an individual patient like M. R. can vividly illustrate the consequences of brain damage, evidence relating to neural mechanisms of attention, and potential interventions for improving attentional deficits. However, generalizations from one case study should be made cautiously.

FIGURE 3.12. Illustration of Performance of Patients With Visual Neglect on Different Assessment Tasks

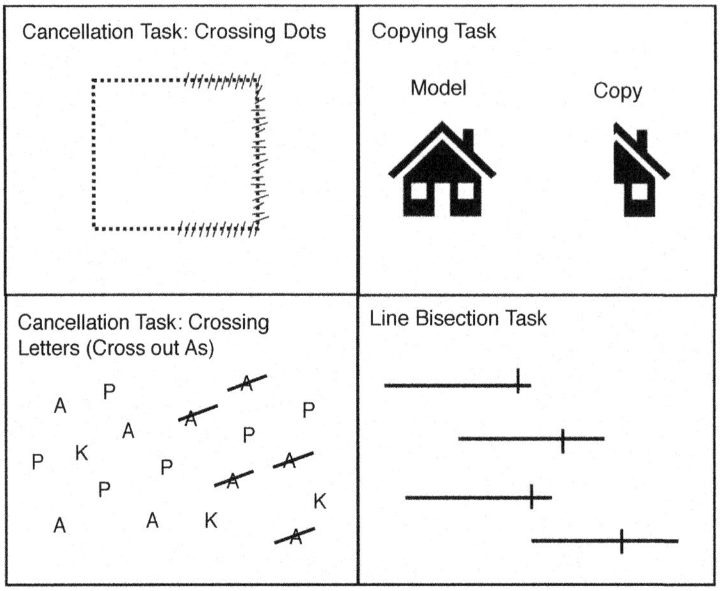

symptoms. Moreover, Ferber and Karnath noted that some neglect patients showed impairment in cancellation tasks but not in line-bisection tasks or vice versa. These findings suggest that multiple tests should be used to identify patients with neglect.

Neglect can manifest not only in the perception but also in the motor behavior of the patient (Bartolomeo, 2021), depending on the location of the lesion. For example, patients may not use the contralesional limb (Parton et al., 2004) or may be slower to initiate and execute actions toward the unattended side (Heilman, Watson, & Valenstein, 1985; Mattingley et al., 1994). As its name implies, spatial neglect is space based; it can occur with respect to position within an object. Patients with right hemispheric damage often fail to include objects located to the left in the original, but they may also fail to draw the left side of objects. Similarly, neglect in reading is demonstrated by missed words at the beginning of each line and by misreading the initial letters of the words that were detected. These findings show that for patients with damage to the right hemisphere, the left side of space and the left side of objects in the right hemifield may be neglected (Driver et al., 1994; Driver & Pouget, 2000).

CHAPTER SUMMARY

Selection is arguably the essence of attention. Knowing what is selected and how and why is a prerequisite for understanding human information processing more generally. Research on selection, perhaps more than any other aspect of attentional processing, has dictated how attention is characterized.

In this chapter, we discussed research that has explored how effectively attention in the auditory and visual modalities can be focused and how the direction and degree of focusing of attention influence stimulus (or response) processing. One of the major findings of this research is that attention can be focused on specific regions of auditory and visual space to give priority to processing stimuli from those locations. Space-based attention can give rise to hemispheric differences in the performance of individuals with and without attentional deficits. The power of selection is notable, although it is not perfect, and some stimuli defined as irrelevant to the task at hand influence performance. This interference comes about largely through the activation of information that competes with the processing of the relevant stimuli, as emphasized in the next chapter. In some cases, the interference may be produced by deep analysis that includes meaning and syntax.

Numerous models and theories have been proposed to characterize aspects of selection since the beginning of the modern era of research on attention in the 1950s. In 1890, William James said that everyone knows what attention is. When it comes to contemporary views of selective attention, there are a variety of models. Although these models differ in details and the range of findings they accommodate, they share many commonalities because they need to fit the same research findings. One shift in recent years has been from debates about early and late selection toward the role played by attention in an integrated view of perception, cognition, and action. A fundamental distinction across theoretical views is the extent to which limited capacity bottlenecks are causes of processing difficulties or consequences of the complexity of coordinating perception, cognition, and action.

KEY POINTS

- **Fact:** Selective attention is essential to being able to function in the physical and virtual worlds.

- **Fact:** People can focus attention on auditory and visual sensory input originating from specific locations.

- **Fact:** People have little awareness or memory of stimuli to which they are not attending, regardless of whether the stimuli are auditory or visual.

- **Phenomenon:** The cocktail-party effect and other attentional phenomena illustrate that people can selectively attend most efficiently based on spatial locations and other sensory properties.

- **Theory:** Filter theory captures the efficient exclusion of unattended stimuli from processing based on physical characteristics.

- **Theory:** Conceiving of visual attention as a spotlight (or zoom lens) that can facilitate the processing of stimuli within it and prevent the processing of stimuli outside of it provides a good heuristic for summarizing a lot of relevant data.

- **Theory:** Theories of selective attention began with the idea that extraneous information can be blocked out entirely but then shifted to allowing unattended information to be processed in specific situations.

- **Theory:** Filter-attenuation and late-selection theories accommodate deep-level processing of unattended stimuli, and perceptual load theory provides a possible explanation of conditions in which selection will tend to be early or late.

- **Theory:** Theories have shifted from emphasizing the locus of architectural bottlenecks in human information processing to a focus on interrelationships between perception and action that promote the efficient performance of specific tasks.

- **Phenomenon:** Right-ear advantage and spatial neglect are phenomena linked to hemispheric dominance in processing related to attention.

4

Orienting and Inhibiting Attention

Selective attention implies that we have considerable control over where attention is directed and to what it is directed. While driving an automobile on the highway, you may decide to take some action relating to the entertainment system, say, to change the music you are listening to. Before interacting with the system, you may assess the immediately surrounding traffic and determine whether you need to keep attending to the task of driving or divert your attention for a brief period to the task of changing the music. In this example, attention is, to a large extent, being controlled by your conscious intentions. But some salient event may occur—a loud noise or flashing lights—that will automatically attract attention to the source. This chapter is devoted to how attention is oriented, voluntarily or involuntarily.

Orienting attention to an object or region increases the efficiency of processing at that location. This fact makes it clear that attention can select some items for preferential processing, but how does this selection occur? As described in Chapter 3, selecting some objects or regions of space may cause nonselected objects or regions to be filtered out or inhibited. In this chapter, we discuss how attention may operate through facilitation or inhibition of processing (or a combination of both) of selected objects and locations relative to baseline performance.

https://doi.org/10.1037/0000317-004
Attention: Selection and Control in Human Information Processing, by R. W. Proctor and K.-P. L. Vu

ORIENTING

When you want to draw someone's attention to an object, you may tell that person to look at a particular location (e.g., "Look up!") or object (e.g., "Look at the dog on the video screen!"). In doing so, you will have made the reasonable assumption that the orientation of one's attention is linked to the direction of gaze (Hunt et al., 2019). Consequently, the person will make head and/or saccadic eye movements to fixate the intended target. However, the assumption that attention will be focused on the point of fixation is not always valid (see Helmholtz's, 1894/1968, demonstration described in Chapter 1, this volume). Even when the eyes are focused on a particular location, it is possible to select only a subset of the available information for perceptual processing (Posner, 1980). For example, in reading a text, you are typically only aware of the information on the current line. But if you focus on a word (e.g., "here"), you will find that it is possible, without changing your focus, to read the words on the lines above and below. Although it is possible to orient attention on items not within the eye's focus, most tasks require overt attention to achieve good performance.

An exception may be found in sports, where covert attention ability is assumed to be associated with good performance. For example, soccer goalkeepers must track the movements and positions of the players and follow where the ball is being passed. Goalkeepers with higher covert visuospatial attention abilities should be better than those with lower abilities (Jeunet et al., 2020). Moreover, dissociations between overt orienting (changes in the position of the eyes or head to improve perception) and covert orienting (changes in attentional focus without moving the eyes) are interesting from a theoretical viewpoint.

Overt and Covert Orienting

Overt movements of the eye (saccades) occur quite frequently—approximately three per second (Land, 2019). As noted in Chapter 2, saccadic eye movements can be either reflexive or controlled (Mulligan et al., 2013). *Reflexive* eye movements are triggered automatically by the sudden appearance of stimulation (through "bottom-up processes"); they are executed mainly by an area of the parietal cortex called the parietal eye fields (Gaymard et al., 2003). *Controlled* eye movements are slow, made voluntarily (through "top-down processes"), and regulated by several areas in the frontal lobes, particularly the frontal eye fields (Pierrot-Deseilligny et al., 2004). The eye movements tend to move toward objects that are informative to the task being performed and to novel, salient objects (Land, 2019). The widespread availability of relatively low-cost eye-tracking systems has made overt fixations and patterns of successive fixations staples in applied studies of attention in human factors and human–computer interaction (Krafka et al., 2016), as well as in studies of social attention (Stephenson et al., 2021).

Covert (hidden) orienting refers to the changes in the focus of attention that are not due to overt orienting. Thus, covert orienting does not affect which information is registered by the sensory receptors but may affect the output of perceptual processes by directing attention to specific locations or items. The relation between covert attention and overt eye movements has been debated. The oculomotor readiness (Klein, 1980) and premotor (Rizzolatti et al., 1987) theories state that there is a direct link between covert attention and eye movements: Attention covertly shifts to a location for which a saccadic eye-movement program has been prepared. However, studies by Ignashchenkova et al. (2004), Thompson et al. (2005), and others found that firing rates of neurons in two areas related to visual attention for cued locations, the superior colliculus and the frontal eye fields, were independent of neural signals for explicit saccadic eye movements. Consequently, in a review, Hunt et al. (2019) concluded, "The weight of evidence suggests that spatial attention does not depend on eye movement programming" (p. 264).

Carrasco (2018) presented evidence that in addition to a type of covert orienting of attention unrelated to eye movements, there is also a type that shifts attention to the target location of an imminent saccade, which she called *presaccadic attention*. The role of covert orienting in selecting information is often studied with "filtering" tasks, in which participants are shown a number of stimuli and asked to attend to just one of them. Filtering tasks are common in everyday life, such as when you search a list of departures to find the gate or time of your flight. Using filtering tasks, Carrasco showed that cuing one of two sinusoidal grating stimuli, called *Gabor patches*, enhanced contrast sensitivity discriminating the orientation of the grating as left or right of vertical. When saccadic eye movements to a target location were required, presaccadic atten-tion shifts also improved performance and enhanced perceived contrast of the saccade target. The results suggested that the effects of voluntary positioning of presaccadic attention are faster than those of covert attention.

A study by Heinze et al. (1990) provides electrophysiological support for the assumption that covert orienting affects early perceptual processing (see also McDonald et al., 2005). These authors examined the effect of attention on the different components of the event-related potential (ERP). Participants were to direct their attention to one side of a display for the duration of a block of trials but to keep their eyes fixed at a central fixation cross. Four-letter arrays that covered an equal part of the left and right visual fields were used as stimuli, and a response was only required when a specific combination of letters occurred on the attended side (this was the case on 25% of the trials). On these trials, the occipital P1 ERP component, which is associated with early stimulus processing, was enhanced on the contralateral side (indicating processing of the attended side) relative to the ipsilateral side (which would indicate processing of the unattended side). Other studies have shown that a spatially uninfor-mative visual cue enhances the brightness contrast of a subsequent target and boosts early cortical processing of the target stimulus starting 100 milliseconds (ms) after stimulus onset (Störmer et al., 2019). The cues in Störmer et al.'s (2019) study also initiated a positive deflection of the ERP that was larger over contralateral than ipsilateral occipital scalp regions, which the authors interpreted as the biasing of visual sensitivity for potential targets at that location.

Exogenous and Endogenous Orienting

Just as overt eye movements may be reflexive or controlled, there are also two ways by which covert orienting can occur. Reflexive covert orienting is commonly denoted as *exogenous* orienting to indicate that it is driven bottom up by stimuli. Controlled orienting is commonly denoted as *endogenous* orienting to indicate that it is controlled by top-down processes within the observer. Because exogenous cues are usually presented in the periphery of the display, they are also called *peripheral cues*. Exogenous cuing effects are found even when observers are aware that the cues do not provide reliable information about where a target will occur. That is, just the onset of an exogenous cue at a specific location will affect responses to other stimuli subsequently presented in the cue's former location. In fact, by definition, the presence of an exogenous cuing effect can only be determined when the cue is uninformative.

Exogenous cuing was demonstrated by Posner (1980, 2016) in a paradigm that has been widely adopted. In that paradigm, participants attend to a fixation point, and a cue occurs at a left or right location. Shortly after the cue, a target stimulus that is to be detected or identified appears at the cued location or the opposite location, with the cue being valid in the former case and invalid in the latter. If the cue is valid on 50% of the trials and invalid on the other 50%, it is uninformative, and any effect it produces can be regarded as unintentional because it is unrelated to the instructed task. If the cue is valid on 20% of the trials and invalid on 80%, there is more reason for participants not to shift attention to the cued location intentionally. Yet, in both cases, responses to a target event at the cued location are facilitated within the first 200 ms after the cue. When 80% of the trials are invalid, the facilitation then shifts at later intervals to the probable location. That is, the cue also has an intentional, endogenous component.

Posner (1980) used central arrows pointing to the left or right as endogenous cues, with the logic being that an arrow pointing a particular direction would not automatically orient attention to the cued location but would require an intentional attention shift. Such endogenous cues also produced facilitation at the signaled location when they were 80% valid but only at longer cue-target intervals than the exogenous cues. An arrow presented in the center of a display might specify where you are to look, but you have to move your attention to the indicated location yourself. However, arrows are unique stimuli in that they have not only semantic properties like the words "left" and "right" but also visuospatial properties like left and right physical locations (Miles & Proctor, 2012). Thus, they can produce an automatic orienting effect as well, which interacts with that of intentional orienting to yield a large benefit at the cued location (Ristic & Kingstone, 2012).

Malienko et al. (2018) compared the effects of an exogenous cue on eye movements and reach movements to one of several possible target locations on a display screen. The cue had no effect on the amplitudes of the saccadic eye movements or reaches, regardless of whether they were performed alone or together. Reaction time also showed no difference between single and combined movements and similar patterns as a function of cue location. However, relative to a no cue condition, the saccades and reaches yielded different patterns of facilitation and inhibition. Reaches showed facilitation when the cue was close to the target stimulus location and no inhibition when the cue was at other locations. In contrast, the saccadic eye movements showed no facilitation when the cue was close but inhibition for cues presented away from the target location. The authors concluded that the results were consistent with both effector-independent and effector-dependent effects operating in parallel.

Exogenous cuing effects reveal that, even when reflexive eye movements are suppressed, attention will move reflexively to the place of onset (or offset) of a stimulus in the visual field. Because sudden changes may not only attract attention but also increase alertness (e.g., Posner, 1978; van der Lubbe et al., 1996), cuing benefits can be measured using a cost–benefit analysis (Jonides & Mack, 1984), as Malienko et al. (2018) did. However, the evidence for effector dependence in Malienko et al.'s study was based on comparing the cuing benefits and costs relative to a no-cue baseline, for which there are many pitfalls (Jonides & Mack, 1984).

Many studies have shown that peripheral cues benefit performance, with the benefit being greatest when the interval between cue onset and target onset (*cue-target asynchrony*) is only about 100 ms (H. J. Müller & Rabbitt, 1989; Posner, 1980; Tsal, 1983). Theeuwes (1991) found that not only stimulus onsets but also offsets can attract attention. The attention-attracting effect of abrupt onsets or offsets may be due to the changes in luminance that they create. Theeuwes (1995) found that abrupt changes in colors of equal luminance do not attract attention. However, luminance changes do not always directly attract attention. Yantis and Hilstrom (1994) showed that whether luminance changes resulted in a cuing effect depended on whether or not there was an object present at the moment of the luminance change. If no object was present, attention was not directed to the location of the luminance change. A more recent study found that stimulus offsets produced cue validity effects for both keypress responses and saccadic eye movements (D. T. Smith & Casteau, 2019). These results are consistent with the hypothesis that exogenous, covert orienting is coupled with preparation for eye movements, as in Carrasco's (2018) presaccadic attention component.

Although exogenous attention shows similar effects to endogenous attention in many cases, there are also differences between the two types of control other than their sources (Carrasco, 2011). Exogenous cues have smaller effects on visual search for targets defined by a single feature than those requiring feature integration, whereas the effects of endogenous cues are similar for the two types of search tasks (e.g., Briand & Klein, 1987). Also, exogenous cues that orient attention involuntarily impair temporal-order discriminations, but endogenous cues that orient attention voluntarily enhance temporal-order discrimination

(Hein et al., 2006). Other differences between endogenous and exogenous attention are discussed by Klein (2009).

ERP studies using exogenous cues with short cue-target intervals have shown an enhancement of the components associated with early stimulus processing when the target is presented at the location of a valid cue. Effects on the P1 component are seen for both nonpredictive (Hopfinger & Mangun, 1998) and predictive (Doallo et al., 2004) exogenous cues. That is, valid exogenous cues enhance the P1 component (see Figure 4.1) when the cue-target interval is short (less than about 300 ms). ERP studies with endogenous, symbolic cues of 75% validity (e.g., Mangun & Hillyard, 1991) have also revealed an enhancement of the P1 component on valid trials at the site contralateral to the target, but this effect is only found with a relatively long cue-target interval (e.g., 800 ms). On the basis of these ERP data, it can be concluded that both endogenous and exogenous cues affect early stages of stimulus processing but that the effects of the respective cues interact with the length of the cue-target interval.

Similar results have been found using functional magnetic resonance imaging (fMRI) analysis. Dugué et al. (2020) obtained findings implying that endogenous and exogenous attention have distinct effects on activity in visuo-occipital areas when orienting based on a cue. They concluded that endogenous attention facilitates both the encoding and the readout of visual information from these areas, whereas exogenous attention only facilitates the encoding of information. Fernández and Carrasco (2020) applied transcranial magnetic stimulation (TMS) over the occipital region while participants performed a visual cuing task, which briefly disrupted the balance of excitation and inhibition. Two pulses of stimulation were applied in rapid succession at target stimulus onset to the cortical hemisphere contralateral to the target (which is the one that would be activated by the target) or the ipsilateral hemisphere (activated by a distractor on the side opposite the target). When the distractor hemisphere was stimulated, exogenous attention yielded performance benefits in the valid-cue condition and costs in the invalid-cue condition compared with a neutral condition. However, when the target hemisphere was stimulated,

FIGURE 4.1. The Difference in the P1 Component of the Event-Related Potential to a Stimulus at a Cued or Uncued Location

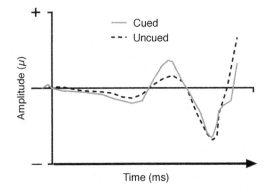
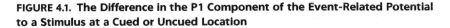

this cuing effect was eliminated. This result suggests that TMS removed the effect of exogenous attention in this situation, establishing a causal link between early visual areas and the effect of exogenous attention on performance.

When the locus of attention varies from trial to trial, which is the case in most studies using peripheral and symbolic cues, transient aspects, or phasic changes of attention can be studied. Sustained attention to a location can be examined by instructing participants to attend to one side of the visual field for the duration of a block of trials. The mechanisms controlling transient and sustained aspects of attention need not be the same. For example, Posner et al. (1980, Experiment 1) compared the costs and benefits of cuing attention in a simple detection task. The attentional cues remained the same for a block of trials or varied from trial to trial. The target could occur in any of four locations. In one condition, each target position was equally likely to be used, and in the other condition, the target was more likely to occur in one position (79% of the trials) and less likely in each of the three remaining locations (7% of the trials per position). When the cued position was blocked, significant costs relative to a neutral cue were found, but there was no significant benefit relative to the neutral cue. In contrast, when the cued side changed on a trial-to-trial basis, both costs and benefits were found. Posner et al. (1980) attributed the absence of benefits in the blocked conditions to an inability or unwillingness of participants to focus their attention at the expected position. However, Heinze et al.'s (1990) study, discussed earlier, in which effects of attending to one side of a display for a block of trials were found, suggests that sustained attention can sometimes be allocated to visual locations.

Whether exogenous orienting is entirely stimulus driven or affected by task set has been debated for more than 25 years (Luck et al., 2021). According to *stimulus-driven* accounts, physically salient stimuli automatically attract attention even when irrelevant to the task goals (Theeuwes, 1993). Yantis and Jonides (1984) found that abrupt onset of a stimulus in a visual search task drew attention to that stimulus independent of whether it was the prespecified target. Theeuwes (1993) provided a theoretical analysis based on this and related results, according to which an initial preattentive parallel process determines how different each object is from the other objects. Attention is then directed automatically to the location with the most distinct object, regardless of the participant's intentions. In contrast to automatic capture accounts, contingent involuntary orienting accounts propose that salient stimuli only capture attention when implicitly enabled by the task set (Folk et al., 1992). Initial evidence for contingent orienting was Folk et al.'s (1992) finding that an invalid abrupt-onset cue at one of five display locations produced interference with detection of an onset target but not with detection of a target color; the opposite pattern was obtained when the cue was a distinct color. These results suggested that attention capture by the cue depends on the task set.

It is difficult to obtain data that uniquely differentiate the automatic capture and contingent capture accounts because both allow for automatic attentional capture, and whether the capture is independent of intention depends on the control settings induced by the task goals, which usually cannot be verified independently. However, Luck et al. (2021) concluded that recent results support an intermediate view that puts emphasis on an inhibitory attentional control setting. An example of such findings is that when participants have to locate a shape (e.g., circle) among other shapes to identify the orientation of a line within it, a single stimulus of distinct color (a color singleton) is less likely to attract attention (overt or covert) initially than the other distractors (Gaspelin et al., 2015, 2017). This suppression is absent when the task is changed to encourage a singleton detection search mode by making the distractor shapes different from the target (e.g., a circle among squares). In this case, a singleton color captures attention and causes interference. These and other findings imply that some stimuli (abrupt onsets and color singletons) will automatically capture attention unless the task includes an inhibitory control process to prevent this capture from occurring (Gaspelin & Luck, 2019).

Casteau and Smith (2020) showed another difference between endogenous and exogenous covert orienting of attention. Exogenous covert orienting was present when stimuli were displayed within the range of saccadic eye movements but absent when stimuli were displayed outside of this range. However, endogenous covert orienting was evident even when stimuli appeared beyond the range of saccadic eye movements. Thus, exogenous covert orienting is restricted to the range of overt saccadic eye movements, but endogenous covert orienting is not. Also, Jefferies et al. (2019) provided evidence that the rate of attentional focusing onto a to-be-attended item, like orienting, is modulated by both exogenous and endogenous mechanisms. They found that contracting attention to a specific stream of items was more rapid when the targets differed in luminance from the distractor items (exogenous) and when there were no task-relevant distractors in the stream opposite the target than when there were (endogenous).

Results of neuroimaging and neuropsychological studies of the parietal cortex are consistent with these distinctions between endogenous and exogenous orienting of attention. Shomstein (2012) reviewed relevant studies and concluded that evidence indicates that the dorsal areas of the parietal cortex, including the superior parietal lobule, are involved in top-down, endogenous attentional orienting. In contrast, ventral areas, including the junction between the temporal and parietal lobes, are involved in bottom-up, exogenous attentional orienting. Thus, the two types of orienting seem to be both functionally and neurally distinct.

Space-Based Versus Object-Based Attention

The early work on cuing attention assumed that attention is allocated to regions of space. However, objects in space might be attended to differently than the regions of space they occupy. An issue in the field of visual attention is the extent to which selection (i.e., orienting of attention) can occur on the basis of features other than spatial location. Many theories assume that selection takes place through a representation of visual space (e.g., Parr & Friston, 2017; Posner et al., 1980; Störmer et al., 2019; Van der Heijden, 1992). However, some theories of visual attention include an assumption that stimulus features (e.g., location, color, form) can also be used as the basis for selection (Baylis & Driver, 1992; Bundesen, 1990; Kahneman, 1973).

Is Space Special?

An early examination of the effects of cuing an aspect other than spatial location was performed by Posner et al. (1980; Experiment 2). In this study, participants monitored a display to detect the appearance of one of 10 uppercase letters presented to the left or right of fixation. On each trial, a cue with 80% validity was presented, with the cue-target interval varying from 800 to 1,200 ms. The cue indicated the identity of the target letter, its location, both the identity and the location, or neither. Knowing the probable location of the target speeded responses when the cue was valid: Reactions were fastest when the cue gave valid location information (249 ms), intermediate when the cue was uninformative (266 ms), and slowest when the cue was invalid (297 ms). However, Posner et al. (1980) found no significant effects of cuing the letter itself.

Similar cuing effects with spatial but not with nonspatial cues were found by Theeuwes (1989), who tested the effects of location and form cues in a discrimination task. The target form was a circle or diamond in which a horizontal or vertical line segment was positioned, and responses were based on the orientation of the line. In different conditions, the most likely target location (left or right) or the most likely target form was cued with 75% validity. The location cue resulted in costs and benefits on performance, but no cuing effects were found with the form cue. Theeuwes and Van der Burg (2007) obtained similar results for cuing target location in a six-position circular array. More recently, Donovan et al. (2020) reported a lack of benefit of exogenous cuing on the color of a target in a circular array of stimuli of different colors, although cuing of location had a beneficial effect at short intervals between the cue and array. However, Kingstone (1992) found effects of position and form expectancies that interacted when the target letter was the only form presented but not when the alternative location was occupied by a letter O. That is, the interaction was evident when the target position was easy to determine but not when it was more difficult to determine. This interaction suggests that when multiple features are cued, location may have no special status.

On the whole, these prior findings support the view that space is more critical for selection than is form or color. However, failures to find effects of form, identity, or color cues in detection and discrimination tasks do not necessarily rule out the possibility that selection can be based on nonspatial features. It could be argued, for example, that the forms or letters were too alike to be effective selection cues. Indeed, a number of studies have shown that efficient selection can take place on the basis of features (e.g., color, form) other than spatial location (e.g., Bundesen et al., 1984; Von Wright, 1968).

Although these latter results support the view that other features may also provide effective selection cues, it may also be the case that selection by color or form takes place by spatial selection. For instance, given a cue to attend to red letters, attention may be automatically directed to the locations containing red letters. Alternatively, selection may also be directly focused on the color red without selecting the location.

As supported by a study conducted by Tsal and Lamy (2000), attending to a nonspatial feature of an object (e.g., its color) implies that its location is also selected (see also Cave & Pashler, 1995). Tsal and Lamy presented participants with circular arrays of six letters of different colors. Three letters were enclosed by or superimposed on a colored shape (e.g., a red, green, blue, or yellow square, circle, or triangle). Participants were asked to report the shape of a given color (e.g., the shape of any yellow objects) and freely report any letters from the array. The results showed that people tended to report letters that shared the location of the target shape rather than preferentially reporting letters that shared the same color as the shape. Thus, attending to an object of a relevant color did not facilitate the identification of objects with the same color but objects that were near the location of the attended object.

In contrast, studies using neurophysiological methods found that feature-based attention was associated with changes of activity within the receptive fields of neurons in visual cortical areas associated with object perception (e.g., Moran & Desimone, 1985), V4 and inferotemporal cortex (IT) of the ventral pathway. Maunsell and Treue's (2006) review of research on single-cell recordings in monkey visual cortex indicated that feature-based attention is associated not only with V4 and IT but also with the middle temporal cortex, associated with motion perception. They concluded that feature-based attention modulates sensory responses throughout the visual field.

Consistent with this view, Andersen et al. (2009) found a benefit for attending to a color in a task for which performance could not be mediated by spatial selection. Participants observed a display of intermingled red and blue dots that rapidly and unpredictably changed positions. They were to detect brief intervals during which 20% of the dots of one color or the other were reduced in luminance. A cue before each trial indicated that the target change was most likely to occur in a specific color or equally likely for both. Hit rates decreased and reaction times increased for detecting changes as cue validity decreased, and electrophysiological measures of steady-state visual evoked potentials during the displays showed attentional modulations of amplitude. The findings of this study indicate that selective attention to a color can produce an enhancement of processing early in the visual cortex that is not dependent on spatial attention.

Attending to an object with a specific color can also affect the processing of a subsequently presented object (a probe stimulus) at the same location. For example, Luck et al. (1993) presented a target, defined by color, in an array of irrelevant stimuli (distractors), with the task of identifying the target. Either the target or one of the distractors was replaced by a probe (which did not have to be responded to) 250 ms after the presentation of the array. ERPs elicited by the probe showed an enhanced P1 component when the probe occurred in the position of the target relative to when the probe was presented in the position of a distractor. This result suggests that the location and not only the color of the target was attended to.

Overall, spatial position does seem to have a special role in visual selection (see also van der Heijden, 1993). In other words, in many cases, attention seems to operate on a spatial representation of visual space. This is not surprising given that attention is generally oriented to a location. However, attention can also be directed to nonspatial features under certain conditions.

Allocating Attention to Objects

According to purely space-based models of selection, attention directly operates on a spatial representation of visual space. For instance, in feature integration theory (see Chapter 1 and later in this chapter), attention is allocated to regions of space and acts to bind features in those regions to form objects. Thus, objects are only identified after attention has been directed to regions of space. However, other models of attention assume that attention selects objects rather than regions of space (e.g., Desimone & Duncan, 1995; G. W. Humphreys & Müller, 1993; for a review, see Goldsmith, 1998). Such object-based theories of visual selection assume that attention only selects regions of space that are occupied by objects. Space-based theories assume that attention can select regions of space whether they are occupied by objects or not.

Several findings suggest that objects may be the target and not just the outcome of attention (Z. Chen, 2012). Duncan (1984) reported a series of influential studies in which participants were presented with two superimposed objects (a small or large rectangular outline box and a superimposed dotted or dashed vertical line tilted clockwise or counterclockwise). They were required to identify either two dimensions of a single object (e.g., line tilt clockwise or counterclockwise, line dotted or dashed) or one dimension on each of the objects (e.g., line tilt clockwise or counterclockwise, box size large or small). Performance was better when both dimensions were on the same object than on different objects.

Duncan (1984) proposed that we attend to objects and not to space and that when judgments are made about two objects, attention must be switched from one object to the other, which takes time. According to this object-based conception of attentional selection, space or spatial proximity is not the dominant factor in the control of attention, but attention operates on objects formed on the basis of earlier perceptual processes. For example, the visual field may be preattentively segmented into separate objects based on gestalt grouping principles such as continuity, proximity, similarity, and movement. After this preattentive stage, focal attention is employed to analyze objects in more detail (e.g., Neisser, 1967).

Virtual objects in a display can be produced using the gestalt principles to create perceptual groups. Prinzmetal (1981) used the proximity principle (objects close together in space are perceived as belonging to a common group) to create displays that would be processed as two groups. An "object" in these displays was a group composed of a row or column of four of five circles; two groups were shown in each display. On each trial, the display was shown briefly, followed by a mask, and participants had to report whether a target was present. Figure 4.2 shows sample displays for the task of determining whether a cross formed by the conjunction of a horizontal and vertical line segment was present in any of the circles in the display.

Prinzmetal (1981) reasoned that if attention is devoted to objects, illusory conjunctions (falsely combining two features to create a nonpresent object) of features on nontarget trials would be more likely to occur when the two features were in the same row of the display (and hence in the same perceptual group) than when each feature was in a different row. This is just what was found. Participants rarely reported seeing a target when the two features in the display were the same (the "target-absent feature displays"; see Figure 4.2). When one horizontal and one vertical line segment were present (the "target-absent conjunction display"), participants were more likely to mistakenly report having seen a target. When the two features were in the same row, illusory conjunctions were reported on nearly 25% of target-absent conjunction trials. However, when the two features were in different rows, illusory conjunctions occurred on about 18% of the trials. These results suggest that people process

FIGURE 4.2. Displays Like Those Used by Prinzmetal (1981)

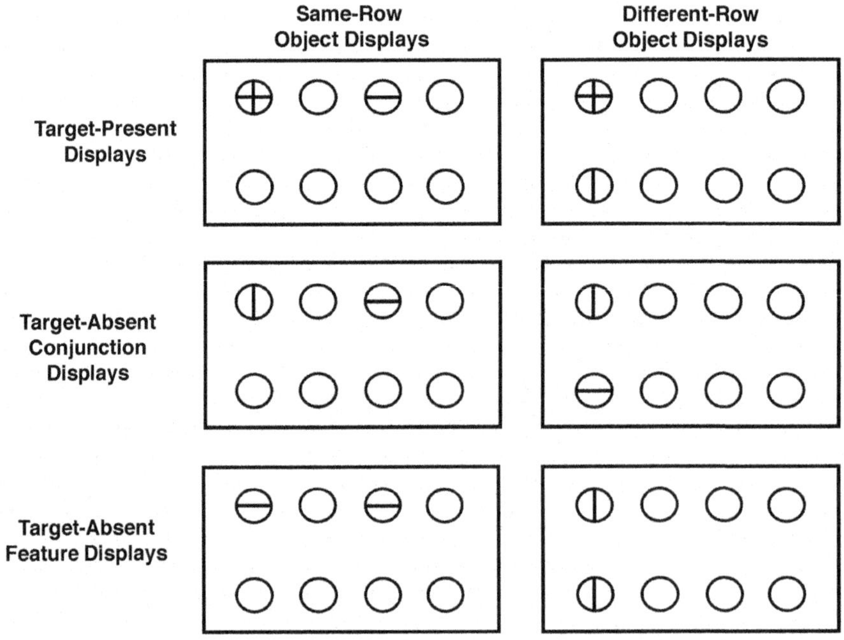

Note. Two rows of four circles were shown; the task was to indicate whether a cross was present.

all the features of a perceptual group at once, as predicted by object-based theories of attention.

One of the most influential studies in this area of research is that of Egly et al. (1994). They had participants make a single button-press response when they detected the onset of a target (dark square) in a display of two bars on opposite sides of fixation (see Figure 4.3). A trial began with the onset of the fixation sign and two vertical bars located at the left and right or two horizontal bars located at the top and bottom. On most trials, the target event was preceded by a cue (brief brightening of the end of one rectangle), which then went off. A target (requiring a response) appeared on two thirds of the trials, and for those trials, it was at the cued position 75% of the time and at one of the uncued positions the remaining 25%. As expected, if the cue directed attention to its location, reaction time was shortest for validly cued trials on which the

FIGURE 4.3. Stimulus Sequence for Egly et al.'s (1994) Cuing Experiment With Vertical and Horizontal Bar Objects

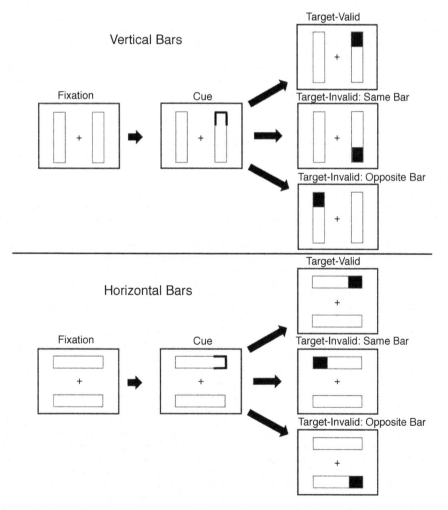

target appeared at the cued location. On invalidly cued trials, reaction time was longer when the target was at the same end of the opposite bar than at the other end of the same bar, even though the locations were equally distant from the cued location. This result suggests that attention to the cued location spread more to the location within the same object than between the two objects.

Pilz et al. (2012) noted that object-based attention effects are small and obtained less reliably than space-based attention effects. They found with Egly et al.'s (1994) methods and similar ones that only horizontally oriented bars showed evidence of object-based attention and that the effect itself was weak at the level of individual participants. Barnas and Greenberg (2016) explored this issue further, using L-shaped objects (see Figure 4.4) for which the vertex was randomly positioned in one screen quadrant to compare changes across the vertical meridian (corresponding to a line extending from top to bottom through the fixation point) and horizontal meridian (corresponding to a line extending left to right through the fixation point). An exogenous cue of high validity appeared briefly around the object vertex. Afterward, a target letter T appeared at the cued position on 60% of trials and an uncued position on 20% of trials (with the remaining two positions containing the letter L). On the remaining 20% of the trials, all three positions contained the letter L, and no response was to be made. Target detection responses showed a horizontal attention-shift advantage (shorter reaction times for horizontal shifts across the vertical meridian than for vertical shifts across the horizontal meridian),

FIGURE 4.4. Trial Sequence in Barnas and Greenberg's (2016) Experiment 1 for a Gray L-Shaped Object With a Cue in the Upper-Left Quadrant

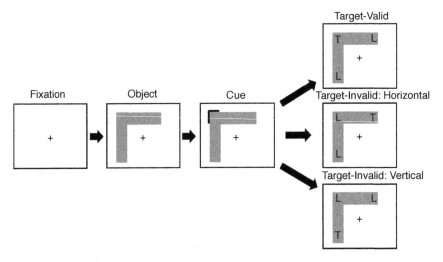

Note. Three possible trial types defined by the location of the target "T" in relation to the cue. From "Visual Field Meridians Modulate the Reallocation of Object-Based Attention," by A. J. Barnas and A. S. Greenberg, 2016, *Attention, Perception, & Psychophysics, 78*(7), p. 1988 (https://doi.org/10.3758/s13414-016-1116-5). Copyright 2016 by Springer Nature. Adapted with permission.

and in other experiments, regardless of whether the shifts were within a cued object or between objects. They hypothesized that this difference is a consequence of the contralateral organization of the visual cortex.

A follow-up study by Barnas and Greenberg (2019) used similar L-shaped objects at various locations relative to fixation and concluded that the difference between horizontal and vertical shifts of attention occurred only when invalid target locations required shifts of object-based attention that crossed the meridians, regardless of object boundary placement. They concluded that this asymmetry is driven by target location relative to the visual field meridians. Thus, object-based attention prioritizes specific target locations and not all target locations within a cued object.

Z. Chen and Cave (2019) took an additional step, based on results from six experiments, and concluded that results from variants of Egly et al.'s (1994) task might not be due to object-based attention at all. Their task required participants to indicate whether two simultaneously presented letters (instances of T and L) were the same or different. In their Experiments 1 to 3, the target stimuli were presented within outlined rectangles, as in Egly et al.'s study, that were oriented either horizontally or vertically. In all the experiments, responses were faster for horizontal target configurations than for vertical configurations. Because the horizontal locations were always on opposite sides of the horizontal meridian, this outcome agrees with Barnas and Greenberg's (2016, 2019) findings. Z. Chen and Cave also found that responses were particularly slow in some conditions when the rectangles were oriented horizontally, but the two targets were configured vertically. In their Experiments 4 to 6, no rectangles were used in any displays, and the target letters were shown on a gray background following a cue that indicated the likely orientation of the target configuration. Even though there were no objects in the display, the horizontal alignment advantage was still evident, as was the cost in responding to vertically arranged targets when cued for a horizontal configuration. Note that these results cannot be attributed to object-based attention. Consequently, Z. Chen and Cave suggested that they could be due to a horizontal advantage and an orientation set cost.

Z. Chen et al. (2020) followed the prior research with a study in which the object had two sides connected in the middle, much like the capital letter H, such that the upper and lower locations on each side were separated by a concavity (see Figure 4.5). Again, participants made the same or different responses to pairs composed from the letters T or L, with one appearing on the screen before the other T or L. Reaction times were longer when the two locations were separated by a concavity in the object and not statistically different from when they were located on two separate objects. Z. Chen et al. concluded that the reaction time reflected the complexity of the region between the two locations and not whether they are on the same or different objects.

The research on object-based attention has shown that numerous factors can influence people's performance with complex displays. The recent findings question the extent to which, in the Egly et al. (1994) paradigm, these factors

FIGURE 4.5. Examples of Trials From Z. Chen et al.'s (2020) Experiment 1

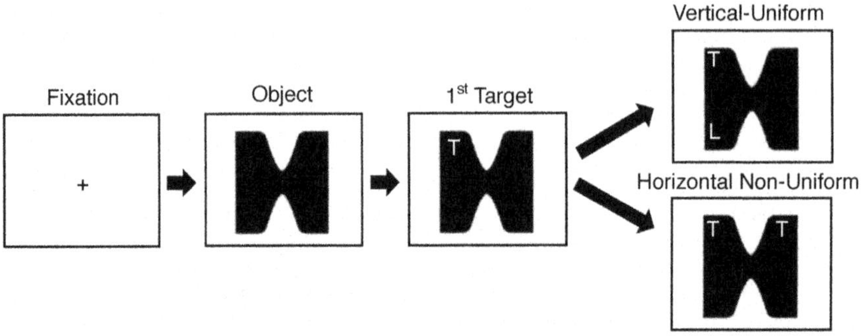

Note. Adapted from "A Region Complexity Effect Masquerading as Object-Based Attention," by Z. Chen, K. R. Cave, D. Basu, S. Suresh, and J. Wiltshire, 2020, *Journal of Vision, 20*(7), p. 3 (https://dx.doi.org/10.1167/jov.20.7.24). CC BY-NC-ND 4.0.

involve object-based attention or are consequences of spatial allocation of attention and attentional set. However, as Z. Chen et al. (2020) pointed out, there is still evidence of object-based attention in other paradigms using perceptual grouping, as in Prinzmetal's (1981) study described earlier, and subjective organization (e.g., Li & Logan, 2008; Pratt & Sekuler, 2001). Thus, the most reasonable conclusion at present is that object-based attention is a real phenomenon but is more limited than often assumed (Z. Chen et al., 2020).

INHIBITION

Inhibition with regard to behavior refers to some aspect of implicit or explicit action that is suppressed. The cuing paradigm has been used to study the prevention of attention from returning to a previously attended location, and a stop-signal paradigm has been used to determine the extent to which intended responses that have been activated can be suppressed.

Inhibition of Return

Recall that when a peripheral cue to the left or right of fixation does not predict where a target stimulus will occur, it produces facilitation of responding to a target that appears at that location within about 250 ms after the cue. Notably, though, a reversal of this benefit occurs when the time interval between cue and target (*stimulus onset asynchrony*, or SOA) is longer (Klein, 2000; Posner & Cohen, 1984). The term *inhibition of return* is based on the idea that the return of attention to the cued location is suppressed.

This result pattern was evident in the initial experiment by Posner and Cohen (1984) that demonstrated the phenomenon. A row of three outline boxes was centered at fixation. The peripheral cue was the brightening of the outline of the left or right box, which was followed at different intervals by the onset of a target in one of the boxes, to which a detection response was required. The target appeared in that box on 60% of the trials and in the peripheral boxes on 20% of the trials (10% for each of the cued or uncued peripheral boxes) to induce participants to return the focus of attention to the center box. The remaining 20% were catch trials with no target stimulus, to ensure that the responses were truly target detections. Even though only a simple detection response was required, reaction times showed the defining reversal from favoring the cued location at short cue-target intervals to favoring the uncued location at the 500-ms interval.

Posner et al. (1985) used a similar method, with the main changes being that after the peripheral cue, the center box was brightened to induce the return of attention to the center. Then, a bright dot occurred in each peripheral box, with an interval between their onsets ranging from 0 to 200 ms. In one task, participants were to keep their eyes at fixation and press a key on the side of the target dot that appeared first. In another task, they were to move their eyes in a direction that seemed most natural. The temporal order judgments showed no inhibition of return, but the eye movements showed a bias to move in the direction opposite the cued location. In another experiment, Posner et al. (1985) also showed longer reaction times for detecting a target in the cued box when eye movements were made to one peripheral box and then back to the center box before target onset. They interpreted their results as showing a link between inhibition of return and the eye-movement system—that is, a bias against returning fixation to the prior location.

Inhibition of return generated large amounts of research in the following years, with variations of the attention shifting account being accepted by many researchers (Klein, 2000). However, the situation is more complex than the consistency in the use of the term and explanations implies (Dukewich & Klein, 2015). This point was made forcefully by Berlucchi (2006) in his article "Inhibition of Return: A Phenomenon in Search of a Mechanism and Better Name." The problem Berlucchi identified is that the name "inhibition of return" for the phenomenon implies an explanation in terms of a specific mechanism, which has been applied by researchers to interpret a variety of results that may have different bases. We will not go into that issue in detail but will discuss instead work by Klein and associates to try to clarify the situation.

Klein and colleagues (Klein & Redden, 2018; Redden et al., 2021) have proposed two forms of inhibition of return that depend on the state of activation of the reflexive oculomotor system. One form is generated when the reflexive oculomotor system is suppressed (when the participant is to maintain fixation on a central focus point) and decreases the salience of sensory inputs. The other form is generated when the reflexive oculomotor system is not suppressed (when eye movements are required) and acts to bias responding. Behavioral evidence for this distinction was provided by Taylor and Klein (2000). Each trial in their study contained two successive signals, either peripheral stimulus onsets or central arrows, separated by 500 ms. Responses were left and right key presses or left and right eye movements. The required responses to the first and second signals were no-response/manual, manual/manual, saccadic/manual, no-response/saccadic, manual/saccadic, and saccadic/saccadic. When the eyes remained at fixation (the no-response/manual, manual/manual conditions), inhibition of return was evident only for peripheral signals, which Taylor and Klein attributed to slowed visual processing. When the eyes moved (the saccadic/manual, no-response/saccadic, manual/saccadic, saccadic/saccadic conditions), inhibition of return was obtained for both peripheral and central signals, which the authors attributed to slowed motor production. The results showed slow responding to peripheral stimuli when the eyes remained fixed (attributed to slowed visual processing) and both peripheral and central signals when the eyes moved (attributed to slowed motor production).

Redden et al. (2021) applied diffusion modeling to results obtained for situations in which the reflexive oculomotor system was active or suppressed and found that two different drift-diffusion parameters accounted for the distinct result sets. Moreover, Satel et al. (2019) provided evidence that the neurological basis of inhibition of return when the reflexive oculomotor system is active is likely in projections from the superior colliculus to cortical areas affecting spatial responses. In contrast, when the reflexive oculomotor system is intentionally suppressed, the input-based form of inhibition of return is generated by affecting early sensory pathways in retinal coordinates. Bisley and Mirpour (2019) summarized evidence indicating that there are priority maps in at least three brain regions. Evidence indicates that (a) the lateral intraparietal area (LIP) of the posterior parietal cortex provides a representation of attentional priority that remaps across each saccade; (b) the LIP provides input to the frontal eye field of the prefrontal cortex, which can suppress the responses to control the eye movements; and (c) the final saccade goal is reflected in the intermediate layers of the superior colliculus.

Klein and colleagues (Klein & Redden, 2018; Redden et al., 2021) stressed that both types of inhibition of return evolved to promote novelty seeking in the environment, as Posner et al.'s (1985) initial account implied. However, Hooge et al. (2005) examined participants' scan patterns in free viewing of pictures and searches for multiple targets and found no tendency for a reduction in revisits to prior locations. Although inhibition of return as a phenomenon is well established, its mechanisms and role in information processing are still subjects of research.

Stopping Task Performance in Response to a Signal

In the study of inhibition of return, effects of inhibition are inferred from the poorer performance at a location to which attention was previously oriented. As noted, a difficulty with attributing the results to inhibition is that alternative explanations are possible. However, there are situations in which an intended response must be inhibited to prevent undesirable outcomes. It is a fact of life that goals change, and actions must sometimes be modified to follow them.

For example, a driver worried about getting to work on time will have to change the priority from speed to safety when a railroad barrier descends in front of him. When the current course of thought or action (get to work fast) is no longer appropriate, it must be replaced by a new one (e.g., stop the car). According to Logan (1994), stopping processes are especially interesting because they provide an unambiguous case of intervention through cognitive control.

The *stop-signal paradigm* was developed to study the stopping process (Logan, 1981, 1994). In this paradigm, people perform a simple task, such as pressing one of two keys when they see an "X" and the other key when an "O" is presented. On trials in which a "stop signal" is presented (e.g., a tone), the response is to be withheld. The use of a detection task for the stop signal minimizes perceptual processes, but after the signal is detected, the "stop" action must be selected and the motor output for the initial task inhibited (Verbruggen & Logan, 2017). The measure of interest is whether people can withhold responses after the stop signal. Although the method seems intuitive, problems can arise in its implementation (Verbruggen et al., 2019).

It has been hypothesized that a stop signal initiates an inhibitory "stop" process that then races against an excitatory "go" process that is set off by the primary task stimulus. In the "race model" of stop-signal performance, these two processes operate independently of each other (Logan & Cowan, 1984). If the stop process finishes before processing on the first task has reached a point of no return (i.e., a point beyond which the response can no longer be withheld), it "wins," and the response is inhibited. The time for this latency of response inhibition, which is not directly observable, can be estimated from the stop-signal reaction time.

Research has focused on finding the point of no return by varying factors known to affect different stages in the initial task and then measuring the effect of these manipulations on stopping time. If a stage before the point of no return is lengthened, there should be more time for the stopping process to finish its course, and thus the percentage of successful stops will be higher. If the process affected is after the point of no return, no change in the percentage of successful stops is expected (see Figure 4.6). For example, stimulus-response compatibility (i.e., having a "natural" stimulus-response mapping) reduces the time required to select a response (Proctor & Vu, 2006b). If response selection and the processes after it are ballistic (i.e., if, once started, they always run to completion), reducing the compatibility of the task would not affect the probability of correctly stopping (see Figure 4.6, Panel C). If response selection is not ballistic, making the response less compatible, thus lengthening the time needed for response selection, it allows the stopping process more time and should lead to a higher percentage of correct stops (see Figure 4.6, Panel B). Logan (1981) found that the latter was the case and concluded that response-selection processes can be interrupted. Given that response selection can be inhibited by stop processes, it is not surprising that increasing stimulus discriminability, which affects perception, an earlier stage of processing, also allows more time for stopping. More surprising is the finding that response complexity, which

FIGURE 4.6. Hypothetical Effects of Prolonging a Stoppable (Panel B) and a Ballistic (Panel C) Process on Stop-Signal Responses Compared With a Control Condition (Panel A)

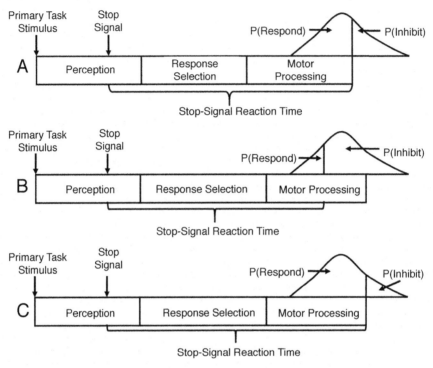

Note. Logan (1981) found that response selection can be stopped when a stop signal is presented.

affects the time required to initiate a movement, affects a stage of motor programming that can be inhibited (Osman et al., 1990). The probability of making a response is lower when response selection is more difficult (see Figure 4.6, Panel B).

Some researchers have argued that there is no point of no return. De Jong et al. (1990) used sophisticated techniques to measure both brain and muscle electrical activity on trials that were successfully stopped and trials that should have been stopped but were not. Initial task responses were made by squeezing a dynamometer (a device that registers the force applied to it). Electrodes placed on the arms recorded the electromyogram from the muscles used in making a response. Finally, electrodes placed on the scalp measured the lateralized readiness potential (LRP), assumed to reflect brain activity associated with the differential involvement of the right and left motor cortex in preparing to make unimanual movements on each trial. Information processes, as measured by LRPs, forearm muscle activation, and even the squeezing of the response meter itself, could all be stopped once begun, providing no evidence of a point of no return.

Stopping Times

A variety of initial tasks and stop signals have been used. Whether the action to be withheld is a button press, a hand movement, speech, or a squeeze, a normal, healthy young adult will be able to stop the response in about 200 ms (Logan & Cowan, 1984). The consistency of stopping times for different tasks and effector systems suggests that stopping relies on a single, central, amodal process. However, one study found that in a two-choice task with left/right responses, eye movements and hand movements were affected differently by central versus peripheral stimulus presentation and whether the stimulus-response mapping was compatible or incompatible (Logan & Irwin, 2000). This outcome suggests that inhibition of eye movements and hand movements are governed by distinct processes (and even these processes are assumed to operate according to the same principles).

The Nature of the Stopping Process

According to the race model, stopping an action depends on a separate sort of processing than selecting and executing an action. Both behavioral and electrophysiological evidence for this assumption has been found. Naito and Matsumura (1996) found that some aspects of motor activation in preparation for a response were unaffected by a stop signal and that the stopping process itself was associated with an independent "no-go" specific electroencephalogram component. Normally, when two stimuli require different responses, the response to the second of the two stimuli is slowed at short SOAs. However, the countermanding action to withhold a response after a stop signal does not show the usual effects found with dual-task performance (see Chapter 6). As Logan and Cowan (1984) asserted, stop signals do not seem to be subject to the same bottlenecks in performance that affect responses to other stimuli.

If the control exercised by the stop process operates outside the system that controls go processes (Logan, 1994), it could be the case that stop processes intervene when it is necessary to stop an action but are not otherwise involved in control. Although the stopping process seems to operate independently of initial-task "go" processes, it may nonetheless influence how these processes operate. For example, for a stop-signal procedure in which only some trials are followed by stop signals, reaction times following stop-signal trials are longer than otherwise. It seems that invoking the stopping process has an inhibitory aftereffect that carries over into the processing of the next trial (M. Rieger & Gauggel, 1999).

Studies using fMRI and other methods to study the neural substrate of control in the stop-signal paradigm have identified a widespread brain network that shows activation. In the cortex, many studies show activation of the right inferior frontal cortex (IFC) associated with inhibitory control, but there is some evidence of bilateral IFC activity playing a role as well (Swick et al., 2008). Numerous other cortical areas have been implicated, as well as regions in the cerebellum. S. V. Clark et al. (2020) reviewed evidence that the cerebellum participates in inhibitory control, suggesting that clusters in the left posterior cerebellum communicate with the cortical right-lateralized inhibitory control network.

In many everyday situations, either stopping an action or a change in action may accompany a change of plan. This raises the question of whether it is necessary to stop an action before a change can be made or whether the changing process has a separate function. The evidence thus far is that stopping is qualitatively different than changing, suggesting that stop processes provide a different sort of control than those needed for go processes.

VISUAL SEARCH

How attention is directed when looking for a target stimulus among multiple distractors can be examined in visual search tasks. Many tasks in the physical and virtual worlds involve visual search. Even in simple detection tasks, such as waiting for a green light at an intersection, the correct signal must be found and attended to. Most search tasks are more complicated, like searching for a tumor in an X-ray film or for a friend in a crowd (see Box 4.1). In laboratory search tasks, the task is usually to search for a particular target (e.g., a white bar) or one of two or more possible targets (a white or black bar) in a display with distractors (e.g., gray bars). With one method, a target is present on some trials but not others, and the task is to detect whether the target was present. With another method, a target is always present, and the task is to identify which target was displayed. A third method entails locating the target. Search performance can be measured by the time needed to detect, identify, or locate the target. Alternatively, the search field can be displayed for only a limited time, and performance accuracy can be measured.

Feature and Conjunction Search

In general, search is easier when the target can be defined by one feature (i.e., a *feature search*), such as a color (see Figure 4.7, left panel), than when it is defined by a conjunction of two or more features, such as color and orientation (see Figure 4.7, right panel). The time to determine whether a target is present depends on the number of items in a display in *conjunction search* but not in feature search (see Figure 4.8). Moreover, in conjunction search, search times are generally shorter when a target is present than when it is not. The fact that conjunction search time depends on the number of items in the display has led some researchers to suppose that such search proceeds serially. That is, each item in the display must be checked to see if it is a target. The shorter search times for target-present than for target-absent trials can be explained by assuming that observers stop searching when the target is found. Because the response can be executed whenever the target is identified, on average,

BOX 4.1 | **WHAT CAN WALLY/WALDO TELL US ABOUT ATTENTION AND VISUAL SEARCH?**

Where's Wally was published in the late 1980s as a series of illustrations in a book where the reader would search for a distinct character, called Wally (or Waldo in the United States; this series was called *Where's Waldo* when published in the United States). Wally/Waldo is a White male cartoon character with brown hair and glasses who wears distinctive clothing (red-and-white striped shirt, red-and-white knit hat with a red pompom, and blue pants). The reader would search for Wally/Waldo in a crowded scene that has other people, animals, and objects sharing his distinctive features. Where's Wally/Waldo is a conjunction search task, where the target shares common features with the distractors in the visual scene. It also reflects search behavior found in real-world settings because eye movements are needed to analyze the features that are often cluttered on a display. Studying how people search for Wally/Waldo can provide information about how attention is allocated when searching for items in complex scenes.

For example, Klein and MacInnes (1999) had participants search for Waldo and, if he was found, continue searching for another character, a wizard. There were eight pictures of Waldo used equally often in the 288 trials. Waldo was present in half of the pictures, and the wizard was never present. On some trials, a probe dot was presented during the search for the wizard after participants made four or more saccades. Participants were instructed to stop searching and fixate on the probe as quickly as possible when it reappeared. On half the trials, the picture remained on the screen until the eyes fixated on the probe, whereas the picture was removed for the other half of the trials. Participants were slower to make saccadic eye fixations to the probes when presented in the general region of preceding fixations of the search task than when presented in a different region. This finding was only evident when the picture (i.e., search scene) was not removed during the presentation of the probe and suggests that inhibitory markers are attached to objects in a scene and used to facilitate search behaviors.

Port et al. (2016) examined saccades of younger and older adults while performing Waldo search tasks, which they referred to as puzzles. They recruited over 300 individuals ranging from 4 to 66 years of age for the study. Participants were given puzzles that varied in difficulty and were asked to find Waldo in the visual scene within a 30-second time limit. An eye tracker was used to measure regular saccades and microsaccades, which involve a narrower region around the fixation point (less than 10–12 arc minute, 0.16°–0.20°). Saccades can be used to indicate where attention is being directed because shifts in attention are often followed by shifts in eye movement in the same direction. Port et al. found that participants of all ages were able to perform the Waldo task, although a few younger participants did quit the task.

(continues)

BOX 4.1 | **WHAT CAN WALLY/WALDO TELL US ABOUT
ATTENTION AND VISUAL SEARCH?** *(Continued)*

The mean time to complete the puzzles was plotted as a function of participants' age, and a U-shape function emerged with the solution time being the shortest for participants around 20 years of age. When performing the task, a large number of saccades were in the 1° to 3° amplitude range, and the frequency of saccades increased as the difficulty increased. Participants made saccades of all sizes along both the horizontal and vertical dimensions, but there was a stronger bias for horizontal than vertical saccades. The percentage of regular and microsaccades made during the search task was similar, but their frequency increased slightly with age. Older adults showed a higher peak velocity per saccade amplitude than younger adults. Together, these findings indicate that, although search efficiencies change with age, being most efficient during young adulthood, the sequence kinematics does not vary much as a function of age. When performing a search task, there is a bias to shift attention horizontally rather than vertically.

Smirl et al. (2016) used transcranial doppler ultrasound to measure cerebral blood velocities of the posterior (PCA) and middle (MCA) cerebral artery when participants performed a Waldo search task, a reading task, or an identification task with color dots on the screen. The Waldo search task is much more complicated than reading text (i.e., it requires longer fixations and more eye saccades), and the images are more complex than color dots presented on a screen. Smirl et al. found that all three tasks resulted in elevations in the PCA velocities compared with baseline measures taken before the task, with the largest elevation evident for the Waldo search task for every participant. There were also smaller elevations in the MCA velocities that were similar for all three visual tasks. The marked differences in PCA elevation for the Waldo task suggest that this task requires a greater level of processing within the PCA-supplied regions associated with complex visual processing and attention shifting between objects in a scene.

The final example by Peltier and Becker (2017) used the Waldo search task to examine the effectiveness of using eye-movement feedback to signal to participants areas where they have already searched in the visual field. Waldo is considered a low prevalence target in a visual display and resembles many real-world search tasks where operators are looking for a target that does not occur often (e.g., screeners looking for a weapon in baggage, radiologists looking for indicators of cancer on an image). For these tasks, eye-movement feedback can mark areas that have been searched from areas that have not been searched to guide the operators' attention to new areas that may contain the target. Unfortunately, Peltier and Becker found weak evidence supporting this type of eye-tracking feedback using the *Where's Waldo* scenes. This finding may be due to the tendency for participants to scan the display rather than to engage in a complete or detailed search of an area. Because target identification in complex scenes requires attention (i.e., longer fixations to analyze the objects in the area), methods that discourage participants from reexamining areas that they quickly scan, such as the eye-movement feedback methods studied by Peltier and Becker, can reduce search performance rather than facilitate it.

FIGURE 4.7. Visual Search Displays for Feature and Conjunction Search

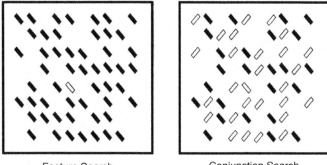

Feature Search   Conjunction Search

Note. From *Attention: Theory and Practice* (p. 82), by A. Johnson and R. W. Proctor, 2004, SAGE (https://doi.org/10.4135/9781483328768). Copyright 2004 by A. W. Johnson and R. W. Proctor. Reprinted with permission.

half the items will need to be checked. However, on target-absent trials, all items will need to be checked to ensure that a target is not present. Consequently, the function relating search time to the number of items in the display should be twice as steep for target-absent trials as for target-present trials (see Figure 4.8).

The notion of *serial self-terminating search* is consistent with many visual search studies. By examining the slope of the function relating search time to the number of items in the display, it is possible to estimate how much time is needed to process each item. For example, if slopes of 70 and 35 ms per item are obtained when the target is absent and present, respectively, the time for each individual comparison can be estimated as 70 ms. Note that this is an application of the subtractive logic, requiring independent comparisons performed in succession, as assumed by the serial model. A limitation is that the results can be mimicked by a model that assumes parallel processing of the stimuli based on a system with limited-capacity processing resources (Townsend,

FIGURE 4.8. The Relation Between Set Size (the Number of Items in the Display) and Reaction Time for Feature and Conjunction Search When a Target Is Present or Absent

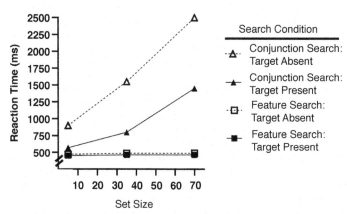

1971, 1972). The point to understand is that in such a case, increasing the number of items in the display will reduce the processing resources devoted to each stimulus, which will yield an effect of set size like that predicted by the serial search model.

Conjunction search is well described by the serial self-terminating search model (although this is not the only model possible), but what about feature search? Initially, it was assumed that feature search could be performed by processing all items in the display in parallel. In fact, feature search is sometimes termed parallel search, whereas conjunction search is termed serial search. The distinction between parallel and serial search formed the basis for theories of visual search (e.g., Treisman & Gelade, 1980). However, this dichotomy has lost importance in some theories (e.g., Treisman, 1998) and is rejected by others (e.g., Wolfe, 1994). Rather than characterizing search as a dichotomy of serial or parallel, it is better described as a continuum of efficiency (from inefficient to efficient; Duncan & Humphreys, 1989; Wolfe, 1998). Very efficient search (e.g., a search for a vertical line among horizontal lines) results in search slopes of zero. Very inefficient search (e.g., a search for a conjunction of two orientations) can take more than 40 ms per item, resulting in a much steeper search slope.

Search Asymmetry

The efficiency of visual search can be influenced by whether one is searching for a basic feature or not. Basic features were initially characterized by efficient search and can be identified through search asymmetry. *Search asymmetry* is evident when searching for Stimulus A among instances of Stimulus B is easier than when searching for Stimulus B among instances of Stimulus A. Treisman and Gormican (1988) argued that search asymmetry can be used to identify basic, preattentive features. For example, in Figure 4.9a, it is easier to find the "C" target among "O" distractors than to find the "O" target among "C"

FIGURE 4.9. Examples of Visual Search Asymmetries

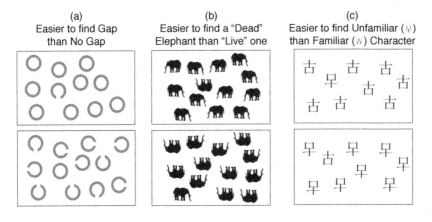

(a)	(b)	(c)
Easier to find Gap than No Gap	Easier to find a "Dead" Elephant than "Live" one	Easier to find Unfamiliar (屮) than Familiar (古) Character

distractors because the presence of a gap is a basic feature, but the absence of a gap is not. Other basic features include color, motion, orientation, and size (including length, spatial frequency, and apparent size; Wolfe & Horowitz, 2017).

However, Treisman and Gormican's (1988) view of search asymmetry was challenged by researchers who argued that the efficiency of search is determined by other factors based on the characteristics of the stimuli used in the search task and the specific experimental procedures (Wolfe, 2001). Rosenholtz (2001) used motion to illustrate that one such factor in producing search asymmetry is distractor heterogeneity. For motion, a large search asymmetry is often obtained when it is easier to find a moving target among stationary distractors than a stationary target among moving distractors. When the target is in motion, the distractors are homogeneously stationary. In contrast, when the target is stationary, the distractors are moving heterogeneously (i.e., in different directions). When the distractors are more heterogenous, search is less efficient, and this property of the search task can give rise to the search asymmetry independent of whether the target is a feature or not. Thus, Rosenholtz cautioned experimenters to avoid generating visual asymmetries from built-in design asymmetries.

Other researchers have argued that novelty plays a role in producing search asymmetries, with search more efficient for a novel or unfamiliar stimulus than for a familiar one. Wolfe (2001) used silhouettes of animals that were upright, or "live," or inverted, or "dead" (see Figure 4.9b). He found that the "dead" elephants were hard to hide. The search was more efficient for the dead elephant because it was in an unfamiliar, inverted orientation. Shen and Reingold (2001) also found that familiarity played a role in producing search asymmetries. In their Experiment 2, the Chinese character for the word "ancient" was used as a familiar stimulus, and the same character was rotated 180° as an unfamiliar stimulus (see Figure 4.9c). Two groups were tested, one with participants unfamiliar with both characters (i.e., only fluent in English) and one with participants familiar with only one of the two characters (i.e., fluent in reading Chinese).

The English-only participants showed more efficient search than the Chinese readers, suggesting that knowing the meaning of the characters can interfere with search. No search asymmetry was observed for the English-only group. For the Chinese readers, search was more efficient when the unfamiliar character was the target and familiar characters were distractors than vice versa. Shen and Reingold (2001) replicated these findings in a third experiment using a different character and its mirror-reverse presentation. Together these experiments indicate that search is more efficient for unfamiliar or novel targets.

However, in their Experiment 4, Shen and Reingold (2001) examined the independent effects of target and distractor familiarity. The Chinese characters for ancient and leaf (similar to the character for ancient but rotated 90°) were used as familiar stimuli for Chinese readers. These two characters were rotated 180° to result in meaningless stimuli that would be unfamiliar to Chinese readers. Again, they had English-only and fluent Chinese readers perform the search task. There were four conditions: the target and distractors were both familiar, the target and distractors were both unfamiliar, the target was familiar and distractors unfamiliar, and the target was unfamiliar and distractors familiar. The English-only participants did not show any search asymmetry. For the Chinese readers, search was more efficient when the distractors were familiar (i.e., had meaning), regardless of whether the target was familiar or not. Thus, Shen and Reingold (2001) concluded that distractor, not target, familiarity was the critical factor.

Preview Benefit and Visual Marking

Conjunction search is effortful and time consuming, with search time increasing as the number of items in the display increases (i.e., there is a display-size effect). If, however, some of the distractors are presented before the entire search display, the display-size effect can be reduced. This phenomenon, called the *preview benefit*, has been found in several studies (D. G. Watson et al., 2003). D. G. Watson and Humphreys (1997) demonstrated the preview benefit in a search task for which participants were to respond whether a blue H target was present or absent among green H's and blue A's. A standard conjunction condition showed a display-size effect in which reaction time was an increasing function of the number of items in the display. For a preview conjunction condition, the green distractor stimuli were presented for 1,000 ms, after which the blue stimuli were added. Reaction times were shorter in the preview condition than in the standard condition, and the display-size effect was similar to that for a condition in which only the same number of blue stimuli were presented. This result implies that participants could restrict search to locations that were not previewed. Other properties of the preview benefit include that the gap between the preview and the rest of the display must be at least 400 ms, and it is reduced when a secondary task is performed during the preview (D. G. Watson et al., 2003).

D. G. Watson and Humphreys (1997, 1998) attributed the preview benefit to a mechanism they called *visual marking*. This marking process is presumed to implement active inhibition of the distractor locations. A finding consistent with this view is that detection of a dim probe dot is impaired when it occurs at the location of an item that was in the preview display (D. G. Watson & Humphreys, 2000). A preview benefit is also found for moving old items (D. G. Watson & Humphreys, 1998). However, static items can be marked even when old and new stimuli contain the same features, but moving items can only be marked when the old items have a unique feature. This suggests that the marking of static items can be location based, whereas the marking of moving items is at the level of a whole feature map (e.g., all green items).

The visual marking account, which attributes the preview benefit to inhibition of the previewed items, is widely accepted but not by all researchers. Donk and Theeuwes (2003) argued that the preview effect results from a bottom-up prioritization for the newly onset items. Among the evidence they provided is that participants prioritized the new items even when the target was more likely to be in the old items. Olivers et al. (2006) reviewed the evidence and concluded that both the top-down inhibition of irrelevant old information through visual marking and bottom-up attentional activation to new stimulus onsets act in combination.

Feature Integration Theory

The most robust finding from decades of visual search research is that search efficiency depends on the nature and combinations of features in the display. On the basis of these findings, many models of visual search and selective attention, in general, assign a special role to the processing of features. Feature integration theory, put forward by Treisman and Gelade (1980), started a revolution in theorizing about visual search that continues to this day. Kristjánsson and Egeth (2020) indicated that "Feature Integration Theory (FIT) is a landmark in cognitive psychology and vision research" (p. 7). They emphasized that Treisman's theory integrated findings from large literatures in the areas of visual perception, visual neurophysiology, and cognitive psychology.

Feature integration theory assumes that features receive preferential processing. In this model (see Figure 4.10), sensory features, such as color, orientation, spatial frequency, brightness, and direction of movement, are assumed to be registered early, automatically, and in parallel across the visual field. In this sense, all the sensory elements present in a display are also present in the early stages of information processing. Feature information must then be combined to recreate the objects of the display. This process of "gluing" features together is assumed to require attention, and attention is allocated on the basis

FIGURE 4.10. Feature Integration Theory

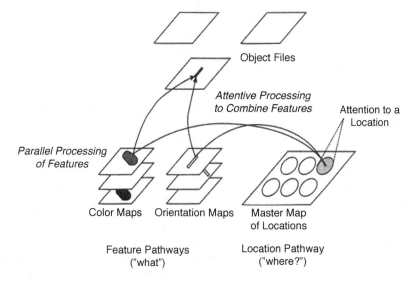

Note. From *Attention: Theory and Practice* (p. 86), by A. Johnson and R. W. Proctor, 2004, SAGE (https://doi.org/10.4135/9781483328768). Copyright 2004 by A. W. Johnson and R. W. Proctor. Reprinted with permission.

of spatial location. Specifically, selection takes place according to a master map of locations, which contains all locations in which features have been detected. Each location within the master map has access to the feature maps (which indicate whether a specific feature is present at that position or not) created during the early, parallel processing of the feature information. Focusing attention at a position automatically activates the features present at that position. These features are then assembled into a temporary object file. Finally, features in the object file are compared with representations of objects in memory (the object frames). Identification occurs when the object file matches an object frame.

Treisman and Gelade (1980) gave focused attention a central role in visual perception. In the absence of attention, feature conjunction is likely to go awry, resulting in objects being incorrectly identified. For example, Treisman and Schmidt (1982) conducted an experiment in which participants searched for a yellow "O" in a display containing letters of different colors. When only the search task was performed, detection accuracy was quite high. However, when attention demands were increased by adding a secondary task (comparing digits presented to the left and right of the search display), detection performance decreased. With attentional distraction, participants were more likely to report that a yellow O had been present when it was not, but a letter O of a different color and another letter with the color yellow were present in the display. In other words, an illusory conjunction of letter and color seemed to take place.

The usefulness of models that contain separate modules or maps for different feature dimensions depends on a means for determining what the basic features are. Treisman and Gelade (1980) suggested an empirical method for defining features: They should pop out in search, mediate texture segregation (i.e., the perception of object boundaries based on texture differences), and hold the possibility of recombining to form illusory conjunctions. Features defined according to these criteria include the obvious ones of orientation and color but less obvious ones such as the perceived direction of lighting (Enns & Rensink, 1990). Wolfe and Utochkin (2019) discussed the criteria proposed by Treisman and Gelade, along with other criteria, and concluded that issues exist with each. Their answer to "What is a preattentive feature?" was "a feature that guides attention in visual search and that cannot be decomposed into simpler features. Thus, color and orientation are features" (Wolfe & Utochkin, 2019, p. 23).

The original version of feature integration theory (Treisman & Gelade, 1980) assumed that features were represented independently of their locations and that locations were only used to bind different features together. Subsequent experiments have shown that features are often localized—as well as identified—even in very efficient feature search. This led Treisman (1998) to conclude that the dissociation between "what" and "where" in feature processing is less extreme than she and Gelade (Treisman & Gelade, 1980) originally supposed. A. Cohen and Ivry (1989) took a stronger stance and maintained that features are preattentively bound to coarsely defined locations.

To account for the fact that conjunction search can sometimes be very efficient (e.g., Nakayama & Silverman, 1986; Wolfe et al., 1989), Treisman and Sato

(1990) proposed that attention may modulate activity in the master map of locations through the feature maps (see Figure 4.11). For example, attention may inhibit irrelevant features and thereby the locations in the master map containing these features so that search can be restricted to locations containing relevant features. Treisman (1991) suggested that such a mechanism can explain why Duncan and Humphreys (1989) found that the difficulty of finding a target depends on both the similarity of the target to the distractors (such that greater target-distractor similarity makes finding the target more difficult) and between the distractors themselves (such that search is more efficient when distractors are similar to each other). According to Treisman, inhibition or activation of feature maps can only influence search when either the target or the distractors activate a unique set of features. Treisman (1998) suggested that attention might also operate by allowing object files to influence the master map of locations. This sort of top-down influence may explain the constancy of objects in the case of movement or changes of the object.

The influence of feature integration theory cannot be overstated. Two special issues of the journal *Attention, Perception, & Psychophysics* containing more than 50 articles were devoted to celebrating 40 years of the theory. In the introduction to the first issue, Wolfe (2020) stated, "FIT has proven to be more than useful. It has shaped the discussion about visual search and much of the discussion about attention more generally for decades" (p. 1).

FIGURE 4.11. Feature Integration Theory Revised to Allow Stimulus-Based Attentional Control

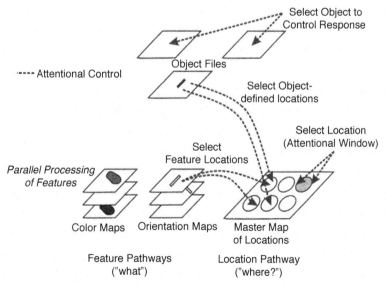

Note. From *Attention: Theory and Practice* (p. 88), by A. Johnson and R. W. Proctor, 2004, SAGE (https://doi.org/10.4135/9781483328768). Copyright 2004 by A. W. Johnson and R. W. Proctor. Reprinted with permission.

Guided Search

In 1989, Wolfe et al. introduced a model called *guided search*, which was intended as an alternative to feature integration theory. It has subsequently gone through many updates, with the most recent version being 6.0 (Wolfe, 2021). The primary basis for the initial model was that the slopes of the functions plotting reaction time against set size were too shallow for conjunction searches to be serial and self-terminating, and reaction times for triple conjunctions (color, size, and form) were faster than for conjunctions of two features. The initial guided search model accounted for these results with parallel processes that use information about simple features to guide attention when searching for

TABLE 4.1. Key Features of Guided Search Versions 2.0 Versus 6.0

Step	Guided Search 2.0	Guided Search 6.0
1	Information from the world is represented in the visual system.	Added eccentricity constraints for a functional visual field (FVF) that considers differences across the retina.
2	Visual representation (features, spatial locations) is available to visual awareness.	Added that the awareness at all points in the field can occur in parallel pathways (i.e., a nonselective pathway).
3	Bottleneck (i.e., selective attention) on the current object for binding.	Emphasis on selective attention to one or a few items.
4	Selected item is bound and recognized as target or distractor.	Access to the bottleneck is guided.
5	Selection is guided by a priority map.	Five types of guidance form the priority map: (a) bottom-up salience, (b) top-down guidance, (c) history (e.g., priming), (d) value (e.g., incentives), and (e) structure and meaning of scenes.
6	One source of priority map guidance comes from bottom-up salience.	Selected object is represented in a working memory template, and search is guided by working memory processes.
7	Another source of priority map guidance comes from top-down guidance.	A second template is held in activated long-term memory, which can hold a larger number of possible targets.
8	Both sources of guidance are combined and weighted; attentional mechanisms such as inhibition of return are employed to facilitate search.	Determining whether an item is a target can be modeled as a diffusion process, with one diffuser for each target template.
9		Each diffuser accumulates toward a threshold; either the target is found or a quitting threshold is reached.
10		Addition of two other FVFs that guide search: attentional and explorational.

conjunctions. The advantage for triple conjunctions was attributed to their having an additional feature that could guide search.

Wolfe (1998) presented Version 2.0 of the model, which made key features of the search process more explicit (see Table 4.1, left column). In the model, visual stimuli are represented by locations and features. Before attention is directed to locations or objects, preattentive processes are at work. In visual search, they guide attention in a bottom-up (stimulus-driven) manner, as when a salient feature pops out of a display and in a top-down (knowledge-driven) way. Stimulus-driven guidance will be strongest when the target is distinct from the distractors and when the distractors are homogeneous (e.g., all the same color). This guidance may occur through a saliency map, which encodes for saliency across the visual field irrespective of the specific feature along which stimuli are salient (Itti & Koch, 2001). Top-down processing can be explicit or implicit and involve where a target may occur or what it may be (Wolfe et al., 2003). In the 2.0 guided search model, information from the top-down and bottom-up analyses of the stimuli are combined in a priority map that ranks items according to their attentional priority. As in feature integration theory, attention is needed to bind features together to identify objects, but the priority weights make search more efficient by directing the application of attention.

Although Wolfe followed guided search 2.0 with several other versions, they were not as influential. Consequently, Wolfe (2021) emphasized that Version 6.0 builds on the main components of Version 2.0 but with additional details (see Table 4.1, right column). The concept of functional visual field is incorporated to consider retinal constraints on visual representation (e.g., acuity), as well as attentional constraints (covert deployment of attention around fixation) and explorational constraints (overt eye movements when exploring the display). Processing can occur along multiple pathways and multiple representations in memory (templates). Sources of activation in the priority map have been expanded to include history (priming effects), value (rewards), and knowledge of structure and meaning of scenes. For naturalistic scenes, people can use their knowledge of structure in the world to guide their search. For example, if the target for which you were looking were a rabbit, you would not direct attention toward the sky. Search can also be modulated by past search history and the value of some items. Brockmole and Henderson (2006) demonstrated that when the location of a target letter (but not its identity) was consistent across repeated presentations of a scene, participants learned the location to look at in the scene. Stimuli previously associated with reward receive increased attentional priority relative to those that have not been, even when they are no longer relevant to the task (B. A. Anderson, 2019). Such evidence has led to the idea that attention can be value driven in a manner that is distinct from goal-directed and stimulus-driven factors.

The 6.0 model incorporates a diffusion decision process of the type described in Chapter 2 to enable predictions of reaction time and accuracy in search tasks. A unique component is that, although initiation of a diffusion process for individual items is serial, several can operate in parallel to classify an item as a target or nontarget. In the diffusion process, items are selected approximately every 50 ms, and each diffusion process takes approximately 300 ms to finish. The evolution of the guided search model is a good illustration of how the understanding of attention is refined through the interplay of data and theory. Feature integration theory captured the essence of findings concerning visual search up to 1980. It triggered research that resulted in findings that it could not explain well, which led to Version 1.0 of the guided search model. As other results have accrued from relevant studies, the guided search model has been updated to incorporate a much larger range of data. Theories will continue to be refined to reflect the empirical data generated as the research on visual search advances.

Can Serial Self-Terminating Search Be Distinguished From Parallel Search?

A study by J. Lee et al. (2021) provides a nice transition into this section, which relies on congruity effects like the Stroop effect, which was described in Chapters 1 and 2. J. Lee et al. reasoned that if search in a task is serial and self-terminating, it should not matter on trials with dual targets whether the targets are the same or different. The logic is that if one target is identified and the search stopped, the other target is never identified. Across several experiments, J. Lee et al. varied set size in search tasks with different characteristics, and participants were to respond according to the first target they identified.

Some of J. Lee et al.'s (2021) experiments yielded a standard congruity effect such that reaction time on dual-target trials was longer on incongruent than congruent trials. These included conjunction search tasks for a green T rotated 90° to the left or right among red T and green O distractors and for a green T among red H and green O distractors. However, others showed no congruity effect. This was the case for the latter task if the same response was to be made regardless of whether the target was T or H. Likewise, there was no congruity effect when the task was to identify whether a target Landolt C (a square stimulus with a gap) had a gap to the left or right among distractors with a top or bottom gap. Finally, the search for a left or right tilted T among Ls yielded a congruity effect, whereas the same task made more difficult by putting small gaps in the Ls showed none. The authors concluded that the lack of congruity effect in several tasks provides evidence that search in those tasks was serial and self-terminating. Thus, this method can distinguish tasks for which the processing is serial and self-terminating from ones for which parallel processing might still apply.

The conclusion of J. Lee et al. (2021) is similar to that made by Klein (1988) in an earlier study of inhibition of return. Klein conducted visual search tasks with displays of two to 10 stimuli, intended to induce set-size functions with steep slopes (thought to reflect serial processing) or shallow slopes (indicative of parallel processing). The key manipulation was to follow the search task immediately with a speeded luminance detection task for which the stimulus occurred at a location previously occupied by a search display item (on probe) or one that was previously empty (off probe). Responses to on-probe stimuli were slower than those to off-probe stimuli but only for the serial-search tasks. This outcome would be expected if participants had searched those locations and applied inhibition to prevent returning to them in the search.

CHAPTER SUMMARY

Visual attention can be overt, where a person looks at the to-be-attended-to object, or covert, where someone directs attention to an object they are not directly looking at. Covert shifts of attention may precede eye movements to the attended locations or be for the purpose of acquiring information from the locations. A separate distinction is that direction of attention can be endogenously or exogenously controlled. Endogenous shifts of attention are controlled by the person's intentions, whereas exogenous ones are controlled by external stimuli such as rapid onsets. Thus, the direction of visual attention is partly under the control of the person's intentions and partly not, and it may coincide with the fixation of the eyes or be distinct from it. Although visual attention is largely spatial, there is evidence to suggest that it may be directed to an object at a specific location and may activate locations within that object relative to ones that are not.

Attention can be directed to new locations and prevented from returning to previously searched locations. Also, stopping an intended response can be accomplished through response selection and even later in the motor stages. Visual search can differ in terms of efficiency. Search is most efficient when a target differs from distractors in terms of a salient feature such as color and least efficient when the target is distinguished by conjunctions of features. Search can be guided to relevant possible targets when several members of the display are distinguished based on target features.

KEY POINTS

- **Fact:** Although visual attention often is paired with the direction of fixation (overt), it can be separated from it (covert).

- **Phenomenon:** A spatial cuing benefit often occurs: Central and peripheral cues improve detection of stimuli at cued locations.

- **Fact:** Locations and objects to which attention is directed receive processing that improves performance and clarity.

- **Theory:** Orientation of attention can occur exogenously (automatically) or endogenously (intentionally).

- **Phenomenon:** *Inhibition of return* refers to the finding that detection or identification of a target stimulus is often delayed at a location that was recently stimulated.

- **Theory:** The most widely accepted explanation of inhibition of return is that attention is inhibited from being directed to a location that was recently attended to.

- **Phenomenon:** People can inhibit an intended response up to reaching a point of no return, and several factors influence the probability of the response being inhibited.

- **Theory:** Most results obtained in the stop-signal paradigm can be attributed to a race between the intended response processes and those associated with the stop action.

- **Fact:** Visual search can vary greatly in efficiency, with there being little set size effect when it is high and much larger effects when efficiency is low.

- **Phenomenon:** Search asymmetry is that search is more efficient when the target contains a basic feature than when it does not or when it is novel compared with when it is familiar.

- **Theory:** Feature integration theory and guided search theory provide useful explanatory frameworks for distinguishing efficient from inefficient search contexts.

5

Attentional Control in Congruity and Negative Priming Tasks

The process of selective attention, described in Chapters 3 and 4, reveals that attending to specific information requires that we control and direct our focus to where and what we need to process and respond to. Equally crucial for successfully completing a task is selecting responses to relevant stimulus information, as defined by the task to be performed, and not to irrelevant information. In binary decisions, reaction time and accuracy are affected by dimensional overlap, or similarity, between the relevant stimulus dimension and response and, if the stimuli vary on an irrelevant dimension, between the relevant and irrelevant stimulus dimensions and between the irrelevant stimulus dimension and the response (Kornblum, 1992). These relations produce congruity effects, for which responses are faster and more accurate when the dimensional relations are congruent than when they are not (Proctor & Reeve, 1990; Proctor & Vu, 2006b).

Kornblum (1992) provided an influential taxonomy that distinguishes eight task types based on all combinations of the three kinds of dimensional overlap. We describe the taxonomy here because it is useful for keeping track of possible sources of the congruity effects in specific studies. For a *Type 1 task*, there is no dimensional overlap, and no congruity effect would be expected. Few situations yield no congruity effect at all, but tasks for which there is no apparent overlap between the dimensions will often yield smaller effects based on more subtle relations (Proctor & Cho, 2006). *Type 2 tasks* are those for which there is only overlap between a relevant stimulus dimension and the response. Such tasks

https://doi.org/10.1037/0000317-005

Attention: Selection and Control in Human Information Processing, by R. W. Proctor and K.-P. L. Vu

are typically called *stimulus–response compatibility tasks*, the term that we use in this chapter, and reaction time is shorter with a congruent mapping of the dimensions than with an incongruent one. Compatibility effects of this type occur for tasks in which stimulus locations are mapped to key press responses. For a two-choice task, responses are substantially faster and more accurate with the mapping of left stimulus to left response and right stimulus to right response than with the opposite mapping.

The remaining task types we mention are those with an irrelevant stimulus dimension. *Type 3 tasks* overlap only on the irrelevant stimulus dimension and the response dimension. The prototype is the *Simon task*, named for J. R. Simon (1990), for which stimulus location varies from trial to trial but is irrelevant to the task. The resulting congruity effect, called the *Simon effect*, is that responses are faster when stimulus and response locations correspond than when they do not (see Lu & Proctor, 1995, for a review). *Type 4 tasks* overlap only on the relevant and irrelevant stimulus dimensions. The exemplar of this category is the *Eriksen flanker task*, named for B. A. and C. W. Eriksen (1974), for which stimuli (e.g., letters) are assigned to a left or right response that is to be made to the stimulus in a centered position but not to the same stimulus when it is in an irrelevant flanking position. Responses are faster when the distractors are congruent with the target than when they are incongruent (i.e., assigned to the same rather than the alternative response), which is the *flanker effect*. The final category we mention is *Type 8 tasks*, for which overlap exists among all three dimensions. For the *Stroop color-naming task*, both relevant and irrelevant stimulus dimensions relate to color, as does the vocal color-name response dimension (MacLeod, 1991; Stroop, 1935/1992). As noted, the *Stroop effect* is that naming responses to the color are slower when the color word is incongruent than when it is not. The other categories of the dimensional-overlap taxonomy include the respective pairwise combinations of dimensional overlap, but they are not as extensively investigated.

Tasks of the sort we described have been studied extensively for what they reveal about attentional control. The Type 2 stimulus–response compatibility tasks, which involve only the relevant stimulus–response mapping, provide insight into intentional selection processes. Sometimes, the term *stimulus–response translation* is used to describe such processes to indicate the intentional selection of the response to the stimulus that appears (Welford, 1976). The Type 3, 4, and 8 tasks enable investigation of the ability to restrict attention to the relevant stimulus dimension and prevent activation by the irrelevant stimulus dimension. Conditions under which information irrelevant to the task produces congruity effects are informative for many aspects of human information processing. We begin with a discussion of Type 2 stimulus–response compatibility effects and their basis in intentional translation processes and then proceed through the Types 3, 4, and 8 tasks, all of which include variability on an irrelevant stimulus dimension that affects performance in a more automatic manner.

COMPATIBILITY EFFECTS FOR RELEVANT STIMULUS INFORMATION

Spatial compatibility effects have been studied since the work of Fitts and Deininger (1954). Of most interest are their conditions in which eight possible stimulus locations were arrayed circularly, as was a corresponding response panel. The task was to move a stylus from a center position on the panel to an assigned target location as soon as a stimulus came on. Responses were much faster and more accurate when the mapping of the eight stimulus locations to the eight response locations was congruent than when it was random. This result illustrates a stimulus–response compatibility effect. Another informative finding is that performance benefited when a mapping rule such as "respond at the mirror-opposite location" could be applied.

We focus here mainly on two-choice compatibility tasks because those have been widely investigated, and almost all studies of Types 3, 4, and 8 tasks have also used two-choice tasks. The two-choice spatial compatibility task uses left and right stimulus locations mapped to left and right responses, typically left and right key presses made with the left and right index fingers. The basic finding, described at the beginning of the chapter, is faster and more accurate responding when the mapping is compatible (or uncrossed; left→left/right→right) than when it is incompatible (or crossed; left→right/right→left). The spatial compatibility effect is not limited to physical stimulus locations because it is obtained with the location words "left" and "right" and left- and right-pointing arrows (Luo & Proctor, 2020; Miles & Proctor, 2012). The responses can be made with fingers on the same hand, unimanual left–right lever movements, and vocal "left"–"right" responses (Heister et al., 1990; Miles & Proctor, 2012). Such results illustrate that the dimensional overlap can be at a conceptual level and not just a physical, perceptual one (Kornblum, 1992).

One thing that does seem essential to obtaining a benefit for the spatially compatible mapping is that the performer has an active task set for that mapping. This is evident from studies in which trials with spatially compatible and incompatible mappings are randomly intermixed, and the mapping on each trial is designated by a mapping signal (e.g., a horizontal or vertical line, red or green stimulus color). When the mapping signal occurs simultaneous with the location stimulus, the benefit for the compatible mapping is absent or reduced substantially (Shaffer, 1965; Vu & Proctor, 2004). However, if the mapping signal precedes the location stimulus by 500 milliseconds (ms), the benefit for the compatible mapping is evident (Shaffer, 1965). Signaling the mapping in advance allows participants to prepare to make the compatible response.

There is widespread agreement that the basis for the spatial compatibility effect is relative *location coding*. When the two possible stimulus locations are designated by outline boxes placed to one side of a fixation point, the compatibility effect still follows the relative left and right stimulus locations. Responses are faster when the left response is to be made to the stimulus in the left box and the right response to the one in the right box (Umiltà & Nicoletti, 1990).

Such a result is also obtained if participants are instructed in terms of the relative positions within a rectangular outline frame that occurs to the left or right, but a compatibility effect with respect to frame location occurs when the instructions are to respond to the frame location (Umiltà & Liotti, 1987). Finally, if participants cross their hands so that the left key is pressed with the right hand and right key with the left hand, the compatibility effect stays with the congruent stimulus and response locations rather than following the hands (Roswarski & Proctor, 2000), implicating the spatial relations and not the anatomical ones as critical to the compatibility effect.

Consistent with the concept of dimensional overlap, compatibility effects occur for nonspatial dimensions. They are found for mappings of stimuli of high and low intensity to responses of greater or lesser force (Romaiguère et al., 1993) and mappings of one or two tones to responses of one or two taps of a response key (J. Miller et al., 2005). Stimulus and response sets that share emotional content also produce compatibility effects. For example, Y. Zhang and Proctor (2008) mapped positive symbols (dove and heart) and negative symbols (skull and crossbones and gun) to vocal "good" and "bad" responses. Responses to these symbols, presented in random order, were faster when participants were to say ''good'' to a stimulus of positive meaning and ''bad'' to a stimulus of negative meaning than for the opposite mapping. Moreover, for mixed mapping conditions in which the spatial mapping (compatible or incompatible) is signaled by a stimulus of positive or negative affect, performance is better with an assignment of positive→compatible and negative→incompatible than with the opposite assignment (Yamaguchi, Chen, et al., 2018). In this case, the compatibility is not between individual stimuli and responses but between the signal stimulus and the mapping that it signals. Thus, compatibility can benefit selection at a higher cognitive level than the final response selection.

CONGRUITY EFFECTS OF IRRELEVANT STIMULUS INFORMATION

Various congruity effects have been investigated in which responses are slower and errors more frequent when an irrelevant stimulus feature conflicts with that of a relevant feature. Such interference was demonstrated by Langfeld (1913) and Geissler (1912) using what they called the method of negative instruction. As summarized by Proctor and Xiong (2017), participants were shown pictures of objects one at a time and were to say the first word that came to mind, except for the object's name. Introspective and behavioral results indicated that the object name was activated automatically and rapidly. It then had to be inhibited and followed by a more intentional selection process. This result is similar to the Stroop effect (Stroop, 1935/1992).

The Simon Effect

The initial demonstration of the Simon effect was by J. R. Simon and Rudell (1967), who had participants press a left or right key corresponding to the word "left" or "right" presented to the left or right ear. Responses were faster when the word occurred in the ear corresponding to the response than in the opposite ear. Although this relation between the irrelevant stimulus location and the response defines a Simon effect, the task was actually a Type 8 task in Kornblum's (1992) taxonomy; that is, all three dimensions involved location. As a consequence, the resulting congruity effect cannot be attributed unambiguously to response selection. In 1969, though, J. R. Simon and Small reported a similar finding for a Type 3 task in which the relevant stimulus dimension was high or low tone pitch, making it clear that the congruity effect was due to the correspondence of the irrelevant stimulus and response dimensions. Like results are obtained when the left and right stimuli are visual and must be classified on a nonlocation dimension such as color (C.-H. Lu & Proctor, 1995; J. R. Simon, 1990). Since the 1990s, the Simon effect has been studied intensively for what it reveals about response activation by irrelevant information.

In the standard Simon task, the left–right response distinction for the task activates left and right locations as part of the task set (Ansorge & Wühr, 2004). Even though the instructions specify stimulus location as irrelevant, the responses make location relevant more generally to the task (see Buetti et al., 2014, for a similar point about the "irrelevant flankers" in the flanker task). A key finding is that the Simon effect based on spatial congruence is found when people cross their arms to press the left key with the right hand and the right key with the left hand (Wallace, 1971), as with the Type 2 stimulus–response compatibility effects. Such results point to the relation of stimulus location to response location as the basis of the Simon effect (Umiltà & Nicoletti, 1990). Hommel (1993) provided evidence that it is not the location of the response key that is crucial but the goal action. When participants were told to turn on a left light (connected to the right key) or a right light (connected to the left key) in response to stimulus color, the Simon effect was a function of congruity between the stimulus location and light location rather than key location. Again, this outcome indicates coding of responses in terms of the goal action.

Explanations of the Simon Effect

J. R. Simon (1969) initially attributed the Simon effect to a natural tendency to respond toward the position of the stimulus. As evidence for this explanation, he reported that the effect was obtained when participants responded unimanually with left–right lever movements, ruling out the necessity of distinguishing left–right effectors or response devices. A Simon effect based on relative location is still obtained when both stimulus positions, designated by square outline boxes, are located to the same side of the body midline (Umiltà & Liotti, 1987), which provides evidence against the orienting account. Thus, it is generally agreed that, like the Type 2 stimulus–response compatibility effect, the Simon effect is a result of spatial coding. Two types of coding accounts have been proposed, attention shifting and referential coding (Hommel, 2011a, 2011b).

The *attention-shifting* account proposes that the spatial stimulus codes are formed relative to the orientation of attention at the time the target stimulus occurs. Stoffer (1991) found that the relative-location Simon effect reported by Umiltà and Liotti (1987) replicated when the potential stimulus locations were designated by separate outline boxes, as in their study, but not when both locations were within a single, larger rectangular box. To explain those results, he postulated that stimulus position is coded relative to the location on which attention was last focused before stimulus onset. According to Stoffer, a spatial Simon effect occurs if the last step in processing before focusing attention on the target stimulus is a horizontal shift. In the case of the rectangular box, the last step is attentional zooming from a global to local level, for which the last step is shifting lower in the image hierarchy and not left or right.

Other evidence consistent with the attention-shifting account comes from Nicoletti and Umiltà (1994), who had participants make a left or right key press to a square or rectangle target stimulus that appeared in one of six outline boxes (see Figure 5.1). Participants fixated on a cross at the far right (or left) of the row of boxes but were to shift the focus of attention to one of the spaces between the boxes when a small cue appeared there. After the cue was removed, the target stimulus appeared in one of the boxes. Responses to the target stimulus showed a Simon effect as a function of location relative to the cue, where attention was focused.

According to the referential coding account (Hommel, 2011a), various stimulus features such as color and location are coded in accord with Kornblum's (1992) emphasis on dimensional overlap. For the location dimension, stimuli are coded relative to multiple frames of reference (Hommel, 1993). One source of evidence for referential coding comes from studies in which a target stimulus can occur in one of eight possible locations, four in the left hemifield (i.e., left of center) and four in the right hemifield. When the hemifield and a pair of adjacent locations within the hemifield are cued in advance of the target stimulus, the size of the Simon effect at the respective locations shows evidence of being determined by multiple spatial codes. That is, the size of the Simon effect is a result of the combination of the left–right congruity relations for the hemifield, pair within the hemifield, and location of the target stimulus within the pair (Lamberts et al., 1992; Yamaguchi & Proctor, 2012). However, if there is no precuing of locations, the Simon effect conforms to coding in

FIGURE 5.1. Illustration of the Type of Displays Used by Nicoletti and Umiltà (1994)

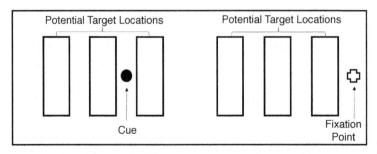

space relative to the center; the farther from the center the target stimulus appears, the larger the effect. More generally, the weightings given to respective codes vary as a function of the saliency of the stimulus dimensions and task instructions (Memelink & Hommel, 2013; Yamaguchi & Proctor, 2012).

Hommel (2011a, 2011b) and Van der Lubbe and Abrahamse (2011) debated the evidence for the referential coding and attention-shifting accounts, but we emphasize that both accounts explain the Simon effect in terms of spatial coding. The referential coding account can handle results that cannot be explained in terms of the attention-shifting account, and it is also consistent with the fact that Simon effects can be obtained for location words, which require no shift of attention to code as left or right, and for stimulus–response dimensions that do not involve location. The focus of attention at the time of stimulus onset seems to be only one of several frames of reference relative to which location can be coded.

Time Course of Code Activation and Dissipation

One finding that has emerged regarding the Simon effect is its change across the reaction-time distribution. This change can be examined by separating the reaction-time distributions for congruent and incongruent trials into bins from fastest to slowest, obtaining a Simon effect for each bin (de Jong et al., 1994). For example, five bins can be created by taking the mean for each condition based on 20% cuts going from the fastest to the slowest and plotting the Simon effect at each bin (called *delta plots*; see Figure 5.2). As depicted in Figure 5.2, the Simon effect is often largest at the first or second bin and then decreases as reaction time lengthens (Proctor et al., 2011). This result is surprising because the Type 2 stimulus–response compatibility effect increases as reaction times get longer (Vu & Proctor, 2004).

The decrease in the Simon effect across the reaction-time distribution has been attributed to the rapid automatic activation of the response corresponding to the stimulus location, followed by dissipation of this activation due to either

FIGURE 5.2. The Simon Effect Across the Reaction-Time (RT) Distribution, From Fastest to Slowest Responses

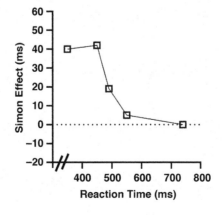

active inhibition or passive decay. This property and others of the Simon effect have been simulated in a diffusion model by Ulrich et al. (2015) called the *diffusion model for conflict task*s (DMC). The DMC distinguishes controlled and automatic processes, for which the change in automatic activation across time determines the shape of the distribution functions. As with any diffusion model, at stimulus onset, information accumulates probabilistically over time toward either of two response thresholds, and a response is executed when one of the thresholds is reached. The superimposition of the automatic activation with the controlled activation causes the response threshold to be reached sooner on a congruent trial than an incongruent trial, for which the two are in opposition.

Given that the Simon effect decreases across the reaction-time distribution, a question is whether this decrease is due to passive decay or cognitive control by inhibition. Hommel (1994) favored a passive decay account. He varied the percentage of incongruent trials (low or high) and the discriminability of the relevant dimension (low or high) in different trial blocks. The basic idea was that responses should take longer when the discriminability was low, allowing more time for the activation of the corresponding response location to dissipate. If this dissipation was due solely to time, it should not interact with the strategy induced by making the incongruent trials highly probable. Results showed effects of both manipulations on the Simon effect: It was smaller when the discriminability of the relevant dimension was low and incongruent trials predominated. However, there was no interaction, suggesting that decay was the major factor resulting from the lower discriminability.

Ridderinkhoff (2002a, 2002b) has advocated an *activation-suppression* account, according to which suppression (or inhibition) increases gradually, making it more effective for slow responses than fast ones. Ridderinkhoff (2002b) reported a study similar to Hommel's (1994), in which he manipulated the percentage of incongruent trials and analyzed the reaction-time distributions. The condition in which incongruent trials predominated showed a reversed Simon effect overall, but, most important, the slopes of the distribution functions for that condition and one in which congruent trials predominated did not interact. However, on the basis of other analyses and individual-difference analyses in other studies, Ridderinkhoff (2002a) concluded that the results support the activation-suppression account. The issue of cognitive control through inhibition will be revisited in the subsequent discussion of sequential effects.

Although the Simon effect decreases across the reaction-time distribution when the irrelevant information is conveyed by physical location, this is not the case for location words and arrow directions. For the latter stimulus types, the effect starts out smallest at the beginning of the distribution and becomes larger as reaction time increases (Luo & Proctor, 2018). However, the DMC can fit these data as well, but with different time courses for the effects (Luo & Proctor, 2020). The results imply that, although activation of the irrelevant information occurs rapidly and then dissipates in the location-based Simon task, it takes longer to build up initially and lasts for a longer time when the irrelevant information is conveyed by arrows or words.

Eriksen Flanker Effect

Stimuli located near a target stimulus can produce interference with responding, as illustrated in a visual search study by C. W. Eriksen and Hoffman (1973). They used 12-letter circular displays composed from the letters A, H, M, and U. Participants were to make a left response if the target letter designated by the black bar indicator was A or U and a right response if the letter was H or M. With the simultaneous onset of the bar and array, reaction time was much longer when the flanking letters were members of the set assigned to the opposite response from the target than when they were of the same set, a finding known as the flanker effect. This result implies that the interference produced by incongruent noise letters is chiefly on response selection rather than letter identification. The interference of opposite-set letters was less when they were more distant from the target in the array, implying a limit to the precision of selective visual attention.

These latter two findings were confirmed in the classic flanker task of B. A. Eriksen and Eriksen (1974), which eliminated visual search. In their experiments, the target stimulus occurred at a known, centered location, and the flankers were six replicas of a letter, three located to the left of the target location and three to the right (see Figure 5.3). The letter H or K as a target required a left response and S or C a right response or vice versa. The overlap in the case of this Type 4 task is between the stimulus dimension of the irrelevant flankers and the stimulus dimension of the relevant target. Even though the participants knew the location of the letter to which they were to respond, reaction time was longer for incongruent flankers (in which the letter was one assigned to a different response from the target) than for congruent flankers (in which the letter was assigned to the same response as the target). The amount of flanker interference was 80 ms when the flankers were close to the target (.06° separation) but negligible when the flankers were separated from the target by 1° (see Figure 5.3). The Eriksens interpreted this result as indicating that the minimum size of the spotlight of attention is 1° of visual angle. Another finding of consequence is that flankers assigned to the same response

FIGURE 5.3. Mean Reaction Time as a Function of Spacing for the Five Flanker Conditions

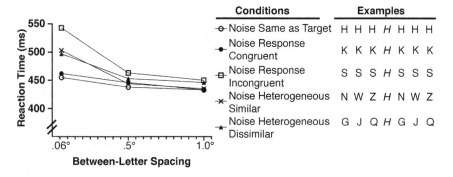

as the target produced little slowing of responses, indicating that the longer reaction times on flanker-incongruent trials are primarily due to the flankers being assigned to the alternative response. C. W. Eriksen (1995) summarized this and related findings: "Research has shown that the reaction-time interference produced by the flankers task arises, at least in large part, from the incipient activation of competing responses" (p. 101).

Selection is most effective when a single region can be selected that includes all possible target locations and excludes possible distractor locations. This region can expand or contract as needed for the task, as suggested by C. W. Eriksen and St. James's (1986) zoom lens model (see Chapter 3). Several factors—including the number of nontarget stimuli, the similarity among stimulus elements, the discriminability of the possible target stimuli, and the discrimination difficulty of a concurrent task—affect this attentional zoom setting. A narrower setting that excludes a distractor will prevent interference from that distractor. Interference from a distractor will be diluted (reduced) by nontarget letters but only if they are within the zoom region.

Because flanker interference occurs only when the distractor letter is assigned to an alternative response than that to the target stimulus, the interference clearly resides in response activation processes. But how peripheral is this response activation? Coles et al. (1985) and Gratton et al. (1988) showed that activation can occur at the level of motor effectors. They had participants respond to the H and S letter stimuli with dynamometer squeezes made by the left or right hand and recorded lateralized readiness potentials and electromyograms (which indicate activity in the muscles that move the hand), in addition to reaction time. The reaction-time measure showed the standard flanker congruity effect, and the other measures provided evidence of activation of the incorrect response hand on incongruent trials, which the authors attributed to activation directly related to the overt response.

It should be noted, though, that the original studies by C. W. Eriksen and Hoffman (1973) and B. A. Eriksen and Eriksen (1974) used unimanual left–right movements of a switch with the right hand. Thus, as emphasized by Proctor and Healy (2021), the interference cannot be due entirely to competing motor activation of the alternative hand. Mattler (2005) conducted two experiments, modeled after those of Coles et al. (1985) and Gratton et al. (1988), that used arrow- and letter-stimulus versions of the flanker task. He found evidence of activation of the incorrect response hand by the flankers on flanker-incongruent trials. However, when Mattler partitioned the trials into a range from those that showed the least incorrect-hand activation to the most activation, he found that the flanker effect for reaction time was essentially independent of the activation. Consequently, Mattler concluded that most if not all of the flanker congruity effect is due to response competition in central processes that are not associated with peripheral motor activation of the responding hands.

Ridderinkhof et al. (1999) used a flanker task within the stop-signal paradigm to determine whether stopping is affected by irrelevant information. The initial task was to press a key corresponding to the direction of a centrally presented arrow. On each trial, four flanker arrows were presented to the left and right of the target arrow. On congruent trials, the flankers pointed in the same direction as the target arrow, and on incongruent trials, the flanker arrows pointed in the opposite direction. Reaction times to the arrow were longer on incongruent trials than congruent trials, showing a flanker effect. Moreover, stopping times were 26 ms longer on incongruent than congruent trials. This finding suggests that the act of suppressing conflicting information uses some of the same processes or resources as those needed for inhibiting a response. Moreover, when a stop signal was presented, but the response was not stopped, the difference in reaction time for the incongruent and congruent trials of 39 ms was larger than that on trials with no stop signal. This result also suggests that suppression of the flankers was less efficient when stop processes were initiated (even though they were not successful) than when they were not initiated. The operation of response competition due to the presence of conflicting flankers in the primary task and response inhibition triggered by the stop signal affect each other negatively, which suggests that the two processes either occur sequentially, such that only one can be exercised at a time, or that they compete for activation.

The Stroop Color-Naming Effect

The Stroop effect has been studied extensively since the 1930s (Algom & Chajut, 2019; MacLeod, 1991; Stroop, 1935/1992) and generated a large amount of psychophysiological and behavioral data (see Box 5.1 at the end of the chapter). Recall that it takes longer to name the font colors of words when the words spelled out incongruent color names than when the font colors were printed in neutral symbols, indicating a failure of selective attention in this Type 8 task. More commonly, the Stroop effect is studied in choice-reaction tasks of two or four choices in which the congruent and incongruent trials of the irrelevant color and relevant color word are mixed.

Possibly because of the overlap among all three dimensions (and the strong association of printed words with their names), the Stroop color-naming effect is often larger than the Simon or flanker effect. For example, Hintzman et al. (1972) found color naming for randomly intermixed stimuli to be 146 ms longer when the color word was incongruent with the font color than when it was congruent, with neutral word and anagram conditions being only 42 ms longer than the congruent trials. Because a congruent color word yielded faster responding than the neutral word and anagram stimuli, they concluded that the Stroop effect is due to response competition.

The Stroop effect also occurs to a reduced extent when the responses are left and right key presses to the relevant stimulus color instead of vocal naming responses (Keele, 1972). This reduction in effect would be expected because the irrelevant color-word dimension overlaps only with the relevant stimulus color dimension (i.e., the key press version is a Type 4 task), much like in the flanker task. In both the flanker and keypress Stroop color-identification tasks, the assignment of letters or colors to key press responses provides a basis for conceptual overlap.

As noted in Chapter 2, Stroop (1935/1992) reported an experiment showing that there was no interference produced for reading a list of words printed in incongruent colors compared with one in a neutral color. This *Stroop asymmetry*—interference of color words with color naming but not vice versa—has been the subject of considerable debate (Sobel et al., 2020). One account of the asymmetry is that it is due to the color-word alternatives being more discriminable than the color alternatives. The best evidence is that the asymmetry is eliminated if the word is made more difficult to identify (Melara & Mounts, 1993). A second alternative is the translation account (Virzi & Egeth, 1985), according to which the asymmetry is due to the color requiring translation from a physical code to a verbal code in order to be named, whereas the color word does not require translation. Durgin (2000) obtained results consistent with this possibility by implementing a task in which attending to the word meaning required translation but attending to the color did not, a reversed Stroop effect. The third possibility, the strength-of-association account, attributes the asymmetry to a stronger association between word meaning and naming than between color and naming. Blais and Besner (2006) showed that translation was not required to obtain results like Durgin's. Moreover, Sobel et al. (2020) found that the reverse Stroop effect was larger for a task requiring localization rather than identification, likely because localization is more strongly associated with visual processing. According to the strength-of-association and translation accounts, the Stroop asymmetry is task dependent.

Summing Up

The key fact conveyed by the flanker, Stroop, and Simon effects is that responding is slowed whenever there is conflict between the response that is to be made to a relevant stimulus attribute and the response signaled by an irrelevant stimulus attribute. This conflict occurs in situations in which there is overlap between an irrelevant stimulus dimension and the relevant stimulus dimension, an irrelevant stimulus dimension and the response dimension, or all three dimensions. Although the core effects have been studied most often with letters, colors, and physical stimulus locations, they occur for many other stimulus types and dimensions as well. As noted, the Simon effect also occurs when the irrelevant left and right location information is conveyed by left- and right-pointing arrows or the location words "left" or "right" (Luo & Proctor, 2018). A widely studied version of the flanker task uses left- or right-pointing arrows as the possible target stimuli, mapped to left and right key presses, with the flanker arrow directions being congruent or incongruent with that of the target (Fan et al., 2002; D. W. Schneider, 2019). Note that this makes the task more similar structurally to the Stroop color-naming task because all three dimensions involve left and right locations (Type 8 task). Such congruity effects occur in a variety of tasks and are expected on the basis of general response activation processes.

SEQUENTIAL AND GLOBAL PERCENTAGE EFFECTS

Much research has been conducted in the 21st century on what is often called cognitive control. Two topics of research involving Simon, flanker, and Stroop tasks in which task-irrelevant information influences performance have been the subject of many studies. These topics are (a) sequential effects of congruent and incongruent trials and (b) global percentage effects (i.e., effects of proportions of congruent and incongruent trials).

The Gratton Sequential Effect Pattern

The predominant sequential effect pattern in congruity tasks is sometimes called the *Gratton effect*, after Gratton et al.'s (1992) study that initially showed the effect. They analyzed sequential effects from a prior flanker-task experiment (Gratton et al., 1988) where participants made a left or right response to a centered letter S or H, flanked by four copies of the same response-compatible letter (HHHHH or SSSSS) or the alternative response-incompatible letter (SSHSS or HHSHH). The reaction times and error rates for congruent and incongruent current trials were analyzed as a function of whether the preceding trial was congruent or incongruent (which yields four data points: congruent-congruent, congruent-incongruent, incongruent-congruent, incongruent-incongruent). The finding of note was that the flanker effect was larger when the prior trial was congruent than when it was incongruent (see Figure 5.4). Gratton et al. (1992) attributed this result pattern to strategic control, with the flanking stimuli weighted more heavily in the choice process when the prior trial was congruent than when it was incongruent.

Botvinick et al. (2001) elaborated this cognitive control account by simulating Gratton et al.'s (1992) sequential effect results with the network model used by J. D. Cohen et al. (1990) for the Stroop effect, modified to explain the flanker effect (see Figure 5.5). The model includes input nodes for each of

FIGURE 5.4. Reaction Time and Error Rate for Each Condition in Gratton et al.'s (1992) Study

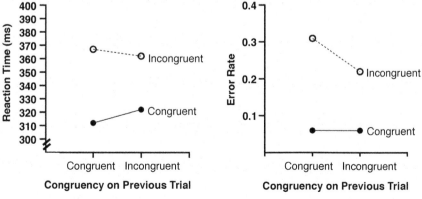

FIGURE 5.5. Structure of Model Used to Simulate the Results of Gratton et al. (1992)

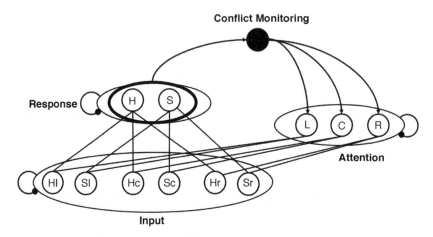

Note. For the input nodes, l = left, c = center, and r = right. The locations are in uppercase letters for the attention module. H and S refer to the stimuli that are to be responded to. Adapted from "Conflict Monitoring and Cognitive Control," by M. M. Botvinick, T. S. Braver, D. M. Barch, C. S. Carter, and J. D. Cohen, 2001, *Psychological Review, 108*(3), p. 640 (https://doi.org/10.1037/0033-295X.108.3.624). Copyright 2001 by the American Psychological Association.

the two possible target letters at the center target location and left and right flanker locations, which feed into an output layer with nodes corresponding to the two letters. The center target node is weighted more in the decision by links from an attention layer that are stronger for that location than for the flanking ones. The major addition to account for sequential effects is a conflict monitoring node that links to the location nodes in the attention layer. This conflict monitoring or control connection allows the weights of the attention layer to be altered from one trial to the next: High levels of conflict (as on incongruent flanker trials) result in a concentration of input to the center attention node, whereas low levels of conflict (as on congruent flanker trials) result in a more even distribution of input to the attention layer. These settings from the prior trial determine that the attention weightings for the current trial allow less or more influence of the flanking letters.

The Gratton sequential effect pattern is obtained not only for the flanker task, as in Gratton et al.'s (1992) study, but also in the Simon and Stroop tasks. For example, Stürmer et al. (2002) had participants press the upper or lower of two keys placed on a tabletop in response to a diamond or square stimulus that could occur in an irrelevant upper or lower screen location. For the standard case in which congruent and incongruent trials were equally likely, the Simon effect was 66 ms following a congruent trial and 0 ms following an incongruent trial. Likewise, Kerns et al. (2004) used a Stroop color-naming task and found a Stroop effect of 120 ms when the prior trial was congruent but only 70 ms when incongruent. Note that in both studies, the respective effects,

Simon and Stroop, were reduced by 50 to 60 ms when the prior trial was incongruent, although the Stroop effect was still evident because it was stronger initially. Stürmer et al. and Kerns et al. interpreted their results in terms of conflict adaptation, with Kerns et al. attributing conflict monitoring and control to the anterior cingulate cortex.

To summarize, the Gratton sequential effect pattern is a generalizable phenomenon that is evident in congruity tasks for which the stimulus display includes irrelevant information that overlaps with the relevant task information. The most widely accepted explanation is cognitive control, in which conflict is detected, and control is then exerted.

Global Percentage Effects

Another widely replicated result pattern obtained in congruity tasks is global probability. Whereas trials with congruent and incongruent relations are presented equally often in most studies, it is possible to vary the probabilities of the two trial types, as in the previously described study of Hommel (1994). Gratton et al. (1992) conducted an experiment in which they varied the global percentage of congruent and incongruent flanker trials so that the flanker-target relation was 75%, 50%, or 25% within a given trial block. The 50% value corresponds to the typical flanker effect study, whereas the 75% and 25% blocks include both trial types, but with congruent trials predominating in the former case and incongruent trials in the latter case. The flanker effect was largest when congruent trials predominated (38 ms), intermediate when both trials were equally likely (33 ms), and smallest when incongruent trials predominated (27 ms).

The influence of global percentage is even more striking for the Simon and Stroop effects. Logan and Zbrodoff (1979) had participants make a left or right key press to the word above or below, with the word occurring in an irrelevant location above or below fixation. When 80% of the trials were congruent, responses were 90 ms faster for trials on which the word and location were congruent than when they were incongruent. This difference decreased to 62 ms when 60% of the trials were congruent and 5 ms when 40% were and reversed to a 58 ms advantage for the incongruent trials when those trials were 80%. Melara et al. (2008) had participants respond with left or right key presses to auditory square-wave and sine-wave tones (which differ in timbre) presented to the left or right ear. The Simon effect was 93 ms when 75% of trials were compatible, 45 ms when 50% were compatible, and 10 ms when 25% were compatible. Thus, the global percentage effect is generalizable across a range of congruity task variations.

Botvinick et al. (2001) showed that the global percentage effects obtained for flanker and Stroop tasks can be simulated similarly with the conflict monitoring or control model, having a cumulative effect. In the model, the conflict monitoring unit detects conflict between the two responses in the response layer and can provide a basis for responding quickly when incongruent trials predominate.

Alternatively, the global percentage effects could be a consequence solely of the sequential effect pattern described in the prior section because congruent trials will follow congruent trials more often when the global percentage of congruent trials is higher than incongruent trials and vice versa.

Questioning Conflict Adaptation

With the success of conflict adaptation models at simulating data for the Gratton sequential effect and the global percentage effect, one might think there would be complete agreement on such accounts. However, Schmidt (2013, 2019) published two review articles in which he argued strongly against conflict adaptation, and Algom and Chajut (2019) have done so specifically with regard to the Stroop task. The argument is that there are alternative ways to account for the phenomena taken as evidence for conflict monitoring and adaptation. Much of the dispute centers on whether the variation of the congruity effects from trial to trial or as a function of global percentages is due to the same activation that produces the core effects.

Schmidt (2013) noted that the Gratton sequential effect pattern can be explained by a confound with feature repetition, whereas the proportion congruent effect is produced by contingency learning. With regard to the former, Mayr et al. (2003) and Hommel et al. (2004) noted, for the flanker and Simon effects, respectively, that when the prior trial is congruent, current congruent trials are complete repetitions or switches of a stimulus and its assigned response from the prior trial. Likewise, when the prior trial is incongruent, current incongruent trials are repetitions or switches of the prior trial. However, when the congruity relation of the current trial is different from that of the prior trial, all the possible changes are partial repetitions or switches. For example, in a Simon task, if the stimulus on the prior trial is green and left and requires a left response to the relevant color, for the next trial to be incongruent, either the stimulus color must change to red (requiring a right response) and the location remain left, or the stimulus color must remain green but the location change to right. It has been known for many years that complete repetitions of stimuli and responses on a trial are facilitated in most choice reaction tasks (Soetens, 1998), and the same may hold as well for complete switches of stimuli and responses (because they signal "different" relative to the prior trial).

Note that according to the feature repetition or switch account, the sequential effects have a distinct basis from the core congruity effects. The sequential effects are due to short-term memory of the prior trial, or what Hommel (2004) called an event file, which is like the object file in Treisman and Gelade's (1980) feature integration theory but with the response also included. This separate memory basis for responding can account entirely for the Gratton sequential effect pattern without assuming conflict monitoring and control. Indeed, Hommel and Frings (2020) presented evidence that event files decay over time.

For the global percentage effect, an account based on learning and memory processes is also viable. Schmidt (2013) emphasized that confounds due to contingency learning might be the source of the global percentage effect. For example, if the color red occurs mainly on congruent Stroop trials, a person may learn to make a quick response, possibly based on the color word, whenever red is detected. Evidence favoring a contingency learning explanation of the global percentage effect is that the effect can occur at the level of individual items. That is, for the Stroop task, when some colors are presented with their congruent words on the majority of trials and others with incongruent words, an item-specific percentage effect still occurs (Jacoby et al., 2003). According to the conflict adaptation account, this should not be the case because, at the level of the entire list, the percentage of congruent and incongruent trials is 50%. In contrast, the item-specific percentage effect is predicted by the contingency learning account. This result opens up the possibility that the global percentage effect at the list level could be due entirely to contingency learning because the item-level and list-level congruencies are confounded.

However, findings from a few studies suggest that item-level percentages cannot account entirely for the list-level effect (e.g., Bugg & Hutchison, 2013), implying that the residual small effect may be due to conflict adaptation. Schmidt (2013) noted that another factor, temporal learning, which occurs with regard to the need to balance speed and accuracy, could account for the residual effect. Participants may learn under what conditions responses can be made faster without a cost in errors. Schmidt (2019) reviewed the research intended to distinguish between the accounts and concluded, "The net results can be more coherently understood in terms of (relatively) simpler learning/memory biases unrelated to conflict or attention that confound the key paradigms" (p. 753). Schmidt (2019) also indicated that future studies intended to examine conflict monitoring need to control for these known biases.

Algom and Chajut (2019) objected to the conflict or control account of the Stroop effect. They noted that the size of the Stroop effect varies based on manipulations such as the relative perceptual salience of the colors and color words, which are not explainable in terms of conflict adaptation but imply that bottom-up processes are important. They also pointed out that because the Stroop task is defined by naming of the color, to which the participant must attend, introducing a correlation between colors and color words renders the "irrelevant" color word relevant (see the similar discussion earlier in the chapter for the Simon and flanker effects). That is, the task no longer requires selective attention to the color. Algom and Chajut concluded, "Against a wealth of studies and emerging consensus, we posit that data-driven selective attention best accounts for the gamut of existing Stroop results" (p. 1).

Where does this leave the status of research on cognitive control? Cognitive control provides a straightforward account with high face validity for much research on the Gratton sequential effect pattern and the global percentage effect. If it is assumed that those effects reflect cognitive control, detailed accounts of the conditions under which such control operates and how it operates can be developed. However, the same data and some additional findings can be explained without invoking the concept of cognitive control. Researchers agree that the Gratton sequential effect and global percentage effect are replicable. But the question of which explanation provides the best account of the results is a topic of ongoing research.

NEGATIVE PRIMING

A type of sequential effect that has also been studied is called *negative priming*. In tasks for which irrelevant information can conflict with relevant information on some trials, selecting a target requires rejecting distractors. For example, in the Stroop color-naming task, words must be ignored—insofar as possible— to be able to name the font colors. Similarly, in the flanker task, responses to distractors must be prevented when they conflict with the response signaled by the target. The negative-priming paradigm was initially developed to examine the nature and time course of the inhibition of distractors from one trial to the next (Lowe, 1979; Neill, 1977; Tipper, 1985). In a common version of this paradigm, participants receive pairs of trials, the first trial called the *prime* and the second the *probe*. One or more distractors typically accompany the target on both the prime and probe trials. Using the flanker task as an example (see Figure 5.6, left panel), a participant is told to identify the central letter and ignore flanking distractor letters (e.g., Neill, 1977). Across trials, the effects of the relation between the distractors on the prime trial to the target on the probe trial are examined. Of most interest are ignored repetition trials, on which the letter that was a distractor on the prime trial is the target on the probe trial, compared with control trials, on which both the relevant and irrelevant stimuli on the probe trial are unrelated to those on the prime trial. Negative priming is said to occur when reaction times to the target are longer on ignored repetition trials (for which the target was present as a distractor on the prime trial) than on control trials. The negative priming effect provides evidence that the requirement not to respond to the target on the prime trial interferes with responding to it on the probe trial.

The task just described requires the identification of the target. Negative priming has also been studied using a task in which participants respond to the location of a stimulus rather than its identity (e.g., Tipper et al., 1990). The task shown in the right panel of Figure 5.6 is to make a spatially compatible key press (with the index or middle finger of the left or right hand) at the location of a specific stimulus (in this case, the number 2) and not to the location of a distractor stimulus. People are slower to respond to the location of a target on the probe trial when it is presented at the location of a distractor from the prime trial, compared with control trials in which the probe target is presented in a previously unoccupied location. Although this task has been used to study negative priming in other studies in the visual modality and studies in the auditory (Eben et al., 2020) and tactile (Wesslein et al., 2016) modalities, a methodological problem has been noted (Christie & Klein, 2001): The task is typically implemented with only a subset of the possible prime-probe

FIGURE 5.6. The Typical Sequence of Events and Trial Types Used by Frings et al. (2015)

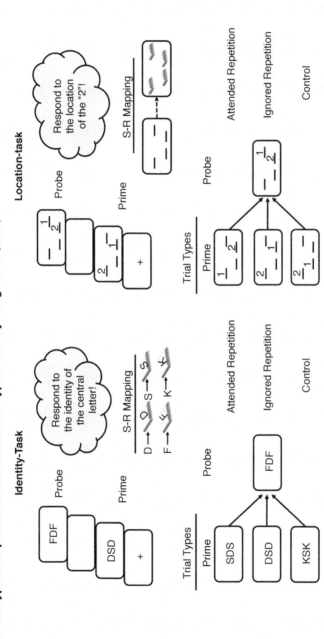

Note. For the stimulus–response (S-R) mappings, the arrows designate the response keys assigned to the stimuli. From "The Negative Priming Paradigm: An Update and Implications for Selective Attention," by C. Frings, K. K. Schneider, and E. Fox, 2015, *Psychonomic Bulletin & Review, 22*(6), p. 159 (https://doi.org/10.3758/s13423-015-0841-4). Copyright 2015 by Springer Nature. Reprinted with permission.

combinations, which means that properties of the probe array are related to the prime layout and might serve as an informative precue. Specifically, the results of two studies that used all the alternatives found that the results may not reflect negative priming but inhibition of return (Christie & Klein, 2001; Milliken et al., 2000).

In the previous task, possible stimulus locations and possible response locations correspond; that is, they are confounded with each other. That correspondence means that the negative priming could be due to the target stimulus on the probe trial being shown at the same location as that of the distractor on the prime trial or to the required response being at the same location as the one that matched the prime distractor location. Studies have tried to dissociate these two variables, and results suggest that the negative priming is linked to stimulus location. Neill and Kleinsmith (2016) had participants press a key corresponding to the ordinal position of a target O in one of four locations, ignoring a distractor X appearing in another location (see Figure 5.7). The location markers were widely or narrowly spaced, with the inner two locations of wide displays corresponding to the outer two locations of narrow displays. This arrangement allowed different responses to be assigned to these identical locations for wide and narrow displays. By varying the wide versus narrow display separately for the prime and probe trials, the contribution of the stimulus location separate from the response could be evaluated. Results showed negative priming when a probe target appeared at the location of the prime distractor, regardless of whether the response was the one associated with the distractor. Also, negative priming did not occur for a probe target that occurred in a different location but required the same response as the distractor. The results imply that negative priming is indeed specific to stimulus location rather than being response specific. Wesslein et al. (2016) obtained similar results for tactile stimuli.

Theories of Negative Priming

From the earliest research on the topic, two types of theories have been prominent. *Inhibition-based* accounts (e.g., Tipper, 1985) assume that the distractor

FIGURE 5.7. Example of Negative Priming With Wide and Narrow Spaces

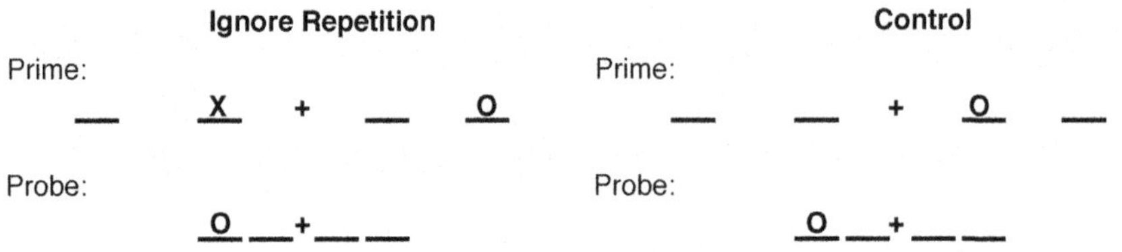

Note. From "Spatial Negative Priming: Location or Response?," by W. T. Neill and A. L. Kleinsmith, 2016, *Attention, Perception & Psychophysics, 78*(8), p. 2414 (https://doi.org/10.3758/s13414-016-1176-6). Copyright 2016 by Springer Nature. Adapted with permission.

activation on a prime trial is actively suppressed and that this suppression carries over to the probe trial. Thus, when the target on the probe trial was a distractor on the prime trial, the suppression must be overcome before a response can be made. *Retrieval-based* accounts attribute negative priming to retrieval from memory of the prime-trial episode during the probe trial (Neill et al., 1992). The distractor on the prime trial has associated with it that no response was made to it, which produces interference with responding on the current probe trial when it is the target. The crucial difference is that the inhibitory account attributes negative priming to control actions taken on the prime trial, whereas the retrieval-based account attributes it to memory of the probe trial.

In a review of the negative priming research, Frings et al. (2015) concluded that several findings are most consistent with the inhibition-based account, such as that the negative priming effect is a positive function of the selection difficulty on the prime trial (e.g., Milliken et al., 1994). MacDonald et al. (1999) had participants view two animal names (e.g., DONKEY and CAMEL) on a computer screen, one printed in red and the other in white. In the "easy-selection" condition, the task was to read the red word. In the "difficult-selection" condition, the larger of the two animals had to be named. When selection was more difficult, much larger negative priming effects were observed. However, Frings et al. noted that other findings seem to favor the retrieval-based account, such as ones of display similarity. For example, Fox and De Fockert (1998) presented letter displays with either high contrast (white against a black background) or low contrast (dark gray against a black background). Negative priming was maximal when the prime and probe displays were of the same intensity contrast, implying that greater similarity between prime and probe displays yielded better retrieval of the prime display information.

Frings et al. (2015) indicated that most researchers now agree that both inhibitory processes and retrieval processes contribute to negative priming. They also highlighted three approaches that attempt to provide more detailed accounts of the findings. The first of these is called *temporal discrimination theory* (Milliken et al., 1998), for which the discrimination is whether the probe stimulus is old or new. When the probe target is a repetition of the prime target (attended repetition in Figure 5.8), the target is quickly classified as "old," and the response from the prime episode is retrieved. If there is no overlap between the stimuli on the prime and probe trials (as in the control trials), the probe display is classified as "new," and the response is then computed. On ignored repetition trials, there is ambiguity in classifying the display as old or new because it contains both old and new elements, which delays classification and responding. Note that the temporal discrimination theory is closer to the retrieval-based account in having a memory component, but it does not include an inhibitory process performed on the prime trial or a memory feature indicating that the distractor was not responded to.

The second account, the stimulus–response retrieval theory, is also a retrieval-based explanation (Rothermund et al., 2005). According to it, the entire prime episode is integrated into an event file. For negative priming, the repetition of

FIGURE 5.8. Sample Prime and Probe Stimuli for Negative Priming Tasks

PRIMES

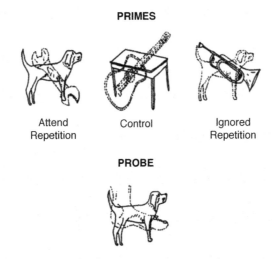

Attend   Control   Ignored
Repetition   Repetition

PROBE

Note. From "The Negative Priming Effect: Inhibitory Priming by Ignored Objects," by S. P. Tipper, 1985, *Quarterly Journal of Experimental Psychology, 37*(4), p. 584 (https://doi.org/ 10.1080/14640748508400920). Copyright 1985 by SAGE Publications. Reprinted with permission.

the prime distractor stimulus in the probe display on ignored repetition trials might be sufficient to retrieve the prior response, which is not the one to be made on the probe trial because that prior distractor is the target. Frings et al. (2015) noted that this account is not based on selective encoding and storing in any form.

The third account is transfer-(in)appropriate processing (Neill, 2007). The basic idea is that a stimulus reinstates processes similar to those applied to it in the past, which is called *transfer appropriate processing* when the processing is relevant to the current task. With respect to negative priming, the processes reinstated when the probe target was the prime distractor are inappropriate for selecting the response to the target, thus causing interference. Again, note that this account is a close relative of the episodic-retrieval account, but it explains negative priming in terms of processes rather than retrieval of a prior episode.

Although negative priming was initially thought to reflect inhibitory processes operating on the prime trial to enable a correct response, this discussion illustrates that the situation is more complex. This complexity is evident in studies examining neural correlates of negative priming that are described in Box 5.1. Inhibition likely is a factor in at least some situations, but most accounts now focus more on processes occurring at the time of the probe stimulus and invoke memory in some form.

Negative Priming in Action Control

D'Angelo et al. (2016) noted that not many studies have examined negative priming in everyday tasks, such as selecting to grasp when other objects are present. One exception is Tipper et al.'s (1992) study that assessed whether

BOX 5.1 | **WHAT CAN NEURAL CORRELATES OF THE STROOP AND NEGATIVE PRIMING EFFECTS TELL US ABOUT THE UNDERLYING ATTENTIONAL MECHANISMS IN CONFLICT RESOLUTION?**

Electroencephalogram (EEG) recordings have high temporal resolution, meaning that an accurate timeline of neural processing can be measured. Although the electrode placements provide some information about what brain regions are activated during task performance, functional magnetic resonance imaging (fMRI) provides higher spatial resolution. Activated brain regions are often referred to as "neural generators." These two methods combined can inform us about attentional processing by examining brain activity that correlates with behavior. Here, we provide an overview of research on EEG and fMRI correlates of the mechanisms for resolving conflict in Stroop and negative priming tasks.

Models of the Stroop effect attribute it to competition between relatively automatic and controlled processing. Based on event-related potential (ERP) markers, Heidlmayr et al. (2020) distinguished three subprocesses of attentional control in the Stroop task: conflict monitoring, interference suppression, and conflict resolution. They noted that conflict monitoring and overcoming of inhibition are associated with the N2 component, with its neural generator being the anterior cingulate cortex (ACC). When participants make errors and receive negative feedback about their performance, a distinct fronto-central negativity is observed. This component is thought to be associated with the processes involved in overcoming inhibition. The N400 component is associated with interference suppression, with possible neural generators being the ACC and prefrontal cortex (PFC). The larger N400 amplitude found in the incongruent compared with congruent and neutral conditions is often interpreted as reflecting the larger cognitive costs associated with processing incongruent stimuli. Finally, Heidlmayr et al. identified another distinct component obtained 550 to 800 ms after stimulus onset, called the late sustained potential (LSP). The LSP is often found in tasks with a linguistic component and is associated with conflict resolution, with neural generators likely being the PFC and frontal cortex (see Figure B5.1).

FIGURE B5.1. Event-Related Potential Components and Associated Brain Regions in the Processing of the Stroop Task

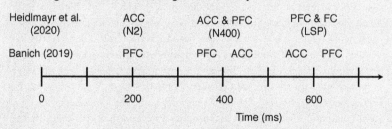

Note. ACC = anterior cingulate cortex; FC = frontal cortex; LSP = late sustained potential; PFC = prefrontal cortex.

(continues)

BOX 5.1 | **WHAT CAN NEURAL CORRELATES OF THE STROOP AND NEGATIVE PRIMING EFFECTS TELL US ABOUT THE UNDERLYING ATTENTIONAL MECHANISMS IN CONFLICT RESOLUTION?** *(Continued)*

Unlike Heidlmayr et al.'s (2020) model favoring a pathway that involves the ACC early in processing and the PFC late in processing, Banich (2019) proposed that the PFC can exert top-down influences before the ACC is involved (see Figure B5.1). Specifically, the dorsal lateral regions of the PFC can bias processing toward task-relevant information and away from task-irrelevant information to establish a task set. The PFC can also activate a selection bias to establish control by allowing task-relevant information to be maintained in working memory. However, if the task set is not well-established initially, the ACC exerts control at later response-selection stages. The final process is evaluating the response selected for appropriateness that stems from the ACC, which can provide feedback to the PFC to adjust attentional control. In other words, if the earlier portions of the cascade involving the PFC do not provide the appropriate task set, later portions of the cascade, those involving the ACC, must exert control to achieve task-relevant goals.

With regard to negative priming, Frings et al. (2015) indicated that the P1 and N1 ERP components, which reflect early sensory and perceptual processes, seem to be modified in the ignored repetition condition for spatial negative priming tasks. Variations in the N2 and P3 components, which reflect later cognitive processes, are observed in identity tasks. D'Angelo et al. (2016) agreed that early and late ERP correlates are evident for both location-based and identity-based negative priming. However, they noted that it is unclear whether these ERP correlates can distinguish between inhibition and retrieval accounts because there is substantial variability across researchers as to how the ERP components are interpreted.

Brain imaging studies using fMRI revealed that negative priming effects are evident in the activation of the right middle frontal gyrus and the left superior temporal gyrus, as well as within the ACC (Frings et al., 2015; Yaple & Arsalidou, 2017). The right middle frontal gyrus is involved in the coordination of sequences and response inhibition, and the left superior temporal gyrus has been implicated as playing a role in inhibitory control and representation of semantic knowledge. However, because both these brain regions appear to play multiple roles in processing, Yaple and Arsalidou (2017) concluded that the activity in them could be accommodated by either inhibition- or retrieval-based accounts of negative priming. Because the ACC is involved in the detection of conflict, a question is whether its activation reflects a contrast of incongruent and congruent trials, as in the Stroop task, rather than negative priming.

In summary, the PFC and ACC are considered the main neural generators for the Stroop effect. The ACC, right middle frontal gyrus, and left superior temporal gyrus are considered the main neural generators for negative priming effects.

BOX 5.1 | **WHAT CAN NEURAL CORRELATES OF THE STROOP AND NEGATIVE PRIMING EFFECTS TELL US ABOUT THE UNDERLYING ATTENTIONAL MECHANISMS IN CONFLICT RESOLUTION?** *(Continued)*

Although fMRI and ERP analyses show systematic activation patterns for both Stroop and negative priming tasks, the data do not necessarily discriminate between the explanations proposed on the basis of behavior. One reason for this limitation is that interpretation of the ERP and fMRI findings is based on assumptions made by the researchers, which means that the same data can be interpreted as supporting alternative models regarding the locus of the Stroop and negative priming effects. That is, inferences made about the type of processing occurring at the time of the enhanced ERP components or activated brain regions are based on models endorsed by the researchers. Also, it should be noted that neurophysiological data are only correlated with behavior, which means that recorded activation may not be causal. Despite these limitations, the use of ERP and fMRI can continue to provide information about the underlying neural mechanisms of attention, and with future advances in technology, these metrics have the potential to help researchers tease apart the processes involved in attentional control for conflict resolution.

the role of negative priming is to facilitate goal-directed action. They developed a selective reaching paradigm in which participants had to reach one of nine targets (see Figure 5.9). Each possible target was marked with two lights, one color indicating a target and another serving as a distractor location that was to be ignored.

In one condition, participants began each trial with their hand on a start button close to their body, at the bottom of the display, and reached toward the target. In this case, the distractor light produced negative priming only when it appeared next to the target along the reach path (e.g., for responses to buttons in the middle row, only front-row targets produced interference; see Figure 5.10). In the other condition, participants started with their hand at the top of the display such that they had to move the hand toward the body to respond. In this case, only distractors in the back row interfered with responses to the middle row (see Figure 5.10). That only distractors on the path for making a response (i.e., distractors over which the hand had to move) caused interference led Tipper et al. (1992) to conclude that negative priming is action centered. When actions are directed at objects in the environment, attention is directed to action-centered representations in which the relation between the target and the effector is prominent.

Tipper et al. (2002) used this same paradigm to test an implication of the inhibition-based account that the negative priming effect should be smaller in a condition that requires less response inhibition. They did this with a

FIGURE 5.9. The Selective Reaching Paradigm of Tipper et al. (1992)

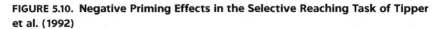

Note. The task is to move the hand to the key corresponding to the target light (shown as the darker circle). Control and ignored-repetition trials occurred with both hand placements. From *Attention: Theory and Practice* (p. 147), by A. Johnson and R. W. Proctor, 2004, SAGE (https://doi.org/10.4135/9781483328768). Copyright 2004 by A. W. Johnson and R. W. Proctor. Adapted with permission.

FIGURE 5.10. Negative Priming Effects in the Selective Reaching Task of Tipper et al. (1992)

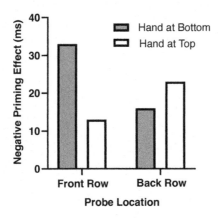

2 × 2 version of the hand-at-bottom arrangement shown in Figure 5.9, for which the near-right location had a transparent plastic "obstacle" between the stimulus lights for it and the response button. The response for this target location required avoiding the obstacle, which necessitated a more complex movement. Negative priming was evident for the control group without the obstacle, as in Tipper et al.'s (1998) study, and for all locations except the near-right one in the obstacle group. Tipper et al. (2002) interpreted this finding as showing that less inhibition must be applied when the distracting light on the prior trial is associated with a more complex movement because that action will not be activated automatically.

CHAPTER SUMMARY

Stimulus–response compatibility effects for mappings of a relevant stimulus dimension to a response dimension (Type 2 tasks) are ubiquitous. Most common is spatial compatibility, for which responses are faster and more accurate when the stimuli are mapped to their congruent responses, but similar effects can be found for any situation in which there is a dimensional overlap between the stimulus and response sets. Such effects can be attributed in large part to intentional processes involved in selecting which response to make to the identified stimulus. Congruity effects also occur when a stimulus dimension is irrelevant to the task, as in the case of Simon (Type 3), flanker (Type 4), and Stroop (Type 8) effects. In those cases, the activation of the corresponding response occurs unintentionally but due to its being primed by the overall task set. Even though the Simon, flanker, and Stroop tasks differ in the nature of the overlap of the irrelevant stimulus dimension with the relevant stimulus and response dimensions, all three effects seem to have their basis primarily in response competition. That is, on incongruent trials, incipient activation of the response corresponding to the distractor competes with the activation produced by the relevant target dimension, slowing response selection.

A common pattern of sequential effects occurs for the Stroop, flanker, and Simon tasks: The congruity effect in each case is larger when the prior trial was congruent than when it was incongruent. Global percentage effects occur, too, for which the particular congruity effect varies as a function of the relative frequency of congruent and incongruent trials. Such sequential and global percentage effects are attributed by many to adaptive cognitive control, but alternative accounts are possible that do not invoke trial-to-trial control modulations. Likewise, effects of irrelevant information in negative priming effects can be interpreted in terms of residual inhibition from the prior trial, but they also can be explained by retrieval-based accounts.

Although it has not been possible to arrive at an unambiguous theoretical explanation of the underlying attentional mechanisms for the phenomena described in this chapter, we again emphasize that they are robust and highly replicable. Also, there is consensus on the most fundamental aspects of the various phenomena, such as that the spatial stimulus–response compatibility and Simon effects are due to spatial coding. The essential message conveyed by the congruity effects is that dimensional overlap among stimulus and response features is incorporated into task sets, which then enables information that is nominally task irrelevant to influence performance. Congruity effects of this type will affect the speed and accuracy of people's choices in many contexts and may have a residual influence on subsequent choices.

KEY POINTS

- **Phenomenon:** Intentional response-selection processes are quicker and more accurate when a stimulus–response mapping is compatible with natural response tendencies.

- **Phenomenon:** Congruity effects (Stroop, flanker, and Simon effects), in which responses to relevant information are influenced by the similarity of nominally irrelevant information, are widespread and occur in a variety of task contexts.

- **Fact:** Evidence indicates that congruity effects are due to dimensional overlap, which often results in response competition.

- **Phenomenon:** The Gratton sequential effect and global percentage effects are reliably obtained across different types of congruity tasks.

- **Theory:** Adaptive cognitive control of activation from distracting information can account for sequential and global percentage effects, although other accounts cannot be ruled out.

- **Phenomenon:** Negative priming effects are obtained in many situations, with people being slower when a previously irrelevant source of stimulus information becomes relevant.

- **Theory:** Negative priming effects likely have an inhibition-based component, but a retrieval-based component contributes to at least a part of the effects.

6

Change Detection and Cross-Modal Attention

Detecting change in the environment is often a precursor to directing attention to that object, event, or location. In baseball, an outfielder must be able to detect the onset of a ball hit in their direction, as well as perceive the trajectory and position at which the ball can be caught. In driving, the driver needs to be able to detect movement in the visual periphery to identify whether the detected event is a relevant one, such as a child ready to dart into the street, for which an action needs to be taken.

Detecting and localizing changes and the events producing the changes often involve multisensory information. The "crack" of the bat hitting the ball can alert the outfielder that the ball has struck the bat, directing attention to pick up visual cues and information, which ultimately produces tactile feedback of having caught the ball through the impact on the glove. Shoulder rumble strips on a roadside can provide vibrotactile and auditory stimulation to alert the driver that the vehicle is leaving the roadway, as well as possibly visual cues induced by the rapid movement of the driver caused by the vibration.

Although detection of changes in sensory stimulation seems straightforward, the perception of change is not so simple. Studies we describe show that without attention, we may not see or hear changes in the visual or auditory scene that are fully registered on the sensory receptors. Moreover, the onset of a stimulus in one modality may draw attention and affect the perception of the multimodal event that caused the changes, as well as aspects of other stimuli in the environment. How change is detected and input integrated across the sensory

https://doi.org/10.1037/0000317-006
Attention: Selection and Control in Human Information Processing, by R. W. Proctor and K.-P. L. Vu

modalities, and the role of attention in the process, are topics relevant to perception and action in everyday life because the world in which we live is multimodal.

CHANGE DETECTION

Detection and identification of changes in the environment for all sensory modalities are crucial, but this section focuses on vision and audition. The tactile modality is covered in a separate section before considering multimodal integration. *Change* can be defined as "the transformation over time of a well-defined, enduring structure" (Rensink, 2002, p. 248). Failure to detect change has been studied in tasks that yield change blindness and change deafness.

Change Blindness

Rapid change of visual displays will often produce transient apparent motion cues or localized changes in intensity (Breitmeyer & Ganz, 1976; Kahneman, 1968). These cues are critical in everyday life, but they must be removed in studies of change detection with visual displays when the researcher does not want such cues to alert the viewer to the change. The elimination of transient cues can be achieved by presenting a masking stimulus between successive displays or by separating the displays by a blank interval. Two variations of such methods are used (Jensen et al., 2011): (a) a one-shot task in which an initial display is viewed, followed by a blank or mask and then the changed display (Simons, 1996) and (b) a flicker task in which the two displays alternate several times (Rensink et al., 1997). With the latter method, the viewer can attend to different regions of the display on successive presentations and often will eventually perceive the changed object. Studies using both methods have shown that notable insensitivity to change occurs in some situations, known as the *change blindness* phenomenon.

Types of Change Blindness

Several types of change can be introduced to visual displays (Rensink, 2002). For one, an item can be added or removed. An example is a study by Mondy and Coltheart (2000). Their first experiment examined participants' accuracy in detecting and identifying changes made to photographs of naturalistic scenes that involved the addition or deletion of objects. On each trial, the first photograph was displayed for 5 seconds, followed by a pattern mask for 1 second. The first photograph or an altered version of it was then displayed for 5 seconds. Participants were to respond, "no change" or "change" and, in the latter case, to describe the type of change. Identification accuracy was higher for deletions of objects from scenes than for additions. A second experiment replicated the advantage for identifying deletions of whole objects, as well as parts of objects, but only when the deletion was of a unique object in the scene. The presence of an identical object eliminated the advantage for deletion identification. Mondy and Coltheart also included trials for which the color of an object changed. Those changes were not detected with as high accuracy as were the object deletions. In general, detection is best when the change is to a unique property or a switch between two objects (e.g., Wheeler & Treisman, 2002).

The semantic identity of an item can be changed by replacing the item with a different one (e.g., D. T. Levin & Simons, 1997; P. Williams & Simons, 2000). If the change maintains the general appearance of the changed item, the change is unlikely to be detected. One of the most compelling examples of this phenomenon was provided by Simons and Levin (1998), who had an experimenter ask a pedestrian for directions while holding a map. During the conversation, two persons (also experimenters) passed between them carrying a wooden door that temporarily blocked the first experimenter from the pedestrian's sight. At that time, the first experimenter switched places with an experimenter who had been carrying the door. This different person then continued discussing directions with the pedestrian. Immediately afterward, the pedestrian was asked whether they noticed anything unusual when the door passed. Eight of the 15 pedestrians tested did not report noticing the change of experimenters.

In D. T. Levin and Simons's (1997) experiment, those who did not notice the change were aged 35 to 60 years, whereas those who did notice the change were aged 20 to 30 years. Thus, Simons and Levin (1998) reasoned that the better change detection for the younger pedestrians might be due to their attending more to the experimenters' features because those pedestrians were from the same age range. Consequently, D. T. Levin and Simon repeated the experiment with 12 pedestrians from the younger age group but with the experimenters dressed as two different construction workers from a nearby work site. In this case, only four of the participants noticed the change, providing evidence consistent with the hypothesis that people are less likely to differentiate individuals from a social group that is distinct from their own.

The fourth type of change is in the spatial layout of display items. Rensink (2002) noted that there are cases in which layout change is easier to detect than feature change (e.g., Simons, 1996), whereas in the Mondy and Coltheart (2000) study discussed previously, it was more difficult. Rensink suggested that the divergence in results may be due to different encoding strategies.

Mechanisms of Change Detection

In general, the mechanisms allowing correct change detection and those resulting in change blindness are reasonably well understood (O'Regan et al., 2000). A sudden change in the environment introduces a local visual transient, which on detection, automatically attracts attention to the change location (Rensink et al., 1997; Turatto & Bridgeman, 2005). When the local visual transient is masked or rendered ineffective by a gap between successive displays, the change location is unattended, and change blindness is the result. Jensen et al. (2011) listed five steps required for successful *change detection* (the opposite of change blindness):

1. Direct attention to the change location.
2. Encode into memory what was at the target location before the change.
3. Encode what is at the target location after the change.
4. Compare what you represented from the target location before the change to what was there after the change.
5. Consciously recognize the discrepancy.

Box 6.1 describes how magicians can induce change blindness by misdirecting attention.

BOX 6.1 | **MAGIC'S RELIANCE ON MISDIRECTION OF ATTENTION AND INATTENTIONAL BLINDNESS**

Many of us have been mesmerized by magicians. What appears as magic, though, can be explained by many perceptual and attentional phenomena. Penn and Teller's (BotoxZombie, 2008) explanation of the "sleight-of-hand" technique, in which a magician skillfully makes objects appear and disappear before the audience, lists misdirection of attention as one of seven key components:

- palm: hold an object in what should be an empty hand.
- ditch: secretly dispose of an unneeded object.
- steal: secretly obtain a needed object.
- load: move the secretly obtained object to where it is needed.
- simulation: give the impression that something has happened.
- misdirection: lead attention away from a secret move.
- switch: secretly exchange one object for another.

When reading the seven task components, one will notice that "magic" is not one of them. Misdirection occurs when the magician leads the audience to focus their attention on a particular area, which leaves them unable to perceive changes that occur in other areas. In the sleight-of-hand technique, magicians use gestures and props to misdirect the audience's attention to one location and then secretly obtain, discard, or exchange objects in another location. Misdirection of the audience's attentional spotlight occurs in terms of where to look, what to look at, and when to look. Of course, good acting skills are also needed for simulating events to make what has not happened look like it has occurred and to accumulate suspense.

BOX 6.1 | **MAGIC'S RELIANCE ON MISDIRECTION OF ATTENTION AND INATTENTIONAL BLINDNESS** *(Continued)*

Macknik et al.'s (2008) perspective is that "magic shows are a manifestation of accomplished magic performers' deep intuition for and understanding of human attention and awareness" (p. 871). Magicians have learned to exploit attentional limitations to generate perceptual and cognitive illusions that leave the audience with no other explanation than magic. In addition to misdirection of attention, inattentional blindness is key to many magic techniques. "Blindness" to changes occurs because our attention is focused on another location, and attention is needed to detect all but salient changes. As demonstrated in an experiment by Simons and Chabris (1999), when our focus is on a basketball that is traveling back and forth between team members wearing white shirts, a large number of individuals will not be able to detect a salient object in the scene: a gorilla walking across the viewing area. Individuals are "blind" to what is happening in front of them because their attention is focused elsewhere. Macknik et al. noted that a successful magician should only perform the same trick once because repeating the trick increases the chances that some members of the audience will identify the method used to perform the trick. They noted that the observers who were shown the basketball video in the gorilla experiment were more likely to see the gorilla in the scene the second time watching the video.

For the vanishing ball illusion, the magician can make a ball disappear with the help of perceptual illusions in addition to misdirection of attention. Macknik et al. (2008) pointed out that all actions of a magician have a purpose. For the vanishing ball trick, the magician performs the same movement of throwing a ball in the air multiple times and catching it. This repetitive action is intended to prime the audience to expect a ball to be thrown into the air. However, on the last "throw," no ball is actually thrown up, but the magician will direct their head and eyes in an upward trajectory as if the ball was actually being thrown. The result is that the audience will report "seeing" a ball fly in the air and then disappear. The success of this trick is likely a result of the attentional spotlight being directed to where the ball was predicted to be (and not at the location where no ball left the magician's hand) and/or by the implied motion based on the magician's actions that activated neural circuits that respond to real movement.

As the examples in this box show, "magic" occurs because our spotlight of attention is limited, it follows objects, and attention is needed to detect changes. Skilled magicians are able to misdirect the audience's attention to achieve their desired perceptual or cognitive illusions.

Notice that the last step of the five refers to conscious recognition, that is, an ability to report the change. However, for cases in which the change cannot be reported, evidence suggests that it may be processed to some extent (Ball et al., 2015; Chetverikov et al., 2018). A recent demonstration of such processing is a study by Xiang (2021) that used a one-shot task. Of interest was the comparison of reaction times for trials on which there was a change but the observer said "same" versus trials on which there was no change and the observer correctly said "same." Results showed that the reaction times were longer on change blindness trials than on the baseline trials in which the two displays were physically the same. This result was found both when the change was a single feature and when it was a conjunction of features. The difference in reaction times between the change blindness and no-change trials was larger with longer exposure durations and intervals between the two display members, implying that processes related to implicit detection of the change were operating throughout the blindness period. This finding is similar to one reported years ago by Pisoni and Tash (1974), for which two speech stimuli that were physically identical were classified as "same" faster than two speech stimuli that were not physically identical but were indistinguishable to participants.

Change Blindness in a Naturalistic Setting

Attwood et al. (2018) demonstrated change blindness for museum artifacts in two testing conditions. In a real-world viewing condition, participants in one group viewed pairs of similar but slightly different artifacts, looking at one and then making head and eye movements to look at the other. Those participants wore a head-mounted camera, and the video captured by that camera was viewed by a paired participant on a video screen. In both cases, the participants were to indicate whether they noticed a difference between the two objects.

Change blindness was similarly evident for both viewing conditions (about 45%), even though the binocular depth cues and intention to move fixation in the real-world condition were absent in the on-screen viewing condition. Combined results from both viewing conditions showed that artifacts that exhibited low versus high levels of change blindness were distinguished mainly by bottom-up, stimulus-driven factors. That is, they had larger and higher contrast changes in the critical area, which would tend to attract attention to them.

Change Deafness

Fewer studies have been conducted on auditory change detection with tasks like those just covered for vision, but they show an analogous phenomenon to change blindness that has been called *change deafness* (Vitevitch, 2003). Eramudugolla et al. (2005) had participants listen to auditory scenes composed of four, six, or eight natural sounds (e.g., birds chirping) at distinct locations.

On a trial, a scene was presented for 5 seconds, and after a 0.5-second interval of a white noise mask (randomly varying intensities across the auditory spectrum), the scene was repeated intact or with one sound missing. The participant was to respond whether there was a missing sound. In a directed attention condition, the name of the object associated with the sound (e.g., birds) was shown at fixation to cue the participant as to which sound, if any, would be missing in the second occurrence. In a nondirected attention condition, no cue was provided. Sound deletions were often missed in the nondirected attention condition, with this number increasing as the scene size increased. In contrast, in the directed attention condition, the change was rarely missed. These results imply that attentional limitations are a major factor in change deafness.

Pavani and Turatto (2008) examined whether the mechanisms underlying change deafness are similar to those that produce change blindness for visual stimuli. Their method was like that just described, except that the pairs of complex auditory scenes were composed only of animal calls for which there could be a maximum of four. Also, in addition to the possibility of a sound deletion, a sound could be added to the second scene, and participants were required to make the same or different judgments. Similar results were obtained with regard to change deafness regardless of whether the scenes were separated by 500 milliseconds (ms) of masking white noise or 500 ms of silence or even whether they were presented with no separation. Because change-related auditory transients should be present in the latter condition but absent in the former, Pavani and Turato concluded that they likely play little role in auditory change detection. Instead, the main cause of auditory change deafness is the limited capacity of auditory short-term memory.

Converging evidence was obtained by Gregg et al. (2017). They presented scenes in a change-detection task composed from naturalistic sounds, spectrally dynamic unrecognizable sounds, tones, and noise rhythms. They assessed the role of memory capacity by varying the number of sounds within each scene and that of memory loss by varying the silent interval between scenes. For all sound types, change detection decreased as scene size increased. For the natural sounds, change detection did not decrease much as the interval between scenes increased up to 2 seconds but did at longer intervals, whereas for artificial sounds, change detection decreased greatly at much shorter intervals. The results imply that change detection is limited by the capacity for all sound types but that auditory memory is more durable for sounds in naturalistic scenes.

MONITORING FOR CHANGE IN ODDBALL TASKS

Detection of auditory change has also been studied extensively in the *oddball task*, in which one or more streams of tones of the same pitch is monitored for a tone of a different pitch, the oddball. This paradigm, introduced in Chapter 2, has received widespread interest for its value in research on attention and other cognitive processes that involve measuring event-related potentials (ERPs).

The Oddball Paradigm

Figure 6.1 depicts the oddball-task paradigm, in which standard stimuli are presented along with an infrequent oddball stimulus. An *oddball* refers to a distinctive or deviant auditory stimulus presented in a channel among a set of standard stimuli. For example, an oddball sound with a relatively high pitch may be periodically interspersed among a stream of standard sounds all with the same low pitch. Although most widely used with auditory stimuli, the oddball task can be used for visual stimuli as well (e.g., a stimulus of lower luminance may be a deviant among higher luminance standards; Güntekin et al., 2008).

One value of the oddball task for studying attention is that physiological measures can be taken separately for standard and oddball stimuli, whether or not a participant is asked to pay attention or respond to those stimuli. Thus, researchers can study the physiological effects of attending to stimuli. The single-channel oddball task has been used extensively to isolate preattentive, or automatic, processes of cognition (Ermutlu et al., 2007).

Detecting change in a uniform environment is thought to be a relatively automatic process. As mentioned earlier, the ability to detect change preattentively would appear necessary for soliciting attention, such as when an abrupt onset of a sound quickly orients us to it (Quinlan & Bailey, 1995). Researchers have been able to study change detection by making separate ERP measurements to standards and oddballs in a single-channel task. The repeated presentation of standards during the task creates a context of regularity relative to which the infrequent appearance of the oddball signals a perceptual change. The average ERP waveform to the oddball stimulus can be compared with the average ERP waveform to the standard to examine the evidence for detecting this change in ERPs. Among the ERP markers that have been shown to be of interest are the mismatch negativity and P300 (P3a and P3b).

Mismatch Negativity

In an early study of auditory mismatch, Sams et al. (1985) presented participants with tones at a rate of one every second. Of these, 80% were standard tones of 1,000 Hz, and an oddball sound of higher frequency (1,004, 1,008,

FIGURE 6.1. The Oddball-Task Paradigm

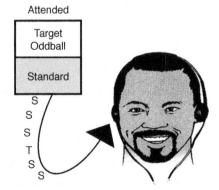

1,016, or 1,032 Hz in different trial blocks) was presented randomly on the remaining 20%. In an inattention condition, participants were asked to read a book during the task so they would not pay attention to the sounds. Recordings were made at frontal and central midline locations on the scalp (Fz and Cz). The results for the Fz location are shown in Figure 6.2. Notice that there is more negativity to the oddball than the standard approximately 200 ms after sound onset. This difference is the *mismatch negativity* (MMN), which reflects the brain's response to a mismatch in the perceptual context established by the standard.

Notice in Figure 6.2 that the magnitude of MMN increased with the physical difference between the standard and the oddball stimulus. The MMN was not present for a 1,004-Hz oddball, was small for a 1,008-Hz oddball, and was visibly evident for the 1,016-Hz and 1,032-Hz oddballs. Sams et al. (1985) showed that participants could not discriminate between the standard and the 1,004-Hz oddball and could barely discriminate the difference with the 1,008-Hz oddball. This correlation of ERP and performance illustrates that the MMN response corresponds with a participant's perceptual discrimination ability.

Other studies have confirmed that this MMN can occur in the absence of attention (Näätänen et al., 2007), even when the participant is asleep (Sabri et al., 2000), under anesthesia (Heinke et al., 2004), or in a coma (Kane et al., 1993). Moreover, it can occur for abstract rules (Näätänen et al., 2019). For example, Carral et al. (2005) had participants listen to tone pairs while attending to the performance of a visual task. For 80% of the pairs, the tones in the pair were the same pitch, but for 20%, the pitch of the second member was higher or lower than that of the first. Both relative changes elicited MMN, and this was of similar size across four amounts of mismatch. Thus, the MMN indicated the detection of the deviation in the rule for the tone pairings.

The MMN is still evident if the participant pays attention to the stimuli, but it is accompanied by another negativity called the N2b (Sams et al., 1985). The change detection reflected in the MMN can also switch attention to a previously unattended stimulus. In Figure 6.2, for example, the MMN is

FIGURE 6.2. Event-Related Potential Results From Sams et al. (1985) Measured From the Fz Location

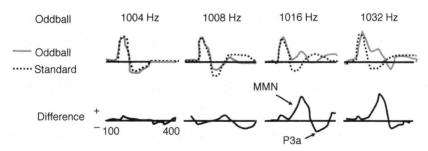

Note. Larger deviants from the 1,000-Hz standard yield larger mismatch negativity (MMN) and P3a responses. Data from Sams et al. (1985). From *Attention: Theory and Practice* (p. 338), by A. Johnson and R. W. Proctor, 2004, SAGE (https://doi.org/10.4135/ 9781483328768). Copyright 2004 by A. W. Johnson and R. W. Proctor. Adapted with permission.

followed by an increased positivity in the ERP to the oddball for the 1,016 Hz and 1,032 Hz tones. This subcomponent, called the P3a, signifies that the deviant oddball not only attracted the observers' attention but also produced an orientation response to it. Thus, the MMN may reflect the implicit detection of change or novelty, which then triggers the explicit awareness of the change, as reflected in P3a (Schröger, 1996).

Insight into the neural generators of MMN and P3a has come from an approach that combines ERPs and functional magnetic resonance imaging (fMRI). Opitz et al. (2002), for example, presented complex tones to participants in an oddball paradigm as they watched a cartoon video. During a tone sequence, three types of oddballs (small, medium, and large deviants) were intermixed with presentations of a standard tone. In one session, the tones were presented while ERP recordings were taken as in the usual study of MMN and P3a. In the other session, the tones were presented while the participants lay on their backs in a scanner and performed the task while fMRI scans were taken. The reconstructed images were *event related*, meaning that a separate functional scan was made of the brain's blood oxygenation level–dependent (BOLD) response to each of the standard and each of the three deviant oddballs. Event-related fMRI scans thus could be meaningfully compared with ERPs because each is a measure of brain activity to a specific stimulus type.

The neural activation to the tone mismatch was measured by taking the difference between the standard and each oddball, using the electrical potentials or the BOLD contrast signal. The ERP differences revealed an MMN response followed by a P3a. The magnitude of each of these ERP components corresponded to the size of the oddball's physical deviance from the standard, a finding similar to that of Sams et al. (1985). The fMRI scans, depicted in Figure 6.3, revealed that tonal mismatch activated regions of the superior temporal gyrus in both hemispheres for small, medium, and large deviants. Näätänen et al. (2019) stressed that this region is different from the region in

FIGURE 6.3. The Neural Activation to Tonal Mismatch

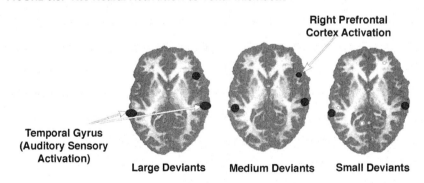

Note. From "Differential Contribution of Frontal and Temporal Cortices to Auditory Change Detection: fMRI and ERP Results," by B. Opitz, T. Rinne, A. Mecklinger, D. Y. von Cramon, and E. Schröger, 2002, *NeuroImage*, *15*(1), p. 171 (https://doi.org/10.1006/nimg.2001.0970). Copyright 2002 by Elsevier. Reprinted with permission.

the superior temporal cortex that receives input from the auditory sensory neurons, which is associated with N1. The authors emphasized that the evidence favors that the MMN is generated by a memory-dependent process sensitive to memory traces. They concluded that the memory traces correspond to stimuli as events represented in auditory memory.

The fMRI scans in Opitz et al.'s (2002) study also revealed that the medium and large oddballs activated a region in the right prefrontal cortex. One interpretation of this finding is that the larger oddballs drew attention to themselves by triggering neural generators in the frontal lobe, which gave rise to the P3a orienting response. Opitz et al.'s study demonstrates how joint use of ERPs and fMRI can be a powerful approach for specifying both the temporal sequence and the spatial location of the neural activation correlated with cognitive processes. For auditory change detection, an automatic response in the auditory cortex 100 to 200 ms after stimulus presentation often is followed by an attentional orienting response in the frontal lobe 100 to 200 ms later.

The MMN has been advocated as a measure for improving understanding and treatment of psychotic illnesses related to attention. Light and Swerdlow (2015) noted that deficits in the MMN account for significant portions of variance in schizophrenia that relate to cognitive and psychosocial functioning. Moreover, MMN measurement has been shown to improve the ability to predict which individuals at high clinical risk will develop a psychotic illness. Tada et al. (2019) reiterated the value of MMN as a tool for translational investigations into early psychosis, noting that several studies have reported reduced MMN amplitude in patients with clinical high risk for psychosis and with first-episode psychosis (Haigh et al., 2017). Näätänen et al. (2019) concluded that the MMN "is a probe of plasticity of the central auditory system and thereby, possibly that of the functional condition of the whole brain" (p. 177).

P3a and P3b

The P3 wave can be decomposed into two subcomponents, both of which show effects in certain oddball tasks. The *P3a*, which we already mentioned, originates in the frontoparietal cortex and has a sharp peak. It is thought to derive from mechanisms that play a role in orienting attention to salient, unexpected stimuli. The *P3b* peaks later than the P3a and does not have as sharp a peak. It is associated with the identification of a task-relevant oddball and originates mainly from parietal lobe sites. For tone sequences, a change in the tone (oddball) should pop out, whereas a nonchange should not, suggesting different underlying mechanisms.

Blundon et al. (2017) evaluated this possibility in five experiments, two using auditory tones of different frequencies as stimuli and three using visual circles of different colors. For the auditory experiments, participants repeatedly listened to runs of five 50-ms tones presented in rapid succession, with each run separated by a slightly longer interval. There were flat runs for which all five tones were of the same frequency and change runs for which the last tone was a different frequency from the first four. Their first experiment used tone frequencies of 500 and 1,000 Hz. The flat runs could all be low frequency with the change to high frequency or vice versa, and either the flat runs or the change runs could be the common standard for the series, with the other being the rare "oddball." The tone discriminations in this experiment were easy, but those in their last experiment were more difficult (tone pairs that differed by 50 Hz).

The visual task was similar except that the stimuli were circles of two different colors (easy discriminations of yellow or blue in one experiment and black or white in another, a difficult discrimination of dark and light gray in a third), presented in runs of five. Participants were to click a mouse whenever the run was the oddball (20% of the runs). Reaction time and detection accuracy (d') were measured and ERPs recorded, with P3 and its components analyzed.

Across both stimulus modalities, results showed that feature-present target stimuli (change oddball among flat runs) were responded to more quickly and accurately than feature-absent targets (flat oddball among change runs). This is an asymmetry like that found in visual search tasks, described in Chapter 4. The ERP results showed a P3 response that peaked between 300 and 500 ms after the onset of the last tone in each run for rare runs (oddballs) but not for common runs. For the simpler tasks, analysis also indicated a longer P3 latency and larger P3a subcomponent in the feature-present condition than in the feature-absent condition, apparently reflecting automatic identification of the oddball feature. However, in the more difficult tasks, which required focused attention, reaction time and P3 latency differences between feature-present and feature-absent trials disappeared, but the P3 amplitude difference was significant. Blundon et al. (2017) interpreted their results in terms of attention strategies. A diffuse attention strategy may be used for tasks in which the target contains a rare or salient feature that automatically activates the stimulus-driven attention-orienting network. However, for tasks in which the target does not contain such a feature, a focused attention strategy must be used.

TACTILE ATTENTION

Most research on attention and change detection has been conducted in the visual and auditory modalities. However, attention is also relevant to the other sensory modalities, particularly the tactile modality. For example, change blindness occurs in the tactile modality as well as in the visual and auditory modalities (Gallace et al., 2006). Because the tactile modality is highly spatial like vision, it has been incorporated into multimodal interfaces, along with vision and audition (e.g., S. A. Lu et al., 2011). Therefore, before discussing multimodal attention, we provide a brief overview of research on attention in the tactile modality.

Several studies have shown that people can direct their tactile spatial attention to the left or right hand in response to an informative endogenous cue.

For example, Forster and Eimer (2005) visually cued the left or right hand or neither with a central cue pointing to the left or right or both directions. The left or right cues were valid on 80% of the trials with regard to which hand subsequently received the vibrotactile stimulus. The task was to respond by saying "yes" if a weak vibration was detected but not if the vibration was strong. Results showed both benefits and costs of the cues relative to the neutral cue, with reaction times shortest on valid trials and longest on invalid trials. Analysis of ERPs provided evidence that costs and benefits contribute equally to attentional modulations of the somatosensory N140 component, which reflects early processing, although later components showed mainly costs on invalid trials.

Lakatos and Shepard (1997) tested participants by presenting air puffs at four of eight possible locations on the body. In each trial of their first experiment, participants attended to one of the eight locations designated by an auditory message. After 2 seconds, a second location was announced simultaneously with the presentation of air puffs at four randomly selected locations, and the participant was to report as quickly as possible with a foot-pedal press whether or not one of the four air puffs had been presented at the second-announced location. Reaction times increased with the distance between the attended and tested locations. Their second experiment was similar to the first, but participants were tested with their arms or legs side-by-side in front or spread out to each side. Reaction times were found to depend more on straight-line distance in space than on distance through the body, indicating that the operative distance was through three-dimensional space rather than through the participants' anatomy. In other words, attention was organized spatially rather than with respect to the body.

The prior studies illustrate the effects of endogenous cuing of tactile location, but exogenous cuing can also occur (Spence & Gallace, 2007). Spence and McGlone (2001) had participants hold cubes in each hand with two vibrators oriented vertically between the thumb (lower position) and forefinger (upper position). They were to respond with movements of the feet placed on pedals, raising the heel of the corresponding foot if the target stimulus location was lower and the toes if it was upper. At a variable interval of 200 to 400 ms before the target, a spatially nonpredictive tactile cue (vibrotactile stimulation at both locations on one hand or the other) occurred. The tactile elevation discrimination responses were more rapid and accurate when the cue and target appeared on the same side than on opposite sides. Because the cues were not predictive of the target location, these results show that tactile spatial attention can be reflexively drawn toward peripheral tactile cues.

The Simon effect occurs for tactile stimuli as it does for visual and auditory stimuli. Hasbroucq and Guiard (1992) stimulated one of two fingertips with a brief mechanical tap of strong or weak intensity. The fingers rested on buttons, one to be pressed if the tap was strong and another if it was weak. Responses were faster when the finger stimulated was the one to which a response was to be made than when it was the alternative finger. Unlike the other sensory modalities, the tactile Simon effect is determined primarily by a somatotopic (body) representation rather than a spatial one. Medina et al. (2014) showed that the tactile Simon effect occurred when the responses to strong and weak stimulation on the fingers were made with the feet, distinct from the stimulated fingers. When the hands or feet were crossed, responses were faster when the effector locations corresponded than when they did not.

As noted, evidence also indicates that tactile change blindness occurs. Riggs and Sarter (2019) had participants perform a task in which a low-intensity vibrotactile stimulus at a location on the back changed to high intensity on some trials. Participants were to respond when they detected the change. As in visual change blindness studies, the concern was the performance on trials for which a 500-ms extraneous activation of all tactors or a random subset occurred just before the time at which the change did or did not occur. Performance at discriminating change from nonchange trials was significantly worse, as reflected by lower d', when either of the interruptions occurred compared with a baseline condition without the intervening stimulus.

CROSS-MODAL ATTENTION: PERFORMANCE WITH UNIMODAL, BIMODAL, AND TRIMODAL CUES

As indicated at the start of the chapter, in daily life, natural and virtual environments are typically multisensory, with many sensory inputs needing to be processed and integrated. Whereas we discussed attentional mechanisms involved in detecting and monitoring changes in the environment in the initial section of the chapter, in this section, we discuss how the different sensory cues influence one another in the processing of information. The driver of a vehicle, for instance, is faced with many sources of visual and auditory information from inside and outside the vehicle, some relevant (e.g., traffic lights and emergency vehicle sirens) and some irrelevant (e.g., dynamic billboard displays and highway noise). Inside the vehicle, there are many visual and auditory displays, and although often outside of awareness, tactile stimulation is coming from multiple sources (e.g., vibration transmitted from the roadway through the vehicle seat to the body, pressure on the foot from stepping on the brake). It is also possible that the driver of the vehicle may detect an odor coming from inside or outside the vehicle and may even eat a snack while driving. Attention is needed to select between and integrate different sensory information for directing appropriate behavior. Thus, recent years have witnessed an increased interest in studies of cross-modal attention (Spence & Soto-Foraco, 2020).

One of the earliest statements in experimental psychology was Titchener's (1908) law of prior entry, introduced in Chapter 1, which says that a stimulus for which a person is prepared takes precedence over another in entering conscious awareness. This law was interpreted by Titchener and others to mean that attending to a sensory modality speeds up the perception of stimuli in that modality compared with those in other modalities. This proposition has been debated for years, but Spence et al. (2001) provided relatively strong evidence in support of it. They presented participants with pairs of visual and tactile stimuli on the left and/or right sides using different interstimulus intervals. The participants were required to indicate which stimulus appeared first without emphasizing response speed. The responses favored the stimulus in the attended modality as the first judged to have occurred, regardless of whether it was visual or tactile, consistent with the idea of multisensory prior entry.

There are enough differences between visual and auditory processing to support the view that auditory attention is distinct from visual attention, both of which differ from tactile attention. However, it has also been argued that substantial interactions exist between the mechanisms that control attention in the respective modalities and that a cross-modal approach is likely to reveal more about attention than within-modality studies (Spence, 2010; Ward et al., 1998). Perhaps the best way to think about cross-modal connections is with regard to the perception of space and the construction of spatial reference frames. Because each sense collects information from only one set of receptors, and because these receptors move about with respect to each other and objects in the environment, connections between different modalities may be necessary to support a stable representation of the environment (Driver & Spence, 1998).

Visual Dominance and Influence on Auditory and Tactile Localization

What happens when the locations of sensory information from the visual, auditory, and tactile modalities conflict? For vision and audition, the relation between processing in the two modalities is asymmetric. In many cases, the visual information gets the upper hand, and *visual dominance* is observed (Colavita, 1974). Visual dominance refers to situations in which, given competing visual and other (e.g., auditory or proprioceptive) stimulation, the visual information captures, as it were, perception.

A common example of visual dominance can be observed in a train or car. If you are parked next to another vehicle (preferably a large one that fills the field of view outside your window), and that vehicle starts to move forward, you will feel as if your vehicle is moving backward. Despite information from other senses (e.g., proprioception) that you are not moving, you believe what your eyes are telling you. Another example is that visual information from a speaker's lip movements can modify the auditory perception of natural speech. If a listener hears the utterance /ipi/ while watching a video of a person uttering /iki/, they are likely to report having heard /iti/ (McGurk & MacDonald, 1976). This phenomenon, called the *McGurk effect*, shows that what a person hears is not determined solely by the speech signal. This effect of vision on speech perception may contribute to the difficulty some people experience in understanding dubbed speech in films. Perhaps not surprisingly, the effect is stronger when the auditory stimulus is degraded and weaker when the visual stimulus is degraded (Alsius et al., 2018).

Anyone who has seen a ventriloquist has also seen the dominance of visual information on the localization of sound. The ventriloquist cannot throw their voice any more than the loudspeakers used in a movie theater can project the voices of actors onto the movie screen. In both cases, however, the location of the sound is perceived as coming from a source other than the actual one—the dummy's mouth in the case of the ventriloquist and the actors' mouths in the case of a movie. This ventriloquism effect illustrates that perception of sound location can be affected by visual information, with the effect being strongest when the actual sound source is difficult to localize. This has implications for the placement of both the ventriloquist's dummy and speakers in the movie theater.

A technique for masking the location of an auditory stimulus was used by Spence and Driver (2000) to show that spatial attention can be cued to the illusory source of a sound. A visual cue (a set of lights arranged in a grid; see Figure 6.4) was combined with an easily localized sound (a burst of white noise from one loudspeaker) or a hard-to-localize sound (a 2,000-Hz pure tone presented simultaneously from multiple locations). After the presentation of the cue in the upper or lower visual field, a second auditory stimulus, the target (four short bursts of white noise), was presented. The target could come from any one of four loudspeakers located at the corners of the display, and the task was to indicate whether it came from a speaker to the right or one to the left by pressing a right or left key. At short cuing intervals, responses to the target were slightly faster when the vertical position of the target (e.g., upper right or upper left) coincided with the vertical position of the visual cue (e.g., upper middle) than when it did not (e.g., upper-right or upper-left target combined with a cue at the lower-middle position)—but only when the auditory cue was hard to localize. This result implies that it was not the visual cue that

FIGURE 6.4. Depiction of Spence and Driver's (2000) Setup for Cuing Ventriloquized Sounds

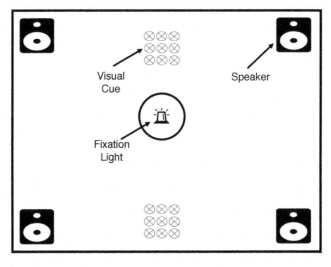

Note. From *Attention: Theory and Practice* (p. 117), by A. Johnson and R. W. Proctor, 2004, SAGE (https://doi.org/10.4135/9781483328768). Copyright 2004 by A. W. Johnson and R. W. Proctor. Adapted with permission.

cued spatial attention to the source of the target but the illusory location of the auditory cue. Spence and Driver concluded that although a visual cue normally does not attract auditory attention to its location, it does do so when the sound is hard to localize. Because the attentional cuing effect depended on the nature of both the visual cue and auditory cues, their study implies that integration of visual and auditory information occurs before the directing of attention.

More evidence that the direction of visual attention can influence the perceived location of sound comes from a study of selective listening by Driver (1996). Here, participants listened to difficult-to-distinguish target and distractor messages and attempted to follow the target message. Both the target (random words) and the distractor (also random words spoken in the same voice) messages were presented from the same loudspeaker. A videotape of a person speaking the words of the target message was played together with the two messages. When this video was presented off to the side of the auditory presentation (above a dummy loudspeaker rather than above the speaker broadcasting the stimuli; see Figure 6.5), selective listening to the target message improved considerably. Presumably, the target sounds were "relocated" by the participant due to ventriloquism. The resulting illusory spatial separation between the target and distractor messages improved selective listening just as actual spatial separation does.

The ventriloquism effect can be used as an indicator of audiovisual binding. Bischoff et al. (2007) presented auditory and visual stimuli that would yield some trials in which participants misperceived the auditory stimulus as emanating from the visual location. fMRI measurements for these trials compared with trials for which no mislocalization occurred showed activation in the superior temporal sulcus, parieto-occipital sulcus, and insula (which separates the temporal from the parietal and frontal lobes). Because these differences in brain activity were a function of the illusion, the authors suggested that they reflect consciousness-related processes.

Visual dominance has been demonstrated in other laboratory tasks, such as making a response with one hand to a tone and to a light with the other hand. On most trials, only the light or the tone is presented. On critical trials, both stimuli are presented, in which case people will generally respond to the visual

FIGURE 6.5. Depiction of the Experimental Setup Used by Driver (1996)

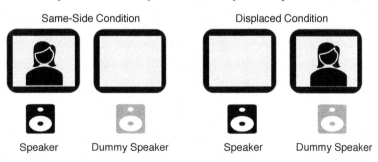

Note. From *Attention: Theory and Practice* (p. 119), by A. Johnson and R. W. Proctor, 2004, SAGE (https://doi.org/10.4135/9781483328768). Copyright 2004 by A. W. Johnson and R. W. Proctor. Adapted with permission.

stimulus and may not even report hearing the tone (Colavita, 1974). Visual information can also disrupt the processing of proprioceptive information of where the limbs are located in space. Although this visual dominance effect was initially thought to be due to directing attention to the visual modality (Posner et al., 1976), research has suggested that a bias to attend to vision cannot account for the effect (Spence et al., 2012).

Visual dominance over audition is also found when participants have to make a corresponding key press response to a left- or right-located stimulus in one modality while ignoring the location of a simultaneously presented stimulus in the other modality. Lukas et al. (2010) used this procedure and signaled the relevant modality on a trial by a centered cue in the same modality. Reactions were faster and errors fewer when the visual stimulus was relevant than when the auditory one was. A spatial congruity effect, indicating cross-modal interference, was observed when responding to either modality, but the effect was larger for auditory-relevant stimuli than for visual-relevant stimuli. In other words, irrelevant visual information had a larger effect than irrelevant auditory information. This finding, replicated by Tomko and Proctor (2017), is robust. Moreover, both Lukas et al. and Tomko and Proctor provided evidence in additional experiments that the congruity effect is a function of the irrelevant and relevant stimulus locations and not of the irrelevant stimulus position and the response position.

Vision can also dominate tactile stimulation. Botvinick and Cohen (1998) reported that when a participant's arm, hidden from view, was stroked with a brush simultaneously with a stroke of a visible rubber arm or hand on the table directly in front of them, the participant reported feeling the stroke at the location of the rubber hand. Pavani et al. (2000) showed similarly that the location of simultaneously presented visual lights could distort the localization of tactile stimulation. In their experiments, people were slower to report whether the finger or the thumb of their own concealed right or left hand was stimulated (by small vibrators located within a cube grasped by the thumb and forefinger) when a visual distractor was presented at a conflicting location (e.g., a light on the upper edge of a cube placed on a shelf presented simultaneously with vibrotactile stimulation at a lower location). The effect was even stronger when rubber hands holding cubes such as those held by the participants were placed on the shelf (see Figure 6.6). Despite knowing that the rubber hands were not their own, participants often reported feeling as if the rubber hands were their own and that the vibration seemed to occur at the location where the rubber hands were seen. These sensations—and the cuing effect—diminished when the rubber hands were placed in an orientation different from (orthogonal to) the participants' hands.

Two distinct aspects of the subjective rubber-hands illusion can be distinguished (Kalckert et al., 2019). One is the experience of the model hand being part of one's body, and the other is the perceptual fusion of vision and touch. Kalckert et al. (2019) examined the influence of relative position (lateral, distal) and distance (13–75 cm) of the model hand relative to the participant's real hand on the illusion experience. Their results showed indications of stronger

FIGURE 6.6. The Experimental Setup Used in the "Rubber Hands" Experiments of Pavani et al. (2000)

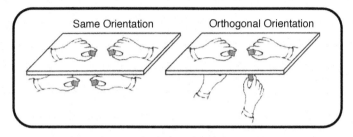

Note. Participant's hands were below the shelf, and the rubber hands were on the shelf. From *Attention: Theory and Practice* (p. 116), by A. Johnson and R. W. Proctor, 2004, SAGE (https://doi.org/10.4135/9781483328768). Copyright 2004 by A. W. Johnson and R. W. Proctor. Reprinted with permission.

illusion experiences in distal than lateral positions, suggesting that alignment of the real hands with the rubber hands is important. The illusion of ownership was restricted to near distances, but the fusion of touch sensations remained stable at farther distances, indicating that these two aspects of fusion of the real and rubber hands can be separated.

Visual dominance is not universal (e.g., Heller, 1992). In a variation of the visual-spatial congruence task described previously, which showed visual dominance, Lukas et al. (2014) found an auditory dominance effect for tasks that required temporal discriminations. An implication is that dominance tends to be shown by the modality best suited for the task. Also, it should be noted that auditory stimuli have a stronger natural tendency to draw attention (Wickens et al., 2016) than do visual stimuli. However, when visual stimuli have equal importance and provide at least as much information as other stimuli present at the time, in many situations, a bias toward the visual information can be expected.

Does Visual Attention Benefit Selection of Auditory Information?

Whether the direction of visual attention affects the selection of auditory information has been a question of interest for some time. Reisberg et al. (1981) reported evidence suggesting that it does. They presented participants with two lists of 30 paired words simultaneously in rapid succession from separate loudspeakers, with one list designated as relevant and the other as irrelevant. More words were recalled from the relevant auditory message, and the number of intrusions from the irrelevant message was less when the participants looked at the loudspeaker that delivered the target message rather than the one delivering the distractor message. However, this finding has proven difficult to replicate (Wolters & Schiano, 1989). Driver and Spence (1994) did not find a difference in location of visual attention when the relevant and irrelevant word streams were presented from left and right located speakers if an assigned visual task was passive (watching alternating Z and O characters). However, when it was active (a rapid sequence of keyboard symbols to which the participant was to stop the task whenever a "+" occurred), there was a recall advantage for the relevant auditory message from visually attending to its location rather than to that of the irrelevant message.

This latter finding, too, proved difficult to replicate, as Soto-Faraco et al. (2005) were unable to do in experiments similar to those of Driver and Spence (2004). Thus, Soto-Faraco et al. concluded, "Despite previous demonstrations about potential synergies in endogenous spatial attention between the auditory and the visual modalities, the link seems to be a fragile one" (p. 456). Best et al. (2020) reported a preliminary finding suggesting a benefit for visually attending to the location of the target auditory message when there are five audio speakers at distinct locations, simulating the noisier conditions of a party. But this result requires confirmation for acceptance as evidence of a condition in which visual attention facilitates auditory selection.

Although most studies of cross-modal attention have focused on the direction of attention and representation of space, some studies have looked at cross-modality effects from the point of view of the processing resources required by auditory and visual information processing. Some studies have suggested that the effects might extend to the sensory receptors. For example, Puel et al. (1988) found that otoacoustic emissions (weak sounds produced by the cochlea in response to external sounds) were smaller when participants performed a visual task (counting the Qs in a stream of Os and infrequent Qs) than when they were just relaxing. This study and some others suggested that performing visual tasks can have a direct (though small) effect on the auditory sensory receptors found in the cochlea. However, a comprehensive study by Beim et al. (2019) found no such evidence. They conducted two experiments using visual and auditory tasks to maximize sustained attention, perceptual load, and cochlear dynamic range. No effects of attention or perceptual load were observed on otoacoustic emissions. The results showed only between-subject variability in the otoacoustic emissions that did not depend on performance in the behavioral tasks. Consequently, Beim et al. interpreted their findings as suggesting that attentional modulation of auditory information arises at stages of processing beyond the cochlea.

Later in processing, visual and auditory stimulation can interact through cross-modal facilitation. Cross-modal facilitation can be studied by comparing the neural responses with each of two unimodal stimuli (e.g., one visual and one auditory) presented alone with the response to the bimodal presentation of both stimuli together. If the bimodal response is greater than the combined response to the two unimodal stimuli, facilitatory intermodal integration can be said to have taken place. Teder-Sälejärvi et al. (2002; see also B. E. Stein & Meredith, 1993) subtracted the ERPs for unimodal visual (a flash of light) and auditory (a burst of noise) targets from the ERP to an audiovisual combination of the two targets. They found an interaction effect beginning around 130 ms and peaking at 160 to 170 ms after stimulus presentation, which appeared to be attributable to regions in the visual cortex that go to the ventral stream.

To summarize, there is some evidence of cross-modal facilitation relatively early in processing. However, for the most part, the benefits of visual attention on auditory processing have been difficult to establish.

Cross-Modal Attention Cuing

The major question addressed in *cross-modal cuing* studies (i.e., presenting a cue in one modality to draw attention to some aspect of a stimulus in another modality) is whether the direction of attention to stimuli in one modality is affected by stimuli in another. Answering this question is complicated because nonattentional factors may be responsible for cross-modal effects. For example, if responses to the location of a visual stimulus are faster when it occurs on the same side as a recent auditory event, one could conclude that visual attention was directed to the location of the auditory stimulus, but it could also be the case that the visual stimulus primed the response associated with the tone. A sound on the left might automatically be coded as "left," and if a left key press response is then to be made to a visual stimulus presented on the left, the response will benefit from this activation of the spatial code (see C.-H. Lu & Proctor, 1995).

To minimize such problems, Spence and Driver (1996; see Driver & Spence, 1998, for a review) developed what they called an *orthogonal cuing paradigm* (see Figure 6.7). In the exogenous cuing version of this paradigm, an uninformative, abrupt onset cue, usually an auditory stimulus, is presented to the right or left. The target stimulus, often visual, may also occur on the right or left but at a high or low vertical position. The participant's task is to judge whether the target was presented in a high or low position, ignoring whether the target was on the right or left. Cross-modal cuing is said to have occurred when responses to the target (i.e., judgments of the elevation of the target) are faster on the cued than the uncued side. By having the auditory cue locations arrayed orthogonally to the relevant visual target locations, the chance that response priming or expectancy effects are the basis for any cross-modal cuing benefit is reduced

FIGURE 6.7. Orthogonal Cuing With Left- and Right-Pointing Endogenous Cues

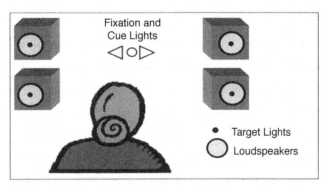

Note. From *Attention: Theory and Practice* (p. 121), by A. Johnson and R. W. Proctor, 2004, SAGE (https://doi.org/10.4135/9781483328768). Copyright 2004 by A. W. Johnson and R. W. Proctor. Reprinted with permission.

but not eliminated (Proctor, Tan, et al., 2005). The same paradigm can be used to study the effects of endogenous cues to direct attention to the probable location of an upcoming target stimulus.

An uninformative, exogenous auditory cue can facilitate responses to a visual stimulus presented on the same side as the auditory cue (Spence & Driver, 1996; but see Ward et al., 2000). Thus, auditory stimuli elicit visual attention at the corresponding location. A nonpredictive auditory cue influences the way people see subsequent visual objects (a) by improving perceptual sensitivity for detection of masked visual stimuli at the cued location, (b) producing earlier awareness of visual stimuli appearing at the cued location, and (c) changing the subjective appearance of visual stimuli at the cued location (McDonald et al., 2012).

Somewhat more debatable is whether visual processing affects the orienting of auditory attention. Spence and Driver (1997), for example, found that visual cues had no effect on auditory discrimination in an orthogonal cuing task. In contrast, Ward (1994) found that spatially uninformative visual cues orient auditory attention in an implicit discrimination task that requires participants to respond to targets at some locations but not others. The different characteristics of the two tasks seem to account for the divergent results of Ward (1994) and Spence and Driver (1996). When both tasks were examined in the same study (Prime et al., 2008), visual cues did not facilitate responses in the orthogonal cuing task. However, they did facilitate responses in the implicit discrimination task to same-side auditory targets presented at the cued location but not above or below that location. Thus, visual cues can cause an involuntary shift of spatial attention in the auditory modality, but this shift affects performance only when the subsequent auditory stimulus occurs within the focus of visual attention.

Störmer (2019) reviewed studies providing evidence that orienting to a salient sound in a peripheral location affects visual processing. Among the relevant findings are those of Störmer et al. (2009), who measured the ERPs elicited by a bilateral pair of equal-contrast Gabor patches (sinusoidal gratings) over the occipital cortex as a function of whether an auditory cue was presented in a left or right location. For trials on which the participants rated the cued visual stimulus as having higher contrast than the uncued one, the visual stimulus elicited an enlarged positive component on the opposite side of the sound's location that began about 90 to 100 ms after stimulus onset. In agreement with the ERP results, Störmer et al. (2016) found that the presentation of a salient auditory cue caused desynchronization of the contralateral occipital alpha rhythm, which is a neural indicator of visual processing and attention. Because the ERP difference was measured over the primary visual cortex, this result suggests that the sound affected the processing of the visual stimulus at an early stage of visual processing.

Evidence indicates that endogenous cues also exert their effects bimodally. Spence and Driver (1996) used central left- and right-pointing arrows as cues in the orthogonal cuing paradigm, with the stimulus occurring 75% of the time on the side signaled by the cue and 25% on the opposite side. The stimulus could be visual or auditory, randomly determined. The cue informed participants on which side they should direct their attention on each trial but not which modality. Both visual and auditory elevation discriminations were faster and more accurate when the stimulus occurred at the validly cued location than when it occurred at the opposite location. This result indicates that the endogenous visual cue enabled attention to be directed to both visual and auditory locations. Similar benefits of endogenous cuing have been found for vision and touch (Spence, Pavani, & Driver, 2000) and audition and touch (Lloyd et al., 2003).

The Simon Effect With Multiple Stimulus Modalities

Rather than controlling for spatial correspondence, as in the orthogonal cuing method, effects of irrelevant stimulus location can be examined with the Simon effect, which occurs in the visual, auditory, and tactile modalities. In addition to occurring as a function of the relevant stimulus location, the Simon effect is also found when the irrelevant stimulus location is conveyed by an auditory stimulus when the task is to respond to a centered visual stimulus. J. R. Simon and Pouraghabagher (1978) initially reported that participants were faster at pressing a left or right key to the centered visual stimulus X or O when the location of a tone presented to the left or right ear corresponded with the response assigned to the visual stimulus. Proctor, Pick, et al. (2005) obtained similar results when the relevant visual discrimination was red or green. Consistent with the results reported in relation to visual dominance, they also found an effect of tone location when the visual task required responding to the location of a visual stimulus.

This location-based Simon effect is also obtained when tones differ randomly in low or high pitch, which produces a separate congruity effect of low pitch with left and high pitch with right (Nishimura & Yokosawa, 2009). Thus, different features of the tones can produce congruity effects. Although the onset of a tone simultaneous with that of the centered visual stimulus produced a Simon effect, the offset of a tone at the onset of the visual stimulus did not (Nishimura & Yokosawa, 2010). A possible interpretation of this result is that only the onset of an auditory stimulus causes a shift of attention to it, producing a left or right location code.

Ruzzoli and Soto-Faraco (2017) focused on the visual and tactile Simon effects obtained under conditions in which only one stimulus modality occurred in a trial, and the stimulus varied in the left or right location, but stimulus modality also varied randomly from trial to trial. With this procedure, the Simon effect for the tactile stimuli was essentially unaffected by the mixing of trial modalities, whereas the visual Simon effect was eliminated. This result pattern was obtained even when the responses were foot presses on left and right pedals, indicating that making the response with the stimulated finger in the tactile trials was not the critical factor.

When performed alone, the tactile Simon effect follows the effector when the hands are crossed: Responses are faster when the left index finger is stimulated regardless of whether the hand is crossed to be on the right side of the participant. This result contrasts with the visual and auditory Simon effects, for which the relative location of the response rather than the effector is crucial. In a final experiment, Ruzzoli and Soto-Faraco (2017) had participants perform mixed trials with visual and auditory stimuli. In this case, where the responses for both modalities are represented in a spatial reference frame when performed alone, Simon effects based on locations were still evident. That a visual Simon effect was evident in this case but not when the mixed stimuli were tactile suggests that specifically being prepared to respond to the stimulation of a finger causes participants not to code the responses spatially.

A Single Supramodal Spatial Attention Controller?

As in the Simon effect, spatial locations of the stimuli affect performance in many situations. Spatial separation in sounds can make it easier to attend to one source and ignore another. It has also been suggested that the proximity of visual and auditory displays can affect monitoring performance. Driver and Spence (1994) found that participants were better at monitoring both a visual and an auditory display when both displays (a speaker and a computer monitor) were located on the same side of the participant, compared with when one display was located to the left of the participant and the other to the right. Although the effects of display location were small, they suggest that some aspect of spatial attention may be supramodal.

A similar conclusion can be reached on the basis of ERP experiments. Eimer and Schröger (1998) found that the direction of spatial attention affected auditory ERPs when hearing was relevant, but there were no effects of cued attention on auditory ERPs when vision was relevant. Tactile attention, however, can influence auditory (as well as visual) processing. Eimer et al. (2001) conducted two experiments in which participants had to focus their attention on their right or left hand to detect infrequent tactile targets. In their first experiment, visual stimuli were also presented in some trials. ERPs were measured, and it was found that a visual target on the tactually attended side elicited enhanced N1 and P2 components at the occipital sites. Similarly, auditory stimuli presented in the second experiment were responded to differently (the N1 component was enhanced) when the sounds were on the side where the participant expected a tactile target. This suggests that cross-modal links exist both between touch and vision and between touch and hearing. Eimer et al. also looked at auditory and visual ERPs when the hands were crossed. In this case, the stimuli in the same physical side of space (and not the same side of the body) showed enhanced responses. This result shows that it is the common external location of the stimuli that determines cross-modal attentional links and not hemispheric projections within the brain.

On the basis of results like these, Driver and Spence (1998) concluded that attention works on cross-modal spatial representations. Ward (1994) interpreted cross-modal cuing effects as evidence for a supramodal representation of space. In this view, the mechanisms underlying visual and auditory shifts of attention are not completely independent but share information at some level of processing. This conclusion is consistent with evidence of visual dominance, such as the ventriloquism effect discussed earlier, the finding that the presentation of a visual stimulus (or the direction of gaze) can affect the localization of auditory signals (e.g., Bertelson & Aschersleben, 1998), and an absence of auditory dominance effects. In agreement with the view that attention is supramodal, Spence, Lloyd, et al. (2000) found that when a random sequence of visual, auditory, and tactile target stimuli was presented to the left or right of central fixation, inhibition of return was evident for targets in all the modalities. Detection of targets in any modality took longer if the prior target had been presented from the left or right location, regardless of the modality in which the prior target was presented.

Neurophysiological evidence is also in agreement with the supramodal attention hypothesis. In a spatial cuing task, responses to invalidly cued contralesional visual targets with auditory cues for patients with lesions in the parietal lobe are slowed (Farah et al., 1989). Neuroimaging studies have shown that cortical regions activated during attention to multiple sensory modalities overlap with the dorsal and ventral frontoparietal regions activated during visual attention tasks. Macaluso (2010) summarized the findings as follows:

(1) most attention control regions in frontal and parietal cortex are multimodal and combine information arising from the different senses;

(2) crossmodal interactions can affect activity in sensory-specific areas and they can do so in a spatially specific manner;

(3) conditions involving multisensory stimuli can trigger stimulus-driven activation of the ventral attention control system irrespective of relevance and task-set factors. (p. 292)

He interpreted such results as supporting the view that supramodal attentional control in the frontoparietal cortex applies top-down influences on sensory-specific areas, which result in the enhancement of the processing of stimuli at the attended location regardless of sensory modality.

Can the finding of cross-modal effects on attention between the visual, auditory, and tactile modalities and for both exogenous and endogenous cues be taken as strong evidence for supramodal attentional control? The fact that the deployment of attention in one modality can modulate attentional effects in another modality does not necessarily imply that attention is directed in a supramodal manner. Cross talk between information processes seems possible at any information-processing level. Although this cross talk may argue against a strict modularity of processing systems, it does not establish the existence of a master controller. Indeed, Klemen and Chambers (2012) suggested that multivoxel pattern analysis, which has higher spatial resolution than typical methods for analyzing fMRI data, might reveal differences between overlapping activations caused by stimuli from various sensory modalities. Kurniawan (2012) performed multivoxel pattern analysis and confirmed this suggestion, leading him to conclude that "both modality-specific and potentially supramodal frontoparietal regions work in concert to selectively bias activity in sensory cortical regions during various states of attention" (p. ii).

CHAPTER SUMMARY

Change detection is fundamental to processing information from the natural and virtual environments, yet people are much less sensitive to detecting change than they might think. This lack of sensitivity to change is evident in numerous examples of change blindness, in which people do not see substantive changes that occur in images at which they are looking. A similar phenomenon called change deafness is obtained for audition. Change blindness and change deafness illustrate that people are unaware of much that goes on in the environment around them.

Evidence from the oddball task indicates that people are sensitive to detecting deviations from regular stimulation at early stages of information processing. A critical difference in the situations that produce blindness and those that produce oddball detection is that there typically is only relatively limited stimulation in an oddball task—that is, a single stream of similar stimuli from which one that is deviant will tend to pop out.

In many contexts in the world, stimulation is multisensory. Input from the senses can be integrated, with possibly one sense dominating another, and attention cued endogenously or exogenously in one sense may influence processing in another sensory modality. The cross-modal cuing effects suggest that modality specificity may be graded or that there may be a supramodal attentional controller. Even if stimuli from different modalities can be attended to independently up to a point, attentional limits involved in the selection of responses are indifferent to whether multiple stimuli originate in the same or different modalities.

KEY POINTS

- **Fact:** People are often unaware of stimulus changes registered by the sensory receptors.

- **Phenomenon:** Inattentional blindness, change blindness, and change deafness refer to the insensitivity that people show with regard to events and changes in their immediate environment to which they are not attending.

- **Fact:** Change detection can be optimized by attending to the change location and consciously encoding what was there before and afterward.

- **Fact:** The oddball task, when paired with ERP and brain-imaging responses, has been an effective tool for studying change detection in a uniform environment.

- **Phenomenon:** Mismatch negativity differentiating an oddball from standard stimuli occurs within about 200 ms of stimulus onset. It appears to reflect automatic detection of the difference.

- **Phenomenon:** P3a and P3b ERP components often occur in oddball tasks and seemingly reflect attentional processes.

- **Fact:** Tactile attention shows many of the same phenomena as visual and auditory attention.

- **Phenomenon:** Visual dominance refers to a tendency for spatial perception to conform more to the visual sense in situations of conflict.

- **Phenomenon:** The rubber hands illusion refers to people attributing stimulation of a hidden hand to the location of a rubber hand that is in view.

- **Fact:** Exogenous and endogenous cuing can be bimodal and prepare people to attend to stimuli in modalities different from that in which the cue occurred.

- **Theory:** Attention may, in part, be supramodal.

7

Divided Attention and Multiple-Task Performance

Dividing attention among multiple sources of information and tasks has become an increasingly prominent feature of modern life. This is sometimes referred to as *multitasking*. People often have multiple screens and multiple electronic devices that they monitor concurrently. It is not uncommon for a student to be engaged in texting or social media while listening to a lecture in class (see Box 7.1). Perhaps most evident is that people engage in conversations on their smartphones in essentially all contexts, including walking through crowds and sometimes even driving, which require locomotion and navigation around obstacles. The extent to which people can truly time-share, as implied by the term "multitasking," has been a source of debate for many years in psychology.

For most people, demands on their attention first become evident when they are required to do several things at once. There is a quick realization that this is difficult to do in many situations. You can carry on a conversation with a passenger under light traffic conditions, but when the driving conditions become difficult, as in heavy traffic, you know intuitively that you cannot do both tasks well and devote most attention to driving. Driving demands processing multiple stimuli, and failure to see a traffic sign, for example, may have an unfortunate outcome. Likewise, becoming skilled in any domain requires the performer to handle and coordinate multiple task demands. For example, skilled musicians must divide their attention between reading a score, playing the instrument, and following the directions of a conductor; tennis players must move to intercept the ball while planning their following shot.

https://doi.org/10.1037/0000317-007
Attention: Selection and Control in Human Information Processing, by R. W. Proctor and K.-P. L. Vu

BOX 7.1 | **MEDIA USE DURING CLASS IS A DISTRACTION**

Media multitasking is the use of two or more media concurrently. Media can include television, computer or laptop, audio player, smartphone, tablet, smartwatch, or game console, to name a few. Multitasking is a divided attention task, involving maintaining more than one task set and switching between tasks. As shown in this chapter, two tasks cannot be performed concurrently without any performance cost unless one or both tasks are automatic and do not require attention or response-selection resources to complete. Usually, a cost of concurrence is obtained with dual-task performance, in which performance on one task is less than single-task performance, even if the person devotes all their attention to that task. Given what we know about the cost of concurrence and task-switching costs, media use during a lecture or even studying can have serious implications for students' learning and academic performance.

Media multitasking is part of many students' daily routines. For example, Calderwood et al. (2014) observed 60 undergraduate students during a 3-hour study period in a laboratory setting. Participants were allowed to bring their laptop, audio player, and smartphone to the session and were told that they could freely interact with any of their devices. The students were distracted by their media devices and engaged in multitasking throughout the session. About 59% of the students listened to music during the study session (i.e., had music playing in the background), with 21% of these students having music playing for most of the session. In addition to listening to music, the students engaged in distractor activities (i.e., surfing the internet, watching videos, emailing, texting, talking on their cellphone) multiple times during the session. On average, the students were engaged in 35 distractor activities taking up about 26 minutes of the session. However, the distribution of the number of distractions other than listening to music (25th percentile = 19 distractions, 75th percentile = 44 distractions) and the total length of engagement in distractor activities (25th percentile = 9 minutes, 75th percentile = 36 minutes) varied widely among the students. Higher task motivation and self-efficacy to concentrate on the task were associated with fewer multitasking behaviors. Although Calderwood et al. did not examine how the use of media impacted the students' learning outcomes, it is clear that media use during studying is a source of distraction for students.

Media multitasking can lead to negative outcomes due to the multiple sources of distraction. The different types of media can attract the learner's attention, and the learner may be predisposed to attend to media (a more pleasant task) over study materials (a less pleasant task). Media multitasking can also lead to depletion of attentional resources due to the need to switch back and forth between media and tasks. Interruptions, in which people suspend the performance of one task to perform another, produce costs that go beyond those associated with task switching (W. Schneider & Dixon, 2009). Interruptions in reading produce costs in reading times and comprehension due to a need to reinstate the context when returning to the text (Foroughi et al., 2015). Similarly, when resuming the performance of a complex cognitive task, reactivation of the task context and goal must occur (Altmann & Trafton, 2007; Hodgetts & Jones, 2006).

BOX 7.1 | **MEDIA USE DURING CLASS IS A DISTRACTION**
(Continued)

Students may argue that engaging in media multitasking makes them more efficient by increasing their cognitive control ability. That is, their use of media multitasking is training that can help them filter interference from distractor tasks and perform tasks more efficiently. However, this is not the case. K. E. May and Elder (2018) conducted a review of 38 articles that examined media multitasking and its relation to the academic performance of college students to determine whether media multitasking is efficient, helpful, or distracting. They found that media multitasking was negatively associated with academic performance: More media multitasking was associated with lower GPAs, lower comprehension of materials, and lower test scores. Specifically, texting during class lectures was correlated with lower test scores; texting during studying was associated with lower GPAs. Students who watched videos or engaged in social media or instant messaging showed higher levels of distraction and obtained lower test scores.

Moreover, using a laptop during a class lecture to multitask not only hindered the student's performance but also the performance of classmates sitting near them. That is, students in direct view of the multitasker scored about 17% lower on a comprehension test than students who were not in direct view of the multitasker. The activities of the multitasker likely caused shifts in the attention of the classmates to the media, making it a distraction to learning. Students tended to underestimate the negative impact of media multitasking, with some believing that they could perform media multitasking during lectures without showing poorer performance (contrary to the data) and others believing that it was less harmful than it actually is. Overall, these findings indicate that media multitasking is a source of distraction, and it is not helpful to engage in media multitasking during class lectures or while studying.

Although information from multiple sources must often be attended to and acted on, only a fraction of the stimulation present in the immediate environment is, as a rule, relevant to current task demands. Thus, most real-world tasks, ranging from reading a book in a crowded waiting room while monitoring the time of one's appointment to taking notes while listening to a lecture and ignoring the activities of fellow students, have both focused and divided attention components. Consequently, several topics from prior chapters come up again in this one.

DIVIDED ATTENTION

Divided attention refers to situations in which you need to process or monitor two or more sources of sensory stimuli simultaneously, both to comprehend the information and take necessary actions. An example is trying to watch a sporting event while talking with someone on your smartphone. As with selective attention, much of the early research in the information-processing revolution used auditory tasks, although visual tasks have predominated more recently. The selectivity observed with the dichotic listening paradigm described in Chapter 3 shows that people can focus attention relatively efficiently on just one source of stimulation when the source is well defined by a basic characteristic such as location. Variations on this paradigm have been used to ask how effectively people are able to distribute their attention across different sources or channels. One such variation, known as the split-span technique, was introduced by Broadbent (1954) to test a prediction of his filter theory.

The Split-Span Technique for Auditory Attention

The *split-span technique* gets its name from the memory span (the number of items that can, on average, be remembered without rehearsal), with the list of to-be-remembered items split into two shorter lists for presentation, one to each ear. In this type of experiment, the listener is instructed to report all items heard in both ears. Broadbent (1954) presented participants with two lists of three spoken digits, one list to each ear, at a rate of two digits per second. He found that listeners tended to report all the items presented to one ear first, followed by the items presented to the other ear (see Figure 7.1) rather than reporting them as pairs grouped by presentation time. This result suggested that selection of information occurs quite early in the course of information processing, at the level of the physical properties of the stimuli (e.g., location, pitch). Broadbent proposed that while the message presented to one ear was attended to, the other was held in a sort of "pre-perceptual" storage. After the items in one ear were reported, the attentional "filter" would switch to the other ear, allowing reporting of those items.

Later experiments showed that the selection of items for report can be based on higher level semantic properties of the stimuli and not just on physical properties such as location or frequency. For example, Bartz et al. (1967) found, consistent with Broadbent (1954), that listeners tended to report lists of digits and nondigit monosyllabic words according to the ear in which the lists were presented. However, when instructed to report the digits first and then the

FIGURE 7.1. A Split-Span Experiment

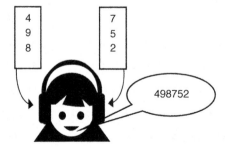

nondigits or vice versa, their recall was at the same level as if they reported by ear. Gray and Wedderburn (1960) found that when a message such as "who-3-there" was played to the right ear and the message "2-goes-9" to the left ear, some people spontaneously reported the familiar phrase, "who goes there," followed by the digits "2 3 9." These results show that, counter to filter theory, selection is not based solely on salient physical features.

Auditory and Visual Monitoring

The split-span technique can be viewed as a special case of a monitoring task. In auditory monitoring, participants listen to streams of auditory stimuli and indicate when they have heard a target. In the split-span technique, all words are targets, and the task is to report everything, but auditory monitoring tasks are usually performed under more noisy conditions. Pohlmann and Sorkin (1976) studied the ability of people to divide their attention using a task in which up to three targets had to be detected in a stream of auditory noise presented to one ear. In a single-channel condition, participants monitored short intervals of noise for the presence of a target of a given pitch. In the multiple-channel condition, one, two, or three targets (of different frequencies) could be presented, which meant that participants had to monitor for different pitches simultaneously. In each condition, a target was present in half the trials.

Pohlmann and Sorkin's (1976) participants performed as well at detecting any one of the three targets in the multiple-target condition as detecting the target in the single-target condition but only when a single target was presented at any given time. Their performance was much worse when two or three targets were presented simultaneously (see also Sorkin et al., 1973). Performance at monitoring information in both ears is quite good as long as only one target is present at a time and the different targets are easy to tell apart. Thus, it seems that auditory attention can be "set" to monitor a number of channels, but limitations on the ability to identify multiple targets simultaneously prevent perfect time-sharing on the multiple channels.

Similar performance results to those of the auditory studies are evident in studies with visual stimuli. Duncan (1980) noted that the number of distractors has little influence on performance when searching for a visual target distinguished by a salient feature (Treisman & Gelade, 1980) or by a learned category such as a letter among digits (W. Schneider & Shiffrin, 1977). In contrast, as in auditory detection, studies of visual detection and identification find considerable performance decrements when two or more targets occur simultaneously. Thus, Duncan interpreted the results for both auditory and visual stimuli as suggesting that only targets have to pass through a limited-capacity system that results in conscious availability for report. Nontarget stimuli can be identified and rejected by earlier parallel, unconscious processes.

Monitoring for single targets cannot always be achieved without costs. This is shown in a study by Ninio and Kahneman (1974) in which two lists of words were presented dichotically, and targets (animal names) could appear in either list. When participants were told to monitor only one list, they were accurate at detecting any animal names (96% hit rate). Performance decreased slightly (to about 90%) if an animal name was presented in the unattended channel shortly before a target was presented in the attended channel, suggesting that excluding the unattended channel was not perfect. When the instructions were to monitor both ears, the hit rate fell to 77%, the false alarm rate rose slightly, and responses were slower, even though only one target was presented at a time. As in visual search (e.g., W. Schneider & Shiffrin, 1977), dividing attention across different channels is more difficult than attending to just one channel.

MULTIPLE-TASK PERFORMANCE

The concept of attention as a bottleneck that can only process one stimulus or object at a time is a variant of a broader range of theories that assume that attention is a limited capacity resource. One can distinguish unitary resource models from multiple resource models of attention. In some terminologies, attention is related to *controlled processing* as distinct from *automatic processing*, which does not require attention. The relation between controlled and automatic processing is a key factor in multitasking performance. Another issue is the role of goals and intentions in guiding the performance of tasks. The interacting roles of memory and attention are taking an increasingly prominent role in models and theories of human performance and are discussed in both this and the following chapter.

Attentional Resources

In part due to issues associated with distinguishing early- and late-selection models of attention, resource models of attention became popular in the 1970s (Posner & Boies, 1971). The best-known unitary-resource model is that of Kahneman (1973), in which attention is viewed as a limited-capacity resource that can be allocated to a variety of processes and tasks (see Figure 7.2). As long as the demands on attentional resources do not exceed the available

FIGURE 7.2. Kahneman's (1973) Unitary-Resource Model of Attention

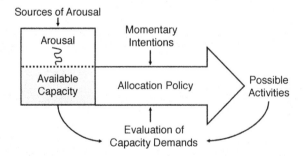

Note. From *Attention: Theory and Practice* (p. 264), by A. Johnson and R. W. Proctor, 2004, SAGE (https://doi.org/10.4135/9781483328768). Copyright 2004 by A. W. Johnson and R. W. Proctor. Reprinted with permission.

capacity, which can vary as a function of arousal level, each process and task will receive the necessary resources for effective performance. However, when demands exceed the supply, there are not enough resources to satisfy the needs of all processes and tasks, so performance will suffer.

The concept of resources that can be devoted at will to various processes and tasks implies that when the demand exceeds the supply, how the resources are allocated to the various tasks will be crucial. Consequently, Kahneman's (1973) model includes an allocation policy for distributing attentional resources. The existence of an allocation policy suggests that there is a sort of "comparator" that assesses current resources and the active intentions and activities of the performer. When performance demands are high, the stability of performance depends on the effectiveness of attentional control in maintaining the current priorities. One example of this is driving a car while talking on a smartphone. When driving demands are routine, the driver is able to carry out a conversation without it interfering with driving. However, when conditions are demanding, such as when the weather is bad or unfamiliar streets have to be navigated, the driver will not be able to do both at the same time and may even terminate the conversation. In many situations, performance must be "protected" from environmental disturbance, and this can be accomplished only through the maintained priority of strong task-oriented goals.

An implication of the unitary-resource model is that as long as peripheral perceptual and motor conflicts are minimized, the main determinant of multiple-task performance should be the amount of attention required for each task when performed alone. Yet, it is easy to find situations in which that relation is violated. For example, the dual-task decrement is dependent on the relation to the input and output modalities, as shown by Wickens (1980). Participants performed a visual tracking task along with a subtraction task in which the difference between successive digits in a series had to be computed and spoken vocally or entered with a key press. The digits were presented auditorily or visually in different conditions. The dual-task decrement was substantially greater for visual versus auditory coding modality and key press versus vocal response modality, even though the content of the subtraction task was identical in these four cases.

Multiple-Resources Framework

The idea that there is just one general resource or capacity for performing all sorts of tasks cannot itself account for some important aspects of task performance, such as the fact that two tasks of apparently equal difficulty may have completely different effects when combined with a third task, with one of the tasks causing interference and the other causing none. Such a finding suggests that the tasks may draw on multiple different resources and that only when the same resources are required by another task will performance show a decrement.

The multiple-resource view is that different sorts of tasks, or different task components, draw on separate resources with their own distinct capacity reserves. This implies that if two tasks draw on different resources, they may be performed together more efficiently, and their combined mental workload may be lower than if they rely on the same resources. Wickens (1980, 1984) proposed that separate processing resources correspond to the basic information-processing stages of perception, central processing, and responding, as well as spatial and verbal processing codes, visual and auditory modalities, and manual and vocal responses. These resources for processing stages, codes, and input and output modalities can be represented as a three-dimensional model (see Figure 7.3). Wickens (2008, 2021) later added a fourth dimension, focal versus ambient, based on evidence that the ventral pathway in the visual system mainly carries focal information for pattern recognition and form perception, whereas the dorsal stream carries ambient information for spatial localization and navigation (see Chapter 2, this volume).

Evidence for distinct visual and auditory attentional resources, reviewed in Chapters 3 to 5, generally supports the proposal that visual and auditory information may be processed independently, at least up to a point. The model is also consistent with the finding that dual-task performance cannot always be predicted on the basis of single-task difficulty. However, the multiple-resource model is only an architecture (Hancock et al., 2007) and therefore is mute on the subject of executive control and possible interactions between codes and modalities. Moreover, interference between particular tasks may be more specific than expected on the basis of the five distinctions in Wickens's (2008) multiple-resource model (Navon & Miller, 1987).

FIGURE 7.3. Wickens's (2008) Multiple-Resources Framework

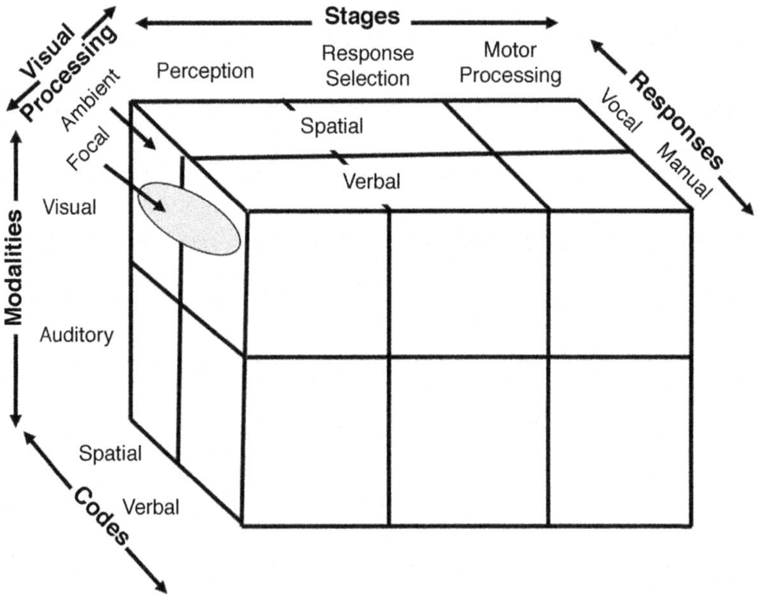

Note. From "Multiple Resources and Mental Workload," by C. D. Wickens, 2008, *Human Factors, 50*(3), p. 450 (https://doi.org/10.1518/001872008X288394). Copyright 2002 by SAGE Publishing. Reprinted with permission.

Although inadequate as a model of attention, the multiple-resources view serves as a useful framework for predicting operator performance in complex tasks. A major strength of this framework is that it allows tasks to be defined in terms that are easy to represent. Researchers can use the framework to develop task combinations that allow the prediction of time-sharing performance. Better time-sharing between two tasks is expected if they use separate rather than common resources because demand increases in one will be less likely to affect the other. A weakness of the framework with regard to modeling performance is its inability to offer clearly defined scales of the amount of demand for resources that generalize across different tasks.

Managing Attentional Resources

Even if a task is well understood from the researcher's point of view when performed singly, taking that task out of isolation and placing it in the context of other tasks means that additional factors will come into play. The need to do two or more things at once brings problems of coordinating task strategies and, often, dividing attention between different aspects of the tasks. In other words, specialized skills are required to become good at performing multiple tasks. One such skill has been called time-sharing (or multitasking). *Time-sharing* refers to efficiently allocating processing resources to component tasks at the appropriate times, and it reflects a basic ability that generalizes across a variety of task combinations (Salthouse & Miles, 2002). Because physicians have to multitask, particularly in emergency settings, it has been noted that an improved understanding of time-sharing and task switching will improve physicians' abilities to help more patients (Benda & Fairbanks, 2017).

Sometimes, however, multiple-task performance improves because performers learn to restructure two or more tasks that are performed together, such that the multiple tasks are treated as a single task (Cheng, 1985). The ability to restructure tasks depends on the components of the tasks to be performed together. For example, task interactions, such as interference in making a manual response for one task and executing a similar response for another task, may prevent two tasks from being combined into a smoothly executable, coherent unit. Although such structural interference may be a major determinant of the ability to perform different tasks together, interference can also arise when senses and effectors used in the two tasks differ.

Given the limited nature of attentional resources, performing a task adequately often depends on the ability to allocate attention appropriately. That is, optimal performance may require devoting less attention to some aspect of the task to devote more attention to a different aspect of the task. It is clear that only some combinations of strategies will lead to optimal performance. For example, moving the head or eyes to collect peripheral information needed for planning can be useful but can also result in accidents, such as tripping when walking or rear-ending the car in front when driving. Optimizing performance requires finding the right combination of attentional strategies (attending to different sources) and perceptual strategies (acting on the minimal effective amount of information). For example, when jogging along a path, it is sufficient to notice that there is a tree in the way; it is not necessary to continue focusing on the tree until one has enough information to know whether it is a maple or an ash.

Erev and Gopher (1999) provided one theoretical account of optimizing performance by changing attentional strategies. They proposed that attention control has two constraints: the cognitive strategies available to the performer and the payoff rule for applying these strategies. At each point, behavior is controlled by a strategy made up of at least two components: an executive control (top-down) component that determines which information will be attended to (according to the payoff rule; see Figure 7.4) and a data-driven perception and action (bottom-up) rule component that controls the execution of a response to the attended information.

Allocation strategies become even more important when there are more than two tasks. These strategies can be studied in what are called *synthetic work environments*. Wang et al. (2007) studied acquisition and transfer of attention allocation strategies in an environment called SYNWORK1, which consists of four concurrent tasks performed with the goal of maximizing the points obtained. The tasks are memory search, addition, visual monitoring of a marker to prevent it from reaching the end of a scale, and auditory monitoring for a high-pitch tone among low-pitch tones (see Figure 7.5). Of concern was whether strategies appropriate to payoffs favoring either the memory search task or the math task would be adopted in an initial day of eight 5-minute sessions and whether the strategies would be modified for four of the sessions on the second day when the relative payoffs were reversed.

The total points participants received increased across the experiment, more so on the first day than the second day. The participants were sensitive to the initial payoff structure in that they performed significantly more instances of the task for which the points were higher (memory or addition). They modified their strategies during the sessions in which the payoffs were reversed on the

FIGURE 7.4. Depiction of Erev and Gopher's (1999) Game-Theoretic Model of Attention and Control

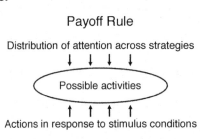

Payoff Rule

Distribution of attention across strategies

↓ ↓ ↓ ↓

Possible activities

↑ ↑ ↑ ↑

Actions in response to stimulus conditions

Perception and Action Rules

Note. From *Attention: Theory and Practice* (p. 165), by A. Johnson and R. W. Proctor, 2004, SAGE (https://doi.org/10.4135/9781483328768). Copyright 2004 by A. W. Johnson and R. W. Proctor. Reprinted with permission.

FIGURE 7.5. Display Screen for SYNWORK1

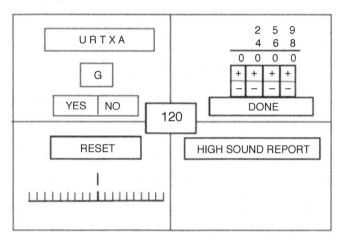

Note. The memory task performed in the upper left, the arithmetic task in the upper right, the visual monitoring task in the lower left, and the auditory monitoring task in the lower right. From "Acquisition and Transfer of Attention Allocation Strategies in a Multiple-Task Work Environment," by D.-Y. D. Wang, R. W. Proctor, and D. F. Pick, 2007, *Human Factors*, *49*(6), p. 997 (https://doi.org/10.1518/001872007X249866). Copyright 2007 by SAGE Publishing. Reprinted with permission.

second day, but residual effects of prior payoffs were evident. The results of this study demonstrate that people can adjust their strategies to accommodate payoffs in a multiple-task environment if the payoffs are explicit, although there is some tendency for strategies to reflect prior as well as current payoffs.

Summary

Attention is typically viewed as a limited capacity to process multiple stimuli. Many models of attention attributed this limitation to one or more limited-capacity resources. When viewed in this manner, strategies for allocating attention to one task or another become important. People are generally flexible at allocating attention but not quite as flexible as a unitary resource account would imply without assuming additional sources of interference. For applied purposes, the multiple resource model provides a useful heuristic for predicting which tasks can be performed together more efficiently than others.

SETTING GOALS AND INTENTIONS

Goal Setting

All experimenters assume that their participants are willing to pursue the goals in which they, themselves, are interested. It is assumed that participants are able to grasp the task instructions and do their best to carry out the assigned tasks. The importance of the instructed task (or *Aufgabe*) was first identified by the Würzburg school of psychologists in the early 20th century (Watt, 1906).

However, participants in even simple experiments cannot always keep the goals of performance current. For example, in an antisaccade experiment (Hallett, 1978), in which a saccadic eye movement is moved to a location opposite to a cued location, participants may lose their concentration or ability to maintain the cue-action relationship and nonetheless allow their eyes to move to the cue. The ability to maintain and modify task goals has received increasing consideration in recent years. These executive control functions have been studied most extensively in situations in which participants must switch from one simple task to another or perform a series of steps in a multistep task.

Task-Set Switching

Efficient, coordinated performance of complex tasks often depends on the ability to switch from one task or task component to another. For example, a baseball player at bat must be prepared to switch quickly from the task of swinging to hit the ball to the task of running to basepaths. *Switching costs*—increases in reaction time and error rates on the task after the switch—have been taken as an index of the control processes involved in reconfiguring and reconnecting various "modules" in the brain so as to perform the correct action with a given stimulus (Monsell & Driver, 2000). Switch costs seem to reflect the time needed by the person to adopt the appropriate task set. For the baseball player, years of practice will have influenced the ability to transition from hitting the ball to running the basepaths. Good players will likely have developed what researchers call *advance reconfiguration* processes to facilitate this transition (Rogers & Monsell, 1995). According to this idea, performers can intentionally prepare for a task switch, thus minimizing any costs of having to change tasks.

Switch costs have most often been studied in paradigms in which participants need to switch between two simple tasks. As you may remember from Chapter 1, such task switching was studied by Jersild (1927). In one study, he compared the time for participants to perform the same arithmetic operation (e.g., addition) on a list of 25 numbers and other conditions in which two operations were mixed (e.g., addition and subtraction) in an alternating manner. The mixed lists required at least 1 second longer per item than the pure lists of a single operation. Nearly 50 years later, Spector and Biederman (1976) followed up this finding, showing that people took more than 400 milliseconds (ms) longer on average to alternate adding or subtracting 3 from each two-digit number in a mixed list, compared with pure lists. The list procedure cannot yield precise estimates of the switch cost because mixed lists require that both tasks be activated in working memory, and participants can look ahead while proceeding through the list.

Contemporary Research on Visual Task Switching

From the mid-1990s to the present, much research has been conducted on task switching (see Kiesel et al., 2010; Koch et al., 2018, and Vandierendonck et al., 2010, for reviews). Most studies during this period have used methods that allow reaction times to be measured for individual trials presented in succession. Rogers and Monsell (1995) used an alternating runs procedure in which the task switched in a fixed sequence. Every two trials, participants switched between classifying the digit member of a pair of characters as even or odd or the letter member as a consonant or vowel. Switch costs reflect poorer performance for task-switch trials (i.e., the first trial after a switch) than for consecutive same-task trials (i.e., trials in which the same task is performed as in the preceding trial). Rogers and Monsell found large switch costs in both reaction time and error rate. When people had sufficient time to prepare for the forthcoming task switch (i.e., when the interval between the response to a previous trial and the presentation of the stimulus for the current trial was long enough), task-switching costs were substantially reduced. However, this preparation for the new task was only partial: Even with 1.2 seconds available for preparation, a large cost in reaction time remained for the first trial of the new task.

Rogers and Monsell's (1995) results illustrate four widely replicated phenomena in the task-switching literature: (a) There is a *switch cost*, when performance is worse on trials for which the task switches from the prior trial than for those on which it repeats. This cost reflects demands associated with switching from the previously performed task to the new task. (b) A *preparation benefit* also exists, for which the switch cost is reduced if the next task is known, as long as adequate time for preparation is allowed. (c) A *residual cost* of reduced size remains even when the time for preparation is provided. The final phenomenon is (d) a *mixing cost*, which is that task-repetition trials in mixed blocks show costs relative to single-task blocks. This cost is presumed to be due to cognitive demands in maintaining two task sets in working memory.

Task switching has also been studied using a cuing procedure in which the two tasks are randomly intermixed and therefore unpredictable. A cue preceding the critical stimulus indicates the task for that trial, and the cue-target interval can be varied to allow different amounts of preparation. Meiran (1996) presented a stimulus (a happy face) in a quadrant of a 2×2 grid that was to be categorized as up or down or left or right with one of two key presses on the diagonal of a number pad (see Figure 7.6). The cues were left–right arrows or up–down arrows presented at the ends of the horizontal or vertical center lines, and the cue-target interval was short (203 ms) or long (1,423 ms). In the example shown in Figure 7.6, the preceding trial was the up–down task, and the response would be "down." The cue for the current trial signaled the left–right task, and the response would be "right," which was the same physical key press as on the prior trial. Results showed a large task-switch cost at the short cuing interval that was reduced substantially at the long interval. Thus, the cuing method typically shows results similar to the alternating runs method.

Rubin and Meiran (2005) demonstrated a mixing cost by comparing the task repetition trials for classifying bivalent stimuli (face or clover in red or blue) according to shape or color with single-task blocks in which only one task was performed (e.g., shape). The task stimulus was preceded by the verbal cue

FIGURE 7.6. Example of Meiran's (1996) Cuing Method for Studying Task Switching

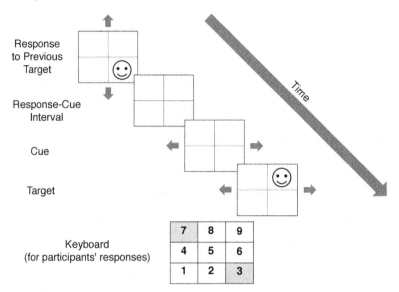

"shape" or "color." With a 1-second cuing interval, which allowed time for preparation, this task showed a mixing cost of 240 ms. A similar difference was not obtained when the irrelevant stimulus dimension varied, but the alternative task was not performed on it.

In Rogers and Monsell's (1995) view, task-set switching depends on two components: a top-down control component and a bottom-up component in which the imperative stimulus triggers the appropriate task set (as reflected in the residual switch costs). Other researchers have argued that residual switch costs reflect a failure to fully discard or inhibit the previous task set (Mayr & Keele, 2000). Common assumptions in models of task-set switching are that (a) task set depends on a configuration of processing pathways or modules in the brain through which some operations are facilitated and others inhibited and thus reflects the degree of "readiness" to perform a task, and (b) the processing system stays in this state of readiness until it is switched again. However, as we have already begun to see, these assumptions are often violated.

The most problematic finding for the view that task set can be preconfigured is that, as noted, even predictable, well-prepared switches show residual switch costs (e.g., Arbuthnott & Frank, 2000). Moreover, the costs are still evident when an alerting signal is presented immediately before the target stimulus to which a response is required. D. W. Schneider (2017) compared conditions with a 2,000-ms interval between the onset of a task cue and the target stimulus that either contained a visual alerting signal 500 ms before the target onset or did not contain one. Although the alerting signal reduced reaction times, the residual switch effect was equally large in the alert and no-alert conditions. Although foreknowledge allows preparation for both repeated and switched tasks, repeating the same task has benefits over task switching regardless of foreknowledge, even when there is plenty of opportunity for preparation.

The suggestion that both attentional control and automatic activation play roles in task switching is consistent with the finding that people cannot "plan away" all switch costs. Attentional control can determine which task will be performed, but readiness to perform the task (and, thus, reaction time) depends on more automatic processes of inhibition and activation from prior trials. One such idea about residual costs in task-set switching is that they primarily reflect competition from earlier stimulus-response mappings. This could be the case whenever the two tasks use the same stimuli but require different responses, although competition may only be a problem when there is a meaning-related similarity between the relevant stimulus dimensions for the two tasks (see Meiran, 2000, for a model that addresses these issues).

For example, Allport and Wylie (2000) reported a series of experiments using Stroop-type stimuli in which participants had to switch between naming the color of the ink in which the color words were printed and reading the color word itself. One finding of note from these experiments was that reading times were greatly increased when the word-reading task had been preceded by the color-naming task. This effect was even more pronounced when the particular word to be read had previously appeared as a color to be named. The size of this negative transfer from the naming-colors to the reading-words task was largest on the first trial of the word-reading blocks of trials. Reading times on the first trial of a block were still relatively long even after several blocks of word-reading trials. This "restart" effect may reflect a general need to reinstate the stimulus-response mapping (e.g., to retrieve it from memory) for the task after any sort of interruption. Thus, traditional estimates of switching costs may be too high: Switching seems certain to contain restart costs and may also reflect negative transfer.

Limitation in the Ability to Prepare or Failure to Engage?

Although most researchers attribute residual switch costs to a limitation in ability to prepare fully for a new task before the presentation of the first stimulus, de Jong (2000) proposed a model that attributes the residual switching costs to a failure to take advantage of opportunities for advance preparation. Unlike accounts of residual switching according to which preparation cannot be completed until the next stimulus appears (e.g., Rogers & Monsell, 1995), de Jong proposed that residual switch costs are due primarily to a "failure to engage" in advance preparation for an upcoming task. Whereas according to an exogenous triggering account, residual switch costs should be present on all switch trials, the failure-to-engage account predicts that residual switch costs should only be observed on trials for which performers fail to prepare for the new task. Because, according to this latter account, the results of any experiment will contain a mixture of prepared and unprepared responses, the results should be able to be modeled by what is called a *mixture distribution*. In a mixture distribution, a distribution of reaction times is assumed to reflect the combined result of two different underlying processes (in this case, a process producing prepared responses and a process producing unprepared responses).

The details of how such a distribution can be fitted are described by de Jong (2000), but the general idea is to estimate the response times for prepared and unprepared trials and then estimate the number of trials in which participants were or were not prepared. An estimate of prepared response time is available by looking at the mean reaction time (RT) on nonswitch trials. An estimate of unprepared response time can be found by looking at switch RTs for trials with little time for preparation (i.e., with a short response–stimulus interval [RSI]). The next step in evaluating the failure-to-engage model is to look at the entire distribution of RTs. This is done by rank ordering all RTs from fastest to slowest and averaging the RTs in each decile (i.e., per 10% of trials) of the distribution. According to the model, very short RTs (e.g., the RTs in the first decile of the RT distribution) for switch trials with long preparation intervals should be just as fast as the fast RTs on nonswitch trials. This is because fast RTs can be assumed to reflect that part of the distribution of RTs that is primarily made up of prepared trials. Because unprepared RTs are longer than prepared RTs, long RTs (e.g., in the 10th decile) should consist mainly (or only) of unprepared RTs and thus be just as slow as RTs in the unprepared (short-RSI) condition. As shown in Figure 7.7, the fast part of the RT distribution for switch trials with a long preparation interval does indeed resemble the distribution of prepared (no-switch) RTs, whereas the slow part of the distribution approaches the distribution of unprepared RTs.

Although it is difficult to distinguish the all-or-none preparation view of de Jong (2000) from the view that preparation can vary in amount (see the exchange between Lien, Ruthruff, et al., 2005, and Lindsen & de Jong, 2010),

FIGURE 7.7. The Cumulative Probability Distributions for Nonswitch, Short-RSI Switch, and Long-RSI Switch Trials From De Jong (2000)

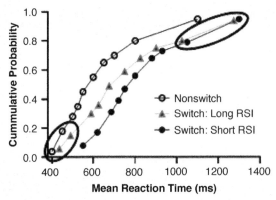

Note. RSI = response-stimulus interval; RT = reaction time. As predicted by the model, RTs of the fastest long-RSI switch trials resemble those of nonswitch trials (lower left); the longer RTs resemble those of the short-RSI trials (upper right). From *Attention: Theory and Practice* (p. 170), by A. Johnson and R. W. Proctor, 2004, SAGE (https://doi.org/10.4135/9781483328768). Copyright 2004 by A. W. Johnson and R. W. Proctor. Adapted with permission.

the evidence tends to be counter to the all-or-none view (Kiesel et al., 2010). For example, an alerting cue should enable the person to prepare on all trials, eliminating the residual switch cost, but it does not (D. W. Schneider, 2017). Koch et al. (2018) pointed out that the mixing costs on task repetition trials also provide evidence that participants are not as prepared to perform the task within the task-switch context as they are if it is the only task performed.

Task Switching in Auditory Selection

We close the discussion of task switching with the mention of a few studies showing that switch costs also occur in the auditory modality. Koch et al. (2011) examined the control of auditory selective attention in a dichotic listening task. Participants were to respond to one of two simultaneously presented number words, one spoken by a female and the other by a male, by performing a numerical size categorization. A visual cue before stimulus onset specified the gender of the task-relevant speaker. The results showed performance costs on trials for which there was a gender switch from the prior trial. Switch costs decreased as the interval between the cue and the number words increased. Interference occurred when the numerical categories for the auditory stimuli were competing, suggesting continued processing of task-relevant information that often leads to responding to the incorrect stimulus. These results imply that there is substantial inertia in intentional control of auditory selection.

Fels et al. (2016) noted that an acoustic scene in natural listening is much more complex than dichotic listening. Therefore, they conducted a similar experiment with a modified paradigm using binaural presentation based on individuals' head-related transfer functions (the acoustic cues at the location of ears created by reflectance off the head). This allowed the presentation of the words at two of eight possible locations arranged in a circle around the azimuth (horizontal plane). Even with this larger number of locations, the effects of attention shift and congruency were comparable to those reported by Koch et al. (2011). In another study, older adults showed longer reaction times and higher error rates than younger adults, but the influence of the spatial switch of the target-speaker was similar for the two groups (Oberem et al., 2017). The congruity effect was also larger for older adults. Thus, the ability to switch auditory attention intentionally to a new cued location was unimpaired, but the older adults had more difficulty suppressing the distractor's speech.

Finally, Eben et al. (2020) examined negative priming in dichotic number judgment tasks like those of Koch et al. (2011). Their experiments included a negative priming condition (in which the distractor on one trial becomes the target on the next), a competitor priming condition (in which the target becomes the distractor), and a no priming condition (in which neither the target nor distractor was related to the previous trial). Results showed longer reaction times for switch trials compared with repetition trials (attention switch costs)—that is, when the internal processing context changed. Reaction times were longer for negative priming trials, but negative priming was not affected by attention switches or decreased switch costs at longer intervals between the response on one trial and the cue on the next. This result suggests that negative priming in auditory attention switching is not sensitive to context or time.

INTENTIONAL CONTROL AND MULTITASKING

Two essential elements in multitasking are keeping current goals active and remembering what to do in the current situation and the future. Such "executive" functions have been attributed to the prefrontal cortex (Yuan & Raz, 2014). Stuss et al. (1995) conducted a study to identify components of the attentional system. They analyzed attentional tasks based on Norman and Shallice's (1986) supervisory control model (described in Chapter 11, this volume), from which they identified five potential component processes related to the attentional system of the prefrontal cortex (Burgess & Stuss, 2017): energizing schemas, inhibiting schemas, adjusting contention scheduling, monitoring goal fulfillment, and exerting control through if–then logic.

Stuss and colleagues (1995) designed a battery of tests to investigate these potential components, called the Rotman-Baycrest Battery to Investigate Attention. The results of numerous studies narrowed the processes from five to three, each of which was related to an anatomically distinct frontal area (Burgess & Stuss, 2017; Stuss & Alexander, 2007). These are *energization*, the process responsible for initiating and sustaining responses, which is linked to the superior medial region; *task setting*, the process responsible for implementing a set to perform a specified task by responding to certain target stimuli with appropriate responses, associated with the left lateral region; and *monitoring*, or checking a task over time, a function of the right lateral region. Note that "inhibiting schemas" was eliminated as a function of the prefrontal lobes. This change is because the performance of the Stroop and related tasks showed that incongruent trials produce activation mainly in the anterior cingulate cortex, which has connections with the left lateral prefrontal region associated with task setting (Floden et al., 2011; see also Box 5.1 in Chapter 5, this volume).

Attention and Skill

According to James (1890/1950), "Habit diminishes the conscious attention with which our acts are performed" (p. 114). Performance becomes automatic in the sense of becoming independent of attentional control. There are two sides to the withdrawal of attention as actions become skilled: reductions in capacity demands, such that skilled operations can operate without experiencing interference from or causing interference to other ongoing operations, and independence of voluntary control, in that, once started, automatic operations run to completion. In some cases, automatic operations also seem to operate outside of conscious awareness.

Automaticity

In terms of resource views of attention, in which attention is viewed as a limited-capacity resource (or, in multiple-resource views, as a collection of limited-capacity attentional resources), two tasks can only be performed together to the extent that sufficient attentional resources are available. Both single- and multiple-resource views imply that if one of two tasks is automatized, such that it does not require any attentional resources, it should be possible to perform the two tasks simultaneously with little or no cost, even if they initially placed overwhelming demands on a common resource. One impressive demonstration of the bypassing of attentional limitations was reported by Allport et al. (1972), who found that skilled pianists showed almost no decrement in playing sight-read music (which should be highly automatized for them) when the requirement to shadow auditorily presented words was added.

For another example of the effects of automatization on dual-task performance, consider the tasks of reading while copying down auditorily presented words or sentences. Although reading is highly automatized, it proceeds more slowly in this dual-task context than when it is done in isolation (Hirst et al., 1980). However, after several weeks of extensive practice, people who practice reading while copying down text have been shown to be able to read equally fast in the dual- and single-task contexts. To test the hypothesis that reading while taking dictation is a skill and not dependent on the specific sort of material read, Hirst et al. (1980) tested the ability of people to read while taking dictation with two types of reading material: short stories and encyclopedia articles. One of the materials was introduced after the other once the performance criterion with one type of material had been met. Excellent transfer to the new type of text was found, suggesting that a general skill at reading while taking dictation had been acquired.

Another impressive illustration of overcoming apparent processing limitations is Underwood's (1974) comparison of the performance of a skilled shadower (the attention researcher Neville Moray) with that of average performers on a dichotic listening task (see Chapter 4, this volume). In this task, which had originally led to the view of the human as a single-channel processor of limited capacity, Moray was able to detect 66.7% of digit targets embedded among letters in the nonshadowed message—nearly seven times as many as that normally found.

On the basis of such results, Spelke et al. (1976) concluded that there are no general limits to attentional skills, and because people are able to develop specialized skills for particular tasks, it may not be possible to identify overall limits on cognitive capacity. However, some researchers have argued the improvements in skill seen in studies like Hirst et al.'s (1980), although impressive, should not be overstated (e.g., Broadbent, 1982). For example, more errors were made in that study when taking dictation while reading than when taking dictation alone.

In most studies of the ability to divide attention across ongoing tasks (or information channels), there is no hard evidence that either task was completely automatized (e.g., Allport et al., 1972; Spelke et al., 1976; Underwood, 1974). In particular, it cannot be ruled out that the primary skill developed by participants in these studies was switching attention between the two tasks (as suggested by Broadbent, 1982; Shaffer, 1975; Welford, 1980). Although switching takes time, it is plausible to suppose that responses to one task can be buffered, and this buffering provides the participant with the chance to select information or responses on the other task. The presence of response buffers (which are assumed to queue both responses and the instructions for emitting the responses) provides the participant with the opportunity to switch central processing resources between the tasks while still giving the impression of continuous performance on both tasks (see Pashler, 1998, for a detailed description of how this might work).

The effects of automaticity on multiple-task performance were tested in a more strictly controlled study by W. Schneider and Fisk (1982). W. Schneider and Fisk used a combination of visual search tasks to examine whether two tasks could be carried out without time-sharing costs when one of them is automatized. They combined a task in which automaticity would be expected to develop (i.e., a visual search task with consistent mapping of items to either the target or distractor sets) with a task in which automaticity would not be expected to develop due to a varied mapping of items to the target and distractor sets. Both tasks were practiced in isolation, with periodic dual-task test sessions in which participants had to monitor two search displays (although only either a consistently mapped or a variably mapped target occurred on any particular trial), and instructions emphasized attending to the varied-mapping task.

It was found that the performance of the consistent-mapping task, in which automaticity had developed as a result of practice, was initially worse in the dual-task condition than in the single-task condition. This finding demonstrates that automatized processes are not entirely immune to interference (e.g., Neumann, 1987). However, with practice in the dual-task setting, the performance of the consistent-mapping task improved to the level of the single-task condition, as did that of the varied-mapping task. Because varied-mapping performance should still be sensitive to available resources, it can be argued that the relative improvement with the varied mapping in the dual-task context was due to a freeing up of resources as the consistently mapped task became automatized. This hypothesis is supported by the results of subsequent experiments in which participants were told to emphasize the consistent-mapping task, which otherwise would be performed without devoting attention to it. In this case, the performance of the varied-mapping task deteriorated in the dual-task context. Hoffman et al. (1983) argued that visual attention is not freed up after large amounts of consistent practice. They found that when a search task that was supposedly automatized was combined with a visual discrimination task, interference between the two tasks was found. Thus, visual attention was still required in the skilled search task.

A Closer Look at Dual-Task Performance

The task-set switching effects discussed earlier in this chapter suggest that it is not possible to prepare fully two separate tasks at the same time. In fact, when people are asked to prepare and execute two tasks at more or less the same time, responses to one or both of the tasks are typically slower than when the respective tasks are performed in isolation. Koch and colleagues (2018) noted this similarity between task switching and performance of dual tasks and provided some evidence to suggest that common cognitive control mechanisms may underlie performance in both paradigms (Hirsch et al., 2018).

Two types of methods have been used to study dual-task performance (Koch et al., 2018). In one, dual-task performance is compared with single-task performance. For example, Huestegge et al. (2014) used left- or right-pointing arrows or left or right tone location stimuli paired with corresponding left or right saccadic eye-movement or "left" or "right" vocal responses. Each combination of stimulus-response modality was performed in single-task trial blocks and dual-task blocks in which congruent responses in both modalities to the same stimulus were required. Results showed dual-response costs in reaction times for saccades and vocal responses of similar size for both stimulus modalities. Because the use of a single stimulus and congruent response relations should have precluded perceptual and memory-related processes for the observed dual-task interference, the authors concluded that it was mainly due to what they called *late central processes*, in which a selected spatial response code is linked to a specific response modality.

The second method is the psychological refractory period (PRP) effect, introduced in Chapter 1, with which a large amount of research has been conducted. The PRP paradigm differs from the first type of method in that two stimuli are presented, each of which requires a response and performance when the interval between stimulus onsets is short is compared with that when the interval is long.

The Psychological Refractory Period Effect

In a typical PRP study, performers are instructed to identify two separate stimuli and make a separate response to each. For example, a high- or low-pitch tone might be followed by a white square shown on the left or right side of the display. The participant's task is to press one response key to indicate whether the tone was high or low in pitch and another response key to indicate whether the square was on the right or left. A robust finding is that reaction time to the second stimulus (the square's location, in this example) is longer than when that stimulus is presented alone. Furthermore, the increase in reaction time is a decreasing function of the interval between the two stimuli. That is, when the interval between the presentations of the two stimuli (i.e., the stimulus onset asynchrony [SOA]) is short, the reaction time to the second stimulus is greater than when the SOA is long. This slowing of the response to the second stimulus is known as the PRP effect (M. C. Smith, 1967; Vince, 1948).

The PRP effect reflects a limitation in the ability to perform two tasks at once. Questions of interest from the information-processing perspective are how and where (and why) these limitations occur. The answers to these questions are still debated, but as discussed later in this section, many researchers agree that the limitation arises relatively late in information processing. The accounts differ, though, in terms of how late the limitation is placed and how much processing precedes it, whether the bottleneck requires serial processing or is more generally of limited capacity, and whether it is an aspect of the cognitive architecture or a consequence of a strategy implemented to control behavior to conform to the task requirements.

The Response-Selection Bottleneck Model

Most accounts of the PRP effect assume that the slowing of the response to the second stimulus occurs because there is some point in the information-processing sequence at which only one stimulus at a time can be processed. Welford (1952) and Davis (1957) proposed that there was indeed a bottleneck in dual-task performance and that this bottleneck was located at response selection. According to this model, the stimuli for two tasks can be processed in parallel, but selecting the appropriate response for Task 2 cannot occur until the response to Task 1 has been selected. The bottleneck model was inspired by the finding that the slope of the function relating Task 2 RT (RT2) to the interval between the onsets of the two stimuli tended to be linear with a slope of −1.0. Thus, it seemed that RT2 could be captured by a model in which (when the SOA is less than or equal to the RT to the first stimulus) $RT2 = RT_n + RT1 - SOA$, where RT_n refers to the time to perform Task 2 in isolation, and RT1 is the mean RT to Task 1. That RT2 is sometimes prolonged even when the SOA is longer than RT1 was explained by Welford as due to the need to process proprioceptive information about the Task 1 response.

Since the introduction of the response-selection bottleneck model, techniques have been developed to test hypotheses about the existence and location of any bottlenecks in dual-task performance. The locus of any processing bottlenecks can be determined by selectively influencing the time it takes to complete the stages involved in performing each task. A pioneering technique for interpreting the effects of selectively influencing stages of processing, Sternberg's (1969) additive factors method, was introduced in Chapter 2. However, it is not always the case that processes are to be carried out in series, as assumed by the additive factors method. In fact, the finding that RT2 in a dual-task situation is often less than RT1 + RT2 when the two tasks are performed in isolation shows that the dual-task condition can result in a savings in total time to do the two tasks and therefore suggests that some parallel processing occurs.

According to the response-selection bottleneck model, the arrangement of processes in a dual-task looks like that depicted in Figure 7.8. Starting and stopping points for each process are shown by the small dark circles (which

FIGURE 7.8. Response-Selection Bottleneck Model

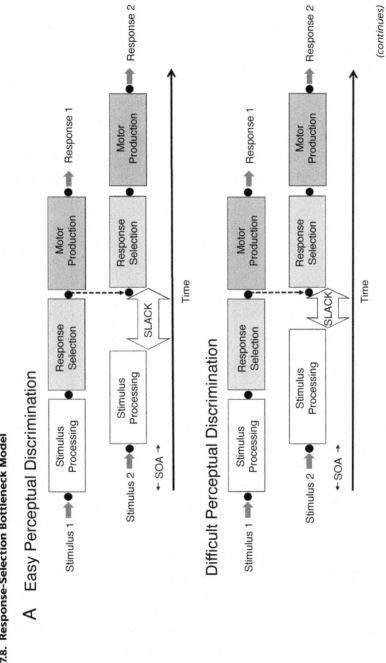

A   Easy Perceptual Discrimination

Difficult Perceptual Discrimination

(continues)

FIGURE 7.8.   Response-Selection Bottleneck Model (*Continued*)

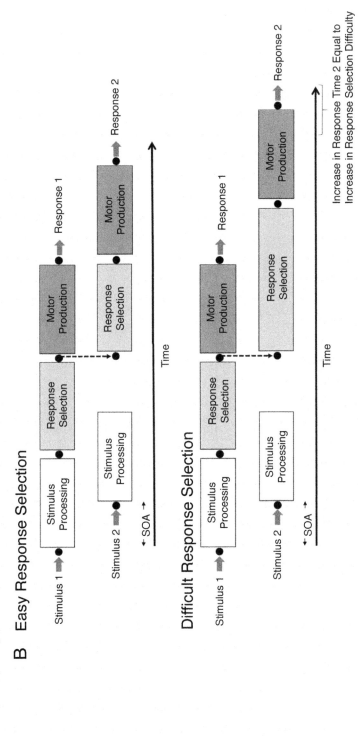

Note. The vertical arrow from Task 1 to Task 2 indicates that Task 2 response selection cannot begin until Task 1 response selection is finished. SOA = stimulus onset asynchrony.

overlap when the end of one process coincides with the beginning of the next). Stimulus and response processing can occur in parallel in this model, but as shown by the arrow from Task 1 to Task 2, response selection for Task 2 cannot be carried out until the response to the first stimulus has been selected.

A key construct for analysis of the response-selection bottleneck model is *slack* (Schweickert, 1978), the time during which task information is not being processed. Slack implies a "downtime" in information processing caused by the need to wait for a bottleneck to be opened. According to the response-selection bottleneck model, slack occurs for Task 2 when the time to identify the Task 1 stimulus and select the response is greater than the SOA plus the time to identify the second stimulus (see Figure 7.8, panel A). Increasing the difficulty of stimulus identification for Task 2 reduces the amount of slack in the network because of the increased identification time. Thus, there will be no observable effect on RT2 until the slack is used up. Because there is no slack in the system after Task 2 response selection begins (see Figure 7.8, panel B), factors influencing Task 2 response-selection difficulty should be additive with SOA.

Pashler and Johnston (1989) had participants respond to low- and high-pitch tones with a left or right key press with the left hand for Task 1 and to a visual letter A, B, or C with a press of one of three fingers on the right hand. The perceptual difficulty for Task 2 was varied by having the letter on any trial be black (easy discrimination) or gray (difficult discrimination) on a white background. SOAs of 50, 100, and 400 ms also varied randomly from trial to trial. Consistent with the response-selection bottleneck model, the effect of reducing discriminability of the Task 2 stimulus, shown at 400-ms SOA, was absent at the 50-ms SOA (see Figure 7.9, left panel).

Another prediction of the bottleneck model is that processes requiring the bottleneck or occurring after it will exert the same effect on RT regardless of the SOA. That is, factors that affect response selection or motor processes should be additive with SOA (see Figure 7.9, right panel). McCann and Johnston (1992) used the PRP paradigm, with Task 1 requiring discrimination of low- and high-pitch tones and Task 2 varying in the compatibility of the mapping of visual stimuli so that response selection would be easy or difficult. Increasing the difficulty of Task 2 response selection by decreasing stimulus-response compatibility resulted in additive effects of compatibility and SOA (see Figure 7.9, right panel), consistent with a bottleneck located at response selection and serial selection of responses in the two tasks.

Modifications of the Response-Selection Bottleneck Model

Distinguishing Response Activation From Response Selection

The response-selection bottleneck model implies that the two tasks in the PRP paradigm are processed in distinct information-processing streams, with the only influence of one task on the other being that response selection for the second task cannot begin until response selection for the first task is completed. However, in the earliest study to use the term "psychological refractory

FIGURE 7.9. Underadditive Effects of Difficulty of Perceptual Discrimination (Pashler & Johnston, 1989) and Additive Effects of Stimulus-Response Mapping (McCann & Johnston, 1992)

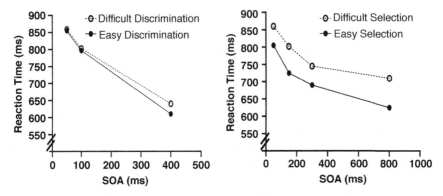

Note. The x-axis is on different scales due to the different stimulus onset asynchronies (SOAs) used in the respective studies. Data from Pashler and Johnston (1989) and McCann and Johnston (1992).

period," Vince (1948) noted the possibility of cross talk between two successive stimuli:

> When a second stimulus is presented within an interval of 0.5 sec. of the first, the beginning of the second response is usually delayed until the completion of the first response, *although there is some evidence that the first response may be modified slightly by the second stimulus* [emphasis added]. (p. 156)

More recent studies have shown that cross talk between the two tasks occurs as a function of the mappings of the stimuli to responses (Hommel, 1998; Lien & Proctor, 2000; Logan & Schulkind, 2000; J. Miller & Durst, 2014). In Hommel's (1998) Experiment 3, a red or green rectangle was presented as the stimulus for Task 1, followed after an SOA of 50, 150, or 650 ms by the stimulus for Task 2, the letter H or S in the same color as the rectangle. For Task 1, participants were to respond to the rectangle color by pressing a left or right key, and for Task 2, they were to respond to the letter identity by saying "red" or "green." The response for Task 2 was conceptually similar to the distinguishing stimulus feature for Task 1. Both Tasks 1 and 2 RT showed cross-talk correspondence effects at the 50-ms SOA, with RT being shorter when the stimulus color for Task 1 corresponded with the response color for Task 2 than when it did not.

Most interest has focused on the backward cross-talk correspondence effect of Task 2 on Task 1 because it implies that some facet of Task 2 responses is activated during Task 1. One way to account for such cross-talk effects is to distinguish subprocesses (response selection, response activation, and response-selection proper), which are not differentiated in the response-selection bottleneck model (Hommel, 1998; Lien & Proctor, 2002). According to this account, stimulus identification and response activation occur in parallel for the two tasks, with the stimulus for one task generating activation in the processing stream for the other task when the tasks are similar, much as for the Stroop and Simon effects in single tasks. The bottleneck in processing is restricted only to the final response selection, requiring that the response for Task 2 cannot be selected until the selection of the response for Task 1 is completed.

J. Miller (2006) showed a similar backward cross-talk effect when Task 2 required a no-go response to one stimulus and a go response to the other. RT to Task 1 was longer on no-go trials for Task 2 than on go trials, suggesting that the "do not respond" signal was leaking through to Task 1 processing. Röttger and Haider (2017) replicated this backward cross-talk effect when the Go/No-go Task 2 was forced choice, as in J. Miller's study, but found only a slight effect for the no-go trials when Task 2 was free choice (i.e., the person decided whether to respond to the stimulus). These results imply that the crucial factor in the slowing of Task 1 responses is whether the Task 2 stimulus explicitly signals not to respond rather than that the response is not selected. The results are consistent with the view that backward cross-talk effects are due to the Task 2 stimulus producing response activation for Task 1.

However, Janczyk et al. (2018) argued against this widely accepted explanation of backward cross-talk effects, providing evidence from a triple-task paradigm suggesting that the backward compatibility effect in their study was not prebottleneck, as the response activation account suggests, nor postbottleneck. Their experiments required two different responses to properties of a second stimulus (R2 to color and R3 to letter identity), with the instruction to make R2 before R3. In one experiment, R2 was a left–right key press and R3 a left–right foot-pedal press. A backward cross-talk effect was evident as faster R2 responses when the R3 response was congruent than when it was incongruent. Because this effect did not interact significantly with SOA, the implication is that it occurred after the bottleneck. Other experiments of Janczyk et al. showed similar results, and still other experiments provided evidence that the locus of the cross-talk effect was not in the motor stage. Consequently, Janczyk et al. concluded that the backward compatibility effect likely has its locus in the capacity-limited stage.

Does Visual Attention Require the Same Bottleneck Mechanism as Response Selection?

Attentional bottlenecks were proposed initially for visual perception, but is visual attention subject to the same bottleneck as is response selection? Reimer et al. (2015) investigated this issue in the PRP paradigm. Task 1 was always a two-choice task (tone-pitch discriminations or color discriminations), and Task 2 was a visual search task requiring the conjunction of visual features to determine whether a target was present or absent. The RT2 analysis revealed an underadditive interaction of SOA and set size, which according to the locus of slack logic, indicates that the performance of visual search occurred simultaneous with Task 1 response selection, regardless of whether that task required pitch or color discrimination.

In a subsequent experiment using tone discrimination for Task 1, Reimer et al. (2017) measured the N2pc event-related potential, which reflects lateralized visual attention processes, in addition to measuring reaction time. If the response selection processes in Task 1 influence the visual attention processes in the Task 2 search task, N2pc latency and amplitude should be delayed and reduced at the short SOAs. However, the N2pc latency and amplitude were uninfluenced by SOA, providing converging evidence with the RT data that visual search operated simultaneously with Task 1 response selection. Thus, visual attention does not seem to require the same bottleneck mechanism as response selection.

Do Ideomotor Compatible Tasks Bypass the Response-Selection Bottleneck?

Greenwald and Shulman (1973) reported a widely cited study from which they concluded, "The psychological refractory period (PRP) effect of interference between 2 choice reaction time tasks at short intertask intervals was eliminated when both of the tasks were ideomotor compatible" (p. 70). *Ideomotor compatibility* refers to tasks in which the stimulus is similar to the sensory feedback from the response. For example, the auditory word *dog* is the sensory feedback from speaking "dog" but not pressing a key. Thus, the spoken response is ideomotor compatible with the stimulus, whereas the key press response is not. In Greenwald and Shulman's study, the ideomotor tasks were to move a switch left or right in response to a left- or right-pointing arrow and speak the letter "A" or "B" in response to the auditory letter A or B. They concluded that Experiment 2 showed no PRP effect, but Experiment 1 showed a statistically significant effect when only RT2 was analyzed, as is standard practice. Moreover, although the concept of ideomotor compatibility seems to imply that the PRP effect should also be eliminated when only one task is ideomotor compatible (because that task bypasses the response-selection bottleneck, leaving it free for the other task), substantial PRP effects were still evident.

In general, the PRP effect has been found in other studies for which one or both tasks could be classified as ideomotor compatible (see Lien & Proctor, 2002, for a review). Lien et al. (2002) conducted four experiments similar to Greenwald and Shulman's (1973) Experiment 2 and obtained a significant PRP effect in all experiments. The reduction of the PRP effect that occurs when Task 1 is ideomotor compatible can be attributed to the bottleneck being "latent" as a consequence of responses for Task 1 being so fast (Lien, McCann, et al., 2005). Although ideomotor compatibility is a factor influencing the magnitude of the PRP effect, its presence for one or both tasks is not sufficient to eliminate the effect when they require discrete responses.

Does Practice Eliminate the Bottleneck?

If the PRP effect results from a fundamental constraint on processing capacity, it would be expected to remain despite long periods of practice. In an early study of the effects of practice on the PRP effect, Gottsdanker and Stelmach

(1971) found that the PRP effect (relative to a single task control) was reduced considerably when extensive practice (lasting 87 days) with one SOA (100 ms) was given. But there was little transfer of this benefit to 50-ms and 200-ms SOAs when several SOAs were randomly intermixed in later sessions. Gottsdanker and Stelmach concluded that the decrease in the PRP effect over the practice was due to a strategy specific to coordinating responses at 100-ms SOA, rather than to a more general improved ability to perform two tasks in rapid succession.

The persistence of the PRP effect has since been demonstrated in a number of experiments using a variety of stimuli, responses, and SOAs. For example, Van Selst et al. (1999) found a large reduction in the PRP effect from 353 to 40 ms over 36 sessions of practice when Task 1 required a vocal response to an auditory stimulus and Task 2 a manual response to a visual stimulus. The reduction in PRP effect with practice was much less when the vocal response for Task 1 was replaced with key presses, like Task 2 (Ruthruff et al., 2001).

One participant in the Van Selst et al. (1999) study showed no PRP effect at the end of practice, but further analysis provided evidence that the bottleneck had not been eliminated but was only latent (Ruthruff et al., 2003). That is, for that participant, reaction times for Task 1 became so short that the bottleneck was no longer occupied when that processing stage was needed for Task 2. Consistent with this interpretation, Ruthruff et al. (2001) provided evidence that the overall reduction in the mean PRP effect with practice in Van Selst et al.'s study was due primarily to improvements in performing Task 1 rather than Task 2. Further, S. J. Thomson et al. (2015) showed that when the duration of the response selection stage in Task 1 was shortened through PRP practice, the size of the backward compatibility effect from Task 2 on Task 1 performance decreased. Those results and others led them to conclude that the backward compatibility effect reflects cross talk of unattended response information for Task 2 acting on the response-selection stage in Task 1. Thus, in general, changes in task performance with practice in the PRP paradigm appear to be due primarily to speeding up Task 1.

A Bottleneck in Response Initiation?

Although evidence for a response-selection bottleneck of some type is compelling, some studies have suggested that there may be additional bottlenecks in performance. For example, not all studies have found additive effects of stimulus-response translation difficulty and SOA. One early study by Karlin and Kestenbaum (1968), the logic of which is described in detail by Keele (1973), manipulated response-selection difficulty for the second task by requiring either a simple or a two-choice reaction. In this study, the number of stimulus–response alternatives had a larger effect at long SOAs than at short SOAs. A model with only one bottleneck—at response selection—cannot explain these results, but as de Jong (1993) showed, the results can be accounted for if there is an additional bottleneck at the stage of response initiation that prevents two responses from being initiated in close succession. Normally, Task 2 response selection lasts longer than Task 1 response initiation, with the result that the response initiation bottleneck is almost always free by the time it is needed for Task 2 processing. However, when Task 2 response selection can be completed quickly (as when there is only one response), the information produced at the response-selection stage may have to wait until the Task 1 response has been initiated before it can be passed along to the motor stage.

De Jong (1993) obtained additional evidence for such a response-initiation bottleneck by combining a go or no-go Task 1 with different second tasks, including simple and choice reaction tasks. He reasoned that the response-initiation bottleneck would not be a factor in performance on no-go trials because no response was required, even though response selection was required to determine whether a response should be made. Thus, any effects of a response-initiation bottleneck should only be apparent on go trials, for which responses for both Task 1 and Task 2 had to be made. Indeed, de Jong found that the difficulty of response selection in Task 2 interacted with SOA on go trials but had additive effects with SOA on no-go trials.

Klapp et al. (2019) presented evidence that the bottleneck is in a process after response selection that is involved in programming the timing of response initiation before responding. They based this hypothesis on two conclusions from recent developments in research. First, studies of the startle response and single-task simple (precued) reaction time indicate that programming the timing of response onsets, which must be delayed until just before responding, is required to enable response initiation. For example, Maslovat et al. (2013) used simple reaction-time tasks requiring a vocal response for Task 1 and a key-lift response for Task 2, with SOAs between 100 and 1,500 ms. The unique aspect of the procedure was that on a few trials, a startling acoustic stimulus occurred simultaneously with the Task 2 stimulus to determine whether it would trigger the response with no cost. However, the PRP effect was evident for both control and startle trials, suggesting that the Task 2 response was not prepared in advance.

Second, studies of concurrent rhythmic movements show that the representation of timing is limited to one temporal frame unless rapid performance enables parallel timing. Evidence that it is not possible to program two temporal codes concurrently comes from studies of rhythmic tapping. Klapp et al. (1998) found that even after training participants to tap different rhythms separately with each hand, they had difficulty tapping the two rhythms concurrently. In other words, they were not able to initiate the responses concurrently. Klapp et al. (2019) made a case that these two limitations, which are general properties of response initiation, combine to produce the PRP bottleneck at the initiation stage of processing.

Alternatives to Architectural Bottleneck Models

No Capacity Limitations
Although the evidence for a true, structural bottleneck in performance is compelling, an argument has been made that the essential aspects of multiple-task performance can be captured by a theoretical framework in which multiple

tasks are executed concurrently, and information processing (including response selection) occurs in parallel (Meyer & Kieras, 1997a, 1997b). Meyer and Kieras's (1997a, 1997b) explanation of the PRP effect is based on an information-processing architecture, the executive-process interactive control (EPIC) framework, which assumes no attentional capacity limitations. Instead, emphasis is placed on executive control functions involved in attentional allocation and task coordination.

Hence, within the EPIC framework, the PRP effect is attributed to a task strategy, specifically one of response deferment for Task 2, without referencing a structural processing bottleneck. According to the strategic response-deferment account, before the start of a trial, the participant adopts a strategy of prioritizing Task 1. In the terminology of the EPIC framework, Task 1 is put into an "immediate" mode, whereas Task 2 is put into a "deferred" mode, for which no information pertaining to response selection will be sent to motor processors. According to this strategic response-deferment view, completion of Task 1 can act as an "unlocking" event that shifts Task 2 to the immediate mode so that motor activation and execution for Task 2 can occur.

Graded Capacity Allocation

A characteristic of the response-selection bottleneck model and the modified version that includes a separate response-activation stage is that response-selection processing is all or none. As long as response selection is performed for one task, it cannot be performed for the other. An alternative view is that although the capacity to perform response selection is limited, it is not necessarily all or none. According to this resource or capacity sharing view, the limited capacity resources required for response selection can be allocated to Task 1 and Task 2 in graded amounts. Detailed analyses of capacity sharing and all-or-none bottleneck models have shown that the capacity sharing models can account for most of the data from the PRP paradigm as well as can the bottleneck models (Navon & Miller, 2002; Tombu & Jolicoeur, 2002, 2005) and thus provide a viable alternative. Moreover, the capacity sharing models predict that RT for Task 1 should increase as SOA increases and should be affected by the difficulty of response selection for Task 2, findings that have been observed in several studies.

From a resource sharing view, serial processing of Task 1 and Task 2 is a strategy that is often adopted because it minimizes the possibility of between-task interference due to cross talk (R. Fischer & Plessow, 2015). However, in some cases, a parallel processing strategy will lead to better performance. J. Miller et al. (2009) performed an optimality analysis suggesting that a serial mode of task performance is more efficient than a parallel mode in many contexts, particularly in the most common PRP methods that include relatively long SOAs. However, they reported results from experiments in which they varied the distribution of SOAs and found evidence of a shift to a more parallel mode as the probability of short SOAs on a trial increases. In other words, with mostly short SOAs, the benefit of allowing parallel rather than serial processing offsets the costs associated with cross talk.

The essential difference between those researchers who favor a response-selection bottleneck account of the PRP effect and those who argue against a fixed bottleneck, therefore, is not whether there is a point in processing at which some operation for the two tasks typically is carried out sequentially but whether this sequential processing is a "built-in" limitation of the basic information-processing architecture or a strategy that participants adopt to comply with the task instructions. The view expressed by de Jong (2000) currently has a lot of adherents:

> Serial organization of activities should perhaps be viewed not as the result of resource scarcity prohibiting a presumably more efficient parallel organization, but as an efficient solution to the problem of getting a powerful parallel processing device, the human brain, to support coherent behavior in environments that provide multiple affordances for action. (p. 357)

CHAPTER SUMMARY

In this chapter, we discussed fundamental limits on performing some aspects of information processing, as well as the way skills in allocating attentional resources can develop. Whether particular tasks can be performed together has been shown to depend on the nature of the tasks, the level of skill attained in each component task, and the relative amount of attention allocated to the respective tasks. People can learn to make trade-offs between certain pairs of tasks that require attentional resources. The ability to time-share is a skill that develops with practice in multiple-task contexts, and if the performance for one of two tasks has been automatized, dual-task performance may show little loss in efficiency.

Although it seems that in multitasking, competing goals can be held active such that different task components can be integrated into smooth performance, some experiments reveal limits on the ability to do two things at once. Even in ostensibly simple tasks such as naming a digit when it is presented on the left in a display and saying whether it is odd or even when presented on the right, people have trouble keeping the instructions straight (i.e., keeping the task goals current). Moreover, when several stimuli, each requiring a speeded response, are presented in close succession, a bottleneck in selecting responses is revealed. Basic limits in doing two or more things at once seem to be a fundamental aspect of human performance.

KEY POINTS

- **Phenomenon:** When dividing attention across messages to the two ears, people often report the stimuli by ear.
- **Fact:** Spatial selectivity and representation tend to predominate.

- **Fact:** Monitoring for multiple targets can be performed effectively, but deficits arise when responding to two targets that occur simultaneously or close in time.

- **Theory:** Unitary resource theories liken attention to a limited-capacity resource that can be devoted to various processes.

- **Theory:** Multiple resource theories liken attention to several distinct pools of resources related to distinctions such as sensory input and type of code.

- **Fact:** Switch costs and mixing costs typically occur when tasks are mixed and can repeat or change from one trial to the next.

- **Fact:** Switch costs can be reduced with time to prepare, but residual switch costs remain.

- **Fact:** The prefrontal lobes of the cerebral cortex are involved in executive control processes.

- **Phenomenon:** The PRP effect is that people are typically slower at responding to a stimulus for a second task when it occurs shortly after the stimulus for a first task.

- **Theory:** The PRP effect is typically attributed to a response-selection bottleneck.

- **Fact:** Some parallel processing occurs between dual tasks as indicated by cross-task cross talk.

- **Fact:** The PRP effect is minimized for ideomotor compatible tasks and highly practiced ones.

- **Theory:** The response-selection bottleneck for dual tasks seems to be a strategic way to optimize task performance rather than an architectural limitation.

8

Memory and Attention

Massaro (1994) noted that two books "set the groundwork for the contemporary study of cognitive psychology and cognitive science" (p. 597). The first was Neisser's (1967) *Cognitive Psychology*, mentioned earlier, and the second was Donald A. Norman's (1969) *Memory and Attention: An Introduction to Human Information Processing*. The latter book makes clear in the title not only that attention is fundamental to human information processing but also that it is closely linked to memory. That link was emphasized again by Nelson Cowan (1997) in his book *Attention and Memory: An Integrated Framework*. Although the connection has been known since at least the dawn of the information-processing revolution, it has become increasingly appreciated (e.g., Logan et al., 2021; Sasin & Fougnie, 2021).

Many of the research findings concerned with attention are, directly or indirectly, dependent on memory. If an observer is able to report what they have seen, we can assume that the information is remembered, however briefly. Sometimes it is difficult to determine whether memory or attention is responsible for a certain effect. For example, some priming effects can be attributed to memory (e.g., semantic priming effects assume the involvement of either an implicit or explicit memory system), whereas others might be attributed to a change in stimulus processing (e.g., a rejected location may be subject to temporary inhibition). This chapter bridges the research on memory and attention, examining in detail the moments at which attention is required for memory and vice versa.

https://doi.org/10.1037/0000317-008
Attention: Selection and Control in Human Information Processing, by R. W. Proctor and K.-P. L. Vu

Without memory, we would be unable to recognize objects, sounds, and smells; experience continuity in an ever-changing world; understand complex sentences; or perform sequences of behavior such as those involved in tying shoelaces or driving a car. Attention plays a prominent role in determining what and how well information is learned immediately and retrieved later. If, while reading this text, your attention is distracted by a conversation being held nearby, you may still be able to read, but your chances of being able to recall what was read decrease. However, if you read a particular segment of the text for a second time, you may recognize parts of it as familiar. These feelings of familiarity indicate that inattention does not always prevent the acquisition of information and that failure to recall information does not necessarily imply that the information has not been stored in memory.

The fact that you may recognize but not recall information indicates that different types of memory tests may be needed to determine whether something was actually stored in memory. Memory tests have in common a learning (or acquisition) phase, during which the to-be-learned information is presented, and a subsequent retrieval phase, during which the learned information is recalled or used in performing a particular task. Also of concern is the extent to which what is learned can transfer to other tasks and contexts (Healy et al., 2014).

One fundamental distinction is between the use of explicit and implicit tests to measure memory (Roediger, 1990). *Explicit* tests rely primarily on declarative knowledge and require a person to intentionally refer to the information presented in the learning phase and report it, as in multiple-choice or essay exams. In contrast, *implicit* tests rely primarily on procedural knowledge and assess memory by showing the effect on the performance of a seemingly unrelated task. For example, an experiment may begin with the task of classifying words as nouns or verbs. An explicit test of memory would ask participants to write down all the words they can remember. An implicit test of memory for these words would have the participants solve anagrams (e.g., "ERTE"). Memory for the words from the learning episode would then be indicated by faster solution times for words (e.g., "TREE") from the prior classification task than for other words. Thus, the primary distinction between explicit and implicit tests is that people intend to retrieve specific information in the former case but not in the latter.

Attention is needed in the forming, retaining, and retrieving of memories. The topics can be organized loosely around Atkinson and Shiffrin's (1968) model of human memory, which is called the *modal model* because it formalized what was known about human memory at that time and continues to provide a framework in which to organize research on memory (Plancher & Barrouillet, 2020). The model distinguishes a sensory register, short-term memory store, and long-term memory store (see Figure 8.1). The first component, more commonly called *sensory memory*, registers incoming information in a sensory format that decays within seconds unless the information is selected and transferred

FIGURE 8.1. Structure of the Memory System in the Modal Model

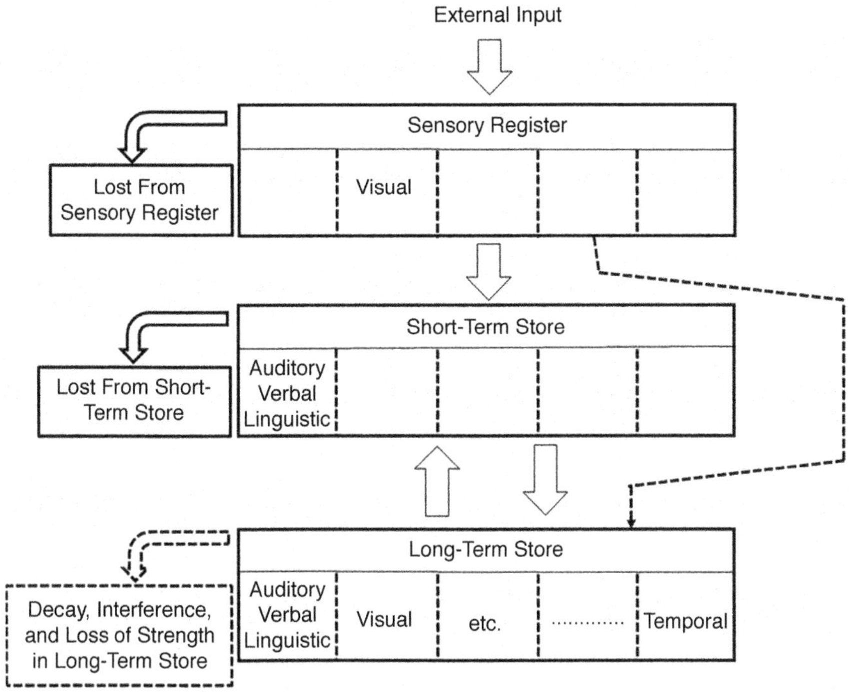

Note. From "Human Memory: A Proposed System and Its Control Processes," by R. C. Atkinson and R. M. Shiffrin, in K. W. Spence and J. T. Spence (Eds.), *The Psychology of Learning and Motivation: Advances in Research and Theory* (Vol. 2, p. 92), 1968, Academic Press/Elsevier. Copyright 1968 by Elsevier. Reprinted with permission.

to the *short-term memory* store. That store is of limited capacity, and the stimuli may be represented in it in a format that is different from the input format (e.g., a visual stimulus may be represented as an auditory name). Information in the short-term store decays within 15 to 30 seconds unless it is maintained through rehearsal. Some of the information in the short-term store is entered into the *long-term memory* store, which is assumed to be relatively permanent but for which the information may lose strength, making it difficult to retrieve.

Attention is incorporated in the modal model through control processes that operate within the constraints of the memory system's architecture. Such processes function on the sensory register by allowing people to select which of two or more simultaneous inputs to process and determine what items are read out from the register into the short-term store. Rehearsal is a crucial control process for the short-term store in governing which items in it are retained versus allowed to decay. The control processes are relevant to memory search, in which the contents of short-term memory must be queried to perform a task. These processes also determine coding, retention, and retrieval of information from the long-term store.

In a 50-year commemorative article, Baddeley et al. (2019) attributed the widespread influence of Atkinson and Shiffrin's (1968) modal model in part to the distinction it made between processes and structure. They concluded,

> The original A&S [Atkinson & Shiffrin] model's well-deserved longevity stems in part from its capacity to crystalize the major advances made in the previous decade in the understanding of human memory and combine them within a well justified theoretical framework, a framework that was broad enough to encompass modifications and additions in the face of new evidence. (p. 584)

In this chapter, we evaluate the extent to which attentional selectivity determines the contents of memory and try to answer the question of whether attentional selection is a prerequisite for remembering information over various periods. Next, we explore how memories of perceived information are formed and stored in such a way that they can be reported. Subsequently, we discuss the attentional demands of the different processes involved in the consolidation and retrieval of previously presented information. The dual-task bottleneck introduced in Chapter 6 is revisited to evaluate whether these processes depend on the same central bottleneck evident in dual-task performance. Finally, we examine the intertwined roles of attention and memory in controlling ongoing behavior, focusing on how they contribute to the adaptability and flexibility of human performance.

SENSORY MEMORY

One way to study the relation among perception, memory, and attention is to design experiments in which information is presented briefly and examine the processes involved in reporting the information. Such research has centered on the amount of information that can be perceived and retained and the rate at which this information decays from memory. As highlighted in the modal model, perceived information may initially be stored in preattentive sensory memory stores from which information that is relevant to current intentions and goals can be selectively attended to. We first discuss the sensory memory research from the visual domain and then turn to a review of auditory sensory memory.

Visual Sensory (Iconic) Memory

Since the work of Hamilton (1859) and Jevons (1871), described in Chapter 1, psychologists have known that the span of apprehension for visual stimuli is limited to four to five items. However, other findings suggested that the actual number processed was larger. Gill and Dallenbach (1926) had three persons trained at introspection rate the clearness of briefly shown displays of various types and numbers of characters. Estimates indicated that array sizes of up to 16, 17, and 35 items for the respective observers were experienced as clear.

In 1960, Sperling devised a method that confirmed objectively that the initial memory for a briefly presented array is closer to what Gill and Dallenbach's

(1926) results suggested. For a briefly flashed 3 × 4 array of letters and digits, he confirmed that whole report averaged four to five items—consistent with the span of apprehension. However, with a partial report procedure, participants were to report only a row of characters in the array, signaled by a high-, middle-, or low-pitch tone. When the cue occurred immediately at display offset, the observers were able to report more than three items on average in the cued row, leading to an estimate of 9.1 stimuli being available. Because the observers did not know in advance which row would be cued, this result shows that almost all the letters were registered and that representations of the letters were available at the time of the cue. At longer intervals between display offset and the cue, this *partial-report superiority effect* disappeared, and performance was no better than with whole report (see Figure 8.2).

The sensory memory store illustrated by partial-report superiority has also been called *iconic memory* (Neisser, 1967). In the standard view, exemplified by the modal model, all items are initially held in the store and then transferred to a more durable short-term store at the time of the cue. According to these assumptions, the relatively small number of items that can be reported in the whole-report condition can be taken to indicate that the transfer process or the durable store is of limited capacity. Sperling (1960) found that increasing the duration of the display from 15 milliseconds (ms) to 500 ms (thus increasing the time available for the transfer of items from the iconic to the durable store) did not affect the number of reported items in a whole-report procedure. Thus, it seems that the locus of this limitation lies in the capacity of the durable store. In contrast, when iconic memory is "erased" by presenting a mask (e.g., rows of Xs) after the letter display, so is the partial-report superiority effect.

The iconic image itself seems to have two stages of representation, a retinal afterimage and a later stage that combines the images from the two eyes (Turvey, 1973). The retinal afterimage is specific to the eye on which the presented information is projected, as is evidenced by the fact that presenting a bright blank field (e.g., a brightness mask) to one eye has no disruptive effect

FIGURE 8.2. Decline in Partial Report Superiority Across Cue Delay

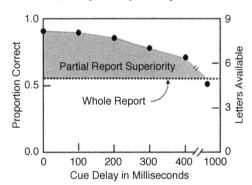

Note. From *Attention: Theory and Practice* (p. 194), by A. Johnson and R. W. Proctor, 2004, SAGE (https://doi.org/10.4135/9781483328768). Copyright 2004 by A. W. Johnson and R. W. Proctor. Reprinted with permission.

on the retinal afterimage retained on the other eye. This early iconic image can be distinguished from a second stage in which the information from both eyes is combined into a single representation that can be used as input for later stages of information processing. Together, these two stages of iconic memory contribute to a memory system that has a relatively large capacity (based on partial report superiority) but a short duration (based on the disappearance of the partial-report superiority effect within less than 1 second).

The partial-report procedure has also been used to assess the level of processing achieved by the information retained in iconic memory. The success of location cues (Sperling, 1960) in increasing the proportion of letters reported indicates that the location of the items is represented in the iconic image. The effectiveness of a number of other cue types has been investigated. Some studies examined whether a difference in color or brightness between the to-be-reported items and the distractor items would result in a partial-report advantage, even though the target items were randomly positioned in the display. In this case, items are originally presented in different colors or luminances, and the cue indicates which items should be reported (e.g., a high tone might be the cue to report the items that were presented in red). Studies using color and luminance to differentiate target and distractor items consistently reveal a partial-report superiority effect (e.g., Van der Heijden, 1992). When the targets and distractors are distinguished by category (e.g., report letters and ignore digits), the results are less consistent. In general, selection by category is only effective when participants know beforehand which category of items should be reported (e.g., Bundesen et al., 1984; Duncan, 1983).

One can ask whether distinct attributes of objects are lost from iconic memory at similar rates. Yi et al. (2018) presented participants with circular displays of eight colored numbers for which they were to remember either color or number in distinct trial blocks. A visual cue signaled the location at which the attribute was to be reported at delays varying from 0 to 1,000 ms. The color attribute was reportable at longer delays than the numerical identity. This result suggests that the attributes that compose an object become unavailable in iconic memory at different rates, possibly due to complexity differences.

Typically, iconic memory has been considered a passive store outside of awareness in which attention plays the role of reading out items into a more durable form. The iconic memory itself has been thought not to demand attention. However, because the observer is attending to the briefly presented display in a typical iconic memory experiment, it is possible that attention could be involved. A debate has emerged as to whether iconic memory requires attention. A study by Persuh et al. (2012) was the first to implicate attention in iconic memory. They had participants perform a visual search task on an array of eight circles inside a larger circular region of the display, centered on fixation (see Figure 8.3). A surrounding array of eight rectangles, each oriented vertically or horizontally, appeared 50 ms after the onset of the circles, and both arrays went off 200 ms later, at which time a yellow bar designated one of the rectangle locations for which the observer was to report the orientation of the rectangle. The idea was to have participants engaged in the visual search

FIGURE 8.3. The Procedure Used by Persuh et al. (2012)

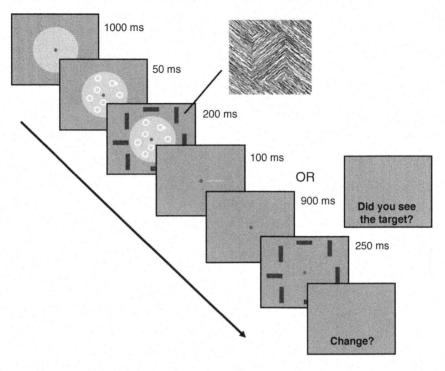

Note. From "Iconic Memory Requires Attention," by M. Persuh, B. Genzer, and R. D. Melara, 2012, *Frontiers in Human Neuroscience*, 6, Article 126, p. 3 (https://doi.org/10.3389/fnhum.2012.00126). CC BY-NC 3.0.

task when the rectangle stimuli for the iconic memory task were presented. Partial report of orientation was relatively accurate when the search task was easy, but it was at chance levels when the search task was difficult. This dependence of partial report accuracy on the amount of attention required for the search task led to the conclusion that the role of attention is more than one of just the transfer from iconic to working memory stores.

Mack et al. (2015, 2016) followed up the study of Persuh et al. (2012) with more compelling results also suggesting that iconic memory demands attention. They conducted a study using the whole versus partial report task of letters in a 3 × 2 matrix. As in the prior experiment, they manipulated attention to the visual array by pairing it with a second task, visual search, that was easy (e.g., find a red circle among green circles) or difficult (among red or green bisected circles, find an oppositely colored one). Only one of the tasks had to be performed on any trial, and the probability of which task was to be performed was varied. When attention was maximally diverted from the array, participants averaged reporting less than a single item, supporting the conclusion that iconic memory requires attention.

Mack et al. (2016) went further. After presenting a series of trials of which 90% were postcued for search and only 10% for partial report, the first nine of the final 10 trials preceding the last were visual search. The last trial was cued for partial report, but no array of letters was presented. However, eight of 15 participants were unaware that the letters on the critical trial were absent, with some trying to report illusory letters. Commentaries between Aru and Bachmann (2017) and Mack et al. (2018) have discussed how to interpret the results of seeing letters that are not in the display, but the results provide evidence that the iconic image of the visual display demands attention if items in it are to be perceived.

Auditory Sensory (Echoic) Memory

The discovery of visual sensory memory led to the question of whether such a sensory memory register also exists for auditory information. Recollect that Broadbent (1958) had already postulated such a memory in his filter theory. Many studies have explored auditory sensory memory, called *echoic memory* (Neisser, 1967), and indicate that there are broad similarities between visual and auditory sensory memory. Analogous to the visual modality, two separate forms of early auditory memory can be distinguished (Cowan, 1984). The first form of auditory sensory memory appears to reflect an ear-specific representation of the physical characteristics of the stimulus (Deatherage & Evans, 1969). This representation can be thought of as an "echo" of the heard information that may last 150 to 350 ms after the auditory stimulation has been terminated. The second form of auditory sensory storage is a representation of information that was previously heard, which may last up to several seconds. In contrast to the initial ear-specific echo, this representation combines the input from both ears and may store multiple items at the same time (Glucksberg & Cowan, 1970).

With regard to the first form, Inui et al. (2010) examined whether a single presentation of a sound can elicit a change-related cortical response, shaping a memory trace enough to separate a subsequent stimulus. Two 300-ms sounds of 800 or 840 Hz were presented in a fixed order at an equal probability, and cortical responses were measured. Sounds were grouped such that a sound was preceded by one, two, or three different sounds or one or two same sounds. The superior temporal gyrus showed greater activation for the different events than the same event, even with only one prior different tone. Thus, a single presentation of a sound was enough to generate a memory trace for comparison with a following physically different sound and elicit a change-related cortical response in the superior temporal gyrus.

Kinukawa et al. (2019) confirmed those results using a procedure like that of Inui et al. (2010) but employing sounds that arrived at the two ears at different times to rule out peripheral factors to the change-related cortical responses. Their results showed a difference in amplitude of the evoked cortical responses for a single prior different stimulus compared with a single same stimulus, implying that one presentation of the sound was sufficient to store the information. No difference in amplitude was found for the second or third of three same stimuli after the different one, implying that the sensory memory of the prior different stimulus was replaced immediately when the brain detected a different sound.

In an attempt to apply the partial-report procedure to auditory sensory memory, Moray et al. (1965) devised an experiment in which participants were presented with four sequences of consonants at a rate of two items per second, with each sequence being presented from a different location (one sequence in front of the participant, one behind, and the other two to the left and right of the participant). In the whole-report conditions, participants were asked to report as many consonants as possible. In the partial-report condition, participants were first presented with the sequences and afterward cued to report the consonants presented from just one location. Although a partial-report superiority effect was observed, it was smaller than that found with visual stimuli. One reason for the relatively small partial-report advantage may be that the location cue used to differentiate between the different sequences may not be as effective in segregating auditory information as it is for visual information (Pashler, 1998). Instead, auditory attention may be more easily directed according to properties such as pitch and frequency than location because of the low spatial resolution of the auditory system (e.g., Scharf & Buus, 1986).

In addition to confirming a significant partial-report superiority effect for auditory information, other studies in which the temporal interval between the offset of the auditory stimulation and the presentation of the cue was varied showed that the advantage for partial report could last as long as 5 seconds, much longer than for visual stimuli (Darwin et al., 1972). Norman (1969) used a dichotic listening task to show that auditory information can be retrieved for several seconds after its presentation. In one experiment, participants were presented with two messages, one to each ear, and were instructed to shadow (i.e., repeat out loud) one of the messages. When asked to report what had been presented to the unattended ear, participants showed virtually no memory for the unattended message. However, when the presentation of the messages was interrupted, and participants were immediately asked to report two digits that had been presented to the unattended ear, they were able to do this accurately. Using a similar procedure, Glucksberg and Cowan (1970) found that the digits presented to the unattended ear could be reported for up to 5 seconds after presentation.

Summing Up

Much evidence supports the existence of memory systems that represent and briefly maintain information generated in the early stages of processing. This information must be attended to, or it is quickly lost. These systems exist in the auditory and visual sensory modalities, and for both modalities, they can be fractionated into ear- or eye-specific sensory aftereffects and a later representation of the combined input from both sensory organs. Evidence that we have not covered in the chapter indicates that sensory memory stores also exist for the senses of touch, taste, and smell (Barker & Weaver, 1983; Bliss et al., 1966; Drewing & Lezkan, 2021). Sensory memory is characterized by a large capacity, susceptibility to masking, and a short life span. By extending the persistence of sensory input, the sensory stores increase the time for attention to select specific items for later processing.

SHORT-TERM AND WORKING MEMORY

Atkinson and Shiffrin (1968) described the short-term memory store as an auditory–verbal–linguistic store because most memory research at the time used verbal materials. Materials were coded in this type of format, even if they were presented visually, and the emphasis was on rehearsal to retain the information active in short-term memory. Atkinson and Shiffrin briefly noted that the short-term store "may be regarded as the subject's 'working memory'" (p. 10). This term has since come to be widely used because it refers to a memory system that holds information relevant to current goals and activities (Postle & Oberauer, in press). The adjective "working" implies that this kind of memory, in contrast to the sensory memory stores, encompasses more than just passive storage of information. *Working memory* can be defined as a system that holds mental representations temporarily for use in cognitive tasks that include understanding, thinking, learning, and action (Baddeley, 1998b; Cowan, 2017; Oberauer et al., 2018). It differs from long-term memory, which is a person's more or less permanent collection of facts, knowledge, and records of experienced events.

Baddeley and Hitch's Working Memory Model

A working memory model proposed initially by Baddeley and Hitch (1974) was dominant for many years and is often just called "the" Working Memory Model. It consists of three components: a visuospatial sketchpad, a phonological (or articulatory) loop, and a central executive (see Figure 8.4). The visuospatial sketchpad and phonological loop are stores that are often described as helper systems. The phonological loop is called on to store and manipulate speech-based information, whereas the visuospatial sketchpad is responsible for storing

FIGURE 8.4. Baddeley and Hitch's (1974) Model of Working Memory

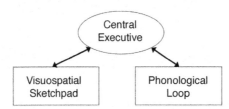

and manipulating visual images. The central executive is an attentional controller that is presumed to supervise and coordinate the work of the two stores.

The Phonological Loop

The *phonological loop* is thought to represent information according to how it sounds. This has implications for measuring memory span (the number of items that can be correctly repeated back 50% of the time) and information processing. People can accurately report back more phonologically dissimilar items than similar items. If memory span for dissimilar words (e.g., mat, fir, nut) is seven items, memory span for phonologically similar words (e.g., top, pop, shop) may be only five items (e.g., Conrad & Hull, 1964). Memory will also be impaired if recall is accompanied by spoken syllables, even when the syllables are irrelevant and should be ignored. It seems that the presentation of speech or speech-like sounds directly interferes with the information held in the phonological loop, and the more similar it is in sound, the greater the interference (e.g., Salamé & Baddeley, 1987).

The phonological loop is unable to deal with multiple sources of conflicting information, indicating that it has limited capacity for processing information. Maintaining the information in the store was postulated to be through subvocal, verbal rehearsal. Requiring participants to repeat a word like "the" or "racket" throughout a trial until a recall signal (a procedure called *articulatory suppression*) impaired performance in short-term memory tasks and seemed to prevent visually presented words from being converted into phonological codes (Murray, 1968). Other research has provided evidence that at least some phonological coding of written words can occur; participants can make rhyme and homophone judgments under conditions of articulatory suppression at better than chance levels (Besner et al., 1981; Norris et al., 2018).

Also, memory span has been shown to depend on the amount of time it takes to pronounce the items that are to be remembered. The more time it takes to pronounce an item (because of the speaker's rate of speech, language used, or type of item), the fewer items can be remembered (e.g., Schweickert & Boruff, 1986). In general, people remember the number of verbal items they can pronounce within about 1.8 seconds (Ricker et al., 2020).

The role of the phonological loop in performing various tasks has also been explored by loading it with words to be remembered and then testing people's ability to perform other tasks. Using concurrent loading tasks or secondary tasks that are thought to interfere selectively with verbal or spatial memory or demand attention, it is possible to investigate whether these different memory processes draw on the same mechanisms or resources. For example, an assumption of the model that has been confirmed is that attentionally demanding tasks will place much more demands on the central executive processes than will tasks that require only maintenance in one of the stores (Baddeley, 2012).

However, even when the phonological loop is heavily loaded, people are still able to comprehend and learn new information (see Baddeley, 1998a; Baddeley

& Hitch, 2019, for reviews). Baddeley and Hitch (2019) described experiments in which they found that a concurrent memory load of six digits or more disrupted a second task involving prose comprehension or long-term learning, but a considerable amount of comprehension and learning was still evident. Thus, although the phonological loop seems crucial for holding and manipulating verbal information, it is only one part of the working memory system. Complex behavior (e.g., solving arithmetic problems while remembering a list of digits) depends heavily on attentional allocation strategies. Keeping information current in the phonological loop requires rehearsal, and rehearsal would seem to require attention. With practice, however, one can learn how long rehearsal can be omitted without losing the information in the phonological loop. In contrast to the emphasis of Baddeley and Hitch (1974) on rehearsal, most researchers accept that a strategy of "refreshing" information periodically by focusing attention on a to-be-remembered item, rather than rehearsing it constantly, can free up resources to allow other tasks to be performed concurrently (Camos et al., 2009).

The Visuospatial Sketchpad

Not all information can be easily represented in a phonological code. For example, Brooks (1968) had participants create a mental image of a block letter F, after which they were to mentally trace the F, starting at the lower left corner and ending at the lower right corner. The task was to indicate whether each corner was "outside" (right turn) or not outside (left turn) the imaged letter. Participants responded in one of three ways: (a) pointing to Y (yes, outside) or N (not outside) in a series of staggered rows, (b) saying "yes" or "no," or (c) pressing one key with a left finger for yes and another key with the right finger for no. The pointing responses took much longer than the two other response modes, but this was not the case when the task was to classify whether each word in a memorized sentence was a noun or not. The results thus suggest that having to attend visually to the response alternatives produces specific interference with the visual image of the letter.

Tasks such as this have been used to study the existence and nature of spatial memory or, in terms of Baddeley and Hitch's (1974) model, the *visuospatial sketchpad*. Such tasks can be efficiently combined with tasks that require verbal memory (e.g., shadowing words) but suffer when a spatial task (e.g., judging whether rotated letters are normal or mirror reversed) must be performed concurrently (see Baddeley, 1998a, for a review). A study by Klauer and Zhao (2004) provided evidence that the visual and spatial components of the sketchpad are distinct. They reported six experiments with German participants, showing that a visual short-term memory task (retention for 10 seconds of one of eight possible Chinese characters) was disrupted more by a visual color-discrimination task performed during the retention interval than by a task requiring discrimination of a nonmoving stimulus among moving ones. The relative disruption was the opposite when the memory task was the location out of eight circular locations where a dot occurred. This double dissociation implies separate stores for what (visual) and where (spatial).

Awh and Jonides (1998; Awh et al., 1998) argued that there is an intimate link between spatial working memory and spatial selective attention. In particular, they argued that the processes involved in keeping a representation active in working memory are the same as those used in selectively attending to locations. In earlier chapters, we saw that there is an interaction of spatial attention and visual processing such that focusing attention on a region of space enhances visual processing at that location (e.g., Carrasco, 2018). That attention to location may be involved in rehearsing information in spatial working memory is suggested by the fact that maintaining locations in memory (e.g., trying to remember where a dot had been presented) results in faster reaction times to another, unrelated visual stimulus when that stimulus is presented at a remembered location than at a location nearby (Awh et al., 1995).

Another line of evidence that there may be a process of rehearsal for spatial memory that resembles spatial selective attention comes from neuroimaging and event-related potential (ERP) studies of brain activity. Imaging studies show a high degree of overlap between the areas involved in spatial working memory and those involved in spatial selective attention (Awh & Jonides, 1998). Similarly, both remembering and attending to specific locations lead to enhancement of the N1 and P1 ERP components (both associated with early stimulus processing) to a probe stimulus (e.g., a checkerboard pattern flashed on a screen) presented at the attended to or remembered location (Awh et al., 2000). Although most evidence suggests a close relation between visual attention and visual working memory, Howard et al. (2020) obtained results for a spatial task suggesting that each involves separate limited-capacity processes.

The Central Executive

In the working memory model, the *central executive* can be viewed as the "controller" of the visuospatial sketchpad and phonological loop. Baddeley (1998a) described the central executive as more of an attentional system than a memory store. Perhaps no issue reflects the interplay between attention and memory as much as how information processing in general and memory specifically are controlled. This issue was addressed in part in Chapters 4 and 5, where we considered the role of facilitation and inhibition in assuring smooth control of information processing. Hasher et al. (2007) specifically linked inhibitory processes to the central executive by stressing that inhibition is likely involved in (a) controlling access of relevant information to working memory, (b) deletion of irrelevant items from working and long-term memory, and (c) restraint in releasing strongly activated response tendencies. Executive control was also discussed in Chapter 7 in relation to goal setting and task-set switching. Here, we consider the processes postulated to mediate between working memory systems or that are responsible for selecting and maintaining strategies.

Much of the research on cognitive control (i.e., executive functioning) in the context of Baddeley and Hitch's (1974) model has been performed with patients who experienced an injury to the frontal lobes. However, even healthy persons often exhibit symptoms of poor cognitive control, particularly when executive aspects of memory are taxed by the requirement to perform a secondary task. G. W. Humphreys et al. (2000) loaded working memory by having participants perform a trails test (Heaton et al., 1991) while performing everyday tasks such as wrapping a gift or making tea. In their version of the trails test, participants had to work their way through the alphabet and count, starting with an arbitrary letter–digit pair. For example, if the experimenter said "B8," the participant would continue with "C9," "D10," "E11," and so forth. This test placed demands on both verbal working memory and executive control because of the requirement to say the letters and digits aloud and keep track of the last letter and digit produced. Participants in an articulatory suppression condition were required to repeat the word "the" as quickly as possible to tax only verbal memory. The reasoning was that the differences in performance between participants in the two conditions should reveal the role of executive control in performing familiar multistep tasks.

Participants in the trails test condition made many more errors on the everyday tasks than those in the articulatory suppression condition—though not nearly as many errors as patients with frontal lobe injuries. Most of the errors involved omitting steps. Unlike patients, these participants rarely added unnecessary steps, repeated actions, or committed spatial (e.g., using too little paper) or semantic (e.g., wrapping the bow instead of the gift) errors. Furthermore, unlike the patients, they were also observed to correct erroneous actions (e.g., stop in mid-reach when reaching for the wrong item). Almost all the observed errors occurred on the step following the commission of an error on the trails test. The correlation between errors on the two tasks suggests, not surprisingly, that executive memory is involved in multistep tasks.

More Recent Additions to the Working Memory Model

Baddeley (2000) added a fourth subsystem, the *episodic buffer*, that accepts input from semantic and episodic long-term memory in addition to information from the other subsystems of working memory, creating multidimensional episodes. Although working memory was assumed to play a role in conscious awareness, the episodic buffer makes that role explicit by its function of integrating knowledge of long-term memory with the contents of the visuospatial sketchpad and phonological loop. Baddeley and Hitch (2019) emphasized that the addition of the episodic buffer clearly differentiates the capacity for passive storage (the buffer) from the attentional function of the central executive. The current version of the model, shown in Figure 8.5, also makes clear that the visuospatial sketchpad and phonological loop each have subsystems, consistent with evidence reviewed in this section, and it includes as well speculative buffers for taste and smell (not illustrated).

FIGURE 8.5. Baddeley's (2000) Working Memory Model

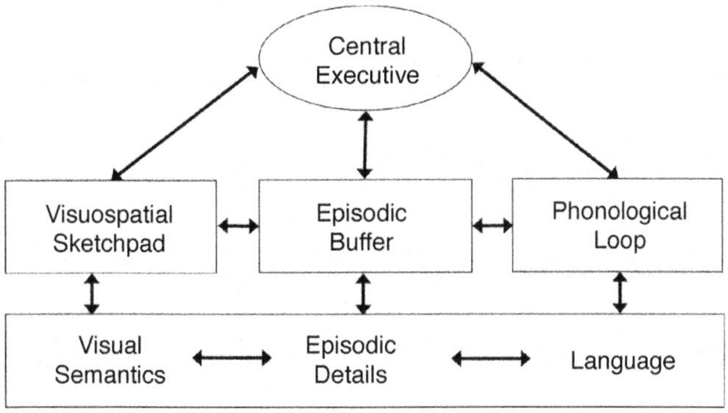

Note. From "The Episodic Buffer: A New Component of Working Memory?," by A. Baddeley, 2000, *Trends in Cognitive Sciences*, 4(11), p. 418 (https://doi.org/10.1016/S1364-6613(00)01538-2). Copyright 2000 by Elsevier. Adapted with permission.

Short-Term Memory as Activated Long-Term Memory

Although Baddeley and Hitch's (1974) working memory model incorporated attention by way of the central executive, most of the emphasis was on the properties of the phonological loop and visuospatial sketchpad. How attention exerted its influence was left rather vague. Beginning in the mid-1990s, models tended to shift from depicting memory in terms of distinct stores to treating short-term memory as activated information from long-term memory (see Baddeley, 2012). This view, in turn, necessitated that attention be brought to the forefront in the study of short-term memory.

Engle (2002) emphasized attention, equating working memory capacity with executive attentional processes. He based this conclusion on studies comparing groups of people who tested low or high on complex memory span tests, which require the performance of an additional task (e.g., verifying numerical equations) between each to-be-remembered item in a list. Memory span measured in this way was found to correlate with performance on tasks used to study attention, including Stroop and dichotic listening tasks, and on everyday life tasks such as learning vocabulary, taking notes, and learning computer coding. These results suggested that the greater working memory capacity indicated by a higher complex span reflected differences in the ability to maintain attention on intended tasks and not be captured by extraneous thoughts and stimuli. Complex memory span is correlated with *fluid intelligence*—the ability to think creatively—which makes it difficult to distinguish which aspect is most critical. More recently, Engle (2018) concluded that complex memory span relates to the ability to maintain information in working memory, whereas fluid intelligence relates to the ability to disengage from that information when needed.

Two influential models that view working memory as activated states of information from long-term memory are the embedded components models of Cowan (1997) and Oberauer (2009). Cowan's model consists of two embedded components, whereas Oberauer's consists of three components.

Cowan's Embedded Components Model of Working Memory

Cowan's (1988, 1997) model views short-term memory as activated memories from the long-term store, a view advocated originally by Norman (1968) in his late-selection model of attention (see Chapter 3, this volume). The focus of attention, which corresponds to a person's immediate awareness, has a capacity of only about four items of unchunked information. Cowan (2001) arrived at this conclusion from a review of studies that met strict conditions to ensure that the estimate of capacity limits was obtained under conditions that did not allow for chunking or other strategies to enhance recall performance. He attributed the capacity limits of short-term memory (following James, 1890/1950) to a limit on the number of items to which attention can be allocated at the same time. Also, following Hebb (1949), he attributed the time limits in retaining information current in memory to limits in the activation of items in memory.

This dichotomy of processes (attention to items and activation of items; see Figure 8.6) allows for separate effects of attention and simple exposure to items. For example, in the dichotic listening paradigm (see Chapter 3), a change in the physical properties of the stimulation on the unattended channel can capture one's attention from the attended channel (Cherry, 1953). In Cowan's (1988, 1997) view, this indicates that physical features of the stimulus activate a part of the memory system outside the current focus of attention.

Oberaurer's Three-Embedded-Components Model of Working Memory

Oberauer (2002, 2009; Oberauer & Hein, 2012) advocated an extension of Cowan's (1988, 1997) embedded components model that also emphasizes a close link between attention and memory but includes three components. The activated part of long-term memory is similar to that in Cowan's model and is represented in Figure 8.7 by the small circles. The region of direct access (also called broad focus), which is comparable to Cowan's focus of attention, is the information depicted by the gray circles. The model also includes a single-item focus of attention that selects one item or chunk as the object of the next cognitive operation, which in the diagram is the object labeled (c).

FIGURE 8.6. Cowan's Embedded-Components Model of Short-Term Memory

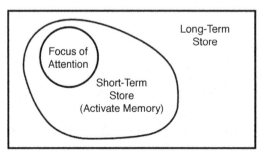

FIGURE 8.7. An Illustration of Oberauer and Hein's (2012) Three-Embedded-Component Model of Working Memory

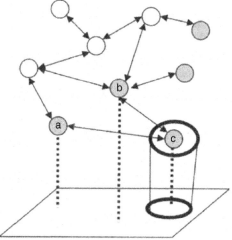

Note. From "Attention to Information in Working Memory," by K. Oberauer and L. Hein, 2012, *Current Directions in Psychological Science*, *21*(3), p. 165 (https://doi.org/10.1177/0963721412444727). Copyright 2012 by SAGE Publishing. Reprinted with permission.

Oberauer (2002, 2009; Oberauer & Hein, 2012) proposed a one-item focus of attention because some studies have demonstrated a unique standing for a single item in working memory. For example, Garavan (1998) showed participants triangle and rectangle figures one at a time, and their task was to count the number of times each shape occurred. The presentation of the figures was self-paced; pressing the spacebar on a computer keyboard removed the current figure and displayed the next one. The figure on a trial could be the same as on the prior trial, in which case the previous mental counter was to be updated again, or the alternative object, in which case the counter from the prior trial had to be switched and that counter then updated. Response times were nearly 500 ms longer on average when the figure switched rather than repeated from the prior trial. This result suggests that the prior object processed is within the focus of attention and does not need to be retrieved if the object is repeated, whereas the new object needs to be retrieved if it is switched from the prior trial.

In sum, Baddeley and Hitch's (1974) model continues in the tradition of regarding the short-term store as a separate system. In contrast, the models of Cowan (1988, 1997) and Oberauer (2002, 2009; Oberauer & Hein, 2012) treat short-term memory as activated long-term memory. Norris (2017) argued that the concept of a distinct short-term store is needed to account for storage of novel combinations of letters or features and multiple tokens of the same type (e.g., two or more instances of the same digit in a password) and for the capability of binding simpler codes. But, as a reply by Cowan (2019) indicates, this issue is far from settled.

MEMORY CONSOLIDATION AND ATTENTION

To interact with the world in which we live, we need to be able to rapidly identify and interpret the objects, events, and information in our environment. This identification is accomplished by linking current percepts of the different items around us, such as objects and faces, to their representations in long-term memory. Matching percepts to their corresponding object representations enables the recognition of objects and people, and we can use the associated knowledge to guide our actions toward or away from them. Given that the input of information from our senses changes almost continuously due to our moving around or to changes in the source of the information itself, interpretations must be integrated over time to experience continuity. Both the activation of representations stored in long-term memory and the integration of currently perceived information with previously perceived information must occur rapidly on a moment-to-moment basis.

Short-Term Conceptual Memory

The processes of identification and categorization have been proposed to be mediated by a *conceptual short-term memory* system (Potter, 1993, 1999). According to Potter (2012), this system differs from and complements other forms of working memory. It enables rapid identification of perceived stimuli in a largely unconscious manner by activating the semantic knowledge associated with the stimulus. Evidence for such fast identification and interpretation comes from studies using *rapid serial visual presentation* (RSVP; for a review, see Potter, 2012). During RSVP, visual items such as letters, words, or pictures are shown rapidly, one after the other, at the same location. This method is intended to mimic the way people perceive the world, as a sequence of brief snapshots (i.e., fixations separated by saccades) but without requiring that the observer make eye movements.

   People are able to detect a picture in an RSVP stream at above chance when provided only with a brief name (e.g., "swan") in advance at durations as short as 13 ms per picture (Potter et al., 2014). Moreover, they are able to read, understand, and recall sentences presented at a similar rate. That people can read sentences presented with RSVP indicates that a presentation duration of 100 ms is sufficient for each word to be identified.

The Attentional Blink

Although people are good at detecting specified targets in an RSVP stream, a limitation is found when a second target occurs shortly after the first: Accuracy of detection of the second target in the stream is notably impaired (Broadbent & Broadbent, 1987). This decrement is called the *attentional blink*, a term coined by Raymond et al. (1992). Their study, and most others, used RSVP sequences in which two targets (denoted T1 and T2) are presented in a stream of distractors, although the effect can be produced by two targets for which a mask follows each one (Duncan et al., 1994; McLaughlin et al., 2001). The number of distractors in the RSVP stream (and, thus, the time interval between the two targets) can be varied to study the time necessary to process the targets (see Figure 8.8). The temporal interval between the first and second target is generally called the *lag* (the number of items that the second target lags behind the first one). At Lag 1, there is no intervening distractor, and the second target follows the first in the RSVP stream. At Lag 2, there is one intervening distractor, and so on. The typical finding is that, although participants are able to identify and report a single target in RSVP, report of the second target often fails (see Dux & Marois, 2009, and Martens & Wyble, 2010, for reviews).

In Raymond et al.'s (1992) experiment, an X (i.e., the probe) had to be detected in a sequence of letters (see Figure 8.8). The study examined the extent to which detection of the probe depended on whether a white letter (i.e., the first target) that had to be identified was presented earlier in the sequence. In one condition, participants were to detect the letter X and to ignore the white letter (unless that letter was X), whereas, in the other condition, they were to both identify the white letter and detect the X. Note that the stimuli were the same for the two conditions; the only difference was whether report of the white letter was required. Probe detection depended on whether the white letter had to be reported, with worse detection accuracy overall for those trials on which the white letter was identified (see Figure 8.9). When the target was identified, detection of the X followed a U-shaped function across lags. Probe detection was good when it was the white letter (as shown by performance at Lag 0) and relatively good when the probe was presented immediately after the target (e.g., at Lag 1). Performance decreased at Lags 2 and 3 and then increased as a function of lag until the level of performance seen in the detect-only condition was again achieved at Lags 7 and 8.

With Raymond et al.'s (1992) method, having to switch from a set to identify the white target to one of detecting an X could be the source of the attentional blink deficit rather than the processing requirements of the first target. Consequently, Chun and Potter (1995) used a method that ruled out a task-switching

FIGURE 8.8. An RSVP Task Used to Study the Attentional Blink

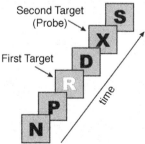

Note. From *Attention: Theory and Practice* (p. 208), by A. Johnson and R. W. Proctor, 2004, SAGE (https://doi.org/10.4135/9781483328768). Copyright 2004 by A. W. Johnson and R. W. Proctor. Reprinted with permission.

FIGURE 8.9. Detection of the Second Target (the Probe) as a Function of Lag and Whether the First Target Had to Be Reported

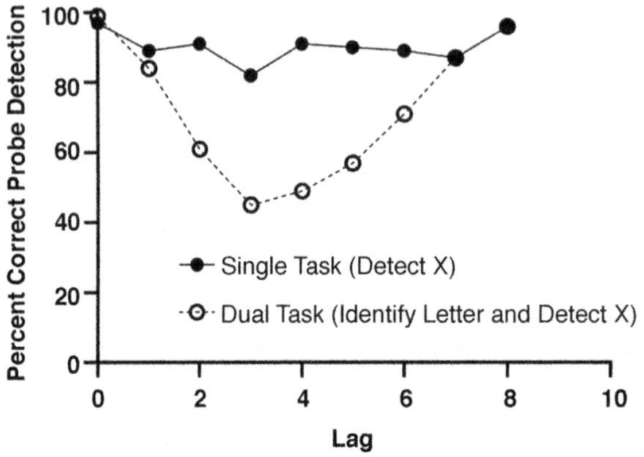

Note. Data from Raymond et al. (1992).

possibility in which participants were required to identify two letters within a stream of digits. Their results were similar to those of Raymond et al., providing stronger evidence that the attentional blink phenomenon is a consequence of processing that is essential to the identification and consolidation in memory of the first target.

The attentional blink has been replicated many times for letters (Grassi et al., 2021). It also has been obtained for spoken and written words (e.g., Duncan et al., 1997) and even pop-out features (Joseph et al., 1997). Several models have been proposed to account for the attentional blink. Consistent with late-selection models of attention (e.g., Deutsch & Deutsch, 1963; see Chapter 3, this volume), these models assume that selection occurs late in processing after the stimuli have been identified and categorized. One influential model is a two-stage model proposed by Chun and Potter (1995).

Following Potter (1993), Chun and Potter (1995) proposed that the first stage of processing the items presented with RSVP consists of identifying the items by the conceptual short-term memory system. This identification should occur rapidly and without attentional limitations; therefore, all items in the RSVP sequence should initially be identified. Indeed, several studies have shown that both the distractors presented in the interval between the two targets, as well as second targets that could not be identified because of the blink, produce priming effects on subsequent implicit memory tests. For example, Maki et al. (1997) showed that when a distractor word that was semantically associated with the second target was presented during the attentional blink, performance on the second target improved relative to a condition in which none of the distractors was related to the second target. The presence of priming effects indicates that these items must have been processed up to a semantic level, even though they were not reported.

The fact that a second target is often not reported when it is presented within half a second of a first indicates that, even though the second target may be processed to a certain extent, the resulting representation requires further processing to be stored in memory. Such further processing occurs in Stage 2 of Chun and Potter's two-stage model and is assumed to draw on limited attentional capacity. Because of this limited capacity, efficient processing requires that only relevant items be transferred into this stage. The selection of relevant items is described as occurring by means of matching the conceptual representation of a perceived item to a target template. If a match is found, the conceptual representation is selected for Stage 2 processing and is stabilized and consolidated into a memory trace that can be reported. However, because Stage 2 processing is limited, if a previous item is still receiving Stage 2 processing, selecting a new item has to wait. As a consequence, the short-lived conceptual representation of a to-be-selected second target is vulnerable to decay and may be overwritten by new information while the first target is being processed in Stage 2.

As shown in Figure 8.10 (left panel), performance on the second target in the RSVP stream is relatively unaffected by the blink when the two targets are presented in direct succession, thereby giving the curve of second target performance across lags its characteristic U-shaped form. The relatively good second target performance at Lag 1, not evident in the two-masked stimuli paradigm (Duncan et al., 1994; McLaughlin et al., 2001), has been termed *Lag-1 sparing.* The two-stage model accounts for Lag-1 sparing by assuming that the selection process that is initiated on detection of the first target is sluggish. Although selection may begin as soon as the first target is detected, it does not shut off fast enough for the item that follows T1 to be excluded from access to Stage 2 processing.

In this regard, the selection process is like an attentional gate that opens rapidly on detection of a target but takes approximately 150 to 200 ms to close. Because the gate is open longer than the actual duration of the first target, the immediately following item may automatically gain access to Stage 2. If this item happens to be the second target, both targets gain access to Stage 2 processing, with the result that the limited capacity for consolidating information is shared between the two targets, with the result that the second target

FIGURE 8.10. Performance in an Attentional Blink Task (Left Panel) in Single-Task (Detect Only Second Target) and Dual-Task (Detect Two Targets) Conditions and the Voltage Differences for Event-Related Potential Components Elicited by the Second Target (Right Panel) at Lags 1, 3, and 7

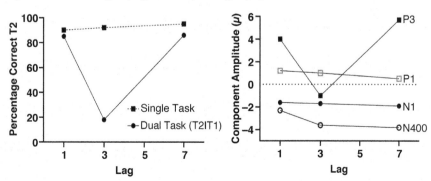

Note. Data from Vogel et al. (1998).

is spared from the attentional blink. However, if a distractor immediately follows the first target, the second target arrives after the gate has been closed. Because this gate remains closed until Stage 2 processing of the first target is completed, the second target is often lost before it can be selected for Stage 2 processing. The gradual increase in T2 performance across longer lags indicates that the chance to gain access to Stage 2 increases as more time elapses.

The two-stage model of the attentional blink (Chun & Potter, 1995) is supported by measurements of the ERPs taken during the performance of an RSVP task. Vogel et al. (1998) examined several ERP components that correspond to different aspects of information processing: the N1 and P1, both of which reflect sensory processing; the N400, which reflects semantic analysis; and the P3, which reflects the updating of working memory. Vogel et al. designed a number of experiments in which an enhanced ERP component would or would not be expected if a stimulus was processed up to the point at which the particular component occurred. By comparing waveforms time-locked to second targets presented at Lag 1, Lag 3, or Lag 7, Vogel et al. showed that only the P3 component was affected by the blink (see Figure 8.10, right panel). That is, whereas the sensory and semantic analysis of the second target proceeded unimpeded by the attentional blink, the ERP component that is assumed to reflect the updating of working memory was significantly attenuated during the attentional blink. These findings are in agreement with the fact that distractors that are presented during the attentional blink facilitate the processing of semantically related targets (Maki et al., 1997) and the assumption of the two-stage model that the attentional blink reflects a deficit in the consolidation phase of storing information in working memory (Chun & Potter, 1995).

Evidence has also been presented that the time elapsing between the two targets in the RSVP sequence is not the only critical timing factor influencing the attentional blink. Shapiro et al. (2017) displayed the stimuli at different entrainment frequencies corresponding to the alpha, beta, theta, and gamma ranges. Their results showed that the attentional blink as a function of time was larger when the frequency of stimuli was in the alpha (8–12 Hz) or beta (13–30 Hz) frequency range than when it was in the theta (4–7 Hz range) or gamma (30–140 Hz) range. This link is critical because the alpha and beta frequencies are thought to reflect processes involved in controlling attention and consciousness (Hanslmayr et al., 2011).

In summary, reporting a particular item briefly presented in an RSVP sequence requires that the item be identified, selected, and consolidated. The attentional blink phenomenon reflects a limitation in the process of consolidating information from an unstable conceptual representation into a stable representation in memory. This limitation is evidenced by the fact that no new inputs can be consolidated while a previous item is being consolidated. However, this limitation does not affect the first stage of identification that is mediated by conceptual short-term memory, as indicated by the finding that items that cannot be reported nonetheless influence performance on implicit memory tests.

The Bottleneck Model Revisited

The RSVP paradigm used to study the attentional blink can be viewed as a dual-task paradigm because at least two targets must be detected and responded to. However, because the responses to both targets are unspeeded, psychological refractory period (PRP) effects like those discussed in Chapter 7 are not generally a factor in performance. Jolicoeur (1999) reasoned that requiring a speeded classification response to the first target in the attentional blink paradigm and thus requiring an immediate response selection would produce a PRP effect on responses to the second target. Jolicoeur showed such a deficit in the identification of the second target (X or Y) when the first target (a large or small letter H or S in red) had to be classified based on letter identity or size. The detrimental effect on the identification of the second target was even larger when the four possible first targets had to be discriminated separately on the basis of the combination of color and size. Jolicoeur et al. (2000) showed similar results when the first target required discrimination of two or four tone frequencies. These results led Jolicoeur and colleagues to conclude that at least one source of interference in the attentional blink effect is the response-selection bottleneck or some later bottleneck.

An explanation for the deficit in the detection of a second target presented shortly after a target requiring a speeded response is that the memory consolidation processes needed to fix the visual target in a reportable form require access to the same central bottleneck that is required to select the appropriate response to the first target. Neural evidence for this joint basis was reported by Marti et al. (2012), who measured brain activity (using a method called magnetoencephalography [MEG]) while participants performed a speeded PRP task. The task required responding as fast as possible to an auditory target as the Task 1 stimulus and a visual target embedded in distractors as the Task 2 stimulus. This method showed slow responses for Task 2 (PRP effect) on some trials and complete misses of the visual target (attentional blink) on others. The MEG data showed similar sensory processing in the visual cortices for the two trial types, but late activation in the frontal cortex was delayed in PRP trials and absent in the blink trials. Thus, evidence implies that the attentional blink has a relatively late processing locus that is the same bottleneck as the one that produces the PRP effect. Even though perceptual processing of the second target occurs, the early perceptual information is lost before it can be established in memory. Consistent with Chun and Potter's (1995) concept of short-term conceptual memory, Jolicoeur and Dell'Acqua (1999) called the process that ensures that the perceived information is remembered *short-term consolidation*.

Short-term consolidation seems to depend on the same limited capacity central bottleneck revealed in studies of dual-task performance. For example, Jolicoeur and Dell'Acqua (1999) combined a memory task (remember one or three letters) with a speeded response to a tone. Participants were first shown one or three letters to remember or one or three digits that did not have to be remembered. After a delay of 350 to 1,600 ms, a high- or low-pitch tone was presented, and a speeded classification response had to be made. Finally, participants reported which letters, if any, had been presented at the start of the trial. The time to make a speeded response to the tone depended on the number of letters encoded and on the stimulus onset asynchrony between the letters and the tone. At the shortest stimulus onset asynchrony (350 ms between the onset of the letters and the tone), reaction times to the tone were elevated for both the one- and three-letter conditions (see Figure 8.11). When three letters had to be remembered, tone reaction time was affected for much longer intervals. This result suggests that the time to complete short-term consolidation depends on the amount of information to be remembered. Short-term consolidation causes interference that delays speeded responses to other stimuli.

Consolidation itself is also subject to interference. Stimuli that are briefly presented during the interval when a response is being made to another stimulus are sometimes remembered less well than if they are presented alone (Jolicoeur & Dell'Acqua, 1999; Experiment 2). Also, a sequence of letters is recalled in the correct order better after the performance of an intervening single task than a dual task, suggesting that the control processes for dual-task performance involve the executive functions of working memory (Otermans et al., 2021).

It is also possible to emphasize reaction time to the second target in the task instructions, which is what Lagroix et al. (2019) did. Participants were to identify one of several vowels that could occur as the first target in a string of RSVP digits and one of several consonants that could occur as the second target. For one group, the instructions emphasized responding as quickly as possible to the second target and reporting the first target only afterward. In a not-masked condition, Target 2 was the last stimulus in the RSVP stream, whereas, in a mask condition, Target 2 was followed by a single digit distractor. The reaction time measure showed an attentional blink effect (longer reaction times at lags

FIGURE 8.11. Mean Reaction Time to a Tone (Task 2) as a Function of the Stimulus Onset Asynchrony Between the Visual Stimulus and the Tone and the Task 1 Stimulus Type (One vs. Three Letters or Digits)

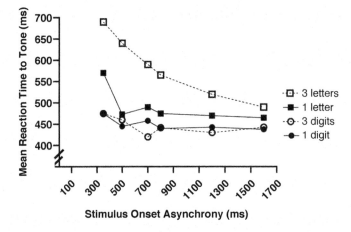

Note. Data from Jolicoeur and Dell'Acqua (1999).

within the blink period). It also showed Lag 1 sparing in the mask condition but a Lag 1 deficit (i.e., the longest reaction times) in the no-mask condition.

Because of the divergence of Lag 1 effects for accuracy and reaction time in the mask condition, Lagroix et al. (2019) proposed a two-bottleneck model to explain the results. The first bottleneck is the same as that in Chun and Potter's (1995) and Jolicoeur and Dell'Acqua's (1999) models. Processing of Target 2 is delayed at the target-selection stage due to the short-term consolidation required for Target 1. This bottleneck results in Lag-1 sparing on the accuracy measure, regardless of whether Target 2 is masked. The second bottleneck occurs at the response-planning stage. If Target 2 arrives after planning the response to Target 1 has been completed, planning of the Target 2 response is not delayed. A delay will result, however, if Target 2 arrives while the planning stage is still occupied with Target 1. Such delays will affect RT but not accuracy.

Predictions of this model were tested in two additional experiments. In Experiment 2, under masked conditions, diverging patterns occurred when Target 2 was presented in a salient red color. Lag-1 sparing occurred on the accuracy measure, whereas a Lag-1 deficit occurred with reaction time. In Experiment 3, a manipulation of stimulus–response compatibility for the response to Target 1 affected the size of Lag-1 sparing when the dependent measure was reaction time but not when it was accuracy. Although Lagroix et al. (2019) cautioned that there may be other bottlenecks, for now, their model nicely captures the relation between the attentional blink and PRP effects.

THE ROLE OF ATTENTION IN ENCODING AND RETRIEVAL

One of the best-known contributions to memory research is the depth-of-processing framework proposed by F. I. M. Craik and Lockhart (1972), according to which retention increases as attention is paid to semantic characteristics of the material rather than the perceptual characteristics. The basic idea of depth of processing is widely accepted, although qualified with what is called *transfer-appropriate processing*, which is that the match between encoding and retrieval is a factor. Morris et al. (1977) reported a study in which they showed that attending to a perceptual feature, the sound of words, led to better performance for a memory test that required recognizing words that rhymed with the study words. Even though Morris et al. emphasized the match of the encoding operations to the retrieval context and F. I. M. Craik and Lockhart (1972) did not, they both emphasized the role of attention.

Bentin et al. (1998) conducted experiments examining the influences of depth of processing and attention on implicit and explicit memory. One experiment presented lists of single-word and nonword stimuli for which a lexical (word or nonword) or color (red or not) decision was made. In another experiment, the lists were pairs of word and nonword stimuli located above or below a fixation, and lexical decisions were to be made on the blue or red word.

In both experiments, the two study conditions were performed in separate trial blocks or intermixed (with the particular judgment or relevant color cued in advance). Notably, both the depth-of-processing and attention manipulations had similar effects on an implicit repetition priming test and an explicit recognition test. Moreover, the difference between deep and shallow processing and attended and unattended stimulus was larger when the conditions were blocked than when they were mixed, apparently because the blocked conditions allowed participants to focus better on the relevant judgment.

Logan and colleagues (e.g., Boronat & Logan, 1997; Logan & Etherton, 1994) also conducted a variety of experiments to show that attention and memory are intertwined. Logan's (1988) instance theory, discussed in more detail in Chapter 11, assumes that attention is necessary and sufficient for the encoding and retrieval of details about presented stimuli. They provided support for this assumption in a number of experiments that show evidence of learning only those attributes that were attended to because they were relevant to task performance. For example, Logan and Etherton (1994) had participants search a set of 32 pairs of words for the presence of words from a particular category—for example, names of countries. This set of words was repeated 16 times during the training phase of the task. Participants were assigned to one of two conditions. In the focused-attention condition, one of the two words was presented in green, and participants were to focus their attention on this word. In the divided-attention condition, both words were presented in the same color, and participants were to search both words for the presence of a word from a particular category. As expected, participants responded faster when they had to attend to only one word.

Following several hours of training with the same 32 pairs of words, the participants were to perform the same task but now with word pairs that consisted of new combinations of previously used words. When comparing performance on these newly combined words with performance in the last block of the training phase, participants trained in the divided-attention condition were markedly slower to respond to the new word pairs than to the old, trained pairs. In contrast, the participants who were trained in the focused-attention condition showed no such difference in reaction times for old and new word pairs. This result was interpreted as indicating that attending to both words had the consequence that both words were stored as a pair, which, in turn, hindered performance when new word pairs were used. The fact that reaction times to new word pairs were similar to those observed with trained word pairs when attention was focused on a single word during training indicates that, in this case, no learning of the unattended material occurred.

Logan et al. (2021) proposed an even stronger hypothesis that memory retrieval is accomplished by the same attentional process that underlies selection from visual and auditory displays, differing only in that attention is directed inward. Their experiments used a variant of the flanker task in which participants had to judge whether a cued letter matched the letter in the cued position of a list previously entered into memory. The results of several experiments showed flanker compatibility and distance effects, as are obtained in visual attention studies. The data were fit well by models from three families of attentional theories—space-based, object-based, and template-based (matching)—indicating that the specific theory of attention was less important than that the results could be accounted for by the sharpness of focus on the target and ability to ignore distraction, much as in visual studies.

Control of Multistep Tasks

Even in laboratory experiments such as pressing a key in response to a light, a goal (e.g., respond as quickly and accurately as possible) must be maintained. In everyday life, the goals (e.g., graduate from college) are generally more complex, as are the steps needed to achieve the goals. Often, subgoals must be created and prioritized to break more complex tasks into manageable parts, and planning is needed to assure the completion of the goals. A number of subgoals must be met if one is to successfully complete college. On a daily level, goals have to be set to direct behavior (e.g., going to class and completing assignments).

Performing sequences of actions is heavily dependent on attentional control. Multistep tasks also place considerable demands on working memory. One aspect of memory in this context is *prospective memory*—remembering to do something at a distant time based on planning in the present (see Box 8.1). For example, while driving, you might remember that you need to email your professor, but you will need to take this action when you are at a computing device. Setting goals, attending to actions and monitoring progress, and remembering to perform acts are all examples of cognitive control.

One approach to studying control of multistep tasks is to embed series of component tasks in a cascaded sequence and study the nature of information processing in these tasks. This approach was taken by Elio (1986) to study the contributions in learning to solve complex mental arithmetic problems of (a) performing intermediate calculations and (b) integrating and combining these intermediate results. Participants practiced solving particular intermediate calculations (e.g., $x = a * (c - d)$, and $y = $ maximum $[(b/2), (a/3)]$) and integrative structures for combining the intermediate results (e.g., $x + y$). They then completed a transfer session with new problems using the same intermediate calculations, the same integrative structure, or neither. Performance was better in the transfer session when either the component steps or the integrative structure was the same, although the benefit was longer lasting for the problems with the same integrative structure. A second experiment showed that the amount of transfer to new problems with the same intermediate components was greater when a familiar integrative structure was used, suggesting that the integrative structure provides a context for applying the component steps that aid learning.

Given that an integrative structure leads to greater transfer of learning of component steps (Elio, 1986), Carlson and Sohn (2000) directly tested the

BOX 8.1 | **PROSPECTIVE MEMORY**

Prospective memory is an intention to perform an intended action at a later time. Attention is needed to maintain goal-directed behaviors and inhibit responding until appropriate. Prospective memory can be event, activity, or time based (S. Walter & Meier, 2014). *Event-based* memory relies on an event that occurs (e.g., remember to get cash from the automatic teller machine when you drive by the bank). *Activity-based* memory is based on the duration of an activity (e.g., remember to attach a document to an email after you compose the message and before you hit the "send" button). *Time-based* memory is based on a particular time (e.g., remember to call your doctor's office at 10 a.m.). Of course, time-based prospective memory can be based on an event, such as setting your alarm clock or calendar reminder at 10 a.m. However, prospective memory is typically measured without the use of aids for reminding the individual to perform the intended task. Performing tasks at the appropriate time is essential in helping individuals complete daily activities efficiently and safely (i.e., remembering to turn off the stove before leaving your house).

Prospective memory is crucial for older adults who need to take their medications at specific times. Cognitive decline occurs with aging, and so does the ability to perform prospective memory tasks. Hering et al. (2018) noted that forgetting intentions and planned actions make up 50% to 80% of memory problems reported by healthy older adults. This large range indicates that there are individual differences, but the large percentage even at the lower range speaks to the prevalence of prospective memory problems experienced by many older adults. To examine the relation between functional ability and prospective memory, Hering et al. had older adults (*M* = 67.5 years) perform a computerized board game called the Virtual Week, which was designed to have participants perform different types of time-based (e.g., go to the grocery store) and event-based (e.g., buy certain items at the grocery store) prospective memory tasks. The older adults' functional ability was assessed by their performance on a timed version of the Instrumental Activities of Daily Living (TIADL) task, where participants had to perform simple tasks such as looking up a telephone number, counting change (coins), and reading directions on a label of a medicine bottle. Hering et al. found that higher scores on the Virtual Week game correlated with faster TIADL performance and that the Virtual Week performance was a significant predictor of TIADL performance. These findings suggest that factors that can enhance prospective memory would increase the functional independence of older adults.

One factor that has been shown to improve prospective memory in healthy adults is attentional allocation strategies. Participants are asked to perform two tasks. The primary task is called the *ongoing task*, and the secondary task is called the *prospective memory task* (Boag et al., 2019). Performance is measured on the ongoing task in single- and dual-task conditions. Attentional focus can be manipulated by providing instructions to emphasize the task importance of the ongoing versus prospective memory task. Prospective memory performance improves if more attention is allocated to that task (Boag et al., 2019).

BOX 8.1 | **PROSPECTIVE MEMORY** *(Continued)*

But other factors can improve prospective memory performance. For example, both extrinsic (e.g., rewards) and intrinsic (e.g., desire to help another person) motivators can improve prospective memory (see S. Walter & Meier, 2014, for a review). But the benefit to prospective memory is often larger with intrinsic motivators, and the enhanced performance does not appear to come at a cost to the other, ongoing task performance. This finding led S. Walter and Meier (2014) to conclude that extrinsic motivators influence participants' attention allocation strategies, but intrinsic motivators strengthen representations, leading to automatic retrieval of the intention. This is similar to what are called *implementation intentions*, which associate anticipated situations with specific, goal-directed actions (Gollwitzer, 1999).

People also can base their attention allocation strategies on factors imposed by the task environment, such as stress. Piefke and Glienke (2017) reviewed the literature on the effects of stress on prospective memory and identified that stressors that induce short, acute stress could improve prospective memory performance in healthy adults, possibly through increasing cortisol levels. In addition, stressors can have differential effects on a time-based versus event-based prospective memory task. Time-based prospective memory tasks appear to be more vulnerable to stress due to greater cognitive demands associated with internally monitoring the prospective memory. Event-based prospective memory tasks are triggered by an external cue, making them less susceptible to stress. Finally, the effect of the stressor also depends on the complexity of the prospective memory task.

Together, these studies show that performance on prospective memory tasks can be altered by employing different attentional allocation strategies. Allocating more attention to the prospective memory task and having the intrinsic motivation to perform the task and the right amount of stress for the type of task can improve performance.

benefit of having formed intentions to perform certain actions. They conducted experiments using cascaded tasks, in which the results of one step are used as input to later steps and in which some steps can begin (e.g., goal formation) before others (e.g., computing a calculation) are completed. Carlson and Sohn compared the effects of giving participants advance knowledge of operands (i.e., digits to be operated on) versus operators (e.g., add, subtract) in multistep arithmetic problems (see Figure 8.12). They found that the solution time was less in the operator-first than in the operand-first condition. Further, the benefit of knowing the operator beforehand did not depend on whether the steps followed in a constant or varied order, suggesting that the effect is not dependent on a strategy for solving a problem but on the instantiation of goals at each step.

FIGURE 8.12. Step 1 in a Multistep Cascaded Problem Such as That Used by Carlson and Sohn (2000)

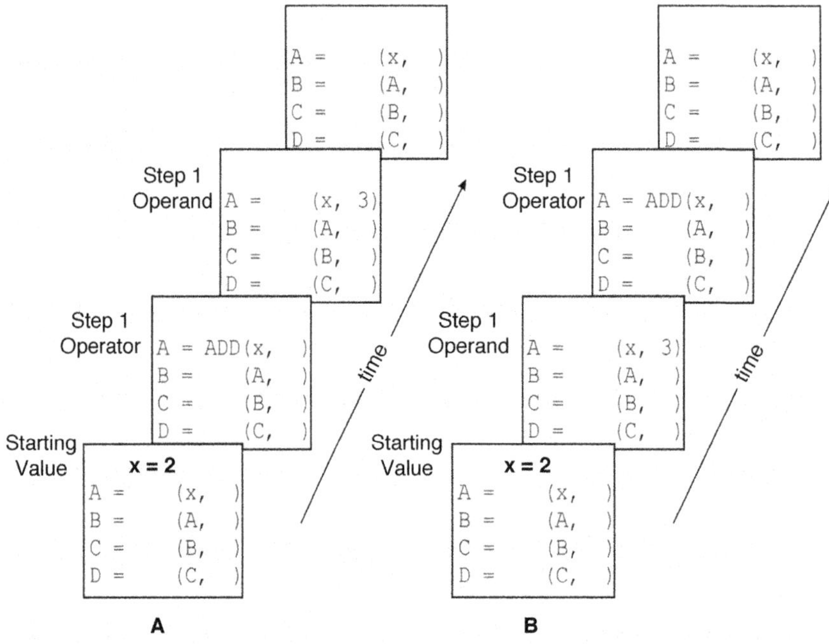

Note. (A) Operator-first condition; (B) operand-first condition. From *Attention: Theory and Practice* (p. 172), by A. Johnson and R. W. Proctor, 2004, SAGE (https://doi.org/10.4135/9781483328768). Copyright 2004 by A. W. Johnson and R. W. Proctor. Reprinted with permission.

Procedural Memory and Implicit Learning

Once you learn how to ride a bike, you will not forget how to do it. A skill such as bicycle riding illustrates that there are different ways of learning and knowing how to do something. Memory may be explicit, based on the conscious directing of attention to the act of recall for remembering facts (e.g., knowing that one should sit on a bicycle or that the front brake should not be used alone at high speeds), or it might, although reflecting past experience, proceed without active attention or conscious recall, as in the performance of a skilled action (e.g., knowledge of how one should balance the bicycle even in turns). *Procedural learning*, or learning evidenced by improvements in the execution of task elements, may involve a different procedural memory system than the declarative memory for facts and instructions.

Procedural memory can be defined as a system that allows people to retain learned associations between stimuli and responses, including complex relationships (Tulving, 1985). It is based on different methods of acquiring, representing, and expressing knowledge than is declarative memory and is characterized by a different kind of awareness. Procedural knowledge can only be overtly expressed, is not available for conscious introspection, and is assumed to provide knowledge that can guide action without containing specific information about the past. This latter assumption is based in part on the fact that amnesiacs can acquire information at a normal rate and maintain performance across delays but not be able to recognize having seen the specific stimuli or task before (Squire, 2009).

Researchers have examined whether and how learning occurs without intention using implicit learning tasks. One of the tasks used to study implicit learning is the serial reaction time task. In this task, the participant presses an assigned key whenever a stimulus appears. The response may be made to the position of the stimulus, its color, or some other stimulus attribute. Two conditions are usually compared: a random condition, in which stimulus position is chosen randomly from trial to trial, and a repeating sequence condition, in which the position of the stimulus is predictable. In a classic study, Nissen and Bullemer (1987) assigned key presses to the spatial location of targets. They compared the performance of participants who practiced the task with a repeating sequence (designating the positions from left to right as A, B, C, and D, the repeating sequence was D-B-C-A-C-B-D-C-B-A) with that of participants who received the stimuli in random order. People who practiced the task with the 10-element repeating sequence showed much more improvement than those who practiced the task with a random presentation of stimuli, even though they were not informed that there was a repeating sequence or instructed to look for repetitions while performing the task.

Although they had not been instructed to look for regularities in the stimulus presentation, participants in the repeated-sequence condition of Nissen and Bullemer's (1987) study reported being aware of the sequence. To determine whether awareness was necessary for learning, Nissen and Bullemer repeated the experiment with patients with Korsakoff's syndrome, individuals characterized by a profound amnesia that prevents them from recognizing and recalling material they have been exposed to. As expected, the patients reported no awareness of the repeating sequence. However, their performance showed learning of the sequence comparable to that of the healthy participants (see Figure 8.13). Apparently, learning can and does occur without awareness, although persons with intact memory function seem to pick up verbalizable knowledge, as well.

Given that learning can occur without awareness, it is interesting to ask whether it also can occur when attention is diverted from the task. One way to assess the role of attention in learning is to compare learning in a single-task condition, where only the task to be learned is performed, with a dual-task condition, in which a secondary task is performed. The requirement to perform a secondary task should take attention away from the primary task. Cohen, Ivry, and Keele (1990) used a serial reaction time task in combination with distractor tasks of different difficulties. The sequences contained either unique associations, in which each stimulus exclusively specified the following (e.g., A always followed by C), ambiguous associations (A might be followed by C when preceded by B and by D when preceded by C), or both. Ambiguous sequences were not learned under the dual-task conditions, but unique associations were. This result suggests that sequence learning depends on two

FIGURE 8.13. Sequence Learning in Control Participants and Patients With Korsakoff's Syndrome

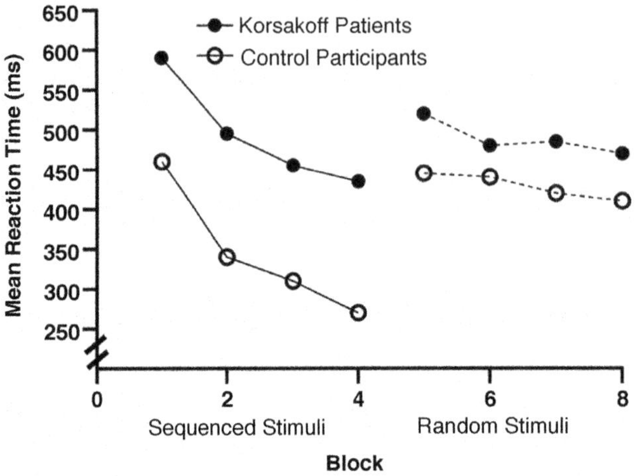

Note. Data from Nissen and Bullemer (1987).

processes, an automatic association that links adjacent items and an attention-demanding process that builds hierarchical codes based on grouping items of the sequence at a higher level.

An issue of interest in implicit sequence learning is the nature of the learned representation. Haider et al. (2020) found evidence that what is learned is an abstract feature code that can be used in responding. Participants first received an induction task in which they responded with compatible key presses to stimuli in a row of six locations. The order of the stimuli for this induction task was random. In a second learning phase, the participants made same–different color judgments to stimuli presented in a repeating sequence of those six locations. In a final test phase, single-digit stimuli 1 to 6 were presented at a central position, to which participants responded with the corresponding left-to-right responses. Reaction times in the test phase showed a benefit of repeating the sequence used for the stimulus locations in the learning phase, indicating that the perceptual sequence shown during the learning phase activated the corresponding response locations to which the stimuli were initially mapped.

The serial reaction time task is only one of several tasks that have been used to study implicit learning. Kalra et al. (2019) examined the performance of four such tasks (the serial reaction task, artificial grammar learning, probabilistic classification, and implicit category learning) by young adults in an initial session and then again about a week later. All tasks except artificial grammar learning showed medium test–retest reliability, indicating relatively stable individual differences in implicit learning. In summary, sequence learning can occur implicitly, at least partly as the result of automatic associative processes that operate independently of mental load but only on active events represented in working memory. Although some simple associative learning can occur automatically, learning involving specific episodic contexts for events depends on attention. As with other aspects of attention and memory, implicit learning varies across individuals.

CHAPTER SUMMARY

This chapter makes it clear that attention and memory are overarching terms for describing complex sets of more or less interrelated functions of information processing. *Memory* refers to representations of information that are retained in different formats and for different durations. Perceptual information is retained briefly in modality-specific sensory stores but must be selectively attended to for further processing to reach conscious awareness. Information is held active and can be operated on in working memory, which is commonly supposed to be capable of processing both spatial and phonological information. Executive control processes couple attention with working and long-term memory to achieve perception, cognition, and action. In other words, the role of attention in memory can be described as that of a selective agent that regulates the flow of information and restricts the operation of memory processes.

Just performing a task is sufficient to learn much about the task. However, some information that we learn escapes awareness. Subtle regularities in the task itself may lead to better performance of the task, even when participants are not able to verbalize what these regularities are. Thus, although successful episodic memory depends on attention to what is being encoded and what is being retrieved, implicit learning can occur in some cases without conscious selection of information. Short-term memory is sometimes defined as that part of memory that is currently available for conscious introspection, but it seems to encompass more than that. Paradoxically, much processing that appears to require retrieval from memory seems to proceed automatically by way of the associations activated by the task set and context.

KEY POINTS

- **Fact:** Attention and memory are closely interrelated.

- **Theory:** Atkinson and Shiffrin's (1968) modal memory model distinguishing sensory, short-term, and long-term stores provided an influential framework for memory research.

- **Phenomenon:** People can report only about four items from a briefly presented array, but they can report almost all items if a cue directs attention to a subset of items at the array offset.

- **Theory:** The limitation of reporting only about four items is attributable to a limited-capacity short-term memory store.

- **Phenomenon:** Attention seems to be essential to the formation of sensory memory though not to the retention of the attended to information represented in it.

- **Fact:** People's short-term retention of information is restricted to about four chunks, and this information will be lost over several seconds if rehearsal is prevented.

- **Theory:** Baddeley and Hitch's (1974) working memory model, which partitioned short-term memory into separate visual-spatial and auditory-verbal stores, along with a central executive module for attentional control, provided the standard for many years.

- **Theory:** More recent models of working memory emphasize activation of information from the long-term store and a limited focus of attention.

- **Phenomenon:** The *attentional blink* is that detection of a target in a stream of stimuli is reduced when it comes shortly after another target.

- **Theory:** The attentional blink seems to arise from the same late-selection bottleneck as the PRP effect.

- **Fact:** Attention plays a major role in encoding stimuli and events for long-term retention.

- **Theory:** Attention may operate similarly when retrieving information from long-term memory as it does when selecting among perceptual stimuli.

- **Phenomenon:** Procedural learning can occur through the repeated execution of a task.

Mental Workload and Situation Awareness

The topic of attention exemplifies the interplay of basic and applied research in making theoretical advances while solving problems encountered in everyday life. As noted in the history of attention in Chapter 1, the need to solve practical problems in the military was at least partly responsible for the resurgence of interest in research on attention in the 1950s. Since then, research on attention has continued to flourish in modern cognitive psychology. Advances in technology have transformed the nature of work in terms of attentional demand and mental workload. Take, for instance, the crew of a commercial aircraft. In the 1950s, five skilled crew members were needed to operate a flight, and by the 1980s, the flight crew was reduced to two, without any decrease in safety, reliability, and performance (Fadden et al., 2015). As technology becomes more advanced, there is interest in reducing the flight crew to a single pilot (Vu et al., 2018). This reduction of work through reliance on advancements in technology, especially to reduce physical, routine, and computational components, can also be seen even in the task of driving. Modern vehicles have automatic rather than manual transmissions, physical maps have been replaced by in-vehicle navigation systems or smartphone navigation applications, and radio tuners have been replaced with voice-controlled operations.

As the examples of the commercial cockpit and driving tasks illustrate, advances in technology can reduce the attentional demands required by an operator in performing a task. However, in most cases, technology also changes

https://doi.org/10.1037/0000317-009
Attention: Selection and Control in Human Information Processing, by R. W. Proctor and K.-P. L. Vu

the nature of the attentional demands required by the task. For example, with autonomous or self-driving vehicles, the driver's task of actively attending to the environment for factors influencing the control and safety of the vehicle is transformed to one of monitoring the automation for proper functioning and intervening when needed. The focus of this chapter is on how attention changes as a function of an operator's mental workload and the role of attention in determining the operator's situation awareness.

MENTAL WORKLOAD

Mental workload is a factor that impacts performance on simple and complex tasks. According to Gopher and Donchin (1986), an individual's *mental workload* reflects "the difference between the capacities of the information-processing system that are required for task performance to satisfy expectations and the capacity available at any given time" (pp. 41–43). Because there are individual differences in cognitive capacity, this definition implies that the mental workload experienced by one individual can be different from that experienced by another, even when performing the same task. Gopher and Donchin also implied that the workload imposed by a task or task combination depends on the cognitive capacities its requires. Thus, when analyzing mental workload, it is essential to specify the types of demands on the resources required by the task.

Unitary resource models (e.g., Kahneman, 1973) attribute high mental workload to situations in which the resources demanded by the task exceed the limited resource capacities. As long as the processing requirements of the tasks are within the resource capacities of the individual, no measurable indications of workload may be present. Moreover, depending on the context, two tasks competing for the same resources can interfere with each other, or one task may interfere with the other but not vice versa (Norman & Bobrow, 1975). According to multiple-resource theory (e.g., Wickens, 1980, 1984), if two tasks draw on different resources, they may be performed together more efficiently, and their combined mental workload may be lower than if they rely on the same resources. From that view, there are two main determinants of mental workload: (a) demands imposed by the tasks (e.g., task difficulty) and the task environment; and (b) the supply of attentional or processing resources to support information processing (perception, cognition, and action), which is modulated by individual factors such as arousal and skill level (Vidulich & Tsang, 2012). The goal is to design systems that demand optimal levels of workload, enough to keep the individual engaged but not too much that it overwhelms the person and prevents them from attending to relevant information.

Arousal and Processing Strategies

Within an individual, resources can change as a function of arousal and effort, a point Kahneman (1973) emphasized in his book *Attention and Effort. Arousal* is the physiological sense of readiness for activity. *Effort* refers to the conscious exertion of resources to perform the task by an individual. The amount of resources available at a given time reflects arousal level and effort being devoted to various activities. Typically, an intermediate level of arousal results in the best performance because too little arousal can lead to boredom and too much to anxiety and stress, following the Yerkes-Dodson law (Yerkes & Dodson, 1908). Like the relation between arousal and performance, performance benefits from an adequate amount of imposed mental workload (see Figure 9.1a).

However, the same amount of arousal can have a different impact depending on the task performed. M. S. Humphreys and Revelle (1984) provided evidence suggesting that the inverted U-shaped function of performance and arousal is a result of two components—sustained information transfer and short-term memory—being influenced in opposite manners by arousal (see Figure 9.1b). According to this model, sustained information transfer resources involved in maintaining attentional focus increase as arousal increases. In contrast, short-term memory resources decrease as arousal increases. Performance on tasks with little or no short-term memory demands, such as many vigilance and sustained attention tasks, should be mainly a function of the sustained information transfer component and, hence, should increase with arousal level. Tasks that depend mainly on short-term memory should show performance deficits with heightened arousal.

Many tasks, even those with heavy working memory demands, such as digit span and operational memory tasks (see Chapter 8), also require focused attention and should reflect both increases in sustained information transfer and decreases in working memory resources. Thus, many tasks follow an inverted U-shaped function of arousal, with optimal performance occurring at intermediate levels. But because, in complex memory tasks, the demands for working memory resources increase more than those for information-transfer resources, the arousal level at which optimal performance is obtained should decrease. This result can lead to the general assumption that greater arousal is

FIGURE 9.1. Hypothetical Relation Between Arousal or Mental Workload and Performance

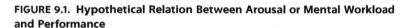

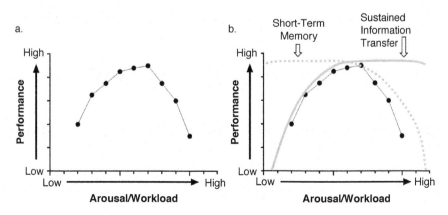

needed for simple than complex tasks (Suedfeld & Landon, 1970). Moreover, according to M. S. Humphreys and Revelle's (1984) model, time of day can affect performance because changes in arousal levels throughout the day can impact the availability of sustained information transfer and short-term memory resources.

Circadian Rhythms

You may be familiar with the sensation of feeling drowsy on awakening despite just having had a night's rest. At awakening, most people still experience the rising portion of the daily cycle of body temperature and readiness for action. Body temperature changes over the course of the day, and arousal level changes with it. Valdez (2019) indicated that four components of attention show variations based on circadian rhythms and sleep–wake patterns: (a) tonic alertness (response to any event in the environment), (b) phasic alertness (responding to an event after a warning signal), (c) selective attention (responding to one event but not others), and (d) sustained attention (maintain attention to an event). For a person who sleeps between the hours of 11 p.m. and 7 a.m., the components of attention are at their lowest levels around 10 p.m. to 10 a.m., reflecting the circadian rhythms and sleep inertia. The attentional components improve from around 10 a.m. to 2 p.m., with a decrease around 2 p.m. to 4 p.m. (often called a postlunch dip), and show higher levels during the late afternoon and evening hours (i.e., 4 p.m.–10 p.m.).

Circadian rhythms of attention can impact cognitive processing and account for poor performance on tasks performed late at night or in the early morning. Valdez (2019) indicated that circadian rhythms in attention influence learning; students might benefit from studying in the later afternoon and evening hours, especially 2 hours before bedtime. But the time course for these attentional components can be modulated by other factors, including sleep deprivation and the person's chronotype (morning or evening person). Sleep deprivation decreases performance throughout the day. Morning-type persons perform better in the morning than in the evening, and the opposite is true for evening-type persons.

The finding that better performance is obtained when participants are tested at times that are synchronized with their peak circadian arousal periods is called a *synchrony effect* (C. P. May & Hasher, 1998). Synchrony effects can be attributed to impairments in inhibitory processes during nonpeak arousal periods of the day. C. P. May (1999) had participants perform problem-solving tasks in which they were to identify a target word that was associated with three cue words. If the cue words were "ship," "crawl," and "outer," the target word was "space." On some trials, distractor information was presented below the cue words, and participants were told to ignore them because they could impact performance. When present, the distractors could be misleading (e.g., ocean with ship) or leading (e.g., rocket with ship), which should interfere or facilitate identification of the target word, respectively, if they were processed.

C. P. May (1999) tested groups of younger and older adults at their peak (i.e., 8 a.m. for older adults and 5 p.m. for younger adults) and nonpeak (i.e., 5 p.m. for older adults and 8 a.m. for younger adults) arousal periods. Both groups performed similarly on the control trials, with no distractors. Younger adults were able to inhibit distractor information (i.e., show no cost in performance with misleading distractors and no benefit with leading distractors) when tested during their peak period. During their nonpeak period, younger adults were impaired in their ability to inhibit the distractors, showing a cost in performance with misleading distractors and a benefit with leading distractors. Older adults were unable to inhibit distracting information completely, showing a cost in performance for misleading distractors and a benefit for leading distractors even during their peak period. This finding suggests that older adults have less inhibitory control than younger adults. However, older adults showed synchrony effects, with the interference effects from distractors being smaller during their peak than nonpeak period.

Energetic Arousal

One aspect of arousal that has been related to attention is subjective feelings of energy versus fatigue, also described as *energetic arousal*. Energetic arousal is moderately correlated with indices of autonomic arousal, as is tense arousal (feelings of tension vs. calmness; Matthews et al., 2010). The relation between performance and energetic arousal does not follow the prediction of the Yerkes-Dodson law, where the simpler the task, the higher the level of optimal arousal. Instead, higher levels of energetic arousal are associated with improvements in performance in a range of tasks, including simple information processing tasks (Matthews, Davies, & Lees, 1990) and more complicated tasks, such as simulated flight (Singh et al., 1993). Moreover, higher levels of energy are more facilitative as task complexity increases (Matthews, Davies, & Lees, 1990). It has been suggested that this effect is directly related to the attentional demands of the task. Specifically, subjective feelings of energy may reflect the availability of attentional resources that can then be allocated to different aspects of task processing.

Matthews and Davies (2001) tested the hypothesis that energetic arousal reflects the availability of general attentional resources by combining a digit-detection task with a secondary *probe reaction-time* task. The digit-detection task required observers to monitor a stream of digits presented visually at a rate of one per second for the presence of a target digit (the digit 0) under low (less-degraded stimuli) or high (more-degraded stimuli) perceptual load. The stimulus for the probe reaction-time task was easy to discriminate, presented either auditorily (a 70-dB tone for 200 milliseconds [ms] over headphones) or visually (a small square in the same location as the digits). Both probes and targets were to be responded to as quickly as possible. To preclude psychological refractory period effects (see Chapter 7), probes appearing directly after targets were not included in the analysis. Energetic arousal was measured using a mood description checklist (the UWIST Mood Adjective Checklist; Matthews, Jones, & Chamberlain, 1990) in which participants rated their current mood in terms of feelings of energy, tenseness, and pleasantness.

Measures of response time and sensitivity to the targets showed that performance was better for individuals reporting high energy rather than low energy. However, this relation held only for the condition in which the digit-detection stimuli were more degraded and the probe was visual—that is, under the highest level of perceptual load within one modality. No effects of energy were found on probe reaction times. These results were interpreted as evidence that high levels of energy lead to greater availability of processing resources. The finding that only performance with the visual probe was influenced by the level of energy of the participants is consistent with other findings of restricted attentional capacity within but not between modalities (Duncan et al., 1996; Wickens, 1984). Of course, it could be argued that perceptual processing rather than general resource availability benefits from high levels of energy.

D. Rieger et al. (2017) investigated whether messages in media can be used to focus the attention of participants and increase energetic arousal after performing a straining cognitive task. Participants performed two cognitively demanding tasks: judging the correctness of a statement and of a mathematic problem. Then, the participants were assigned to watch a video clip with a positive or negative affective valence or to a control condition with no video clip. Finally, the participants performed the cognitive tasks again to measure whether there was recovery from the cognitive strain after watching the videos. Participants showed about a 10% error rate after performing the first round of the cognitive tasks, with no significant difference between the three groups. The error rate decreased to 8% after the second round of cognitive tasks for the groups who viewed the videos during the break but increased to 12% for the control group. Moreover, the video with negative valence led to increases in measures of energetic arousal, whereas the video with positive valence led to increases in measures of relaxation. These findings led D. Rieger et al. to conclude that exposure to media can redirect participants' attention via two different routes (increasing energetic arousal or increasing relaxation) for recovering from a straining cognitive task.

Processing Strategies

The need to learn efficient attentional control strategies is illustrated by the fact that too much information can lead to worse performance (Gopher & Barzilai, 1993). For example, the introduction of new procedures or tools designed to improve performance may actually reduce performance initially because operators must learn how attention should be allocated using the new procedures or tools. The ability to monitor attentional resources and demands allows protection strategies to be used to reduce an operator's experience of overload or fatigue. Protecting the operator's functional state depends on many factors, including workload level, environmental conditions, current operator arousal level, operator characteristics (e.g., skill level), and strategies for task prioritization and effort management (Hockey, 2003). It should be noted that performance-protection strategies or other types of compensatory control can make it difficult to demonstrate overt decrements in primary task performance.

Compensatory costs can be examined by metrics relating to sympathetic nervous system activation or subjective reports of effort, workload, and strain. Studies have shown that people who make more mistakes under stressful conditions show less evidence of compensatory costs (e.g., a relatively low production of catecholamines, a group of hormones commonly used as measures of workload and stress, or reporting less effort), whereas people who perform well show more evidence of such costs (e.g., Lundberg & Frankenhaeuser, 1978; Wilkinson, 1962). These studies imply that sloppy performance may be a protective strategy employed by individuals.

Another possible indicator of stress or high workload is *strategy adjustment*. When demands are high, some individuals will switch to using less effortful strategies for performing a task. Sometimes strategy adjustments occur without intention, as in, for example, attentional narrowing. *Attentional narrowing* refers to the tendency of people in high-stress situations to restrict their attention to a small set of displays or information sources. Attentional narrowing can explain the *weapon focus effect*, where the presence of a weapon attracts the attention of the individual, resulting in an accurate memory of the weapon but inaccurate memory of other details of the event (Fawcett et al., 2013). Attentional narrowing can also explain why eyewitness testimony may not match details captured by videos filmed of an incident. Dahl et al. (2018) interviewed eyewitnesses of a shooting and compared the descriptions of the incidents with videos of the incident filmed on two mobile phones. Dahl et al. found differences between the witnesses' descriptions and the events shown in the film. Witnesses were relatively accurate about the elements associated with the threat (e.g., the assailant's weapon and the number of shots fired by the police) but were inaccurate in details relating to the progression of events.

Other serious consequences of attentional narrowing can occur in environments such as aircraft cockpits, where pilots experiencing a problem with an indicator will focus their attention on that display, ignoring other indicators that are necessary for flight (Wickens et al., 2016). Such attentional narrowing has likely been responsible for more than one "controlled flight into terrain." Even people who only think they are going to experience a stressful situation (e.g., those told that they were going to experience the conditions of a deep dive in a pressure chamber) have been shown to restrict their attention to central cues, ignoring peripheral stimuli in a detection task (Weltman et al., 1971). This strategy allows more capacity to process information within the narrow window of attention by limiting the processing of information outside the window.

A final possible side effect of protecting performance is fatigue aftereffects. Fan and Smith (2020) had 19 participants of a railway company keep a diary of their workload and performance and measured their performance on two cognitive tests, one involving visual search and the other logical reasoning. The diary had participants record information about their workload, effort, fatigue, stress, break duration, and so forth. The cognitive performance measures included time and accuracy for the two tasks. Not surprisingly, Fan and Smith found fatigue to increase from before to after work, but there were individual differences. The group with higher fatigue was less accurate on the visual search and logical reasoning tasks than the group with lower fatigue. After experiencing a fatiguing or stressful day or task, people may show a fatigue aftereffect, preferring to use low-cost strategies for performing other tasks (see Hockey, 1993).

Strategy shifts can also be used to manage mental workload demands. When a task is complex and consists of multiple concurrent processing demands, there are many ways different task components can be scheduled and carried out. The possible variations in the scheduling and execution of tasks mean that operator strategies may vary from one person or situation to another. Baethge et al. (2016) found that nurses who engaged in selective optimization (prioritizing specific goals to optimize resource allocation) with compensation (i.e., the flexibility of resource allocation) were able to maintain better performance under high levels of workload, compared with nurses who did not engage in these strategies. Training and experience can influence the strategies adopted by an individual and lead to fundamental changes in how stimuli are processed. Skilled operators often show evidence of automaticity of processing, such that processing is "rapid, parallel, and effortless" (Eggemeier et al., 1991, p. 212) and not subject to capacity or resource limits normally associated with performance.

In sum, multiple processing strategies can complicate the measurement of mental workload because task demands can be met in different ways, thereby modifying the workload or resource expenditure involved in performance. Strategy shifts themselves can be used to indicate changes in mental workload. For example, higher time demands might lead to a speed-accuracy trade-off. Finally, tasks that have been automatized through extensive, consistent training can show high levels of time-sharing with other tasks (e.g., Strayer & Kramer, 1990). Therefore, it is essential to assess the performance of individuals who possess a level of skill representative of that of the target population when evaluating mental workload.

Measuring Mental Workload

Meeting the goal of maintaining mental workload at an optimal level depends on designing environments and tasks that make appropriate demands on the operator. To determine whether one design or another is better, it is necessary to measure the mental workload of the operator. Three classes of techniques have been developed and extensively tested for these purposes: physiological, performance-based, and subjective measures.

Physiological Measures

Physiological measures of mental workload are measurements of various body or brain responses to task performance. There are two classes of physiological measures, those that presume to measure general arousal and those that reflect brain activity associated with specific processing (Gopher, 1994). The assumption underlying the use of general arousal measures is that various bodily systems are activated whenever mental effort increases. Increases in arousal lead to cardiovascular and respiratory changes and influence brain electrical activity. Charles and Nixon (2019) noted that the technologies used to measure physiological responses are constantly advancing, making physiological measures cheaper and more flexible (i.e., mobile). They identified six such measures: ocular activity, electrocardiac activity, blood pressure, respiration, skin-based measures, and electrical brain activity.

Ocular measures include pupil size and eye blinks (rate, duration, and latency). Parasympathetic activation in the autonomic nervous system is reflected in changes in pupil diameter. Pupil diameter has been shown to be sensitive to a variety of sources of mental workload, including memory load, classification requirements, and motor-response difficulty (Beatty, 1982). The greater the workload demands, the larger the size of the pupil. Marinescu et al. (2018) found pupil diameter to be strongly correlated with subjective reports of workload, indicating convergent validity. However, using pupil diameter as a mental workload measure has limitations. For example, older adults can show lower sensitivity of the pupil to small changes in workload, which may be related to limited ranges with age (Ranchet et al., 2017).

Blink rate is the number of eye closures in a specified amount of time, and *blink duration* is the interval of closure or time spent blinking. S. Miller (2001) noted that increases in eye blinks and blink duration correlate with higher levels of workload; however, it is difficult to separate whether the workload is due to visual or mental demands. Also, when measuring eye blinks and eye blink duration in complex settings such as driving, environmental factors (e.g., lighting levels) impact the measure. Thus, the use of ocular measures as an indicator of workload requires not only precise measurement techniques but also strict environmental and stimulus control.

The functioning of the autonomic nervous system also affects the cardiovascular system measures of heart rate, heart rate variability, and blood pressure. *Electrocardiac activity* includes heart rate and heart rate variability. It is one of the most commonly used physiological measures of workload (Charles & Nixon, 2019). Increases in parasympathetic activity and decreases in sympathetic activity lead to increased heart rate. Cardiovascular changes are associated with arousal levels and both mental and physical work. Heart rate increases with increased task demands and when individuals are multitasking or when additional memory load is placed on the individual. Differences in heart rates of pilots have been found to correlate with the workload associated with different phases of flight (Wilson, 2002).

As parasympathetic activity decreases and sympathetic activity increases, heart rate becomes more regular. *Heart-rate variability*, the changes in heart rate within brief time intervals, is characterized by three frequency bands (low: 0.02–0.06 Hz; medium: 0.07–0.14 Hz; high: 0.15–0.50 Hz). Veltman and

Gaillard (1998) found the frequencies of 0.07 to 0.14 Hz (mid-frequency band) to be the most sensitive to changes in mental workload. However, the mid-frequency bands tend to be more sensitive at detecting low to intermediate levels of workload with shorter tasks but not necessarily high levels of workload for longer tasks in which fatigue plays a role (Charles & Nixon, 2019).

Blood pressure is used to indicate the amount of pressure exerted on the wall of the blood vessels. *Systolic* (contraction of the heart) and *diastolic* (relaxation of the heart) blood pressure are often reported. Although both systolic and diastolic blood pressure were found to be positively correlated with workload, systolic blood pressure tends to be the more reliable measure (Ranchet et al., 2017). Stuiver et al. (2014) had participants drive in a simulator under high or low traffic density, with and without fog during specific segments. They found higher systolic blood pressure in the high traffic density condition compared with the low-density condition. In addition, Stuiver et al. found decreased heart rate variability and decreased systolic blood pressure variability during the fog segments and in higher traffic density, which they attributed to higher workload. Interestingly, the lowest values for heart rate variability and blood pressure variability were found in the low traffic density with fog condition. This latter finding suggests that these cardiovascular measures may be more sensitive at distinguishing between low and high workload than between different levels of workload when it is already high.

Respiration metrics include respiratory rate, airflow, and volume, with respiratory rate being the most useful metric of the three due to its ease of measurement and sensitivity to changes in workload (Roscoe, 1992). Hidalgo-Muñoz et al. (2019) examined how heart rate and respiratory rate change with different cognitive workload levels associated with driving. They had young adults drive in a simulator under single- and dual-task conditions. For the dual task, the workload for the secondary task was low or high. Heart rate was higher and heart rate variability lower in the dual-task than single-task conditions, reflecting higher workload. Heart rate variability decreased in high workload conditions for the low-frequency bands. Breathing rate increased while driving, and it increased for the high compared with the low workload condition under single-task performance. On the basis of these findings, Hidalgo-Muñoz et al. indicated that breathing rate is sensitive to different levels of workload under nondriving conditions, whereas cardiovascular metrics are sensitive to both driving and mental workload.

Skin-based measures have also been used to measure mental workload. These metrics are based on the notion that changes in electrical activity in the sweat glands, found in the palms of the hands or soles of the feet, are controlled by the sympathetic nervous system. Thus, skin conductance is positively correlated with workload. For example, Collet et al. (2014) found that electrodermal response duration increased during a driving task when participants had to brake suddenly. Fairclough and Venables (2006) observed that skin conductance increased from baseline measures during the first 20 minutes on a multitasking task, but the levels decreased as the task progressed. These findings suggest that skin-based measures may be more sensitive at detecting abrupt changes in workload rather than changes over time. Other researchers have shown the galvanic skin response to be sensitive at distinguishing between no load (rest) and load conditions but not different levels of mental workload (e.g., Widyanti et al., 2017).

Event-related potentials (ERPs) have been shown to be effective indicators of mental load. Variations in task properties, demands, and difficulty are correlated with certain ERP components. Solís-Marcos and Kircher (2019) found N1 and P3 components to be sensitive to multitasking. Participants performed an auditory oddball monitoring task alone (single task), paired with a tracking task (keeping a car on a simulated road—dual task), or paired with two tasks (the tracking task plus monitoring a preview display that would alert the participants of future roadside conditions such as a curved path—triple task). Participants showed lower detection accuracy for the auditory task and reported higher ratings of workload in the dual- and triple-task conditions compared with single-task conditions. As shown in Figure 9.2, the amplitudes of the N1 and P3 components in response to the oddballs were smaller for the higher workload conditions (dual and triple tasks) relative to the low workload condition (single task).

M. W. Miller et al. (2011) had participants play a videogame while listening to the game's music. At random intervals, the participants were probed with a set of familiar stimuli. Task difficulty was determined by the level of the game, ranging from Level 1 (easy) to Level 11 (difficult). They found the amplitudes of the N1, P2, and P3 components to the probed stimuli to be inversely related to the level of difficulty: Smaller amplitudes were indicative of higher workload. The smaller N1 and P2 amplitudes with higher difficulty levels likely represent a reduction in the allocation of attention to the probe stimuli. The P3 component also showed a reduced amplitude that can be interpreted as resulting from a reduction in attentional resources available when the game was at a higher level of difficulty.

Performance-Based Measures

One way to assess the mental workload imposed by a task is to measure some aspect or aspects of task performance. In this *primary-task technique*, performance will suffer when task demands exceed available resources. Although overall performance is often what designers consider in assessing a system, when difficulty is below a certain level, primary-task performance will not show any decrements even though the operator may experience feelings of workload. For example, experienced drivers may show no difference in driving performance in light and heavy traffic, even though they may experience higher workload in the latter scenario. Longo (2015) noted that primary-task measures do not represent reliable measures of workload and suggested that they be used with other techniques. For this reason, it is often preferable to use a secondary-task methodology, in which a second task is to be performed at the same time as the primary task to the extent that it can while maintaining

FIGURE 9.2. Global Waveforms of (a) N1 at Fz and (b) P3 at Pz Components in the Single, Dual, and Triple Conditions of Solís-Marcos and Kircher's (2019) Driving Study

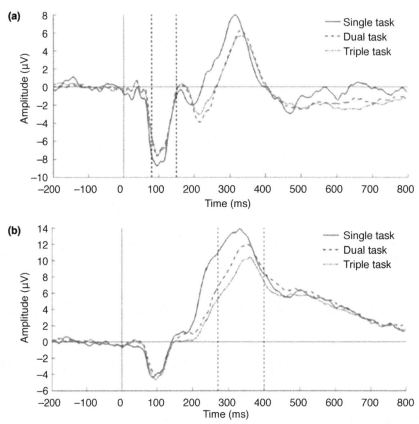

Note. From "Event-Related Potentials as Indices of Mental Workload While Using an In-Vehicle Information System," by I. Solís-Marcos and K. Kircher, 2019, *Cognition Technology and Work*, *21*(1), p. 62 (https://doi.org/10.1007/s10111-018-0485-z). CC BY 4.0.

primary-task performance. The extent to which secondary-task performance is degraded provides the measure of primary-task workload.

For example, operators might be asked to press a key as quickly as possible whenever they hear a tone. This is a simple reaction time task because the participant needs only to decide whether the tone has been heard and then make a key press response. Despite the simplicity of the task, reaction time to the probe tone has been shown to depend on the processing resources required in the primary task, as illustrated by the study of Matthews and Davies (2001) described earlier in the section Energetic Arousal. Posner and Klein (1973) used this *probe-reaction time* task to examine capacity limits in a letter-comparison task. In this task, a warning signal was followed by the presentation of a letter. After a short interval, a second letter was presented. In one condition, participants had to indicate, by pressing one of two keys, whether the two letters were the same or different. In another condition, they made a similar judgment: whether the second letter matched the letter three forward (add three) in the alphabet from the first letter. There were large differences in reaction time depending on when the probe was presented, with reaction times being much longer and occurring earlier for the Add 3 condition than the match condition (see Figure 9.3). This result shows the sensitivity of the probe-reaction time to the processing demands of the primary task.

From a multiple-resource perspective, it is also possible to measure the load or resource demands on specific components using different types of secondary tasks. In a laboratory study using a simulated driving task, Nijboer et al. (2016) found a U-shaped pattern for the interference of a secondary task, where drivers performed just as well or better when they engaged in a listening task (listening to a radio talk show) or an audio quiz of the talk show compared with driving alone. This was especially the case in no-traffic conditions. However, when drivers engaged in the same quiz presented as text on a tablet, they performed worse than driving alone, especially when traffic was present. The worst performance with the tablet condition can be explained by the overlap in attentional resources required by the driving and tablet task. One reason driving with the two auditory tasks was not detrimental may be that the tasks helped reduce drivers' tendency to let their minds wander when engaged in a monotonous driving task.

Some frequently used secondary tasks are choice-reaction time (similar to the probe-reaction time technique but with two or more probes each requiring a different response), time estimation (judging the duration of a specified time interval) or time-interval production (e.g., tapping regularly—tap a key every 15 seconds), memory search (i.e., indicating whether a probe is a member of a memory set), signal detection performance, and mental arithmetic (e.g., perform sums; see Vidulich & Tsang, 2012; Wickens et al., 1986, for reviews). Although each of these tasks has been shown to be sensitive to the workload imposed by different task conditions, they are not interchangeable. For example, time estimation is more sensitive to demand manipulations than is time-interval

FIGURE 9.3. Probe Reaction Time During a Letter Matching Task

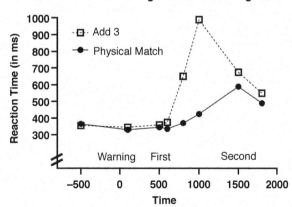

Note. Data from Posner and Klein (1973).

production, but time-interval production is a better indicator of workload in tasks with a high degree of motor output (Eggemeier & Wilson, 1991).

Because many factors may contribute to mental workload, it is beneficial to use several secondary tasks to form a complete picture of the mental load involved in performance. By pairing the task of interest with a variety of secondary tasks, it is possible to construct a load profile of the primary task that gives more complete information about the load imposed by a task than any one measure can. In general, secondary tasks should be chosen based on their overlap with the information resources required for the primary task (e.g., in accordance with the multiple-resources framework; Wickens, 1980, 1984).

Instead of designating one task as primary and the other as secondary, task instructions can be varied to emphasize the relative importance of the two tasks in different sessions. The extent to which the two tasks can be performed together can be graphically represented as a *performance operating characteristic* (POC; Navon & Gopher, 1979), also called an *attention operating characteristic* (Sperling & Melchner, 1978). As shown in Figure 9.4, the POC depicts the combined influences on the performance of the relative allocation of attention to the two tasks.

To plot a POC, it is first necessary to measure single-task performance for both tasks. Performance on the single task is considered to have a score of 100%, and dual-task performance is measured relative to single-task performance. For example, if a single-task score on a task is 52, this score would be considered 100% even though actual scores could be higher; if performance on the same task receives a score of 44 in a dual-task condition, this would be scored as $(44/52) \times 100 = 85\%$. The two tasks are then performed under different priority conditions, in which the emphasis placed on the two tasks is varied (e.g., 80% emphasis on Task A, equal emphasis on both tasks, or 80% emphasis on Task B).

FIGURE 9.4. A Hypothetical Performance Operating Characteristic Showing the Trade-Off Between Two Tasks

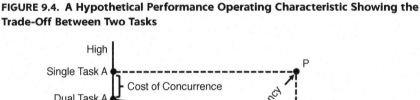
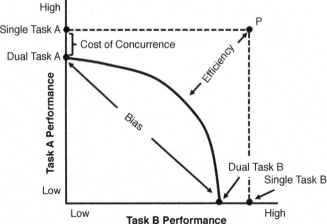

If the tasks compete with each other for a limited pool of resources, the more difficult a task, the harder it will be to combine with a second task and the more performance will suffer to the extent that resources are withdrawn from it and allocated to the other task. If two tasks can be perfectly time-shared, performance on both tasks will remain at single-task levels despite instructions to emphasize one task or the other, and performance will fall at the so-called independence point, P. A diagonal line from the upper left corner to the lower right corner indicates that any allocation of resources to Task B will detract from the performance on Task A and vice versa. Most task combinations will result in a more or less gradual decrease in the performance of one of the tasks as more and more resources are allocated to the other task. In this case, performance at different allocation policies (e.g., "devote 50% of resources to Task A and 50% to Task B") falls along a curve, the POC. The distance of the POC from the independence point reflects the efficiency with which two tasks can be combined.

With appropriate feedback and training, performers can learn to prioritize their performance of two tasks such that one is performed better at the cost of the other (e.g., Gopher et al., 1982). However, augmented feedback, in which details of the nature of the performance are given, may be required to learn to trade-off performance and allocate attention according to instructions (Spitz, 1988). The training of attentional allocation and prioritization strategies can have a strong and long-lasting influence on performance. It seems that dual-task performance can be improved by training with variable priority settings (e.g., Task 1 priority of 25%, 50%, or 75%), relative to training without priority instructions or with only one priority (e.g., 50%). Performers who train under variable priorities become better at detecting changes in task difficulty and are able to better adjust their efforts to cope with changing task demands (Gopher, 1993).

Thropp et al. (2004) used POCs to examine resource sharing between a task that requires spatial processing and one that requires temporal processing. For the spatial discrimination task, participants had to differentiate between lengths of vertical lines. The length difference was 3 mm in the easy condition and 1 mm in the difficult condition. For the temporal discrimination task, participants had to differentiate between lines presented for short versus long durations, and the time difference was 150 ms in the easy condition and 50 ms in the difficult condition. Performance was measured under baseline (100–0) and dual-task conditions. For the dual-task conditions, the prioritization was 90:Spatial/10:Temporal, 50/50, and 10:Spatial/90:Temporal.

Thropp et al. (2004) found the POC to be more efficient for the easy task than the difficult task (i.e., closer to the independence point) when performance was averaged across all participants. The spatial task was more vulnerable to the attention allocation scheme than the temporal task. Allocating more attention to the temporal task (i.e., the 10:Spatial/90:Temporal condition) did not improve performance on the temporal task beyond the 50/50 condition. This finding suggests that spatial tasks draw on resources shared with temporal tasks, but temporal tasks draw on resources that are separate from the spatial task. However, when examining individual POCs, Thropp et al. noted differences in ability that could have contributed to the pattern of results: (a) time-sharing, (b) attentional control, (c) spatial discrimination, and (d) temporal discrimination. They recommended that researchers look at individual POCs in addition to the averaged function when interpreting research findings.

Subjective Measures

The most popular form of workload measurement is to have people rate their subject level of workload, with the assumption that they can accurately report how much workload they are experiencing. Performers may rate different aspects of tasks on a scale or compare tasks to report which one has higher workload demands. These *subjective measures* are relatively easy to implement, nonintrusive, and inexpensive, and they have high face validity.

One of the most widely used measures is the National Aeronautics and Space Administration Task Load Index (NASA-TLX; Hart & Staveland, 1988; see Box 9.1). The NASA-TLX is an example of a multidimensional workload measure. It consists of six different scales, each of which has been shown in preliminary research to make an independent contribution to the subjective impression of workload (see Table 9.1). The overall score can be obtained simply by combining the subscale scores or using a weighting scheme (i.e., weights are applied to the different dimensions to account for individual differences about which of the six dimensions are more related to the individual's definition of workload). Although the weighting scheme can increase the sensitivity of the NASA-TLX (i.e., make it more relevant to the variables being examined; but see Hendy et al., 1993) and decrease interrater variability (Hart, 2006), the weighted and unweighted (raw) scores are highly correlated (e.g., $r = 0.94$; Moroney et al., 1992), and many studies simply report the raw scores (Hart, 2006).

The Subjective Workload Assessment Technique (SWAT; Reid et al., 1981) is another multidimensional measure, which has only three load dimensions: time, mental effort, and stress load. Each of these dimensions has three levels. Participants are asked to rank order the workload that would be assumed to result from all combinations and levels of the SWAT load dimensions. Then, a scaling technique is used to create an individualized workload scale for the rater. One possible benefit of the SWAT over other subjective measures is that the ratings have interval-scale properties, which makes comparisons between different ratings more meaningful.

Gopher (1994) pointed out that the "emotional" components of the NASA-TLX and SWAT ("frustration" and "stress load," respectively) cannot easily be related to any theory of processing capacity. Perhaps partly for this reason, some researchers have argued that simpler, unidimensional measures are just as appropriate as, or better than, multidimensional methods. A simple unidimensional method is to ask people to rate the degree of effort they experienced. This method is essentially equivalent to just looking at one of the scales of the NASA-TLX, the "effort" scale. For example, the Rating Scale Mental Effort

BOX 9.1 | THE NASA-TLX: AN EASY-TO-ADMINISTER AND VALID WORKLOAD MEASURE

The NASA-TLX was originally designed to measure the mental workload of human operators (i.e., flight crews) working in aviation (Hart & Staveland, 1988). It has since become one of the most widely used methods of measuring mental workload. Hart (2006) reported 82,900 citations for the NASA-TLX from Google, and Grier (2015) found more than 10,000 search results for studies with the term "NASA-TLX" on Google Scholar. The NASA-TLX provides workload scores on six subscales, Mental Demand, Physical Demand, Temporal Demand, Frustration, Effort, and Performance, that can be examined separately or combined into a composite or overall workload score. The NASA-TLX is also easy to administer and is available in paper-based and electronic formats.

Akyeampong et al. (2014) used the NASA-TLX to provide a workload profile to evaluate three types of interface designs (two heads-up displays and a monitor display) for a hydraulic excavator. The NASA-TLX profiles showed that the operation of the excavator was high in mental demand across all three interfaces, but the two heads-up displays yielded lower levels of workload than the monitor display. Hoonakker et al. (2011) used the NASA-TLX to measure the workload of nurses. They found that the NASA-TLX was highly correlated with two other perceived workload measures, the RSME and a perceived workload scale, but not with the nurse–patient ratio and only moderately with the nursing activity scores, which are other measures of workload. These findings indicate that the NASA-TLX shows convergent and discriminant validity as a metric of perceived workload. Analysis of the NASA-TLX scores showed that nurses reported experiencing a higher workload when working the night shift, in larger hospitals, and in intensive care units (ICUs). For different ICUs, a higher workload was reported by nurses working in adult and cardiac ICUs compared with the neuro and neonatal ones. Hoonakker et al. concluded that the NASA-TLX is an easy-to-administer workload measure that can be used in work settings to identify areas of high workload.

The NASA-TLX overall scores range from 0 to 100. However, there is no standard benchmark for the NASA-TLX to indicate what is generally considered to be high versus low workload. Grier (2015) analyzed NASA-TLX scores from over 200 publications to help identify "how high is high." Grier found that overall NASA-TLX scores ranged from 6.21 (low) to 88.5 (high), with half of the overall scores falling between the range of 36.77 and 60. Interestingly, the workload scores found for two studies that only had participants wait and not engage in any task were 12 and 14.8, which are numerically higher than the minimum of 6.21 found for the air traffic control task. The ranges of scores also varied for the different types of tasks examined (see Table B9.1 for some examples). Thus, in addition to comparing NASA-TLX scores across different tasks, environments, and interfaces within a study, practitioners can use the ranges of scores found for the same task category to benchmark workload.

(continues)

BOX 9.1 | **THE NASA-TLX: AN EASY-TO-ADMINISTER AND VALID WORKLOAD MEASURE *(Continued)***

TABLE B9.1. Minimum, Median, and Maximum NASA-TLX Scores in Different Task Domains

Task	Min	Median	Max
Air traffic control	6.21	52.44	85.00
Computer activities	7.46	54.00	78.00
Driving a car	15.00	41.52	68.50
Monitoring	20.00	52.24	77.00
Tracking	19.08	51.00	88.50
Video game	14.08	56.50	78.00
Visual search	28.98	57.89	79.23

TABLE 9.1. The NASA-TLX Rating Scales and Definitions

	Scale description
Mental demand	How much mental and perceptual activity was required (e.g., thinking, deciding, calculating, remembering, looking, searching)? Was the task easy or demanding, simple or complex, exacting or forgiving?
Physical demand	How much physical activity was required (e.g., pushing, pulling, turning, controlling, activating)? Was the task easy or demanding, slow or brisk, slack or strenuous, restful or laborious?
Temporal demand	How much time pressure did you feel due to the rate or pace at which the tasks or task elements occurred? Was the pace slow and leisurely or rapid and frantic?
Performance	How successful do you think you were in accomplishing the goals of the task set by the experimenter (or yourself)? How satisfied were you with your performance in accomplishing these goals?
Effort	How hard did you have to work (mentally and physically) to accomplish your level of performance?
Frustration level	How insecure, discouraged, irritated, stressed, and annoyed versus secure, gratified, content, relaxed, and complacent did you feel during the task?

Note. Adapted from *NASA task load index (TLX)* (Version 1.0, p. 13), by Human Performance Research Group, n.d., NASA Ames Research Center, Moffett Field, California (https://humansystems.arc.nasa.gov/groups/tlx/downloads/TLX_pappen_manual.pdf). In the public domain.

(RSME; Van Doorn & Zijlstra, 1988) uses a univariate rating scale with a range of 0 (*no effort*) to 150 (> *extreme effort*). Likewise, the Air Traffic Workload Input Technique (ATWIT; E. Stein, 1985) has operators rate their workload from low to high on a 7-point or 10-point scale. Loft et al. (2015) found the NASA-TLX to be positively correlated with ATWIT ratings. However, Veltman and Gaillard (1993) found low correlations between the NASA-TLX effort scale and ratings on a different unidimensional scale. Verwey and Veltman (1996) found that the SWAT and RSME yielded similar findings for a driving task.

A critical factor that must be considered when using subjective measures is the range of conditions the raters experienced during a session. Subjective measures are based on judgments and are therefore subject to the judgmental tendencies of the raters. A general finding is that raters are influenced by both the range and frequency of different possible stimuli. People seem to divide the stimulus range into categorical intervals and use all categories equally often (Parducci, 1965). Thus, even when stimulus variability is relatively low, raters still tend to use the whole rating scale. This means that ratings of a task with a relatively restricted range of difficulty conditions will tend to overestimate workload, whereas a high range of task difficulties will result in an under-estimation of task difficulty.

Colle and Reid (1999) verified this prediction using both the SWAT and NASA-TLX to measure workload in a categorization task (deciding whether two words belonged to the same category). They manipulated the task load by varying the presentation rate of the stimuli. Using a small range of presentation rates led to higher mental workload ratings for a given rate than when the same rate was embedded in the context of greater variability of presentation rates (e.g., the SWAT rating of a presentation rate of 22 word pairs per minute was 6 in the high-variability condition and 33 in the low-variability condition). Fortunately, Colle and Reid also presented a possible solution to this problem. When all possible conditions were first presented in a practice session, along with the instruction to use the whole scale, the effect of task variability disappeared. Just as it is necessary to describe the rating scales before using subjective measures, it may also be necessary to give raters examples or practice with the task to be rated.

Measure Selection and Use of Multiple Measures

All workload measures have advantages and disadvantages. Thus, several criteria have been identified to determine the workload metric that would be most suitable for use in a particular situation (Moustafa et al., 2017). A workload measure must be reliable and valid to be useful, yielding accurate measures and resulting in similar values with repeated measures under similar situations. Another factor in choosing a measure is the ease of use or implementation. This factor may be a major reason why subjective measures are a popular choice—they are cheap and easy to implement. Sensitivity is also vital. A workload measure is sensitive when ratings made with it reflect significant variations in the workload imposed by a task. A measure is diagnostic when it not only reflects changes in load but also discriminates between the amounts of load imposed on various operator capacities or resources (e.g., perceptual vs. memory load). Finally, intrusiveness refers to any disruption in the performance of the task of interest as a result of the application of the mental workload measurement technique. Depending on the situation, a given measure of workload can be more or less intrusive.

Many studies use multiple methods for measuring workload. Stapel et al. (2019) had inexperienced and experienced Tesla owners perform an on-road driving task. The vehicle was equipped with autopilot hardware that combines adaptive cruise control with automated lane keeping. Participants drove two highway sections selected to be engaging (high traffic density with 10–13 on- or off-ramps) or monotonous (low density with a straight two-lane highway and no on- or off-ramps). Multiple techniques were used to measure workload. For a secondary task, participants performed an auditory detection task while driving. Cardiovascular activity was measured in terms of heart rate and heart-rate variability. Finally, subjective measures of workload were recorded using the NASA-TLX and customized questions.

Stapel et al. (2019) found that reaction times were longer and miss rates higher in the detection task for the more engaging driving scenarios than the monotonous ones. Moreover, automation tended to increase the reaction time in the engaging scenarios, suggesting that automation increases mental workload in more complex driving conditions. Ratings from the NASA-TLX supported this assessment: Workload was rated higher in the engaging condition than the monotonous one. Although workload was rated as lower during automated than manual driving, this was mainly due to the experienced group of Tesla drivers. The inexperienced drivers showed no difference in NASA-TLX ratings for the manual and automated driving conditions. The cardiovascular data did not yield any differences across conditions, suggesting insensitivity of this measure with real-world driving. Based on their findings, Stapel et al. concluded that drivers might underestimate the level of workload when monitoring automation, and they advocated the use of multiple measures of workload.

SITUATION AWARENESS

Whereas high levels of workload can lead to errors, a low level of situation awareness is often the cause of human error. Thus, another characteristic of skilled performance is the ability to maintain good situation awareness. As an experienced driver, you can get from a starting point to your destination without exerting much workload or effort, but driving is a complex and dynamic task in which the environment is constantly changing. Objects come in and out of view as you go past them. Cars change lanes as they pass your vehicle, or you change lanes to pass other vehicles. You try to keep your goal of driving safely in mind as you avoid unexpected obstacles in the road or sudden braking by a vehicle in front of you, look for bicyclists and pedestrians to avoid, and follow traffic signs and signals. To safely get from your origin to destination, you must maintain a dynamic situation model. Such a model includes all the information necessary for task performance, as well as the processes of perceiving and comprehending this information and using it to predict what is likely to happen next. The result of maintaining an accurate dynamic picture of the situation has been called *situation awareness.*

Endsley (1995b) defined *situation awareness* as "the perception of the elements in the environment within a volume of time and space, the comprehension of their meaning, and the projection of their status in the near future" (p. 36). According to this definition, an individual has situation awareness if they are aware of and understand both the current situation and how it is evolving, such that appropriate decisions can be made or actions taken. For example, a driver must be aware of road conditions, the presence of other cars or obstacles, and the rate of change of the traffic in the area to predict whether it is safe to change lanes or pass another vehicle. Two leading causes of driving accidents, "improper lookout" and "inattention" (Treat et al., 1979), can be described as failures to maintain situation awareness. Unfortunately, people often fail to "look ahead" (and behind) and to keep track of traffic and environmental changes. In fact, the ability to shift attention is a good predictor of driving ability (Elander et al., 1993).

Situation awareness is supported by attention, working memory, and long-term memory, but it cannot be equated with any of these processes (Durso et al., 2006). Situation awareness is as difficult to describe as consciousness— it is the awareness that arises when attention is paid to relevant information and when working and long-term memory support the interpretation and maintenance of the attended information (Vu & Chiappe, 2015). Situation awareness can also be decoupled from response processes. Sometimes situation awareness seems low, yet responses continue to occur appropriately, such as when a driver suddenly realizes that they cannot remember traveling a stretch of road.

Moreover, although situation awareness may suffer when workload is so high that necessary information cannot be processed or so low that operators lose vigilance (e.g., Endsley & Kiris, 1995), it is a distinct construct from mental workload. Design changes intended to increase situation awareness do not necessarily reduce mental workload and vice versa. In a review of 15 studies in which both situation awareness and mental workload were measured before and after the implementation of a new interface, Vidulich (2000) found that situation awareness was improved in 80% of the studies, but mental workload was reduced in only 47%.

Like workload measures, there are multiple metrics for situation awareness. Salmon et al. (2009) identified about 30 different types of measures for situation awareness, but the most commonly used methods are the probe techniques and subjective ratings.

Probe Techniques

Situation awareness probes ask the operator to provide answers about information related to the task. Some probe techniques, such as the Situation Awareness Global Assessment Technique (SAGAT; Endsley, 1995a), are memory based and involve pausing task performance (usually in a simulator) and asking performers various questions about their current perception of the situation. The questions asked using SAGAT are based on an in-depth, goal-based task analysis in which the goals of the particular activity are identified, as are the subgoals that support the achievement of the goal. The questions are also directed at the different levels of situation awareness (i.e., Level 1: perception, Level 2: comprehension, Level 3: projection).

SAGAT allows multiple questions to be asked during the pauses in simulator action related to the task goals and subgoals and levels of situation awareness. For example, air traffic controllers have the goals of avoiding losses of separation and landing aircraft safely. Subgoals involve collecting information about each aircraft in the controlled space. SAGAT questions might include reporting details, such as the airspeed and heading of aircraft in the controlled space. Accuracy of responses to SAGAT probes is used to measure situation awareness, where higher accuracy is indicative of better situation awareness. SAGAT has been shown to be a valid measure of situation awareness, and variants of the method have been adapted for specific purposes (Endsley, 2020). However, one limitation of SAGAT is that it can only assess declarative knowledge that is memory based (i.e., information is recalled from working memory or calculated from a situation model that is being held in memory; Chiappe et al., 2016).

Online probe techniques, such as the Situation Present Assessment Method (SPAM; Durso & Dattel, 2004), do not require pausing the scenarios but ask operators to answer specific questions in real time as they are performing the task. SPAM probes allow for a broader analysis than SAGAT by recognizing that operators may not store all task-relevant information in memory but can off-load information into the task environment and only access the information when needed. An example of off-loading is to "flag" a task that needs to be attended to later. However, because SPAM probes are administered while operators are performing the task, it is considered a secondary task that imposes additional workload.

To address the workload issue, the technique uses a "ready" prompt to identify when the workload is manageable for the operator to accept a SPAM query. The probe question is only presented once the operator indicates that they have enough capacity to answer a question; thus, the latency from when the ready prompt is presented to when the operator indicates being ready is a measure of workload. Response time and accuracy to the probe question can be used as an indicator of situation awareness, where shorter response time and higher accuracy indicate greater awareness. Because the SPAM technique does not blank the screen, the operator has access to the task environment to answer a question. This reduces the dependency of probe question accuracy on memory because the operator may off-load information to their display to reduce workload but maintain awareness by knowing where to look for information needed at a specific time. SPAM has been shown to be a valid measure of situation awareness, but it has also been found to be intrusive to performance.

Chiappe et al. (2016) compared the critical differences between SAGAT and SPAM—freezing or pausing the task and blanking the display. They had students studying to become air traffic controllers engage in a simulated air traffic control task under four different conditions that varied in terms of whether the scenario was paused and whether the air traffic control displays were blanked when the situation awareness probe was administered. The condition where the scenarios were paused and screens were blanked is similar to SAGAT; the condition where the scenarios were not paused and screens were not blanked represents SPAM-like queries. The remaining two conditions represented novel situations (scenario paused, screen not blanked; scenario not paused, screen blanked) that allowed researchers to dissociate the effects of display visibility and scenario pausing on the intrusiveness of probe methods. Workload was also measured with ATWIT probes during the scenario and the NASA-TLX post scenario.

Results showed that not pausing the scenarios led to higher workload ratings for both subjective (ATWIT and NASA-TLX) and objective (ready latencies) measures and reduced performance under some situations. Blanking the display had little effect on performance or workload. On the basis of their findings, Chiappe et al. (2016) concluded that a technique in which the scenarios are paused and displays are not blanked during the probe query would be able to capture the operator's situation awareness without being intrusive on performance.

Subjective Ratings

The Situation Awareness Rating Technique (SART; Selcon & Taylor, 1990) is the most commonly used subjective measure (Endsley, 2020). SART is a multidimensional scale that has the operator rate statements relevant to their understanding of the situation (e.g., the amount of knowledge received and understood) and their supply and demand of attentional resources (e.g., how much mental capacity you have to spare in the situation and how complicated the situation is, respectively). The Crew Awareness Rating Scale (CARS; McGuinness & Foy, 2000) includes ratings for three dimensions of situation awareness (perception, comprehension, and projection), along with an overall rating. The Situation Awareness Behavioral Rating System (SABARS; Strater et al., 2001) uses a subject matter expert to rate the situation awareness of operators while they are performing the task using a set of behaviors associated with good situation awareness. It should be noted that judged situation awareness does not necessarily reflect actual situation awareness, and operators' ratings of their own situation awareness can be influenced by their confidence in performance or workload.

Endsley's (2020) review of 37 studies that incorporated both objective and subjective measures of situation awareness showed the divergence of the two types of metrics. She found the correlation between SART and probe measures (SAGAT and SPAM) to be low to none and suggested that SART ratings may be influenced by workload in addition to situation awareness. More generally, the divergence of the metrics can be attributed to poor operator metacognition (i.e., knowledge of their own situation awareness), underestimation or over-estimation of situation awareness due to other factors (e.g., confidence), and confounds with workload in metrics such as SART. However, Endsley noted that the Quantitative Assessment of Situation Awareness (Edgar et al., 2003) metric, which uses probes along with a subjective assessment of confidence in responses, is highly correlated with other situation awareness metrics, including SAGAT (objective) and CARS (subjective).

When selecting a metric for situation awareness, the same criteria described earlier for mental workload also apply: sensitivity, diagnosticity, validity and reliability, intrusiveness, acceptance, and ease of use. There is no preferred situation awareness metric, and researchers are encouraged to examine the advantages and disadvantages of each metric, along with practical considerations such as cost and ease of implementation or use in deciding which measure to employ.

CHAPTER SUMMARY

Our ability to pay attention depends on several factors, including time of day and subjective energy level. Performance is also influenced by individuals' workload and situation awareness. Human errors tend to occur when mental workload is high because demands exceed attentional capacity, as well as when situation awareness is low because attention is not oriented to the relevant information required to perform the tasks. It is essential to measure resource demands to determine whether the mental workload imposed by a particular task is within tolerable limits. The cognitive demands placed on the users can be evaluated by system and product designers, developers of training programs, and accident investigators using techniques ranging from self-report to physiological variables.

Situation awareness goes beyond mental workload in addressing the operator's understanding of the dynamic aspects of a situation. Maintaining a dynamic model requires attending to the relevant cues in the environment and continually updating one's situation assessment. A variety of techniques are available that allow designers to assess operators' situation awareness in specific contexts. However, it should be noted that some of the same factors that improve routine performance have a negative effect on situation awareness. For example, displays designed to support routine tasks may not present enough information to allow the operator to maintain situation awareness (Wickens, 1999).

KEY POINTS

- **Fact:** Circadian rhythms and energetic arousal affect the performance of many aspects of attention.

- **Phenomenon:** Attentional narrowing, a restriction of attention salient stimuli, tends to occur in high-stress and high-workload situations.

- **Fact:** Unitary and multiple resource theories of attention capture the fact that attention can often be traded off in various amounts between tasks.

- **Fact:** Mental workload can be affected by the information-processing resources available, task demands, and individual differences in attentional control strategies.

- **Fact:** Mental workload can be measured in several ways using physiological, performance-based, and subjective techniques.

- **Theory:** Resource theories of attention provide the rationale for the concept of mental workload.

- **Fact:** Lack of situation awareness is a major determinant of human error in many accidents.

- **Theory:** The initial definition of the term *situation awareness* implied conscious experience that is reportable, but other views also allow for an influence of activated knowledge that is outside of awareness.

10

Attention and Displays

The role of attention in processing the information provided by visual and auditory displays has been a topic of interest to applied researchers for nearly a century. Display types are often chosen on the basis of their information support properties, and the success of a display can be measured by whether it can provide the information needed by the operators to support their task and whether it attracts and holds the attention of the operator when alerted. Rather than being just an application of research on attention, display design has driven and continues to guide research on attention. For example, the development of displays that need to be monitored for long periods (e.g., radar displays) led to the discovery of the *vigilance decrement* (Mackworth, 1948). This decrement refers to a decrease in the detection of infrequent target stimuli over the first half hour of performance. More recently, interest in vigilance decrements has been due to the development of automated systems that are found in advance vehicles, cockpits, hospitals, and other operational settings. In addition, developments in three-dimensional (3D) displays and virtual reality have inspired research on spatial representation and spatial cognition and have led to improvements in the visualization process needed for complex product design.

Issues in display design include providing operators with required information, alerting and holding attention, supporting both the ability to selectively attend to a critical display and to integrate information across displays, and maintaining situation awareness. Other issues include the ability to orient

https://doi.org/10.1037/0000317-010
Attention: Selection and Control in Human Information Processing, by R. W. Proctor and K.-P. L. Vu

attention in three dimensions and moving attention between "real" and virtual display spaces. This chapter focuses on the role of attention in display design for improving operator performance, reducing workload, and increasing situation awareness.

ROLE OF SELECTIVE AND DIVIDED ATTENTION

Technological advances have allowed many tasks that were typically performed manually by operators to be automated. This automation has resulted in many jobs being transformed from ones of active involvement to ones of monitoring whether the automated tasks are performed correctly. Monitoring displays can result in vigilance decrements, and a reduction in situation awareness can lead to serious consequences if the operator needs to regain control when the automation fails. Moreover, operators often monitor more than one display or a single display consisting of complex components. Because the components of the display are usually more than the operator can attend to at any given moment, he or she must selectively attend to important or relevant features of the display while filtering out features irrelevant to the current task.

Operators must also learn to divide their attention across multiple displays and attend to the one that will provide the most information to support their task at a given moment in time. For example, driving a vehicle is a task in which attention must be time-shared between the road and in-car tasks such as monitoring the speedometer and other instruments; operating a navigation system or radio, CD, or music streaming service; or using voice commands or manual inputs to access features of a mobile phone. Because the driver needs to attend to visual information from outside the vehicle to keep the vehicle from going off the road or colliding with moving vehicles or other obstacles, increases in the time for which gaze is directed toward the interior will increase the likelihood of accident. To drive effectively while performing secondary tasks, the driver must employ appropriate strategies regarding when and for how long they can divert attention from the roadway to one of the other tasks to accomplish that task while not placing the vehicle at risk. Glances of less than 0.5 seconds are probably too short to gather information about most in-car tasks, but glances longer than 2 seconds keep attention away from the road for too long (e.g., Zwahlen et al., 1988). Thus, displays in vehicles must provide the information the driver needs in the shortest time possible.

Displays often cover a large portion of the visual field, but high visual acuity of operators is restricted to only a small area around the fixation point (see Chapters 2 and 3). Thus, the control of eye movements is essential. *Pursuit eye movements* (those in which the eyes move together to track a visual target) are important in tasks such as driving that require following a road. *Saccadic eye movements* (those for which the eye shifts fixation rapidly from one fixed position to another) occur when an operator checks individual instruments on a display panel (e.g., speedometer). Saccades can be triggered automatically by a salient event (e.g., a vehicle changing into your lane) or intentionally as a consequence of the operator's goals (e.g., checking the rearview mirror in anticipation of a lane change). Although the spotlight of attention can be directed toward a location other than the fixated location, the two often coincide, and the gaze patterns can be used as measures about which displayed information the observer is attending to.

Selective attention has been studied for supervisory control tasks in which the operator must attend to specific instruments on a complex display panel. A skilled operator will select relevant display information at appropriate times. Highly overlearned skills, as well as task requirements and goals, contribute to sampling and search from complex displays. Several factors influence an operator's sampling strategies. For example, experienced drivers have higher sampling rates (i.e., more fixations) and shorter fixation durations and show a broader scanning of the road than inexperienced drivers (Konstantopoulos et al., 2010). Wikman et al. (1998) also found that novice drivers show less adequate cognitive control strategies than more experienced drivers, as would be expected if the strategies were learned. The novice drivers in their study showed more variability in their glance durations than did the experts (i.e., they showed larger numbers of glances that were too short to be effective and too long to be safe), which resulted in larger lateral displacements of the vehicle.

MENTAL MODELS

Displays that are designed to be consistent with the operators' mental models will allow operators to perform their tasks more quickly and make fewer errors by reducing attentional demands. The concept of *mental model* refers to a representation of some aspect of the world (e.g., a system) that reflects the individual's understanding of it. The concept is somewhat abstract, but mental models are presumed to allow operators to use past experiences to simulate the behavior of the system of interest and make predictions about future events. When interacting with a system, operators interpret the information provided by the display in terms of their expectancies and use their knowledge to direct sampling behavior. The operators have mental models of how the system with which they are interacting operates, what displayed information is relevant to the current situation, and where and how that information is displayed.

An example using a web browser is as follows. If an operator must perform tasks using a browser, they would expect the layout of the webpage to match "typical" webpages: The homepage hyperlink is located at the top left corner, the major navigation controls or links for the major sections of the site are located across the top of the page, the local navigation within each major section is along the left side of the page, and so on (see Vu et al., 2021). The user also understands how the browser operates and takes actions dependent on this understanding. Because the operator is likely to have considerable experience with websites and to have developed a strong mental model for them, webpages within a site that are not formatted in a manner consistent with the operator's mental model may lead to poorer performance. For instance, a user expects text that is colored and underlined to be hyperlinks, for which a click on the text will "take them" to information relating to the text. Displays that underline and color text solely to emphasize a word or concept that is not hyperlinked may cause confusion for the user.

Mode Errors

A *mode error* occurs when users perform an action that does not produce the desired response due to the system being in a different mode (Sarter & Woods, 1995). Having an inaccurate mental model of how a system works can lead to low levels of situation awareness and mode errors. Endsley (2017) recorded her experience with the autonomous driving features of a Tesla Model S over a 6-month period. Endsley had difficulty developing an accurate mental model of how the automation worked because (a) the training she received from the sales representative was brief and ad hoc (i.e., driven by the questions she asked the representative), (b) the description of features in the manual was not comprehensive, and (c) the rapid rate of software updates (often with insufficient description of the changes) required constant updating of her mental model. Endsley recorded automation-related problems on 30% of her trips, with mode errors being the most frequent problem. For example, the adaptive cruise control was still on when Endsley thought that she took manual control:

> When the driver presses the brakes, the ACC [adaptive cruise control] and auto-steer will turn off; however, if the driver turns the steering wheel, only autosteer is canceled, and the ACC remains on. When I turned the wheel to exit the freeway at an off-ramp, for example, I was surprised that I was still traveling very fast and needed to brake as well to disconnect the ACC. This problem also occurred on a sharp curve when I took over manual steering; I was surprised that the ACC was still engaged and that the car was going too fast for the curve. (p. 232)

Endsley (2017) observed that some of the mode errors were a result of the lever controlling the adaptive cruise control and autosteer functions being located directly below the lever for the turn signal and that she would accidently perform the desired action on the wrong lever. However, she was able to notice the mode error and make corrections before an accident happened. In other situations, fatal accidents can occur if the display does not provide the operator with a salient indicator of the mode. Sarter (2000) noted that a reason why pilots may miss automated mode changes when monitoring automated flight deck systems is because the transition is signaled by a box that appears around the new flight mode for a short period and then disappears. Thus, if pilots are not looking directly at the display, they will miss the warning of a mode change. Fortunately, under most circumstances, pilots are able to realize at a later time on the basis of feedback from subsequent interactions with the system that the mode has changed. However, Sarter described one case where this correction was not made:

> The crew did not realize that due to the coupling of lateral and vertical modes, their selection of a new lateral mode had the indirect unintended effect of a transition

from the flight path angle to the vertical speed mode. When a target descent rate was subsequently entered, the systems interpreted the pilot-entered digits, 33, to mean 3,300 fpm instead of the desired 3.3° angle of descent . . . the [team] members approached and ultimately crashed into a mountainside. (p. 234)

Sarter (2008) suggested several countermeasures to mode errors, with the first being to use other modalities, such as tactual cues, to capture the pilots' attention and signal mode changes. The second is to inform pilots about changes in the mode status directly in the display (highlight the current mode and available controls). Other countermeasures are to redesign the displays so that they provide information that support pilots' understanding of the system (i.e., have an automated display provide a preview of future instructions) and provide better training.

Pictorial Realism and Moving Parts

A user's mental model may not contain complete information about the system, and it may include concepts that are not part of the system (G. Fischer, 1991). To format the display in a manner consistent with the operator's mental model, Wickens et al. (2004) suggested that three design principles should be incorporated: pictorial realism, moving components, and ecological interface design. The *principle of pictorial realism* is that the display should visually depict the item it is supposed to represent. As illustrated in Figure 10.1A, when a laptop is plugged in, a good display would show a plug icon next to a battery icon to represent that the device is plugged in, and a lighting symbol should appear in the battery icon to signify that the laptop is charging. Karimi et al. (2011) found that participants were faster to respond and more accurate with the pictorial display than with the symbolic or textual display for identifying seven parameters of an agricultural air seeder.

The *principle of moving components* refers to the notion that moving elements of a display should be in the direction consistent with the user's mental model. For example, when displaying how much battery is left (see Figure 10.1), the battery indicator bar should move from bottom (low charge) to top (full charge) or from left (low charge) to right (full charge). The principle of moving components suggests that the animation of processes and diagrams should

FIGURE 10.1. Illustration of the Principles of Pictorial Realism and Moving Components

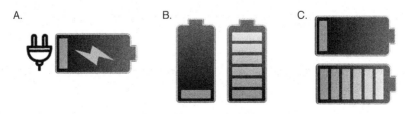

Note. Pictorial realism (A) and moving components from low to high, going bottom to top (B) and left to right (C).

be better than static images. Ploetzner et al. (2021) found that animation was more effective at teaching students to identify motions of a gear, whereas a static image was more effective at teaching students to identify its spatial arrangement. However, I. Wagner and Schnotz (2017) showed that students did not learn more about horse gaits or synaptic transmission processes from animation sequences that illustrated the movements than from static images. Thus, whether the moving component or animation aids learning depends on the task.

A *schema* is similar to a mental model in that it is also a representation of a concept, but the term typically is used to refer to the long-term knowledge about a category or concept. Hurtienne (2017) found that people tend to make responses consistent with image-schematic metaphors such as "more is big" and "less is small," "more is heavy" and "less is light," and "important is central" and "unimportant is peripheral." Displays that are designed to be consistent with users' schemas should lead to better performance by reducing cognitive load.

Although the principle of pictorial realism makes intuitive sense and has been enthusiastically endorsed by the design community and end users, Smallman and St. John (2005) indicated that, in many of their studies, the use of realistic 3D displays led to poor performance, especially for tasks requiring relative position and distance judgments. They noted that a reason that realistic displays may not benefit performance is that they contain too many details. These details can make many objects appear similar or overload the operator in search of the relevant one. Moreover, use of both symbolic and spatial information in 3D displays can lead to ambiguity and difficulty in discrimination and identification. Thus, designers should consider the type of tasks and the level of realism needed for end users to perform the task effectively rather than just striving for pictorial realism in all cases.

Grouping and Proximity Compatibility Principles

When organizing the components of a display, the way individual elements are grouped is important, and when these elements are grouped in an optimal manner, performance will be better and the attentional demands will be less. Displays can be grouped by following the gestalt perceptual-organization principles (Palmer, 2003). These include, among others, (a) components in close spatial proximity tend to be grouped together (*proximity*), (b) components that are similar in appearance tend to be grouped together (*similarity*), (c) components that follow a continuous contour tend to be grouped together (*continuity*), (d) gaps between contours tend to be filled in (*closure*), and (e) components that move in the same direction or at the same speed will tend to be grouped together (*common fate*). With a good display organization, when the operator wants information regarding a certain aspect of a task, the operator will be able to focus attention on one area of the display rather than switching between multiple areas. Elements of a display should be grouped together when they (a) are related, (b) are usually monitored in sequence, or (c) can be clustered together in a way that allows the operator to attend to particular groups of elements at once.

The benefit of a good perceptual grouping is illustrated in studies conducted by Banks and Prinzmetal (1976; Prinzmetal & Banks, 1977). In their experiments, participants judged whether a T or F was presented among hybrid T-F distractors. They found that performance was worse when the target letter was clustered into the same group as the distractors than when it was not. For example, one experiment demonstrated an effect of continuity. In all cases, the target was presented among five distractors. In one condition the target was placed in a line with four of the distractors so that continuity grouped it as part of the line (as in Figure 10.2, left configuration). In a second condition, the target was placed separately from the line of five distractors so that they were grouped separately from it (as in Figure 10.2, right configuration). Reaction times to identify the target were longer in the former case than in the latter.

Wickens and colleagues (Wickens & Andre, 1990; Wickens & Carswell, 1995) developed the *proximity compatibility principle* to emphasize that there is a relation between different types of displays and how information from the displays has to be used. According to Wickens and Andre (1990), the proximity compatibility principle asserts that tasks in which "close mental proximity" is required (i.e., information integration) will be best served by more proximate displays, whereas tasks that require "low mental proximity" (i.e., independent processing of two or more variables) will benefit from more separate displays.

Wickens and colleagues (Wickens & Andre, 1990; Wickens & Carswell, 1995) specified two types of proximity: perceptual and processing. *Perceptual proximity* refers to the perceptual similarity that exists between different display components. This type of proximity includes spatial (distance), chromatic (color), form (shapes), measurement (physical dimensions), and perceptual

FIGURE 10.2. Displays Used by Prinzmetal and Banks (1977)

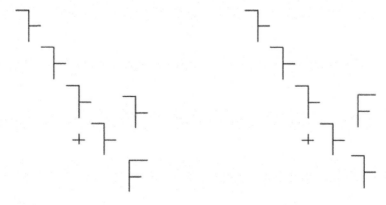

Note. From "Good Continuation Affects Visual Detection," by W. Prinzmetal and W. P. Banks, 1977, *Perception & Psychophysics, 21*(5), p. 390 (https://doi.org/10.3758/BF03199491). Copyright 1977 by Springer Nature. Reprinted with permission.

codes (verbal vs. manual). *Spatial proximity* refers to distances between items. For example, the flanker congruity effect (B. A. Eriksen & Eriksen, 1974; see Chapter 4, this volume) demonstrates an effect of spatial proximity in that reaction time to the target stimulus is affected most when the flankers are in close spatial proximity.

Processing proximity refers to how much attention must be focused on the different components of a display to obtain the information necessary to complete a task (Wickens & Carswell, 1995). Processing proximity can be characterized by three different categories: integrative, nonintegrative, and independent. *Integrative processing* involves active integration of the components through *computational integration* (using mathematical operations) or *Boolean integration* (meeting more than one parameter, e.g., X "and" Y). *Nonintegrative processing* involves similarity among the components of the display, such as *metric similarity* (displays that are measured in the same units), *covariance similarity* (changes in one display can predict changes in another), and *functional similarity* (multiple displays that yield information about a class of information). Finally, *independent processing* does not require processing of components together. Separate decisions are made for each display component (e.g., determining the vehicle's speed from a speedometer and whether there is enough gas from the gas gauge).

In some cases, multiple elements of a display or multiple displays can be arranged or grouped in a way that certain properties of the monitoring task will emerge. An emergent display or feature can reduce the attentional demands because the operator can monitor the global property rather than the individual components. Emergent displays can be classified into integral and configural displays (Bennett & Flach, 1992; Garner, 1976), which are often compared to separable displays. *Separable displays* allow each component to maintain its unique perceptual properties so that the processing of these components can be done independently. *Integral displays* refer to emergent properties of the components being so strong that the perceptual properties of the individual components are not distinguishable. Although this type of display provides a good depiction of a system's overall status, it affects the operator's ability to selectively attend to an individual component or divide attention to monitor components of the system. *Configural displays* have emergent features but maintain the individual perceptual properties of the components. For example, the emergent features can be of vertical symmetry (e.g., as in brackets [ ]), but the individual components can be maintained. With configural displays, there is a smaller cost of divided attention but a larger cost of selective attention.

Signaling Action Through Perceived Affordances and Display-Control Mappings

In display design, *perceived affordances* allow the user to perceive the action that should be taken based on the how the real item is displayed or represented on an interface (Norman, 2013). When looking at a physical display that contains a button, the button affords a push response. Using a mouse to move a cursor on the screen affords pointing and clicking of objects. More generally, the visual information provided by the environment needs to be designed to accommodate the position of the body to maximize effective responses (Reed & Hartley, 2021). Displays that take advantage of such relations can improve operator performance by signaling the desired actions, thus reducing attentional demands and working memory load.

Wickens et al. (2004) suggested three memory principles that should be incorporated into display design. First, the display should anticipate the actions of the operators so that when operators are overloaded, they know what action to take without much effort. Second, the display should match what the operator is seeing in the environment. Third, the display should be consistent with the operator's actions as constrained by the physical environment. These points are illustrated in Figure 10.3, which shows two types of push bars for opening doors. Both are designed anticipating that the user will push the door to open it. But only the one on the right visually signals unambiguously which side of the bar to push to allow the door to be opened based on the side that is hinged. The difference between the designs may seem trivial, but when people need to exit the building quickly, as when there is a fire, a good design can save lives.

For a display to be arranged for optimal selection, its arrangement should also correspond to the configuration of the controls (e.g., Fitts & Seeger, 1953). In a classic study of stove-top configurations, Chapanis and Lindenbaum (1959) evaluated four control-burner arrangements (see Figure 10.4). The experimenter demonstrated the individual pairings of burners to controls for one of the four stoves and then instructed participants to push the control assigned to the burner that was lit. Participants responded more quickly with Design 1, for which congruity between the horizontal locations of the burners and controls was maintained, than with Designs 2 to 4, for which it was not. Furthermore, no errors were made with Design 1, whereas the overall error rates were 6%, 10%, and 11% for Designs 2, 3, and 4, respectively. Practice significantly reduced response time and errors for Design 2 compared with Designs 3 and 4, but performance was still worse than with Design 1. This study illustrates the importance of both display arrangement and how the display maps into any responses that must be made.

FIGURE 10.3. Illustration of Perceived Affordances for Pushing a Door to Open

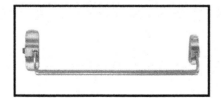 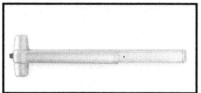

Note. The left handle does not indicate which side of the door to push, but the right one does.

FIGURE 10.4. Stove Configurations With Different Mappings of Burners to Control Knobs

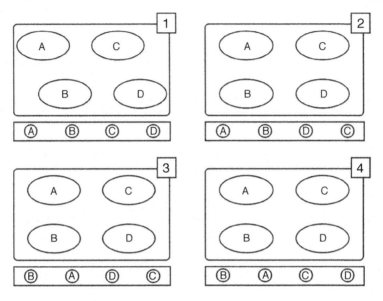

Note. From *Attention: Theory and Practice* (p. 239), by A. Johnson and R. W. Proctor, 2004, SAGE (https://doi.org/10.4135/9781483328768). Copyright 2004 by A. W. Johnson and R. W. Proctor. Reprinted with permission.

The salient features of the display can also predict what response will be made to the stimuli (Reeve & Proctor, 1990). As noted earlier in the book, *stimulus–response compatibility* refers to the fact that people respond faster and more accurately to some mappings of displays to controls than others (Proctor & Vu, 2006b). The role of salience can be illustrated for situations in which stimuli and responses vary along both horizontal and vertical dimensions, thus allowing compatibility to be maintained for both, one, or neither of the dimensions (Vu & Proctor, 2001).

Figure 10.5 illustrates situations of this type examined in a study by Nicoletti and Umiltà (1985). The stimuli could occur in the upper-left or lower-right

FIGURE 10.5. Stimulus-Response Configurations Used by Nicoletti and Umiltà (1985)

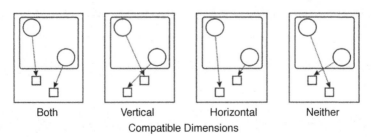

Note. From *Attention: Theory and Practice* (p. 240), by A. Johnson and R. W. Proctor, 2004, SAGE (https://doi.org/10.4135/9781483328768). Copyright 2004 by A. W. Johnson and R. W. Proctor. Reprinted with permission.

corners of the display panel, and responses were made by pressing one of two buttons with the left or right thumb. The two response alternatives were arrayed along the same diagonal as the stimuli (upper left, lower right) or the opposite diagonal (upper right, lower left). When aligned on the same diagonal, the mapping of stimuli to responses was compatible on both the horizontal and vertical dimensions or on neither dimension. When located on opposite diagonals, the mapping of stimuli to responses was compatible on only the horizontal dimension or only the vertical dimension. Not surprisingly, performance was best when both dimensions were mapped compatibly and worst when both were mapped incompatibly. More important, performance was better when compatibility was maintained along the horizontal dimension than along the vertical dimension, a phenomenon called the *right–left prevalence effect* (Nicoletti & Umiltà, 1985; Rubichi et al., 2006).

On the basis of these results, Andre and Wickens (1990) concluded that the horizontal dimension preferentially attracts attention at the cost of the vertical dimension. However, studies demonstrate that right–left prevalence only occurs for situations in which the environment provides a horizontal frame of reference for response coding. When responses were made by the contralateral hand and foot (e.g., right hand, left foot), a right–left prevalence effect was obtained. However, with ipsilateral hand and foot responses (e.g., right hand, right foot), a top–bottom prevalence effect was evident (Vu & Proctor, 2002). Thus, the salient reference frame for location coding determines the relative weightings of the horizontal and vertical dimensions.

Another factor that can influence performance is anticipated effects produced by responses. Control-display *population stereotypes*, known for many years, are of this type. Responses to turn a knob to move a display element in a particular direction, for example, will be faster and more accurate if the mapping corresponds to stereotypical relations (Vu & Sun, 2019). Kunde (2001) provided the first experimental demonstration of such *response-effect compatibility* effects, showing shorter reaction times when key press responses based on task instructions produced "effect" stimuli at locations congruent with the key locations rather than incongruent with them. J. Chen and Proctor (2013) offered evidence that response-effect compatibility influenced performance in a simulated scrolling task. For that task, participants were to bring a target stimulus into view from the top or bottom of a display screen by pressing the up or down arrow key on a computer keyboard. Responses were faster when the key direction was incongruent with the initial stimulus location but congruent with the intended stimulus movement direction. However, Janczyk et al. (2019) found only a negligible influence of response-effect compatibility in a similar task for which the responses were touchless upward and downward gestures, suggesting context-dependent results.

Ecological Interface Design

Ecological interface design focuses on the idea that displays should not be arbitrary symbolic representations of the "real" environment but should impose lawful constraints that are representative of the actual environment (Flach, 2001;

Vicente & Rasmussen, 1992). Ecological interface design begins by considering the constraints in the task environment that are relevant to the user (Bennett et al., 2018). It is based on Rasmussen's (1986) behavioral taxonomy that distinguishes three modes of behavior: skill, rule, and knowledge based. The *skill-based* mode is relatively automatic behavior that occurs when the situation is a familiar one in which overlearned procedures are applicable. For example, after driving for years, a driver is highly experienced at the basic operation of a car and can automatically execute the required actions (i.e., perform a lane change or brake for a stoplight) under normal driving conditions. Behavior is *rule based* when a rare event occurs, but the event is one for which a previously learned rule can be retrieved from memory and applied. Rule-based behavior may occur for the driver when a siren is detected, and the driver moves over to the side to let the emergency vehicle pass.

Finally, behavior is *knowledge based* when an event is unfamiliar, no simple rule applies, and the user must engage in problem solving. Knowledge-based behavior may occur for the driver if the check engine light comes on, and the driver needs to engage in problem solving to determine the cause and what can be done to fix the problem. Another example is when a driver is following a navigation system, but the map on the system is old or inaccurate. The navigation gives a direction (i.e., turn left on Maple Street) that is inconsistent with the environment, and the driver must engage in problem solving. For example, if there was an island or road divider that was preventing a left turn at Maple Street, the driver can decide to make a U-turn at the next possible location to make a right on Maple Street. If the map is not accurate and the driver realizes that Maple Street becomes Elm Street as the driver crosses between the boundaries of two cities, they can decide to make a left turn at Elm Street.

The basic idea behind ecological interface design is that the information that needs to be represented in a good display varies as a function of the appropriate behavior mode. The display should highlight the goal-relevant information in a way that changes dynamically to reflect the physical world. For skill-based behavior, the user should be able to respond directly to the display, with the structure of the displayed information matching the required actions. For rule-based behavior, the interface should signal the appropriate rules to be retrieved and applied with a consistent mapping between constraints of the work environment and the displayed information. For knowledge-based behavior, the work environment should be represented in a form that provides an externalized mental model in support of problem solving.

Bennett et al. (2018) used ecological interface design principles to develop a prototype computer network defense system designed to protect sensitive information stored on computer networks by alerting operators of the system's state. The prototype employed three design principles of ecological interface design: *direct perception* (ability to perceive the state of the system by the patterns being displayed on the interface), *direct manipulation* (the ability to directly manipulate objects on the screen and not through menus), and *visual momentum* (helps the user find the "right" screen to support the current task goals). Ecological interface design predicts that operator performance will be better when the display follows a design principle that is consistent with type of processing that is most appropriate for the task.

For example, if the task requires determining the exact value of transmissions by a single host or internet protocol (IP) address, an alphanumeric display should be effective. For tasks that require comparing transmission rates across two different hosts or IPs, a bar graph display should be effective. A *treemap display*, which is a contingency table that includes rectangles of different areas to represent aggregate transmission, should be effective at conveying global transmission levels. Sushereba et al. (2020) examined these ecological interface design predictions and found some evidence consistent with the predictions. However, across all tasks they found the alphanumeric display to be the most effective and the treemap display to be the least effective. Although Sushereba et al. indicated that the poorer performance associated with the treemap display may have been due to the type of questions that were used for assessing performance, it may be the case that the treemap display was too complex for users.

Multiple design principles, including grouping principles and ecological interface design, can be combined to help designers determine the optimal arrangements of display elements on a panel for automotive instrument display panels (Shmueli et al., 2013). Take, for example, a road management display where operators need to respond to alerts, gather information, and make decisions about courses of action to take (e.g., post a message on a sign about traffic situations and/or propose detours due to traffic congestion). Baber et al. (2019) evaluated two displays designed for road traffic management, one designed using only ecological interface design principles and another combining them with proximity compatibility principles. Although both principles state that related information should be grouped together, the proximity compatibility principle is more specific in how proximity is defined: task versus display.

Baber et al. (2019) indicated that task proximity is similar to the principle of ecological interface design. However, the distinction between integrative and separate displays is unique to the proximity compatibility principle. Thus, Baber et al.'s two displays varied in terms of whether the key information sources were presented in separate windows of the display or overlaid and integrated into one view. The time to submit decisions was shorter with the separate windows, but time to gather information and the total task time were shorter with the integrative display. From these findings, Baber et al. concluded that there is an added benefit for applying the proximity compatibility principle when following the ecological interface design approach. Integrative displays can support gathering information to determine the state of the system to increase operators' situation awareness.

TYPES OF DISPLAYS

Many factors influence the effectiveness of a display. Even something as basic as whether text is best presented electronically or printed on paper can influence performance, attention to the material, and even preference (see Box 10.1).

BOX 10.1 | **READING ON ELECTRONIC DISPLAYS OF DIFFERENT SIZES**

During the COVID-19 pandemic, school closures forced many students to learn remotely. While technology made remote learning possible, some studies have shown a negative impact of computer displays on learners' attention and comprehension of material (e.g., Delgado & Salmerón, 2021). As illustrated in Box 7.1 in Chapter 7, students often engage in multitasking with different media displays during study, decreasing their test scores and grades (K. E. May & Elder, 2018). However, even when students are not distracted, the display medium of the information can impact students' comprehension and retention of the learning material.

Mayes et al. (2001) found that students took about 30% longer to read the same article when it was presented on a computer screen than when it was printed on paper. However, the students' test scores on a comprehension test did not differ between the two mediums. Delgado and Salmerón (2021) indicated that the lack of comprehension differences when reading on a computer screen versus on paper is a common finding when the reading tasks are based on narrative (e.g., stories) text and were self-paced. However, they found that students did differ in reading comprehension scores for more expository (i.e., educational) text under time pressure.

Delgado and Salmerón (2021) had students read a long article on human learning and artificial intelligence on a computer screen or paper and with or without time pressure. The time pressure group were alloted 75% of the average time that students likely would have spent reading the task under no time pressure. In addition to testing the students' comprehension of the reading material, they also captured students' self-reported mind-wandering behaviors during the task. Mind wandering is considered to be a failure of sustained attention to a task where attention wanders to unrelated task thoughts. Delgado and Salmerón found the time pressure manipulation to be effective; about half the participants in that condition reported not being able to finish the article (equally distributed across the computer screen and paper conditions).

For students assigned to read the article on the computer screen, those in the time pressure group scored lower on the comprehension test than students who read the article at their own pace. However, for students assigned to read the article on paper, the test scores were not different for the group with time pressure and the one without. Also, participants in the computer screen with time pressure condition reported more mind wandering than participants in the other three conditions. Delgado and Salmerón (2021) attributed their findings to inattentive reading that occurs when the information is displayed on a computer screen compared with paper and the inability of participants to engage in attention control to suppress mind-wandering tendencies under time pressure in the computer screen condition.

BOX 10.1 | READING ON ELECTRONIC DISPLAYS OF DIFFERENT SIZES *(Continued)*

E. Park et al. (2018) examined students' comprehension of video lecture material when the lectures were viewed on mobile devices. Three screen sizes of 3.5 inches (small), 7 inches (medium), and 10.1 inches (large) were examined to reflect viewing the lectures on a phone and tablet devices. Students watched six lectures on European history, lasting 1 hour each, over 6 consecutive days in a laboratory setting. On the last day, students were tested on their comprehension of the lecture material and were asked to rate their satisfaction with the course materials. There was a significant effect of screen size on the participants' comprehension and satisfaction scores.

Performance on the comprehension test was the best for the large display group, intermediate for the medium display group, and worst for the small display group. Students also reported greater satisfaction with the course material when the lectures were viewed on large screens than medium and small screens. A subset of the students returned to the lab after 2 months and was tested on the lecture materials using different test questions. At this longer retention interval, there was no difference in test scores for all three groups, and the comprehension level was at that for the small screen group for the immediate test. E. Park et al. (2018) attributed the decline in performance for the large and medium displays to the visual attention benefits for the larger screens decaying rapidly over time. That is, the larger screen size allowed for better visual quality of the material and better encoding of the material, which allows learners to attend to details that are not as visible on the small display. This benefited the participants in the larger display groups at the immediate test.

In this section, we consider several types of displays and how attention and performance are impacted by their designs.

Search Displays

When a target differs from distractors by a basic feature such as color, reaction time and error rate often show little increase as the number of distractors increases (Treisman & Gelade, 1980). As discussed in Chapter 4, this is because features are analyzed preattentively, allowing the target feature to "pop out" and search to be efficient (Wolfe, 2001). Thus, when feature search is possible, little benefit of providing structure to the display is expected. When two or more features must be combined to distinguish the target from distractors (conjunction search), search is less efficient: Reaction time and error rate typically increase sharply as the number of distractors increases. A limited capacity attentional process is required for conjunction search because responses cannot be based on the detection of a single feature, and each location must be examined until a target is detected or all items present have been searched.

In this situation, structuring the array can improve performance significantly by allowing the operator to direct attention to the locations most likely to contain the relevant information.

According to Wolfe's (2021) guided search model, activation produced by individual features (e.g., color, orientation) is summed in an activation map, and the relative amounts of activation at different locations can be used to guide where attention is directed. Consequently, attention-demanding conjunction search will be easier when the display is structured such that the similarity of the potential targets to distractors is low and similarity among the distractors high. As an example, Rauschenberger et al. (2009) had participants search for a target icon on a display with other icons. The icons were classified by spatial frequency as high (detailed) or low (global shapes). Participants were able to find high frequency targets fast, regardless of set size, if all the distractors were low in spatial frequency and vice versa due to pop-out. When the display had a mixed presentation of high- and low-frequency items, and the target was known to be either high or low in spatial frequency, participants were able to narrow the subset of searched items based on spatial frequency. In this case, search through low frequency icons was more efficient than search through high frequency icons. Rauschenberger et al. cautioned designers that the use of spatial frequency as a search strategy to reduce the set size is only effective if the user realizes this meaningful distinction between targets and distractors.

When targets are rare, they are missed at a higher rate than when the targets are prevalent, a finding known as a *low prevalence effect* (e.g., Hout et al., 2015). Hout et al. (2015) indicated that three factors could lead to the low prevalence effect: perceptual errors, early termination of search bias (i.e., criterion shift), and motor errors (i.e., make habitual responses consistent with the prevalence rates). To test between these accounts, Hout et al. had participants search for two targets and manipulated the prevalence rate for each target to be unbalanced (10% vs. 40%), near balanced (20% vs. 30%), or extreme (5% vs. 45%) but kept the overall prevalence rate at 50%. The participants were instructed to respond that a target was present if they found either target. Participants' detection of rare targets remained low even though the task was set up so that the overall prevalence rate was 50% (ruling out the motor pattern errors). In subsequent experiments, Hout et al. used Rapid Serial Visual Search (RSVP; see Chapter 8, this volume) to ensure that participants could not terminate the search on their own without seeing all stimuli and still found the low prevalence effect. These findings imply that the low prevalence effect is due to perceptual identification errors.

Structuring the display so that the critical information will appear where the operator is most likely to look can also improve performance. Mudd and McCormick (1960) conducted a study in which they asked participants to perform a visual search of a 32-dial display to locate a deviant dial with and without the assistance of auditory cues. Their study showed that participants tend to use a systematic pattern of visual search (i.e., participants tended to search the quadrants of the display panel in a similar order), which could delay search times of targets in the quadrants that participants tend to search last.

Structuring search can also be beneficial for navigating through menus (Paap & Cooke, 1997). This change in the interface may be the desired output or may allow the user to obtain the desired output. A good menu should be composed from unambiguous descriptors that accurately convey each option to the user, with the options organized in a manner that will lead to short search times. When a user intends to execute a goal, they direct their fixation at an option on the display and evaluate whether selecting that option would help them achieve the goal. If the user decides to select the option, it is executed; if not, they must redirect their attention to searching other options. When the user knows exactly what option to search for, *identity matching* can be used, and search time is fastest. When the users need to find an option that is classified within a main menu, *inclusion matching* occurs in which the user must decide under which class a specific option would be categorized. Finally, a user can also engage in *equivalence search* in which they know what option should be executed but do not know how the option is labeled. To structure the options of menus in an optimal manner, designers must consider the type of search in which the user would most likely be engaged. Designers may also want to be aware that many users want a search feature to quickly find information and hyperlink to it rather than search through menus in a display for navigation.

Alerting Displays

When an operator must monitor various components of a display, a warning signal can be used to capture the operator's attention. Tao et al. (2017) examined whether warning icons (e.g., an exclamation mark, skull, no smoking sign) are better at capturing attention than ordinary icons (e.g., house, airplane, garbage bin). Participants searched for a target letter in an array of six letters presented on an invisible circle. For a subset of the search trials, a much larger warning icon or an ordinary icon was presented outside the search array. The icons were successful in capturing attention: Search time was longer when an icon was present than when one was not. Because the warning icons had a larger effect than ordinary icons, Tao et al. concluded that warning-symbol icons are more effective at capturing attention than ordinary icons.

Warning and alerting systems should help individuals make decisions to improve their task performance, such as providing the users with information that lets them know when or whether a particular action will exceed safety thresholds or reduce task accuracy. Phansalkar et al. (2010) indicated that several features make alerting systems effective in medical environments. Some features an alerting system should include are (a) specifying the categories of alerts and their prioritization scheme, (b) prioritizing the alert levels (e.g., for visual displays, color progression such as yellow to orange to red can be used to indicate increasing hazard levels; for auditory displays, urgency can be communicated by decreasing the interpulse interval), (c) producing a low level of false alarms, (d) being placed where the alert is likely to be seen or heard by the user, and (e) being consistent with the user's mental model (i.e., provide data that support users' assessment of the risks associated with the task).

Because most displays are visual, auditory warning stimuli are often effective. First, auditory cues do not impose additional demands on the visual system. Second, auditory cues can be perceived regardless of the operator's current orientation, whereas if the warning signal is visual, the operator must be directly looking at the visual display to benefit from it. Properties of the auditory alert can also be manipulated to promote prioritization through perceptions of urgency. For example, increases in the fundamental frequency and decreases in interpulse intervals can produce higher levels of perceived urgency (Baldwin & Lewis, 2014). Marshall et al. (2007) found that characteristics of alerts that promote higher levels of urgency also increase users' rated annoyance. This may be problematic because users may disable the alert if they are annoyed by it. Fortunately, Marshall et al. also found that, for a simulated driving task, increasing pulse duration and interpulse interval increased perceived urgency more than annoyance.

Multisensory Displays

Auditory spatial cuing can reduce visual search time because the cue directs attention to the target (e.g., Vu et al., 2006). Such benefits of auditory spatial cues in reducing visual search time depend on the factors surrounding the environment, such as target distance from fixation, distractor density, and size of the display (Strybel et al., 1995). Auditory spatial cuing effects have also been examined with simulated 2D and 3D cues, and both types of cues are equally beneficial in reducing search time (Perrott & Saberi, 1990). Perrott and Saberi (1990) attributed this reduction in search time to the auditory spatial cues signaling the general area in which the target is located, limiting the visual information that needs to be searched to locate the target.

Although auditory cues are excellent for warning signals, having operators monitor both auditory and visual information at the same time may not be a good idea. Spence and Driver (1996) showed that, although it is possible to direct auditory and visual attention to different locations, there is a cost associated with shifting attention between visual and auditory modalities (see Chapter 6, this volume). Spence and Driver proposed a "separable-but-linked" hypothesis to explain these cross-modal interactions. In their study, an orthogonal cuing method was used, in which participants were asked to make up or down discriminations of targets that were presented to the left or right side of fixation. Participants were instructed to direct either their auditory or visual attention to one side of fixation. Results showed that reaction times for the elevation judgments were shorter when the targets appeared on the cued side than when they appeared on the uncued side, even if the target was in a different sensory modality. This finding indicates that when attention for one modality is directed to one side of fixation, there is a corresponding shift of attention for the other modality to that location. Spence and Driver also included an experiment in which participants were instructed to direct their auditory attention to one side of fixation and their visual attention to the other side for a block of trials. Results showed reduced effects of spatial expectancies for both modalities. This finding indicates that participants were able to split auditory and visual attention when the targets for the two modalities were expected on opposite sides of fixation, but this splitting reduced the cuing effects within each modality.

When selective attention is not required—that is, when the task does not require attending exclusively to one feature while ignoring others—a redundant signal in a different modality can improve performance (see Opoku-Baah et al., 2021, for a review). For example, if participants are required to respond to a tone, they will perform more quickly when the tone is accompanied by a light (and to a light when accompanied by a tone; e.g., B. E. Stein et al., 1996). Just as with the speeded classification task discussed earlier, this redundancy gain depends on the relation between the stimuli. If stimuli are coded along some similar dimension, the effect of signal redundancy will depend on the particular pairings of the two signals. For example, both positions of visual stimuli and auditory pitch are coded along a vertical spatial dimension (see Walker & Ehrenstein, 2000). J. Miller (1991) found a redundancy gain for presenting a tone along with a visual signal when the task was to indicate the position of the visual stimulus, and the benefit of the auditory cue was greater when a high-pitched cue accompanied a high spatial location and a low-pitched cue accompanied a low spatial location than when these relations were reversed.

Multifunctional Displays

Multifunctional displays consist of multiple display options with which users interact. Early research on multifunctional displays focused on evaluating the *glass cockpit*, a term used in reference to the switch made in the aviation industry from the use of multiple dials and gauges to display information to the use of multifunctional displays (e.g., Sarter & Woods, 1992). A glass cockpit provides the operator with different types of information on the same display, allowing for flexibility of what is presented on the screen without taking up space for each information display element on the display panel. More recently, multifunctional displays have been examined to support operator performance in driving (e.g., J. Park & Park, 2019) and medical settings (e.g., Tremper et al., 2018). For example, a multifunctional infotainment display can provide drivers with audio player status (the device playing music, song title, artist), phone call–related information (calls, connection to mobile phone, access to phone apps), and other in-vehicle entertainment options. Similarly, a multifunctional display used in a hospital can extract real-time data from a variety of a hospital's systems (e.g., admission or discharge system, physiological data, labs) and display pertinent information about a patient to the appropriate health care provider through menus of a single display.

Because of the many options and combinations of options that multifunctional displays provide users, the use of a hierarchical structure (deep design) is preferred to reduce search time when using a menu interface for the display (E. Lee & MacGregor, 1985). Francis (2000) introduced a computational method of mapping labels to buttons (used to execute functions) optimal for hierarchical multifunctional displays. According to Francis, two steps are involved in creating an optimal mapping of labels to buttons: (a) the development of a quantitative model of the time needed to search through the hierarchy and (b) the application of an optimization algorithm to determine the best mapping according to the model. The model assumes that the time needed to reach a target is a function of the button-path time (sequence of buttons that need to be executed, including the time for the user to reach the button) and the label time (time that is needed in addition to button-path time). Francis optimized the design using a hill-climbing method in which the costs of different mappings are calculated by the computer, and if the new cost is smaller than the old, the new mapping is adopted. Using this method to model user search time and obtain parameters for the model, Francis tested the optimized mappings against a random assignment of labels to button paths and found that the optimized mapping resulted in a 32% reduction in search time.

Head-Up Displays

Head-up displays (HUDs) superimpose a virtual image of the information display (the near domain) on the central area in which the outside world (the far domain) is viewed to place important display information in close proximity (Weintraub & Ensing, 1992). HUDs allow the operator to access information without looking away from the primary viewing area (e.g., windshield). They were initially developed for use in aircraft, where the pilot must maintain visual contact with the external environment and monitor displays at the same time. However, automotive vehicles have included HUDs as an advanced feature (J. Park & Park, 2019). The basic idea for using HUDs is that superimposing the displays for the near and far domains will allow more parallel processing of the two images, reducing the need for scanning. HUDs have many uses due to their advantages, but they also have disadvantages (Newman, 2017). The advantages of HUDs are that (a) they allow both the environment and display to be monitored simultaneously, minimizing "head-down" time during which the pilot or driver is looking away from the outside environment; (b) a display can be aligned with its counterpart in the environment; and (c) the display can be collimated to appear at "optical infinity" to match that of the environment with the intent that the lens does not have to refocus for accommodation when switching focus between the environment and display. The drawbacks of HUDs are that they (a) create clutter, (b) may not be seen against the environmental background, and (c) reduce the visibility of environmental objects that are located behind them.

According to Weintraub and Ensing (1992), the costs and benefits of HUDs must be based on the three dimensions by which they differ from conventional head-down displays: their optical distance, location, and symbology. Figure 10.6 shows that the tasks can require focusing on the far domain (1) or near domain (2) or integrating information across the two (3). Attention may thus be focused on one domain, divided between the two domains, or switched between the domains. A supposed benefit of HUDs is to minimize cognitive switching because the eyes do not need to be moved or refocused. However, Weintraub and Ensing noted that all the cues that a switch is occurring with a head-down display are absent with a HUD: looking up, changing focus, and changing convergence. Consequently, a HUD may produce *cognitive capture* (or *cognitive tunneling*) and make it difficult to shift attention to the environment. Cognitive tunneling has been shown to occur in pilots for unexpected events (Wickens & Long, 1995), but it can be eliminated in certain situations. For example, Foyle et al. (2001) found that placing the HUD at least 8° away from the out-of-window path information eliminated cognitive tunneling.

For HUDs in automobiles, the problems of *positive misaccommodation*, where outside objects appear smaller than they are, could be exacerbated due to the closer focal distances used for automotive displays (Tufano, 1997). Tufano (1997) noted, "One of the paradoxes of HUDs is that they may do their job too well. Their salience, legibility, and head-up location may command too much of the operator's visual attention" (p. 306), consistent with the earlier description of cognitive tunneling. Thus, the benefits and costs of HUDs should be evaluated in their implementation in automobiles.

J. Park and Park (2019) reviewed the information regarding HUDs for commercially available vehicles. They found that the existing automotive HUDs provided drivers with 27 information types relating to the vehicle's state, safety, navigation, communication and infotainment, and the outside environment. They found that none of the information types were created specifically for the automotive HUD. That is, the HUDs provided the same information that

FIGURE 10.6. Representation of Pilots' Attention Processing Between Near and Far Domains Using Head-Up (HUD) and Head-Down (HDD) Displays

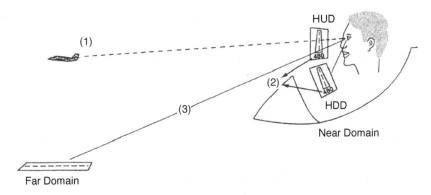

Note. From "Object Versus Space-Based Models of Visual Attention: Implications for the Design of Head-Up Displays," by C. D. Wickens and J. Long, 1995, *Journal of Experimental Psychology: Applied*, *1*(3), p. 180 (https://doi.org/10.1037/1076-898X.1.3.179). Copyright 1995 by the American Psychological Association.

can be found in conventional in-vehicle displays. Thus, the HUDS displayed completely redundant information found in the conventional display. However, being able to reconfigure the display and present information that may be more relevant to the primary driving task (i.e., navigation and detection of hazards) within the primary field of view may be beneficial to the driver and must be considered along with the known drawbacks of HUDs.

SUSTAINED ATTENTION AND VIGILANCE

Vigilance tasks have become more frequent in the work environment with the increasing automation of many jobs. A *vigilance task* requires an individual to monitor a display or environment to detect a rare target stimulus or event. For example, a baggage screener at an airport checkpoint views a large volume of images of luggage contents on a display to identify whether any of them contain weapons or other restricted items. Similarly, an operator of a self-driving vehicle must monitor the automation to ensure safety and intervene (i.e., takeover driving) when necessary. Performing a vigilance task requires sustained attention, which can be challenging for individuals. The most common finding for vigilance tasks is called the *vigilance decrement*: The hit rate at detecting target events decreases as the time on the vigil increases.

The Vigilance Decrement

The vigilance decrement was first noticed during World War II. After 30 minutes in a shift, radar operators in the Royal Air Force began to miss the signals on their screens that indicated possible enemy submarines (Mackworth, 1948). Mackworth (1950/1961) developed a clock test in which a pointer moved around a blank clock face, jumping 0.3 inches every second. Occasionally, the pointer would make a double jump of 0.6 inches, and the participant was to respond to this target event by pressing a key. About 85% of the targets were detected early in the session, but this decreased to about 75% over the first 30 minutes and continued to decrease slightly more after that time. This decrement in performance has been confirmed numerous times with a variety of tasks in subsequent research.

The vigilance decrement is affected by several factors that can be classified into three broad categories: task parameters, environmental or situational factors, and participant characteristics (Ballard, 1996; Neigel et al., 2019). Performance usually declines less when the target event is salient than when it is not. Detection performance also varies inversely with the background event rate and directly with signal event frequency. When spatial uncertainty exists about where a signal event may occur, performance is worse than when the event can occur in only a single location. Similar results are obtained when the number of displays that must be monitored increases. Performance also improves if participants are cued verbally that a signal will occur soon, just before the occurrence of one.

Gartenberg et al. (2018) found that the vigilance decrement occurred to the same degree for tasks performed successively and simultaneously if no response deadlines are used. However, imposing deadlines enhanced the vigilance decrement for successive tasks. Other factors that influence the vigilance decrement include environmental factors such as noise, heat, and vibration and subject characteristics such as age, with performance being an inverted U-shaped function of age across the life span.

Accounts for the Vigilance Decrement

Several accounts for the vigilance decrement have been proposed that are related but focus on different aspects of the situation. The first is that the decrement is due to underarousal (i.e., a low level of alertness and preparation; e.g., Frankmann & Adams, 1962). According to this account, because the task is monotonous, the operator cannot maintain a sufficient level of alertness. Second, being underaroused can lead to boredom or mindlessness, decreasing task performance (Manly et al., 1999) and increasing mind wandering (D. R. Thomson et al., 2015). Third, maintaining focus on the vigilance task is effortful and mentally demanding, which depletes attentional resources over the period of the vigil (Dillard et al., 2019; Warm et al., 1996). This latter view emphasizes that vigilance tasks can be demanding and stressful to the operator (Warm et al., 1996, 2008).

Warm et al. (1996) used the National Aeronautics and Space Administration Task Load Index (NASA-TLX; Hart & Staveland, 1988) as a measure of mental workload demands (see Chapter 9). Perceptual sensitivity (i.e., responding to the target event and not to nontarget events) was greater when the target was of high salience than when it was of low salience, and the former condition was judged to be less demanding than the latter. Moreover, ratings on the mental demand subscale of the NASA-TLX increased linearly over the period of the vigil. In a series of other experiments, Warm et al. showed other variables that reduce vigilance performance (e.g., low background event rate, spatial uncertainty) also lead to higher ratings of mental effort.

In a later study, Warm et al. (2008) used transcranial Doppler sonography to measure cerebral blood flow velocity in the medial artery to examine whether the amount of blood flow correlated with vigilance performance. They found that increases in task demands were correlated with increases in blood flow early in the vigil and a more rapid decrease over the course of the vigil. This finding suggests that the cerebral blood flow velocity in the medial artery can be used as an objective indicator of resource utilization and depletion for vigilance tasks.

Dillard et al. (2019) examined whether perceived time on task influenced the vigilance decrement. Perceived time was manipulated by telling participants that the session was longer (i.e., the perception that time flew by) or shorter (i.e., the perception that time lagged) than the actual session length. Dillard et al.'s manipulation successfully induced the intended perception of time, but even when "time flies by," participants rated the vigilance task as unpleasant, mentally demanding, and stressful. These findings are counter to the boredom accounts and consistent with resource depletion accounts of the vigilance decrement.

Change in Perceptual Sensitivity or a Shift in Response Bias?

One issue of concern in the research on vigilance has been whether the decrease in signal detection across time is due to a change in perceptual sensitivity or a shift in response bias (see Chapter 2). This issue can be addressed by examining the frequency of false detection responses on noise trials and performing a signal detection analysis. If the proportion of correct detections decreases across the vigil, but the proportion of incorrect detections does not, the decrement reflects a decrease in perceptual sensitivity. If, however, the proportion of incorrect detections also decreases, a shift to a more conservative response criterion is implicated. Parasuraman and Davies (1977) concluded that, for many situations, signal detection analyses show little change in d' across time but a shift in β to a more conservative response criterion. That is, the false alarms, as well as the correct detections, decrease as a function of time on task. However, perceptual sensitivity also seems to be affected as well when the task requires the participant to compare rapidly presented events with information in memory to identify the events as signals or nonsignals. Signal discriminability and task type (cognitive vs. sensory) can also influence the type of decrement observed (See et al., 1995).

McCarley and Yamani (2021) reported a vigilance task in which they tried to maximize the possibility of obtaining a sensitivity decrement. Working memory was required by presenting stimuli without a standard for comparison, time stress was imposed by presenting trials at a rapid rate, and the stimuli were embedded in visual noise. Using a detailed method of analysis, McCarley and Yamani found evidence of both a shift toward a more conservative response criterion and a decrease in perceptual sensitivity, as well as a tendency for participants to have mental lapses. However, they pointed out that criterion shifts accounted for the largest change in performance across the task. Thus, even for tasks that maximize the possibility of sensitivity decreases and mental lapses, the vigilance decrement is due largely to a criterion shift.

Individual Differences in Size of the Vigilance Decrement and Interventions

Neigel et al. (2019) examined whether individual differences in state motivation influenced vigilance performance when participants had to monitor one, two, or four different displays for targets that required perceptual (i.e., bolded font) or cognitive (i.e., a derived difference based on an arithmetic calculation) processes. Workload was measured using the NASA-TLX, and stress was measured using the Dundee Stress State Questionnaire (DSSQ; see Matthews, 2021, for a review). The DSSQ has two subscales, success motivation to excel on the task and intrinsic motivation from interest in the content of the task. Performance was measured using correct detection and false alarm performance and measures of sensitivity (*d'*) and bias.

Participants performed better when they had to monitor a single display or two displays than when they had to monitor four displays and reported workload to increase as the number of monitored displays increased. These results are more consistent with the resource accounts than the mindlessness or mind-wandering accounts because the one and two display conditions should be lower in load than the four displays condition. Neigel et al. (2019) also found that pretask state success motivation was related to sensitivity: As pretask success motivation increased, sensitivity increased. Posttask intrinsic motivation was also related to correct detection performance: As posttask motivation increased, correct detections increased. The latter findings suggest that facilitating intrinsic motivation of operators can help offset the vigilance decrement.

Over the years, many researchers have examined interventions to reduce the vigilance decrement. These interventions include behavioral (e.g., training and exercise) and physiological (e.g., caffeine and transcranial stimulation) techniques. For monitoring tasks, Al-Shargie et al. (2019) found the following to reduce reaction times by an average of 10% or more: video game playing and cognitive workload modulation, transcranial and haptic stimulation, taking caffeine and modafinil (a medication that promotes wakefulness), chewing gum, and listening to music. The effects of these interventions are reduced for more complex vigilance tasks that require comprehension and working memory, with some techniques showing little (e.g., cognitive workload modulation) or negative (e.g., listening to music) effects on performance.

VIRTUAL REALITY ENVIRONMENTS

Virtual reality (VR) environments manipulate sensory stimuli, such as visual, auditory, and haptic stimuli, to provide the observer with a sensation of interacting with the actual world. Research has shown that participants are able to orient their attention to locations in VR. For example, Quinlivan et al. (2016) had participants wear a head-mounted display to complete head movements toward peripherally located visual targets in VR. They found that participants showed orienting effects in VR, where they initiated head turns 57 ms earlier when given a valid rather than invalid cue. Thus, attention can be directed to locations within a VR environment.

If the VR is designed optimally, the observer will report a strong "presence of reality." When interacting with the system, the observers must focus on the coherent set of stimuli simulated by the environment. Thus, the amount of attention allocated to the VR environment is critical in determining the degree of presence a user will feel (Nash et al., 2000). Harjunen et al. (2017) showed that presence in VR can be enhanced when participants are able to see their body parts depicted in the display. Harjunen et al. examined the effect of presence on cross-modal spatial attention by having participants count the number of visual or tactile stimuli presented on one side (e.g., count the number of white filled circles flashed on the left side) when streams of tactile and visual stimuli were presented to both sides. Counting the relevant target in the designated modality should enhance early processing of the other stimulus modality when that stimulus is presented on the same side. Presence was studied in three viewing conditions. In the VR hands condition, motion tracking sensors were used to simulate the participants' hand positions so that participants could see an image of their hands through the head-mounted display. In the VR no-hands condition, participants used the head-mounted display but were not shown their simulated hands, and in the control condition, participants performed the task without the head-mounted display and their actual hands were visible.

Harjunen et al. (2017) recorded participants' EEGs and examined somato-sensory evoked potentials for the tactile stimuli and visual evoked potentials for the visual stimuli. When the tactile stimuli were to be counted, early negativity was found for tactile stimuli at N140. This component indicates early inter-modal attentional processing of relevant tactile stimuli and was evident for all three displays. The amplitude of the N140 was greater when the tactile stimuli were presented on the irrelevant side rather than the relevant side, regardless of whether the relevant task was counting the visual or tactile stimuli. However, this enhanced attentional effect was only evident for the control and VR hands display conditions. This finding suggests that when the hands are visible, tactile stimuli presented to the hands are more distracting. When the real or virtual hands were visible, tactile stimuli on the relevant side also produced larger P200 components, indicative of inhibition, regardless of whether the relevant stimuli were visual or tactile. The visibility of the hands did not influence the visual-evoked N200 or the later P3 components. These findings suggest that in VR environments, being able to see one's body (i.e., hands) could induce presence and influence early attentional processing.

One benefit of head-mounted displays and VR applications is that they can help users visualize the world around them. This feature can be used for entertainment purposes, such as allowing users to visit different places. In this case, users must also be able to navigate through the VR application to reach a desired location or object. The quality of the user experience will be determined by whether the VR application is able to provide the user with a high-fidelity simulation of the location they are visiting and whether the cues in the VR application would reduce disorientation and simulation sickness. In addition to the entertainment value, VR can help designers perform tasks that require intensive visualization, such as in the construction industry (Han & Leite, 2021).

Han and Leite (2021) had novice construction engineers (i.e., graduate students) and expert construction professionals perform tasks relevant to construction design using an Oculus Rift VR system with a head-mounted display or a regular desktop computer. Participants performed four tasks. The first task was to detect design errors in a piping system. The second task required the participants to color code nine work packages that could be used to sequence the installation of the piping system. For both Tasks 1 and 2, the expert VR group performed the best, followed by the novice VR group, expert desktop group, and novice desktop group.

The third task required the participants to review the completeness of the work packages (i.e., to identify "leftover" objects located in the test bed that did not belong there). All participants were able to complete this task at 100% accuracy. The final task was a memory task where participants had to recall objects located between the work packages and other systems that were displayed. For this task, the expert VR group performed the worst, followed by the novice VR group, expert desktop group, and novice desktop group. These findings, taken together, show the advantages and disadvantages of using head-mounted VR displays to perform specific construction design review procedures. Han and Leite (2021) recommended that the construction industry take advantage of specific benefits that VR can bring to their design process.

CHAPTER SUMMARY

Many tasks in everyday life require directing attention to critical aspects of information at appropriate points. Displays designed to be consistent with human attention capabilities will be easier to use than ones that are not. We showed that strategies and control processes play a critical role in the sampling of displayed information. For a display to be effective, it must take advantage of task constraints and automatic response tendencies, as well as users' expectancies and mental models. Search of a complex display can be facilitated by structuring the display so that the most important information will be examined first and by using cues to signal locations of relevant visual information.

Vigilance performance is a function of the features of a task, situational factors, and participant characteristics. In many cases, the vigilance decrement appears to reflect an increasingly conservative response bias or a bias to sample information for a shorter period before making a decision. The full capabilities of new display technologies such as VR will be realized only if they are designed to be consistent with the characteristics of human attention and implemented in a way that takes advantage of the specific attributes of the display.

KEY POINTS

- **Fact:** Monitoring displays requires selective and divided attention.

- **Fact:** Displays designed to be consistent with the user's mental model allow faster and more accurate task performance, with reduced attentional demands.

- **Fact:** Having an inaccurate mental model of how a system works can result in mode errors.

- **Fact:** Maintaining realism of symbols and their movements limits user confusion.

- **Fact:** Displays intended to depict the physical environment should act in a manner that is representative of that environment.

- **Theory:** Ecological interface design is an approach that emphasizes the match of the interface with a person's mental representation of the environment.

- **Phenomenon:** Display-control compatibility effects, population stereotypes, and response-effect compatibility effects reflect natural or learned response tendencies.

- **Fact:** Displays should be designed to allow the user to perceive the appropriate action to take.

- **Fact:** Designing and grouping displays to maintain proximity compatibility and to be spatially compatible with controls will typically benefit performance.

- **Phenomenon:** The vigilance decrement refers to a decrease in detection of infrequently occurring target events over a watch or vigil.

- **Theory:** Evidence most strongly supports resource depletion accounts of the vigilance decrement, according to which the decrement is a consequence of the demands of maintaining attentional focus on the task.

- **Fact:** Designers of automation should be aware of the vigilance decrement and factors that reduce it and allow operators to stay "in the loop."

- **Fact:** Virtual environments are becoming an increasingly available means for developing programs to train users to make effective use of their attentional capabilities.

11

Individual and Group Differences in Attention

Although human performance is inherently variable, cognitive psychologists have tended to emphasize mean performance. Commonalities are taken to the extreme in engineering models of human performance, where designers use estimates of mean time (sometimes including a parameter for variability) to model performance in real-world tasks (see Weyers et al., 2017). However, there are individual differences in the ability to pay attention to the task at hand and other aspects of performance. For example, in the classroom, some students are better able to focus on relevant information (what the teacher is saying) and filter out irrelevant stimulation (e.g., what a student seated nearby is doing) than others. The ability to focus attention on the current task may depend on a multitude of social, motivational, and cognitive factors.

Failures to consider individual differences in the knowledge and training of human operators can have disastrous effects in some technical applications. In October 2018 (Lion Air Flight 610) and March 2019 (Ethiopian Airlines Flight 302), there were two fatal accidents involving the Boeing 737 Max 8 (Kitroeff et al., 2019). Like many accidents, the cause was due to several factors. But lack of training on the aircrafts' new Maneuvering Characteristics Augmentation System (MCAS) was considered a major factor responsible for the varied actions taken by the pilots in response to the MCAS alerts. One day before the fatal accident of the Lion Air flight, the pilots of the same aircraft encountered the exact malfunction experienced by Flight 610, which caused the aircraft to nosedive soon after takeoff. However, the pilots from that flight were able to

https://doi.org/10.1037/0000317-011

Attention: Selection and Control in Human Information Processing, by R. W. Proctor and K.-P. L. Vu

recover from the error because an extra off-duty pilot in the cockpit helped the flight crew resolve the problem (A. Levin & Suhartono, 2019). Unfortunately, the next day, that same alert from MCAS came on, and the Flight 610 crew was unable to attend correctly to the relevant cues and did not have the knowledge to prevent their fatal descent.

In this chapter, we examine the development of attention during childhood and how it changes due to aging. Although differences in performance and attentional control between groups of different ages have been mentioned throughout the book, we highlight key changes in attention across the lifespan in the present chapter. We also discuss how attentional skills change as one gains expertise in an area, highlighting the role of automaticity in skilled performance and the types of errors that occur in highly practiced tasks. Finally, the chapter ends with a few examples of group differences in the performance of attentional tasks.

ATTENTION ACROSS THE LIFESPAN

Cognitive capacity is known to increase from childhood to adulthood, but in later adulthood, it declines. The age-related decline in late adulthood is typically associated with frontal lobe atrophy (F. I. M. Craik & Grady, 2002). Although there is still debate about which cognitive processes are impaired due to frontal lobe atrophy, there is a clear relation between it and a decline in executive functioning (e.g., McAvinue et al., 2012). In the following sections, we discuss some key changes in attention across the lifespan, from childhood to old age.

Development of Attention

Many aspects of attention we take for granted (e.g., moving our eyes to an object of interest) cannot be performed by very young infants. Their visual attentional capabilities are restricted by the maturational status of the primary visual cortex (M. H. Johnson, 1990). Thus, a 1-month-old infant tends to exhibit behavior that seems unnatural, such as "obligatory attention," when the infant maintains fixation on an object for minutes. Eye movements at that age are controlled mainly through a subcortical pathway from the retina through the superior colliculus as the cortical pathways develop. But by about 6 months of age, the cortical pathways involved in the control of overt visual attention have developed (M. H. Johnson, 1990).

Somewhat less obvious are differences in attentional resources or abilities between older children and adults. One factor complicating the study of the development of attentional processes is that other cognitive processes, such as short-term memory, are also subject to developmental changes. Moreover, developmental disorders can manifest in childhood, leading to cognitive or behavioral problems for those children.

Typically Developing Children

Understanding changes in attentional processing across development is essential because even at an early age, attention determines what aspects of the environment will shape the child's behavior. As attention develops, children become better able to monitor their performance and events in their environment. Considering how to direct attention to relevant information at different ages can be of value in developing effective educational techniques (Markant & Amso, 2014). Effortful cognitive abilities that mature relatively late in childhood are often the first to weaken in old age. Studying attentional processes in children allows us to understand changes in attention in adulthood and even deficits of attention in old age.

Attentional Focus

According to Colombo's (2001) model of attention, there are significant changes in infants' alertness, visuospatial orienting mechanisms, and attention to object features. *Alertness*, the ability to attain an alert state, typically develops over the first 2 to 3 months after birth, mirroring cortical developments in the brain. Newborns spend less than 20% of the day in alert states, but this percentage increases across the first 3 months, correlating with their sleep–wake cycle. In infancy, spatial orienting ability is associated with the development of the "where" system, involving the thalamus (engagement of attention), posterior parietal lobe (disengagement of attention), and superior colliculus (shifting of attention). Up to about 6 months of age, control of eye movements develops as infants become increasingly able to inhibit automatic saccades, produce anticipatory saccades, and delay planned saccades. Covert shifts of visual attention first emerge around 4 to 5 months of age. In terms of attention to object features, Colombo's review indicated that infants can attend to color and form, but they do not perceive multidimensional stimuli (i.e., a compound of color and form) until 4 to 5 months of age. Infants are also able to scan objects early in life, but infants older than 2 months show more extensive scanning than infants under 2 months. Finally, infants can orient to novel objects, but 6- to 9-month-old infants showed stronger orienting responses to novel stimuli than 3-month-old infants.

The ability to keep task instructions in mind and sustain attention in a task also changes radically throughout childhood. In one study (Levy, 1980), it was found that the percentage of children who could perform a relatively simple go/no-go vigilance task (pressing a key on the relatively few occasions when the letter x is shown, ignoring all other letters) increased monotonically from just 27% of children between 3 years and 3 years 5 months of age to 100% of children 4 years 6 months of age and older. The speed and accuracy of responding continued to improve up to 7 years, the oldest group tested. Although a number of abilities change throughout childhood, studies that control for other cognitive abilities show clear differences in many aspects of attention, ranging from the development of covert orienting in infants to the final stages of the development of cognitive control in adolescence.

Studies using the dichotic listening paradigm have shown that selective attention improves during childhood. For example, Geffen and Sexton (1978) found that 10-year-old children were better able to select relevant auditory information than were 7-year-old children (i.e., they were able to selectively listen to one of a male and female voice spoken together and a voice presented in one ear rather than the other ear). The older children in this study also showed better divided attention, as evidenced by higher target detection rates when both channels had to be monitored. Not all researchers have found that older children are better able to divide attention than younger children. When single-task performance is equated for the groups studied, a common finding is that younger and older children perform equally well when two tasks are performed with equal priority. However, even when performance on the component tasks is equated, older children are better able to allocate attention to the two tasks differentially. That is, older children are better able to vary the amount of attention they place on one task at the cost of another (Irwin-Chase & Burns, 2000).

Many studies have also shown that children are more sensitive to interfering information than are adults (Lane & Pearson, 1982). For example, younger children (6–8 years old) are more sensitive to the spatial separation of two stimuli when they are required to ignore one spatially distinct stimulus to make a judgment about another than are older children (9–11 years). That is, they show more interference than older children when the stimuli are closer together. When the judgment requires attending to both stimuli, younger children's performance is worse with greater spatial separation. Together, these results suggest that the ability to narrow or broaden the attentional focus is still developing in this period of childhood (Enns & Girgus, 1985).

Executive Control

The most robust effects of attention across the lifespan are evident in tasks requiring executive control of attention, which includes selection, scheduling, and coordination of perception, cognition, and action. Control is needed for resource allocation whenever more than one task must be carried out at a time and when different task goals must be kept active. Hughes's (2011) review of executive control functions throughout development indicates that it emerges during the first year. When an object is moved from one location to another, 5-month-old infants show persistence in searching for the object at the original location, whereas infants 8 months or older show search at the new location. More advanced functions of executive attention, such as anticipatory looking, begin to emerge around 6 to 7 months and are clearly evident by 2 years. During preschool years, children show age-related improvements in attention, inhibitory control, and coordination, but the level of development depends on the child's environment and verbal ability. During ages 6 to 7 years, children show improved ability to shift their task set, and from age 8 to 12, they show marked improvements in planning, organizing, and strategic thinking. These skills are further improved throughout adolescence.

During puberty, structural changes in the brain occur, especially those involving the frontal cortex areas associated with inhibitory control, working memory, and decision making. All these executive function abilities influence adolescents' behaviors. Adolescents may pay more attention to rewards valued by their peers (Hughes, 2011). Adolescents with lower working memory capacity tend to be more impulsive and may have difficulty sustaining attention. Although many executive functions plateau by late adolescence, the ability to switch between tasks does not fully develop until early adulthood (Karayanidis & McKewen, 2021). Adolescents show poorer performance on switch trials than young adults, but the larger switch costs may result from the strategies employed by the adolescents. That is, adolescents tend to emphasize speed over accuracy, making more errors on switch trials. The speed-accuracy tradeoff may be related to the impulsivity shown by adolescents. Executive control processes, especially those involved in task switching, continue to be fine-tuned in adulthood.

Developmental Attention Disorders

Developmental disorders can be relatively specific, affecting one cognitive function (e.g., dyslexia on reading), but often they are more generalized and affect a broad spectrum of cognitive functions (e.g., Bishop, 1992). Development disorders such as attention-deficit/hyperactivity disorder (ADHD) and autism spectrum disorder can exert financial and emotional costs on the individuals and their families (Cakir et al., 2020; Sciberras et al., 2022), and early identification can allow for interventions that may reduce the severity of the impact.

Attention-Deficit/Hyperactivity Disorder

One of the most well-known attentional disorders that occurs during child development is ADHD. This disorder is characterized by severe impairments in attention (e.g., difficulty sustaining attention, avoidance of tasks requiring sustained effort) and control of behavior (e.g., fidgets, interrupts or intrudes on others, has difficulty waiting for their turn). The Centers for Disease Control and Prevention (CDC; n.d.) reported that, according to a 2016 parent survey, 9.4% of children have ADHD, with the rate being higher for boys (12.9%) than girls (5.6%). According to this survey, six out of 10 children diagnosed with ADHD have mental, emotional, or behavioral problems, making it critical to determine which children have ADHD to allow them to receive help. Because individuals with ADHD often have comorbidity with other clinical disorders (Nigg et al., 2020), it is difficult to specify the causal factors for ADHD.

Diagnosis of ADHD should be made by a health professional, usually following the criteria listed in the fifth edition of the *Diagnostic and Statistical Manual of Mental Disorders* (*DSM-5*; American Psychiatric Association, 2013). The *DSM-5* specifies that a number of ADHD symptoms of inattention and hyperactivity or impulsivity need to be met within a period (see Table 11.1 for example characteristics). Moreover, because reports of symptoms are subjective, it is necessary to confirm that the symptoms occur across multiple settings. Individuals with

TABLE 11.1. Example Characteristics of Inattention and Hyperactivity and Impulsivity

Inattention	Hyperactivity and impulsivity
Making careless mistakes	Frequently fidgeting or tapping the hands or feet
Being easily distracted	Showing restlessness
Having difficulty organizing tasks and activities	Frequently interrupting others
Having difficulty following instructions	Responding before a question has been completed
Not finishing schoolwork, chores, or duties in the workplace	Talking excessively
Being forgetful in completing daily activities	Being impatient with waiting for a turn
Showing difficulty paying attention to details	Constantly being "on the move"

ADHD often show problems with cognition, emotion regulation, and social skills in childhood that can persist into adulthood.

Research on the cognitive basis of ADHD began in the 1970s. The vigilance task was used to determine how children with ADHD would perform at detecting visual targets that occur infrequently compared with their non-ADHD peers (Sykes et al., 1973). Children with ADHD performed worse on vigilance tests (i.e., showing both more misses and more false alarms than their peers). The increases in misses and false alarms suggest that children with ADHD had problems with sustained attention. Subsequent studies have provided evidence that basic information processes such as stimulus encoding, comparison, and response selection are relatively unimpaired in children with ADHD (see Logan et al., 1997, for a review). Instead, children with ADHD exhibited deficits compared with typically developing peers in measures of planning, working memory, inhibition, and vigilance (see Willcutt et al., 2005, for a meta-analysis).

Researchers have also focused on exploring processes that control basic information processes, such as inhibition (Senderecka et al., 2012) and cognitive control (Craig et al., 2016). For inhibitory processes, studies using the stop-signal paradigm found that children with ADHD were slower to respond to the stop signal than children without ADHD, and this impairment to inhibit responding was observed for both boys and girls (Nigg, 1999). Moreover, when they are able to stop their responses, it takes children with ADHD longer to do so (Schachar & Logan, 1990). Finally, participants with ADHD had greater variability in responding, which Nigg (1999) suggested could be related to non-inhibitory mechanisms such as arousal or effort.

Janssen et al. (2018) investigated event-related potential (ERP) components of children with ADHD and typically developing children. They found no difference in stop-signal response times between the two groups in early perceptual processing (i.e., no difference in the amplitude of the N1 and P2 components). However, the children with ADHD showed reduced N2 and P3 amplitudes compared with the typically developing children. Because N2 is associated with inhibition and ventral attention networks and P3 with the monitoring network, Janssen et al. suggested that children with ADHD may partially compensate for inhibitory and/or attentional difficulties by intensifying sensory processing and that disruptions in the ventral attentional network contribute to the poorer performance on the stop-signal task.

Fosco et al. (2019) examined whether the longer response times to stop signals shown by children with ADHD is due to the deliberate slowing of responding to increase accuracy or the dual-task requirements of the task (i.e., quickly responding to a go signal but withholding responding to a stop signal), which can slow overall responding due to strategic adjustments to maximize accuracy. Children with and without ADHD showed slower responding on go trials when stop signals were presented intermittently. But drift diffusion modeling (see Chapter 3) showed that the presence of stop-signal trials did not alter the rate of information accumulation on the go trials or the nondecision time (i.e., encoding and response execution time). Fosco et al. attributed the slowing of go-trial responses to a deliberate strategy of performance adjustment made by children to maximize accuracy regardless of whether they had ADHD. This finding suggests that children with ADHD have intact self-regulation processes involved in speed-accuracy criteria, and difficulties shown in other studies are specific to the task demands.

Many factors contribute to the development of ADHD, including genetics, mothers' use of cigarettes and alcohol, exposure to other environmental toxins during pregnancy, and the child's exposure to environmental toxins (CDC, n.d.). Currently, there are treatments available to help improve individuals' functioning, which include medication and behavioral training (Nigg et al., 2020). Medications are available to reduce symptoms of hyperactivity, impulsivity, and inattention. There is evidence for a dysfunctional neurotransmitter system that results in lower catecholamine levels in the brain (e.g., Todd & Botteron, 2001). This evidence is in line with the fact that the most common types of medications used for treating ADHD are stimulants (e.g., methylphenidate and amphetamine) that increase levels of dopamine and norepinephrine, neurotransmitters associated with motivation, attention, and movement. Nonstimulant medications (e.g., atomoxetine, guanfacine, clonidine) are also available to help alleviate symptoms of ADHD for children who may not tolerate stimulants.

In addition to medication, behavioral therapy techniques can also be used to help improve individuals' attentional processes and reduce disruptive behavior. Interventions that lead to promotive (i.e., self-perceptions of competence) and protective (i.e., goal-directed solitary play) strategies for the individual and parental training to promote resilience and a positive environment for the child can also be beneficial (Dvorsky & Langberg, 2016).

Autism Spectrum Disorder

Autism spectrum disorder (ASD) can cause significant disruption to a child's life. According to the CDC (n.d.), ASD has been identified in about one in every 45 children. Like ADHD, ASD is more common in boys than in girls by a factor of four. Early signs of ASD can be identified around 18 months to 2 years of age. As with ADHD, a diagnosis of ASD is made by health professionals by comparing the child's behavior with that of typically developing children (see Table 11.2 for some examples). Because children with ASD miss many developmental milestones, early identification can lead to timely intervention.

Children with ASD differ in how they interact with others socially and attend to social cues. Mundy et al. (2016) indicated that information processing during joint attention may be atypical in children with ASD. *Joint attention* refers to changes in stimulus encoding that occur from social-attention coordination (see Chapter 12). For adults, memory for pictures is better when an avatar's gaze follows the participant's gaze shifts during encoding of the pictures than when the participant's gaze follows the gaze shifts of the avatar (Kim & Mundy, 2012). Mundy et al. found that children without ASD showed this result, but those with ASD did not.

Using a basic divided attention task, Boxhoorn et al. (2018) found that children with ASD made more omission errors (i.e., failure to respond) than

TABLE 11.2. Examples of Developmental Milestones by Age for Typically Developing Children

Developmental feature	Age	
	18 months	**2 years**
Social and emotional	• Likes to hand items to others • May be afraid of strangers • May cling to caregivers in new situations	• Copies others • Gets excited when with other children • Shows defiant behavior
Language and communication	• Says several single words • Says no and shakes head • Points to show a desired item	• Points to things when they are named • Says sentences with two to four words • Knows names of familiar people
Cognitive	• Points to get attention of others • Can follow one-step verbal commands (e.g., sit down) • Knows use of ordinary items (e.g., brush)	• Likes to hand items to others • Can follow two-step verbal commands (e.g., pick up your toy and put in toy chest) • Names items in a picture book
Movement and physical	• Walks alone • Drinks from a cup • Eats with a spoon	• Begins to run • Climbs onto and down from furniture without help • Kicks a ball

Note. Example items are from those listed on the Centers for Disease Control and Prevention website (CDC, 2021).

typically developing children. In this task, they had to simultaneously monitor visual items moving in a 4×4 matrix for a pattern and an alternating sequence of low- and high-pitched tones for deviations in the alternations. However, Boxhoorn et al. did not find any differences between the two groups on other basic attentional functions, including tonic alertness and selective attention. Furthermore, other studies have shown children with ASD outperforming children without ASD on some tasks.

Children with ASD who were matched with typically developing controls on a variety of demographic variables, including verbal ability (Plaisted et al., 1998) and nonverbal abilities (O'Riordan et al., 2001), showed similar responding in feature search tasks but faster responding in conjunctive search tasks. For the conjunctive search, the increase in search times as the number of distractors increased was less for children with ASD than typically developing controls. O'Riordan et al. (2001) also found that when searching for a tilted line among vertical lines or vice versa, typically developing children show standard search asymmetry effects (see Chapter 4, this volume), where it is easier to find a tilted line among vertical lines than a vertical line among tilted lines. Children with ASD performed like the typically developing children on the easier task of finding the tilted line but had more efficient search performance on the more difficult vertical-line task. Thus, children with ASD did not show a visual search asymmetry effect.

O'Riordan (2004) found that adults with ASD showed similar visual search benefits as those found for children with ASD. In addition, she found that adults with ASD were more efficient than their controls on search tasks with more similar targets and distractors, suggesting that adults with ASD had better stimulus discriminability. Shirama et al. (2017) examined whether the visual search advantage was due to better target discriminability or reduced susceptibility to crowding (decreased ability to identify a target when other items are in close proximity). Adults with ASD and a matched control group performed visual search tasks that varied the target characteristics (e.g., luminance and shape) and crowding (proximity of items in the display). They used a procedure that replaced the search display with a noise mask, which disrupts serial search but not nonsearch processing (i.e., bottom-up processing of multiple stimuli across the visual field). Participants in the ASD group showed shorter search times than the control group. Also, retinal eccentricity did not impact the search performance of the participants with ASD, which would have been expected if their search benefit result from a reduced crowding effect. Thus, Shirama et al. concluded that participants with ASD were better at simultaneously discriminating between multiple visual stimuli than participants without ASD.

Burack et al. (2016) noted that individuals with ASD tend to perform better than typically developing peers on other tasks such as those involving embedded figures and block design. In contrast, they perform worse on theory of mind tasks, where participants are asked to place themselves in a viewpoint of another person and respond appropriately. However, Burack et al. argued that researchers should not focus on how well individuals with and without ASD perform on tasks but rather on how the individuals process the information. Burack et al. pointed to a study by Russo et al. (2012) to illustrate differences in the information processing of participants with ASD and those without. In that study, participants were presented with an image of an animal and a sound that matched (a barking sound and image of a dog) or mismatched (a meow sound and image of a dog). There were no differences between groups in reaction time and accuracy. ERP waveforms showed a difference between congruent (i.e., matched) and incongruent (i.e., mismatched) responses around 150 milliseconds (ms) for adults with ASD, but the difference was not evident with adults without ASD until 350 ms. Early differentiation of the waveforms suggests that participants with ASD rely more on perceptual processing to complete the task, whereas participants without ASD rely more on cognitive processing.

Like ADHD, several interventions for ASD have been shown to be effective in helping individuals function in society. These interventions include medication and behavioral therapy designed to improve cognitive functioning, daily communication, and living skills. Some researchers have suggested that ADHD and ASD have the same genetic basis. Craig et al.'s (2016) review indicated that there is significant overlap (50%–72%) of the contributing genetic factors for both disorders. This can explain why the co-occurrence of both disorders in the same individual is also high, and similar medication and behavioral interventions have been used to treat individuals diagnosed with the two disorders.

Craig et al. (2016) examined 26 studies that investigated deficits in executive functioning (e.g., inhibition, working memory, attention, planning) for children diagnosed with ASD, ADHD, or both. They found that, although the results of the individual studies may have differed (due to differences in the characteristics of the sample of participants studied), several themes emerged. First, all groups show similarities in neurocognitive profiles. Second, in terms of specific executive functions, the group with both ASD and ADHD share more impairments relating to flexibility and planning with the ASD group but share more impairments relating to response inhibition with the ADHD group. However, the working memory, fluency, and concept formation performances were similar across all three groups. Craig et al. noted that being able to identify the unique characteristics associated with each group of children is key to enabling practitioners to develop treatments and interventions to help the children.

Aging

Attentional control capabilities developed in childhood are refined during adulthood, except in severe cases of development disorders. However, there are some age-related declines in attentional processes in old age. With normal aging, older adults show poorer performance than younger adults on some attentional measures but not others. For example, McAvinue et al. (2012) found large age-related declines in measures of attentional capacity but smaller reductions in tasks related to selective and sustained attention. In a review of attentional alerting and orienting, Erel and Levy (2016) concluded that older adults show reduced alerting abilities and overt shifts of attention, but they do not show impaired performance on tasks involving covert attention shifts. Moreover, older adults shift their attention less rapidly to endogenous cues but show no deficit in shifting attention to exogenous cues. In their literature review, McDonough et al. (2019) also concluded that normal aging impacts attentional processes involved in alerting but not orienting.

The performance of older adults can be influenced by individual capabilities and contextual factors that make it difficult to predict performance in any one individual. Methodological differences also exist between studies, causing the literature to show mixed findings using similar tasks (e.g., Rey-Mermet & Gade, 2018). That said, understanding why attention-related declines occur in old age is a major topic of research due to the extended lifespan in the 21st century. In this section, we briefly review the research on aging in two areas thought to be most impacted by aging: executive control and inhibition.

Executive Control

F. I. M. Craik (1977) concluded, "One of the clearest results in the experimental psychology of aging is the finding that older people are more penalized when they must divide their attention" (p. 391). Although the underlying mechanisms for this finding have been debated, the basic result has been replicated many times (e.g., Crossley & Hiscock, 1992; Korteling, 1991, 1993). Studies have shown that older people experience more difficulty than younger people in rapidly redeploying attention among two or more tasks or processes (e.g., Korteling, 1991) and exhibit less flexibility than younger adults in varying their speed-accuracy criteria (e.g., Strayer et al., 1987). Moreover, older adults have particular difficulty with time-sharing, or allocating resources to different tasks at the same time (McDowd, 1986).

However, Kramer et al. (1999) found that older adults can show reduced task-switching costs after brief amounts of practice. They compared the performance of younger (18–25 years old) and older (60–75 years old) adults on two tasks: an element number task (i.e., counting the number of digits [222] presented and determining whether it was greater or less than 5) or a digit value task (i.e., identifying if the digits presented [88] were greater or less than 5). The digits presented on a trial could be congruent (i.e., 222 would lead to the less-than-5 response for both tasks) or incongruent (i.e., 222222 would lead to a greater-than-5 response for the element number task but a less-than-5 response for the digit value task). At the beginning of each block, participants were told whether they would be performing the same task for the entire block or whether they would have to switch between tasks during the block. Participants performed three sessions lasting 1.5 hours each and came back 2 months later for a fourth session to test retention.

In the first session, the older adults showed much larger switch costs than the younger adults (switch costs were about 850 ms for older adults and

220 ms for younger adults). But by the second session, the switch costs for older and younger adults were more similar (switch costs of about 350 ms for older adults and 220 ms for younger adults). By the third session, there was no difference in switch costs between the two groups, and no age-related deficits were observed in the retention session 2 months later. The congruity effects were larger following task-switch trials, but this effect did not differ between younger and older adults. In a subsequent experiment, working memory load was increased by requiring participants to keep track of the number of trials and switch between tasks every fifth trial. In this experiment, age-related differences in switch costs were evident across the two sessions tested. Thus, Kramer et al.'s (1999) findings suggest that there is an age-related decline in the ability to switch tasks, especially when the tasks are unpracticed or more complex (e.g., require higher memory demands).

Rhodes et al. (2019) examined whether the dual-task performance decrement associated with aging is a consequence of storage or processing demands competing for attention. Storage demands are those placed on memory, whereas processing demands are those placed on executive control. Thus, if memory and processing tasks are performed together, will older adults experience more conflict than younger adults, leading to larger dual-task decrements? Baddeley and Hitch's (1974) working memory model attributes storage and processing to different components (the visuospatial sketchpad and phonological loop) that are distinct from the central executive (see Chapter 8, this volume). Consequently, it would predict no or small differences. In contrast, shared or embedded resource working memory models, such as Cowan's (1988), predict that storage and processing demands should compete for attention, resulting in larger age-related effects.

Rhodes et al. (2019) had participants, aged 18 to 81 years (binned into five age groups), perform single and dual tasks. A letter-span task was used for the memory task and a single-digit math verification task for the processing task. The stimuli for the letter-span task were presented visually for typed recall and auditorily for oral recall. For the processing task, participants indicated whether the math equation was correct (5 + 7 = 12) or incorrect (3 + 8 = 12). Each task was adjusted for difficulty to ensure that both tasks were equivalent in terms of difficulty to the participants. Participants were given different incentives by way of points received (90, 70, 50, 30, or 10 points) for correctly performing the memory or processing task to examine prioritization of the individual tasks in the dual-task conditions.

For both the memory and processing tasks, participants in all age groups were able to follow the prioritization scheme, performing better on the task that was assigned more points. For the memory task, the difference between single- and dual-task performance at the maximum priority (90 points) was larger for older than younger adults. This cost of concurrence appeared to increase linearly with age. However, this cost was not evident with the processing task. Overall, the results of this study suggest that older adults have more difficulty than younger adults storing and maintaining information in memory, but they are just as efficient at shifting priority between storage and processing based on the incentives provided.

McDonough et al.'s (2019) review of studies on attentional processes in executive control found that aging had little impact on executive control until about 80 years of age, when age-related deficits started to emerge. One reason for a lack of an age-related deficit in executive control shown by older adults is that a lifetime of experience and knowledge can result in the use of compensatory strategies (see Chapter 9) to offset age-related declines in basic cognitive functions for healthy older adults up to a point (Reuter-Lorenz & Cappell, 2008).

Inhibition of Irrelevant Information

One notable effect of aging is a general slowing in information-processing speed. It has been hypothesized that this general slowing is in part due to declines in the control of inhibitory processes (Connelly & Hasher, 1993). Studies examining changes in the ability to inhibit information with age have shown mixed results (see Rey-Mermet & Gade, 2018, for a review). Part of the reason for mixed results is that inhibition is multifaceted, with various studies using different types of tasks. For example, Kramer et al. (1994) compared the performance of younger and older adults on (a) the stop-signal task, (b) learning new rules in a categorization task (which requires inhibiting previously learned rules), and (c) negative priming. They found older adults performed worse than younger adults on the stop-signal and categorization tasks but not the negative priming task. Kramer et al. also found low correlations between the different tasks, which may reflect the nonunitary nature of inhibition.

For the Stroop color-naming task, Verhaeghen and De Meersman (1998) showed no age-related differences in the interference from color words. But West and Baylis (1998) found a larger Stroop effect for older adults when the percentage of incongruent trials was high. Recall from Chapter 5 that increasing the percentage of incongruent trials decreases the size of the Stroop effect because the global percentage provides relevant information for the task. Thus, West and Baylis's result suggests that older adults may have a decreased ability to take advantage of the global percentage information rather than a general deficit in inhibition.

For the Simon task, older adults show larger Simon effects for both the visual and auditory modalities (Pick & Proctor, 1999; van der Lubbe & Verleger, 2002). However, Proctor, Pick, et al. (2005) found no age-related difference in the Simon effect when an accessory version of the Simon task was used, for which the irrelevant accessory stimulus was presented to the left or right of the centered, relevant stimulus for which responses were assigned to left and right key presses based on the stimulus color. This latter finding suggests that older adults have more difficulty inhibiting irrelevant location information when the task requires that attention be directed to the stimulus's location to perform the relevant task.

Rey-Mermet and Gade (2018) reviewed the aging literature and inhibition that used the following tasks: stop-signal, go/no-go, Stroop, flanker, Simon, global–local tasks (i.e., stimuli where smaller elements [local] are arranged to form bigger elements [global]), positive priming effects, inhibition of return, and task-switching. They performed a meta-analysis of 191 studies and found that there were age-related deficits in the performance of older adults for the stop-signal and go/no-go tasks, but no age-related deficits for the Stroop, flanker, local element, and task-switching tasks. The results were inconclusive for the Simon, global elements, positive priming, and inhibition of return tasks. Rey-Mermet and Gade indicated that these findings do not support a general age-related deficit in inhibition. Rather, the findings support the notion that aging decreases a person's ability to suppress an activated response but not necessarily the ability to prevent influences of irrelevant or distracting information.

Summary and Other Considerations

Studies on age-related deficits in attentional processes have shown mixed findings, which can be due to individual differences in capabilities or method-ological differences used by various researchers. Reviews and a meta-analysis of the literature show that there are age-related deficits in alerting and inhibi-tion of activated responses. However, there seem to be little or no age-related deficits relating to orienting or the ability to prevent irrelevant information from influencing performance. Age-related deficits in executive control can be compensated through strategies, which can result in a nonobservable age-related difference, except for high-workload tasks. However, it should be noted that individuals with clinical conditions, such as Alzheimer's, show age-related declines in alerting, orienting, and executive control earlier in adulthood that worsen with age (McDonough et al., 2019).

Although chronological age is used as the indicator for aging, factors such as medical condition and stress can negatively impact aging. Individuals may perform "younger" or "older" than their chronological age. Wiesman et al. (2020) used blood samples and a procedure called methylation analysis to determine biological indicators of age. The resulting metric, DNA methylation-age, was used to estimate acceleration or deceleration of chronological age. Using the flanker task to measure selective attention, they found that DNA methylation-age predicted performance. Moreover, it mediated the relation between chrono-logical age and flanker task performance. Although DNA methylation-age can be used in future studies of aging along with chronological age, not enough data have been collected to show the ultimate value of this metric.

Skilled Performance

In the prior section, we discussed changes in attention and performance throughout childhood and late in adulthood. However, much of one's life is spent developing skills in early and middle adulthood. For example, working in a domain for years allows one to develop expertise and/or elite performance in that domain. An individual is typically considered an expert after 10 years of deliberate practice with techniques in that domain (A. Johnson & Proctor,

2017). In this section, we discuss how attentional control changes as one becomes skilled in an area and the types of errors that result from these changes.

Automaticity With Skilled Performance

People who are instructed to emphasize some aspects of task performance over others are able to do this, and their ability to do so improves with practice (Brickner & Gopher, 1981; Rhodes et al., 2019), approaching a level that is "automatic." For motor skills, Lewthwaite and Wulf (2017) stressed that practice and performance benefit from an external focus of attention on the action goal rather than an internal focus on the body mechanics. More generally, automaticity is presumed to develop gradually with practice, freeing up resources that then can be allocated to additional tasks (Fitts, 1964). Thus, research has aimed to identify when and how components of complex tasks become automatized. Research directed toward understanding the proposed shift from controlled to automatic processing used tasks in which a display is searched for one or more targets held in memory (W. Schneider & Shiffrin, 1977; Shiffrin & Schneider, 1977). As shown in Figure 11.1, with a consistent mapping, the items in the memory set on the current trial (Trial N) are never distractors on other trials (e.g., Trial $N + 1$). With a varied mapping, the items in the memory set on the current trial can be distractors in the search array on another trial.

Varying memory set size on a given trial can allow determining when search becomes essentially automatic. Figure 11.2 shows typical results, for which the impact of set size is reduced with practice for consistent mappings but not

FIGURE 11.1. Visual Search Using Consistent Versus Varied Mapping

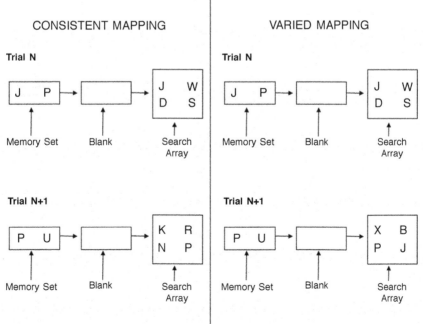

FIGURE 11.2. Automatic Processing Occurs With Practice for Consistent Mapping but Not Varied Mapping

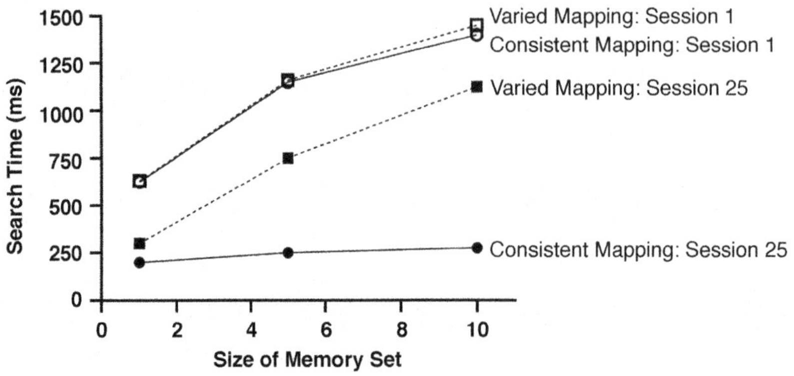

varied mappings. Consistent mappings show little set-size effect after practice because participants know the set of target items and have developed procedures for identifying them without explicit search.

In a more naturalistic task, Castillo et al. (2018) compared the performance of novices (surgery residents and interns) and laparoscopy experts on completing laparoscopic stitches (primary task). A secondary task procedure measured spare capacity by having the operators concurrently respond to a target pattern on a visual display screen (visual–spatial secondary task). The novices were proficient with the primary task and were extensively trained (given 100–200 repetitions). The quality of primary-task performance was evaluated by subject-matter experts who viewed videos of the participants' performance and rated them on operation time and objective skills scales. The visual–spatial secondary task performance was measured by a detectability index (the ratio between right and wrong answers; a higher ratio reflects better performance). Castillo et al. found that experts achieved a detectability index of .78, and novices were able to achieve that level after extensive training (preassessment index .48; postassessment index .78). Moreover, novices who achieved detection indexes of .65 or higher on the secondary task performed better on the laparoscopic stitch task (i.e., lower operative times and higher scores on the objective assessment skills scales). These findings led Castillo et al. to suggest a detection index of .65 as a cutoff point for achieving automaticity in this task.

The work by W. Schneider and Shiffrin (1977; Shiffrin & Schneider, 1977) and Castillo et al. (2018) focused on when automaticity is achieved, and there has also been work on how it is achieved. Fitts and Posner (1967) characterized the acquisition of perceptual–motor skill as proceeding through three distinct phases. When first learning a task, the individual enters the *declarative phase*, where the task components are verbalizable and held in working memory. With practice, the components become linked or connected in the *associative phase*. Expertise is achieved in the *autonomous phase* when the task is performed automatically. J. R. Anderson (1982) incorporated this three-phase framework for skill acquisition in his adaptive control of thought (ACT) cognitive architecture. According to J. R. Anderson, the transition from the cognitive to the associative phase with practice is due to the declarative components of a task and its associations being compiled into a *procedural memory* (i.e., the retrieval of learned answers). The change from the associative to the autonomous phase is through the establishment of task-specific production rules (i.e., if . . . then pairings) that generate implicit or explicit actions when their conditions are met.

Tenison et al. (2016) employed the ACT-R (rational) cognitive architecture to model how participants solve complex math problems, called *pyramid problems*. These problems involve a specified base digit (e.g., 7) and a number of terms to add (e.g., 3), with each term being one less than the prior one. In this example, the answer would be $7 + 6 + 5 = 18$. Some of the problems were performed repeatedly throughout the session, which allowed the examination of the three learning phases, which they called computation, retrieval, and autonomous. Within each learning phase, Tenison et al. simulated the contributions of three processing stages (encoding, solving, and responding) using functional magnetic resonance imaging (fMRI) and behavioral data. For the first phase of practice, the *computation* phase, the solving stage took the longest and was a function of the number of terms to be added because participants had to carry out the sequence of arithmetic operations. In the second phase, *retrieval*, computation was no longer needed because the correct answer could be retrieved from memory, resulting in a negligible duration of the solving process. Finally, in the *autonomous* phase, after more practice, the duration of the encoding process also became negligible because participants could recognize the entire problem as a single unit and respond on that basis. However, even after considerable practice, there were individual differences in the extent to which participants relied on holistic recognition of the problem.

Fitts's (1964) framework attributes automaticity to changes in cognitive processes across the three learning phases, but others have argued that automaticity reflects the same process used in the first two phases, just performed more efficiently. Logan's (1988) instance theory of automaticity describes the development of skill as the acquisition of instances rather than the buildup of procedural knowledge (J. R. Anderson, 1982). Instances are episodes in which attention was directed to relevant information, with the result being that the information was encoded into memory. Moreover, attention must be paid to the relevant cues if associations dependent on those cues are to be retrieved (Logan & Etherton, 1994). Thus, attention is needed at both the time of encoding and time of retrieval. In instance theory, there is a race between retrieval from short- and long-term memory, and automaticity is achieved with fast and effortless retrieval from long-term memory after practice. Thus, automatic processing is presumed to be based on the efficient retrieval of instances rather than the execution of learned procedures.

Both the ACT-R model of skill acquisition (J. R. Anderson, 1982) and the instance theory (Logan, 1988) predict that performance follows a power law of practice: The time to perform a task decreases as a power function of the number of practice trials (see Figure 11.3). The power law has been shown to

FIGURE 11.3. Power Law of Practice for Reaction Times on Target Present and Target Absent Trials

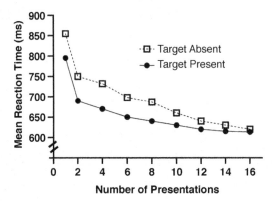

hold for group performance across a variety of domains. Note, though, that the practice function for individuals may fit a different function better (e.g., exponential) because averaging data sets produces a bias toward a power function (Heathcote et al., 2000).

Both models also predict a shift in reliance on working memory to long-term memory as skill is acquired. Servant et al. (2018) examined ERP components to determine whether there was evidence for such a switch. Participants in their study determined whether one of two pictures of everyday items, one displayed to the left of central fixation and the other to the right, matched a target item that was centrally displayed on the next screen. Pictures of items in the memory set were always presented with a distractor item on the other side. Only a consistent mapping was used, for which items in the memory set and distractors did not overlap, allowing participants to learn the memory set. After practice, participants were faster at responding to targets (i.e., items in the memory set) than distractors. The ERP data showed patterns consistent with that predicted by a switch to long-term memory retrieval: The contralateral delay activity, which correlates with visual working memory, decreased in amplitude with practice. The N400, which correlates with semantic processing in long-term memory, became more positive with practice. Although this pattern of ERP shifts points to retrieval from long-term memory after practice, it does not differentiate whether this retrieval is by way of instances or procedures.

In sum, there is little doubt that there is a shift from heavy demands on working memory when starting to learn a task to reliance on less-effortful retrieval from long-term memory once skill is acquired. However, there is an ongoing debate as to whether the development of automaticity reflects a change from declarative to procedural knowledge or more efficient processing of instances. The transition occurs gradually, and there are individual differences.

Action Slips and Supervisory Attentional System

Skilled performance is not immune to errors. In fact, it has been argued that error arises according to the same principles that are responsible for skilled performance. Reason (1990) developed a well-known taxonomy of unsafe acts in which the primary distinction is between ones for which the action is intended and ones for which it is not. We focus here on the unintended errors directly related to lapses of attention due to action slips, given their prevalence in well-learned or skilled performance. For example, take a task of making a pot of coffee from coffee beans every morning and the error of meaning to do one thing but doing something else. The individual opens a package of coffee beans with the intention of filling the grinder, but instead of pouring the coffee into the grinder, pours the beans into the coffeemaker rather than grinding them first. In this case, the correct action was performed (pouring), but the object of the action (the coffeemaker) was the inappropriate one for grinding the beans. Reason (1979) was one of the first researchers to systematically describe this kind of error, which he called a *slip of action*. Such errors arise because much of our behavior is performed more or less automatically, without conscious mediation or monitoring. In other words, slips occur because of how action is organized and automated (Reason, 2017).

Slips of action occur most often during the automatic execution of highly practiced, routine actions. Action slips can be described as failures of attention, with slips occurring either because the wrong action plan is maintained or because attention is switched to the wrong elements of a plan or aspects of the environment. Reason (1979) identified five main types of action slips: (a) program assembly failure (e.g., unwrapping a piece of candy and throwing the candy in the wastebasket and the wrapper in one's mouth), (b) discrimination failure (e.g., putting shaving cream on a toothbrush), (c) subroutine failure (e.g., reaching for your sunglasses to take them off as you enter a building but realizing that you were not wearing sunglasses when your fingers reached your face), (d) test failure or monitoring the progress of an action (e.g., going into the bedroom to change into clothes for going out to dinner and, instead, putting on pajamas and going to bed), and (e) storage failure (e.g., pouring hot water into a freshly made pot of tea).

Lapses of attention that give rise to action slips are common even for healthy adults. Jónsdóttir et al. (2007) had 189 adults, 20 to 60 years old, record signs of absentmindedness (i.e., action slips) in a diary over 1 week. The participants recorded an average of 6.4 action slips over the week (range = 0–30, $SD = 4.9$). Jónsdóttir et al. found that participants recorded action slips in all five of Reason's main categories, with most action slips from the storage failure category. There were no gender differences in the number of slips and only a weak negative correlation between the number of slips and age ($r = -.20$).

Norman (1981) extended the work of Reason (1979) and used his analysis of action slips as the basis for a theory about how intentions are represented and acted on. Norman based his theory on the idea that actions are based on schemas that embody the procedural knowledge needed for carrying out an act. Action schemas are generalized procedures for carrying out actions; they embody both motor programs and rules for selecting between specific versions of motor programs. According to Norman, any complicated act requires a number of schemas arranged in a particular control structure. For actions to be performed correctly, the appropriate schemas must be activated at the right time and with the right information. Norman's activation-trigger-schema system assumes that actions are governed by high-level parent schemas. For skilled actions, once the parent schema is activated, the child schemas that control component parts of the action are initiated automatically. Thus, intention can be equated with the activation of the parent schema, and attention is only needed when critical choice points are reached.

Because a number of schemas may be active at any one time, a means of triggering the appropriate schema for a particular act is needed. For example, most drivers have a schema for "drive home from work." Deviations from the schema, such as "pick up groceries on the way home," require a separate sub-schema that must be triggered at the appropriate time. Once on the way, the task of driving occurs more or less automatically. The driver, however, must pay sufficient attention to the errand schema if it is to be activated at the appropriate moment. If the activation for the schema is not sufficiently high, the better-known "drive home" schema will prevail, and the grocery shopping will be forgotten. Exhibit 11.1 summarizes the types of action slips that occur due to errors in the formation of intentions or activation or triggering of schemas.

Norman and Shallice (1986) proposed two systems that influence schema activation: a contention-scheduling system and a supervisory attention system. The basic mechanism of action control, according to Norman and Shallice, is *contention scheduling*, a passive process that emerges naturally because of the way schemas are learned and performed. The contention-scheduling system can directly activate and order action schemas linked to each other with inhibitory and excitatory connections (see Figure 11.4). For example, a schema for tying shoelaces might have inhibitory connections to other schemas involving fine motor control of the hands but excitatory connections to a schema for pulling down pant cuffs. The precise timing of schema activation occurs through "triggers." A schema is triggered for execution when environmental conditions match the triggering conditions incorporated in the schema. The notion of triggering provides an explanation for the capture errors described earlier: When intentions are not actively maintained, schemas can become activated simply because their triggering conditions are present in the environment.

Schemas operate whenever their activation exceeds a threshold, whether this activation comes from contention scheduling, the activation of other schemas, or environmental conditions. Top-down mechanisms also play an important role in schema activation and action control. In Norman and Shallice's (1986) model, top-down control of action is performed by the *supervisory attention system*. The supervisory attention system works by modulating the contention-scheduling system, as is necessary whenever a less familiar version of an action

EXHIBIT 11.1

Classification of Action Slips

Slips Due to Errors in the Formation of Intentions

Mistakes in Goal Determination or Cognition

- **mode errors:** erroneous classification or interpretation of the situation
- **description errors:** ambiguous or incomplete specification of the intention

Slips That Result From Faulty Activation of Schema

Unintentional Activation (activation of schemas that are not part of a current action plan)

- **capture errors:** capture of control by a better learned, but currently inappropriate, schema
- **data-driven activation:** schemas inappropriately triggered by outside events
- **associative activation:** activation by another, currently active schema

Loss of Activation

- forgetting an intention (but continuing to perform the action)
- misordering the components of an action sequence
- skipping steps in an action sequence
- repeating steps in an action sequence

Slips That Result From the Faulty Triggering of Schemas

False Triggering (correct schema triggered at inappropriate time)

- **spoonerisms:** reversal of event components
- **blends:** combinations of components from two competing schemas
- **thoughts leading to actions:** triggering of schemas only meant to be thought, not executed
- premature triggering

Failure to Trigger (when an active schema never gets invoked for the following reasons)

- action preempted by competing schemas
- insufficient activation as a result of forgetting or because initial activation was too low
- trigger condition does not match due to insufficient or faulty specification

Note. From *Attention: Theory and Practice* (p. 287), by A. Johnson and R. W. Proctor, 2004, SAGE (https://doi.org/10.4135/9781483328768). Copyright 2004 by A. W. Johnson and R. W. Proctor. Reprinted with permission.

FIGURE 11.4. Norman and Shallice's (1986) Model of Action Control

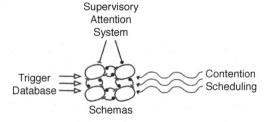

Note. Small black circles depict excitatory connections; short lines depict inhibitory connections. From *Attention: Theory and Practice* (p. 288), by A. Johnson and R. W. Proctor, 2004, SAGE (https://doi.org/10.4135/9781483328768). Copyright 2004 by A. W. Johnson and R. W. Proctor. Reprinted with permission.

sequence must be performed in place of a more familiar one. The supervisory attention system can directly activate or inhibit schemas but cannot select them directly. Control always proceeds through the process of contention scheduling, with the supervisory attention system biasing selection by inhibiting some schemas and activating others. Attentional resources are needed for stopping actions as well as initiating them. For example, driving is a familiar task, for which many schemas (e.g., behaviors at a traffic signal, behaviors to change lanes, behaviors to respond to emergency vehicles) are triggered by environmental cues (e.g., a red traffic light triggers a braking response, a signal triggers a changing-lane response, sirens and blinking lights trigger a "pull over" response). However, when an unexpected event occurs, such as your exit ramp being blocked, the supervisory system and contention scheduler need to inhibit certain schemas (e.g., merging on the exit ramp) and activate others needed to get you to your destination.

If the supervisory attention system is not intact or not functioning properly, as in the case of patients with frontal-lobe lesions, different types of disorders may result. Perseveration may occur due to strong schemas remaining active too long. This results in prolongation or repeated application of a schema where the patient shows an inability to switch from a current action or goal to a newer, more appropriate action. Another disorder, *utilization behavior*, can also occur when the patients grasp and attempt to use an object placed in front of them without being asked or expected to interact with the object. Utilization behavior can occur because the object can be the trigger that activates an action schema and its contention scheduling. Finally, heightened distractibility can occur because many schemas of similar activation values may be competing for control, producing disorganized behavior.

P. Watson et al. (2018) used fMRI to examine the brain regions that are activated when slips-of-action tasks are performed. Participants were trained to discriminate between cues associated with reward. During the test phase, some of the cues were devalued by the task instructions, and participants had to quickly respond to cues that resulted in "still-valuable" outcomes and refrain from responding to cues that resulted in "devalued" outcomes. The trials that resulted in devalued outcomes should show evidence for competition between goal-directed and habitual processes. Moreover, action slips occur when participants are not able to successfully refrain from responding on devalued trials. The devalued trials showed increased activation in the anterior cingulate cortex, paracingulate gyrus, lateral orbitofrontal cortex, insula, and inferior frontal gyrus extending into the premotor cortex. Also, activation in the premotor cortex correlated with action slips. Increased activation in lateral regions of the premotor cortex and cerebellum during training was predictive of more action slips on devalued trials. Increased activation in the caudate nucleus, dorsolateral prefrontal cortex, and frontal pole during training was predictive of good goal-directed action on still-valued trials. Because different regions of the brain activated during task performance were indicative of habitual versus goal-directed control, P. Watson et al. interpreted their findings as supporting the notion that action slips result from competition between goal-directed and habitual control.

In sum, action slips are errors due to lapses of attention or the breakdown of attentional control. Unlike errors that occur through lack of knowledge or practice (i.e., mistakes), action slips cannot be reduced through training and are more prevalent in skilled performance. Neurophysiological data showed that the regions of the brain activated during actions slips are those typically involved in the planning and execution of habitual and goal-direct actions, suggesting a competition between those processes.

GROUP DIFFERENCES: SELECTED EXAMPLES

Many tasks have been developed to test the limits of our attentional processing capabilities. Most of these studies have been devoted to describing common-alities in the ability for selective and divided attention to characterize human performance. When differences are examined, comparisons are usually made between groups, such as males versus females, people classified as having high versus low working memory capacity, monolinguals versus bilinguals, and so forth. The groups selected for comparison are typically based on theoretical assumptions about how attentional processing occurs for each group.

For some groups, differences in performance on attentional tasks are small. For example, gender differences may be expected due to laterality effects. That is, it is often assumed that men tend to outperform women on visual–spatial tasks (right hemispheric functions), but women tend to do better on verbal tasks (left hemispheric functions). However, hemispheric differences are not a major factor contributing to gender differences in cognitive performance (see Hirnstein et al., 2019). Voyer (2011) found only a small laterality effect for men in a meta-analysis of studies using the dichotic listening task. Given that the effect was so small, Voyer concluded that there might not be any practical implications of this finding. Moreover, some group comparisons may yield null effects if the phenomenon or experimental manipulation has large, but opposite, effects for specific individuals in the sample (J. Miller & Schwarz, 2018).

Other groups, such as those that differ on working memory capacity, show larger differences in performance (see Chapter 8). For example, Kane et al. (2001) found that observers with a high working memory capacity were better able to resist attentional capture (i.e., made fewer saccades to the cue in an anti-saccade condition) than those with a low working memory capacity. Colflesh and Conway (2007) found that individuals with a higher working memory capacity were better able to divide their attention. They had partici-pants shadow the message in the attended ear while explicitly listening for their name in the other channel, pressing the space bar when they detected it. In this divided attention scenario, 67% of the participants classified as having a high working memory capacity were able to detect their name compared with 35% of the participants classified as having a low working memory capacity.

In this section, we examine group differences in performance in three areas in which discrepant findings have been observed: bilingualism, video game experience, and mindlessness. The mixed results from the different studies examining similar groups may be related to the different methodological variations in tasks and procedures used in the specific studies. These areas were selected as examples for illustrating the research on group differences in attention.

Is There a Bilingual Advantage in Executive Control Processes?

Bilinguals spend their life straddling between two languages, so it is plausible to think that this requirement to mediate between languages results in better executive, or cognitive, control functions compared with monolinguals. For the past quarter-century, considerable research has been devoted to this possibility. Bialystok et al. (2004) initiated the intensive research on the topic. Their Experiment 1 compared performance on a Simon task of monolingual English participants living in Canada with that of bilingual participants fluent in English and Tamil (a southern Indian language) who were living in India. The bilinguals showed a smaller Simon effect (a correspondence effect for irrelevant stimulus locations with left–right key presses) than monolinguals for both middle-age (40 ms vs. 535 ms) and older adults (748 ms vs. 1,723 ms). The authors attributed the smaller Simon effect size for bilinguals to better attentional processes in general and inhibitory processes in particular.

Other studies reported superior performance of bilinguals compared with monolinguals on other tasks assumed to rely heavily on executive control processes, including task-switching (e.g., Bialystok et al., 2008) and negative priming (Treccani et al., 2009). As an example of the former, Prior and MacWhinney (2010) had groups of monolingual and bilingual students perform two tasks in which they had to respond based on the color or shape of a stimulus. Both single-task and mixed task performance were measured in separate blocks of trials, with the task in the mixed trials being cued before the onset of the imperative stimulus. The bilinguals and monolinguals showed similar overall costs in reaction time of mixed-task over single-task blocks, but the bilinguals evidenced smaller task-switching costs (i.e., differences in reaction time between task switch and nonswitch trials) in the mixed-task blocks than the monolinguals. Prior and MacWhinney interpreted the finding of a bilingual advantage for the local task-switch but not the global mixing cost as evidence that the bilingual advantage in executive control processes extends beyond inhibition to include flexibility in switching between task sets.

For negative priming, Treccani et al. (2009) had bilingual and monolingual participants perform a four-choice task in which the stimuli and responses were arrayed congruently in a trapezoid shape. On each trial pair, a target stimulus (e.g., the letter X) was presented in one location with an irrelevant stimulus (e.g., the letter O) in one of the other locations. Shortly after responding to the current array, a second target stimulus was presented. For the negative priming trials, the second target corresponded to the location of the distractor on the prime trial. Reaction times showed large negative priming effects for both monolinguals and bilinguals but no significant difference in effect size. However, bilinguals showed a smaller increase in error rates than monolinguals for trials with distractors than those without, coupled with a larger negative priming effect. Treccani et al. interpreted these results as consistent with bilinguals being better at inhibiting irrelevant location information, which can produce benefits or costs.

The strength of the evidence from these and other studies can be questioned. In Bialystok et al.'s (2004) experiment, the reported Simon effects for all except the middle-aged bilingual persons were larger than those typically obtained. Also, their Experiment 3, conducted with middle-aged French–English bilinguals and English monolinguals, only showed a smaller Simon effect for the bilinguals than the monolinguals (23 ms vs. 234 ms) in the first of 10 trial blocks and not in the last block (8 ms vs. 12 ms). Thus, any benefit for the bilingual group was short-lived. As noted, Prior and MacWhinney (2010) showed no overall advantage for bilinguals in dealing with the mixing of trial types, and the executive control function implied by a task-switching benefit is different from the inhibition function suggested in the other two studies. Finally, Treccani et al.'s (2009) results showed up in the error data rather than the reaction times and in inferior not better performance of the bilinguals on negative priming trials. Those authors later stated that they did not report results of other tasks that had failed to show evidence for presumed inhibitory processes (in Simon, color negative priming, and spatial precuing tasks; de Bruin et al., 2015).

Given that state of affairs, it should not be surprising that other studies have reported no significant differences between bilinguals and monolinguals in tasks of executive control. For example, Desjardins and Fernandez (2018) examined the effects of age and bilingual experience on inhibitory control using Bialystok et al.'s (2004) Simon task and a dichotic listening task. They tested younger and older adult English monolinguals and Spanish–English bilinguals. Unlike Bialystok et al., they found no difference in the Simon effect between bilinguals and monolinguals for either age group, with effect sizes in the more typical range. Similarly, they found no bilingual advantage for the dichotic listening task.

Several factors have led to relatively widespread agreement that there is no clear evidence for a general cognitive control benefit for bilinguals (de Bruin et al., 2015; Paap et al., 2015; Valian, 2015). Findings have been difficult to replicate, and many nonsignificant tests of a bilingual advantage apparently have not been published, either due to decisions of editors or the researchers themselves (de Bruin et al., 2015). Also, numerous other individual-difference factors are correlated with bilingualism, including socioeconomic status, culture, and immigrant status (which are associated with educational differences and differences in age of onset of dementia; Paap et al., 2015). These intercorrelations make it difficult to ensure that bilingual and monolingual groups are matched on all other differentiating factors. Exactly what constitutes executive control processes has not been specified clearly, and accounts have shifted between emphases on various subsets of processes. The tasks themselves have been a mélange that may be tapping different processes. Moreover, some evidence for differences between bilinguals and monolinguals comes from psychophysiological studies of brain functioning that show no performance advantage for bilinguals. Without a performance difference, what to make of differences in brain activity is unclear (Hilchey & Klein, 2011; Paap, 2019).

Although there is widespread agreement that the current evidence does not allow a firm conclusion as to whether there is a bilingual advantage in executive control and, if so, what the control mechanisms are, a difference of opinion exists about whether there is a true benefit of bilingualism that is being hidden by other factors that influence performance (Valian, 2015) or whether there is no bilingual advantage in executive processing at all (de Bruin et al., 2015; Hilchey & Klein, 2011; Paap et al., 2015). Due to the noisiness of research on this topic, some of which is inherent to the topic itself, resolution of this debate is not likely to occur soon.

Video Gamers and Nongamers

There have been many studies in the literature showing a relation between video game experience (especially with action video games) and multitasking ability (e.g., Boot et al., 2008; Cardoso-Leite et al., 2016; Chiappe et al., 2013). In this section, we look at differences between participants with specified amounts of video game experience (no, low, high) and within participants as they practice video games. Also, there is interest in action video games compared with other types of games due to the type of practice that players receive dealing with multiple demands and overlapping game components. C. S. Green and Bavelier (2003) examined the performance of action video game players and nonplayers on four attention tasks. The flanker task was used to provide an indicator of spare attentional resources. Video game players showed a larger flanker congruity effect than nonplayers, especially when the task was difficult. C. S. Green and Bavelier attributed the benefit in the performance of the gamers to having more spare resources for attending to a larger field of view.

C. S. Green and Bavelier (2003) used an enumeration task to indicate the participants' span of apprehension, where participants had to report how many squares (between one and 10) were briefly flashed on a display. Video game players performed better at this task than nonplayers when the number of items flashed was more than four squares. A task designed to measure attention over space showed that video game players were able to identify visual targets better than nonplayers at 10°, 20°, and 30° eccentricities, suggesting that they could attend to a larger field of view. Finally, video game players had better attention over time, showing smaller attentional blink effects than nonplayers for Lags 1 to 5. The authors interpreted this latter finding as gamers having better task-switching or multitasking capabilities.

Kowal et al. (2018) found a positive correlation between action video game experience and task-switching performance. They also found that action video gamers showed shorter reaction time on a Stroop task than nongamers but a larger Stroop effect for errors. This finding suggests that gamers may adopt a strategy of speed over accuracy and not necessarily have better inhibitory skills. There have also been some data from fMRI studies indicating that different brain regions are activated in gamers versus nongamers. Bavelier et al. (2012) had participants perform an attentional task in which they maintained fixation on a central point while identifying a specific target under different levels of perceptual load and in the presence of moving distractors presented centrally or peripherally. Gamers had less activation in the middle temporal and medial superior temporal gyri compared with nongamers in response to the moving distractors. Because these regions are correlated with motion detection and attentional modulation of visuoperceptual processing, Bavelier et al. suggested that gamers are better at early filtering of irrelevant information. Also, non-gamers showed an increase in the activation of the frontoparietal network as a function of perceptual load that was not evident for gamers. The authors attributed this to the gamers being able to allocate attentional resources with less effort than nongamers.

Some studies showed no difference between action video gamers and nongamers or context-dependent effects. Klaffehn et al. (2018) compared the performance of participants experienced with first-person shooter games and video gamers who engaged in real-time strategy games with a control group of chess and go players without extensive video game experience. They indicated that action video games, such as first-person shooter games, emphasize fast responding to elements on the screen. In contrast, real-time strategy games involve more resource management and coordination, which may be more reflective of attentional control processes. If video game playing produces bene-fits in cognitive control, both types of video gamers should perform better on dual-task and task-switching tasks than the chess and go (a game that does not have a rapid task-switching component) players. Klaffehn et al. found that neither type of video game experience resulted in performance benefits for task-switching or dual-task performance. That is, all groups performed similarly on the tested cognitive tasks.

Cardoso-Leite et al. (2016) compared the performance of action video gamers with different levels of media multitasking experience with nongamers. Unlike video game experience, which is associated with better attentional control, media multitasking, or using two or more types of media simultaneously, is associated with deficits in attentional control. Action gamers and nongamers were classified as high, intermediate, or low in terms of media multitasking based on self-report. When averaged across all groups, gamers did not perform better than nongamers. Gamers outperformed nongamers on both memory and task-switching tasks but only when they were classified as intermediate media multitaskers. Based on these findings, Cardoso-Leite et al. concluded that the attentional control skills gained by playing video games can be counter-acted by other experience, such as media multitasking.

In addition to examining differences between gamers and nongamers, researchers have also assessed whether video game training improves attentional skills. Because the differences in the performance of gamers versus nongamers could be related to personality differences, group differences could be due to factors other than the video game training. C. S. Green and Bavelier (2003) trained a group of nongamers on action video games or a control puzzle game that would promote visuospatial skills but not multitasking skills. Training nongamers for 1 hour a day over 10 days was effective in improving their performance on the game. That is, training on the action video game led to greater improvements on attentional tasks relating to the capacity of visual attention, spatial distribution, and spatial resolution compared with training on the puzzle game.

Whether there is a benefit of video game training to general cognitive skills such as attentional focus and control has also been examined. For example, Franceschini et al. (2013) compared the performance of two matched groups of children with dyslexia before and after they received nine 80-minute training sessions with action or nonaction video games. Reading performance was measured by examining the speed and accuracy of the phonological decoding of pseudowords and words in text. Spatial attention was measured by having the children focus on a red dot and report items appearing above it. Temporal attention was measured by the time it took the children to localize a target stimulus at short versus long cue intervals. Only the group that received action video games showed improved reading efficiency (i.e., increased reading speed without a cost to accuracy), spatial attention (i.e., greater accuracy), and temporal attention (i.e., larger cuing effects). This finding led Franceschini et al. to conclude that action video games can improve the attention of children with dyslexia.

Other studies provided video game training to participants and examined multitask performance before and after training (e.g., Boot et al., 2008; Chiappe et al., 2013). Boot et al. (2008) had nongamer participants play video games, classified as fast-paced action (visual and attentional skills), strategy (executive control skills), or puzzle (spatial skills), to evaluate whether video game training improves specific skills or broad skills. Participants' visual attention, memory, reasoning, and executive control performance were measured before and after 10 or 21 hours of game playing over a 4- to 5-week period and compared with a control group and an expert gamer group that did not receive any video game training. Practice playing the games improved game performance for all groups across the training period. Also, the expert gamers performed better than nongamers on many tasks (e.g., tracking of objects and visual short-term memory). However, Boot et al. found that 21 hours of playing time was not enough to improve performance significantly on many transfer tasks. The type of game played also had little impact. That is, the video game playing groups performed similarly to each other and did not outperform the nongamer control group.

Although Boot et al. (2008) found no general transfer effect with 21 hours of game playing, other studies that have included more training have shown transfer effects of video game training to multitasking skills. Chiappe et al. (2013) had nongamers perform 10 weeks of training with first-person shooter video games for at least 5 hours a week. Participants were tested on four tasks of a multiattribute task battery before and after training. The tasks included two primary tasks (tracking and fuel management) and two secondary tasks (systems monitoring and communication). Playing the video games improved performance on the secondary tasks that was not evident with the control group. Moreover, the improvements in secondary task performance for the video game group did not come at a cost to performance on the two primary tasks.

In sum, video game training does appear to have some benefit for improving attentional focus (Franceschini et al., 2013) and multitasking performance (Chiappe et al., 2013). The magnitude of the benefit is likely to depend on the extent of the video game training and how much the training matches the task being tested (Strobach & Schubert, 2021). Thus, there does not seem to be a general benefit of video game training on attentional control capabilities (see Box 11.1 for similar conclusions for visual training in sports).

Individuals Prone to Mind Wandering

As noted earlier, driving is a task that requires monitoring the environment for obstacles and traffic signs and/or signals and controlling the vehicle through steering, accelerating or braking, or maintaining speed. For most individuals, driving is a highly practiced task, and many components of driving can be carried out without much attention being devoted to them. The routine nature of driving, especially along familiar routes, can be related to everyday absent-mindedness and lapses of attention. There has been a lot of research on the relation between lapses of attention and attentional control, working memory capacity, personality variables (i.e., boredom proneness), current motivation levels, and level of arousal or alertness (see Unsworth et al., 2021, for a review). These studies used different methods to measure lapses in attention. Unsworth et al. (2021) showed that different behavioral measures (e.g., reaction times, error rates) and subjective reports of task-unrelated thoughts (i.e., mind wandering) are distinct but correlated ($r = .44$) and that these metrics capture an individual's general susceptibility to lapses of attention. In this section, we provide a few examples of studies that focused on lapses of attention and mind wandering.

Models of attentional modulation of action planning (e.g., Norman & Shallice, 1986) suggest that there may be a positive relation between the ability to ignore irrelevant stimuli and to avoid making everyday errors. Larson and Perry (1999) administered the Cognitive Failures Questionnaire (Broadbent et al., 1982), in which individuals are asked how often they make certain types of errors, such as misplacing keys or forgetting why they entered a particular room, to group participants low or high in terms of "cognitive failures" based

BOX 11.1 | **LIMITS OF GENERAL TRAINING: AN EXAMPLE
IN SPORTS**

In sports, athletes are required to perform many perceptual-cognitive tasks. From earlier chapters, we know that attending to an object allows for better processing of the object's features. Sports vision training is based on developing the general visual skills of athletes, such as depth perception, ocular tracking, static and dynamic acuity, and peripheral detection and sensitivity. According to Hadlow et al. (2018), a defining characteristic of sports visual training is the use of generic stimuli (i.e., symbols, patterns, and shapes) to simulate the types of visual targets that the players would encounter in the specific sport. The general idea is that if the athletes practice attending to key features of the target, they will be able to identify it more quickly and respond to it faster and more effectively in the context of the sport.

Hadlow et al. (2018) indicated that the practice tasks should be based on a representative learning design, where the training should have learners attend to three interacting factors: (a) perceptual processes linking (b) information to (c) action. Moreover, focusing attention on the consequences of actions rather than the body movements to execute them may be most beneficial in some tasks. For example, skilled dart throwing results from attending to the trajectory of the dart and not on the motion of the arm involved in throwing the dart (Lohse et al., 2010). Because most complex, real-world tasks require selectively attending to different information sources, the ability to allocate attention to the appropriate cues might be a good predictor of successful task performance in many situations. Schumacher et al. (2020) noted that for sports such as soccer, the players must attend to both the ball and other players, teammates and opponents, on the field. Thus, in addition to reducing the processing time for stimuli in central vision, shortening reaction time to visual stimuli in the periphery should benefit players' performance. Schumacher et al. found that a sport-specific form of perceptual-cognitive training, consisting of two exercises promoting hand–eye coordination and peripheral reaction, reduced players' reaction time on visual detection tasks. However, the players' performance in a real game was not examined.

Deveau et al. (2014) had baseball players perform visual training for 30 sessions of 25 minutes each. The training included presenting the players with visual targets of varying spatial frequencies and orientations at visual thresholds for detection. The players given the visual training and a control group of untrained players were assessed for visual acuity before and after the training period. Those given the visual training showed 31% improvement in binocular acuity, as well as improvements in near vision and contrast sensitivity. The players who received the visual training also reported that it benefited their performance in ball games: They said they were able to see the ball better and see farther and had greater peripheral vision. The untrained players did not show the observed or reported benefits in vision. Analysis of performance for the trained players 4 months before training and 2 months afterward suggested that their performance did, in fact, benefit from the visual training. They had a 4% decrease in

BOX 11.1 | **LIMITS OF GENERAL TRAINING: AN EXAMPLE IN SPORTS** *(Continued)*

strikeouts, which was significantly better than the 1% decrease shown by other players in the league during that time. These data suggest that visual training may be beneficial, but the findings must be interpreted with caution because the training literature shows that improvements on laboratory tasks typically do not tend to generalize broadly (Healy & Bourne, 2012).

This latter point is illustrated in a study by Maman et al. (2011), who evaluated the performance of university-level tennis players after 8 weeks of just daily practice or training plus daily practice. The training group received 30 minutes of visual training for 3 days a week, a placebo group read and watched televised tennis matches for 30 minutes 3 days a week, and a control group received only the daily practice. Participants' choice reaction time, movement time, depth perception and accommodation ability, and saccadic eye movements in the vertical and horizontal planes were measured pre- and post-training. Tennis playing performance was also evaluated before and after the 8 weeks. The visual training led to significant improvement in basic visual skills and motor skills. This improvement was larger than for the placebo group, which showed only slight improvement, and the control group, which showed no improvement. Despite this difference, the three groups did not differ in tennis playing performance, providing no evidence that the visual training had a measurable impact on the court.

In sum, although some evidence suggests that there are benefits to training athletes to attend to perceptual features (e.g., Deveau et al., 2014), other studies have found no evidence of benefits in the field (e.g., Maman et al., 2011). Renshaw et al. (2019) cautioned that trainers should not rely too much on a process training approach, such as visual training. They noted that training of isolated processes, such as attention, memory, and visual processing, at most would provide some transfer of general skills but typically not be sufficiently specific to enhance performance significantly in the field. For elite athletes, skilled performance is only achieved after extensive practice on techniques specific to the sport. Further, some skills, such as archery, are only evident in the narrow contexts in which the training takes place (Nabavinik et al., 2018).

on action slips and attentional or memory lapses. They found that participants performed similarly in a visual discrimination task with valid spatial cues regardless of whether they scored high or low on the questionnaire. However, individuals with high scores on the questionnaire showed more difficulty inhibiting reflexive saccades in the direction of a distracting cue. Although the questionnaire scores accounted for only a small amount of the variance in capture errors ($r = .3$), Larson and Perry suggested that the antisaccade task could be useful in screening individuals for tasks in which capture errors are likely and have serious consequences.

S. Lange and Süß (2014) used a mobile app version of the Questionnaire for Cognitive Failures in Everyday Life to measure slips (e.g., took salt instead of sugar) and lapses (e.g., greeted someone twice) in older adults. Although scores on this questionnaire did not significantly correlate with mixing costs (i.e., the difference between single-task and task-switch blocks), they showed a significant negative correlation ($r = -.24$) with task-switching performance. Individuals who scored higher on the questionnaire showed poorer task-switching performance.

Self-report and electroencephalogram (EEG) measures have also been used to examine whether drivers' minds wander during a driving task. Baldwin et al. (2017) had participants drive on a monotonous simulated road. At various intervals, they were probed by an auditory tone to self-report whether they were mind wandering or focused on the driving task. Periods of driving when mind wandering were compared with periods when participants were focused on driving. Participants reported mind wandering on about 70% of the probes. During periods of mind wandering, participants drove at lower speeds and showed reduced lane variability compared with periods when they reported being focused on the task. EEG measures taken during the task showed greater magnitudes in the alpha band over parietal regions during periods of mind wandering, which is often correlated with inattentiveness. Analysis of participants' responses at the time the auditory probe was presented showed the P3a component over Fz and Cz sites to be smaller in amplitude when participants reported mind wandering relative to when they reported being focused on the task. The smaller P3a amplitude suggests that participants' attention to the driving task was diminished during periods of mind wandering.

Ju and Lien (2018) examined how working memory capacity and mindfulness are related to mind wandering. For working memory, participants performed an *N*-back task where they had to recall items presented several trials (*N*) previously. For the low-load condition, recall was based on the digit presented on the current trial (0-back), and for the high-load condition, recall was based on the digit presented two trials previously (2-back). Participants were probed about their mind wandering behavior after a block of several trials. The participants reported engaging in mind wandering more when the load was low than when it was high and in later blocks of trials than earlier blocks. Most participants said that their mind wandering was unintentional, and some were aware of their mind wandering behavior. Participants reported more awareness of mind wandering in the low-load than high-load condition, likely because they had more attentional resources available in low-load than high-load conditions. Also, participants who scored higher on a complex working-memory span test reported less mind wandering but only under conditions of high-task load. Participants who scored high on a mindfulness scale also showed less mind wandering regardless of whether the task load was high or low.

It is known that mind wandering can lead to decrements in performance. Techniques aimed at improving focused attention should decrease mind wandering and increase performance. For example, meditators who had practiced concentrative or focused attention meditation for an average of 6.6 years showed fewer lapses on a response-switching task than nonmeditators (Badart et al., 2018). Although this finding suggests that meditation may enhance sustained attention and cognitive control, other factors should be accounted for before making any firm conclusions about the effectiveness of proposed interventions.

CHAPTER SUMMARY

As for any other cognitive ability, differences in attention between and within individuals over time can be observed. The literature on individual differences in attention is complex and is complicated by the facts that attention itself is multifaceted and researchers use different terms to describe similar aspects of attention. Robust differences between individuals have been found for selective attention, divided attention, and attention control, and they change throughout a person's lifespan and with their varied experiences.

Skilled performance takes years to develop. Although general perceptual, cognitive, and video game training can improve performance on the trained tasks and other tasks that involve similar processes, there is little evidence of this training generalizing to skilled performance in the field. Thus, skilled performance is a result of extensive, domain-specific training rather than general visual or cognitive training. Automaticity is a defining feature of skilled performance, and current views of automaticity involve attention as a mediator of processing efficiency rather than processing without attention. Errors occur in skilled performance when lapses of attention result in action slips or the activation of inappropriate action plans.

We also evaluated group differences in the performance of bilinguals versus monolinguals, video gamers versus nongamers, and individuals prone to mind wandering versus those who are not, and the literature showed mixed results. Few differences were seen between monolingual and bilingual persons when other factors were controlled. Video game experience does apparently lead to some benefit in performance, but the magnitude of the benefit is specific to the types of skills developed by playing the games. Finally, individuals prone to mind wandering tend to perform worse than those less prone to mind wandering. We acknowledge that there is research on group differences in other areas, such as personality (e.g., Matthews, 2021) and culture (e.g., Shell & Flowerday, 2019), that were not covered in the chapter. Readers should look up the literature on other groups of interest.

KEY POINTS

- **Fact:** Many aspects of attention develop over the first 2 years of life, with attentional skills continuing to develop through adolescence.

- **Fact:** Attention-deficit/hyperactivity disorder and autism spectrum disorder are relatively widespread developmental problems that have long-lasting influences throughout life.

- **Fact:** In older adults, cognitive processes linked to frontal lobe function—memory, attentional capacity, and possibly inhibitory processes—tend to show deficits for adults aged 65 years and beyond, whereas functions relating to attentional control show less deficit.

- **Fact:** Older adults have the advantage of crystallized intelligence and knowledge and skills acquired through years of experience.

- **Fact:** Automaticity tends to develop when the mapping of stimuli to task categories is consistent.

- **Fact:** Performance improvements with practice follow a power law at the group level.

- **Theory:** Power law improvement with practice can be generated by models that assume either the acquisition of task-specific procedures or memories of many instances of the events.

- **Phenomenon:** Action slips are common errors that occur when routine tasks are to be performed.

- **Fact:** Training attentional skills and practice at video games show some benefits but with limited transfer to performance of everyday tasks.

- **Fact:** Working memory capacity, as measured by operation span tasks, correlates with the performance of many tasks requiring working memory and attentional control.

- **Fact:** Bilinguals do not necessarily show better executive control processes than monolinguals.

12

Social Attention and Team Performance

Attention places emphasis on the individual. Attention is directed exogenously by events in the environment and endogenously according to the goals and strategies of the person. Individuals read books, watch movies, listen to music, determine the sources from which to obtain the news, and so on. Individuals' knowledge gained from prior experiences and its activation in working memory determine what they are prepared to process and how they will comprehend ongoing events. However, people live in social environments and, nowadays, virtual environments in which they interact and engage with other people in person or online and, increasingly, with robots and other forms of automation. The direction of attention and the tasks to which people devote their cognitive resources can be determined, at least in part, by other people. This is true not just for social interactions with friends and relatives but also with marketing interactions in which website designers, telemarketers, politicians, and the like may try to direct individuals' attention to particular products or news stories. There are also many situations in which people need to cooperate or compete in teams of two or more persons. Attentional processes also play key roles in these cooperative and competitive interactions. Cooperative teamwork may even involve automation as a team member.

The topic of social attention is one part of social cognition (Happé et al., 2017). There is no doubt that social factors influence various aspects of attention. What is less clear is the extent to which this influence is enacted through the general properties of attention we described in prior chapters, which Heyes

https://doi.org/10.1037/0000317-012
Attention: Selection and Control in Human Information Processing, by R. W. Proctor and K.-P. L. Vu

(2014) described as *submentalizing* or rooted in processes that are more specifically social in nature, which she called *implicit mentalizing*. This latter term comes from the emphasis of social cognition on implicit, or automatic, processes and the closely linked theory of mind view, according to which representation of the mental states of others is fundamental to humans (Frith & Frith, 2005). The issue of social, mentalizing accounts versus information-processing, submentalizing accounts recurs repeatedly with regard to phenomena discussed in this chapter. The basic point to understand is that just because a certain phenomenon occurs in a social context or with people as stimuli does not necessarily mean that the phenomenon is due to social processes per se. Proponents of the social-processes view often include control experiments intended to rule out nonsocial alternatives, whereas proponents of the general-processes view conduct similar experiments intended to show that the phenomena occur when social aspects are eliminated. Because the task contexts typically differ in many ways, it is difficult to rule conclusively one way or another in most situations.

SHARED ATTENTION

We begin our consideration of social factors with *shared attention*, which was defined by Stephenson et al. (2021): "When two people look at the same object in the environment and are aware of each other's attentional state, they find themselves in a shared-attention episode" (p. 553). By this definition, shared attention is used to convey intentions and thoughts between the two persons, as well as to provide a basis for coordinating thinking and behavior. The emphasis on awareness of each other's attentional state in this definition distinguishes shared attention from joint attention, which is basically the same but lacks the awareness component. Shteynberg (2015) defined shared attention more broadly to encompass a broader range of activities, including watching the same sporting event, watching the same movie, and engaging in the same social media groups. There is nothing in either definition of shared attention to indicate that mechanisms unique to social interactions are involved.

The Shared Attention System

Let us first consider the approach of Stephenson et al. (2021), which emphasizes two people looking at the same object. In a two-person interaction, gaze perception is a critical part of both joint and shared attention. The visual system contains multiple neural channels that analyze the horizontal direction of another's eye gaze (Calder et al., 2008) and horizontal and vertical orientations of head direction (Lawson et al., 2011). Consequently, people are relatively sensitive at detecting another person's gaze direction. A distinction can be made between the *initiator* of the interaction, who starts the shared attention episode, and the *responder*, whose attention follows that of the initiator.

The initiator often begins by looking directly at the responder and making eye contact. After eye contact is established, the initiator's gaze moves elsewhere, causing the responder to shift their gaze to the same location or object. The gaze direction is a cue to where and what the responder should attend to. Because shared attention is a cooperative process, it must be studied from both the initiator's and responder's viewpoints.

Stephenson et al. (2021) incorporated much of the research of the past 20 years into the shared-attention system (see Figure 12.1), which they explicitly indicated includes components of social cognition. The model distinguishes three levels of processes: first, second, and third order. The *first-order* processes derive meaning from the social signals offered by others and include detecting gaze and encoding its direction. The *second-order* processes establish joint attention by reorienting attention (which, for simplification, is assumed to involve an overt gaze shift) and generating an appropriate response, taking into consideration that one's actions may cause changes in the cognitive, emotional, or physical state of the person with whom joint attention is engaged. The *third-order* processes are those devoted specifically to shared attention; they are related to determining and processing the social consequences of one's actions.

Gaze Perception and Orientation of Attention

The first-order processes of gaze detection lead to the reorientation of attention to the gaze location. In experimental settings, this process has been studied under the topic of *gaze cuing* (Frischen et al., 2007), which focuses on the responder's responses to social cues. Indeed, Dalmaso et al. (2020) noted that the number of studies on the topic of gaze-mediated orienting has increased dramatically since the introduction of the gaze-cuing task by Friesen and Kingstone (1998). The research paradigm is a variant of the Posner (1980, 2016) location cuing task described in Chapter 4, this volume. It involves presenting a centered face photograph or schematic with eyes looking to the left or right. A stimulus appears later at a left or right location, corresponding or not with the gaze direction, which is to be detected or identified as quickly as possible, depending on task requirements. Most studies focus on situations in which gaze direction is not predictive of the location of the target stimulus. The gaze cue is considered to be valid when the stimulus occurs to the side indicated by the gaze and invalid when it occurs to the opposite side. Figure 12.2 shows a trial sequence for a validly cued trial in which a neutral face is replaced with the same face looking to the participant's left, going from left to right. Following that (after an interval), the stimulus to which the participant is to respond appears in the left location (designated by the asterisk). For an invalid cue, the stimulus would appear to the right of the gaze cue.

As indicated, Friesen and Kingstone (1998) reported the first study of this type with adults, cuing participants with faces like those in Figure 12.2. The target stimulus was the letter T or F, which could appear 105, 300, 600, and 1,005 milliseconds (ms) after the onset of the gaze cue. Participants were told

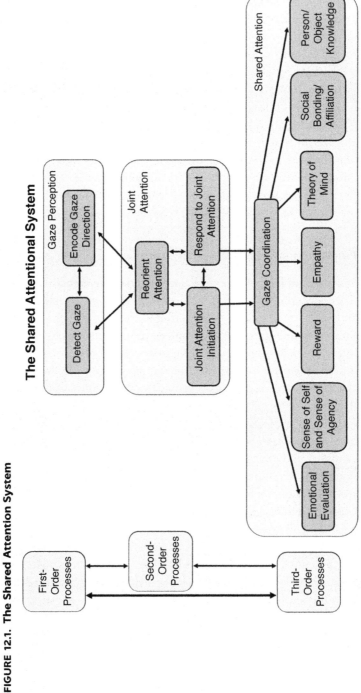

FIGURE 12.1. The Shared Attention System

FIGURE 12.2. Gaze-Cuing Paradigm Using a Schematic Drawing

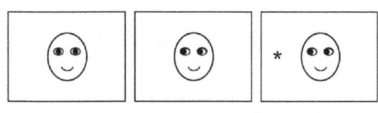

that the gaze cue was uninformative as to the location in which the target stimulus would occur. In different sets of trials, each participant performed three tasks: detection (indicated by pressing the space bar), localization (pressing a left or right key corresponding to the left or right stimulus location), and identification (pressing one key for the letter F and another for T). For all three tasks, reaction time was shorter when the stimulus occurred on the side consistent with the gaze cue than when it occurred on the opposite side. Because the gaze cue was uninformative, the authors concluded that their results provided evidence for covert, reflexive orienting of attention to peripheral locations. Driver et al. (1999) obtained a similar benefit of gaze direction in a letter-identification task when a digitized face-gaze cue preceded the letter by at least 300 ms. The reflexive nature of this orienting effect was illustrated by the fact that this benefit was evident even when the letter was 4 times more likely to occur on the opposite side, although it reversed at a 700-ms interval when there was more time to prepare.

Although both the initial groups of authors interpreted their results as unique to eye gaze—due to its biological and social relevance—an obvious question is whether similar results are obtained with other directional stimuli, specifically arrows. Two studies confirmed that they are. Tipples (2002) reported experiments with pairs of arrows, both pointing to the left or both pointing to the right, that showed cuing effects on identification of one or two target letters like the effects found by Friesen and Kingstone (1998) and Driver et al. (1999). Ristic et al. (2002) conducted a detection task with the schematic face-gaze cues for half of the experiment and left- or right-pointing arrow-direction cues for the other half. The cuing effect was as large for the arrow-direction cues as for the gaze cues, implying that the eye-gaze cues are not special.

Despite the similarity of results for gaze-direction and arrow-direction cues, Ristic et al. (2002) argued that the effects were subserved by different brain systems. Their argument was based on a prior result obtained for two split-brain patients, who had their cerebral hemispheres disconnected because of intractable epilepsy (Kingstone et al., 2000). Those patients showed a gaze-direction cuing effect when the stimuli were presented in the left visual field and went to the right hemisphere, which is known to have areas sensitive to faces and eyes, but not when the stimuli were presented in the right visual field and went to the left hemisphere. Ristic et al. placed considerable emphasis on the data from these two split-brain patients, but other researchers weight the evidence from the neurologically intact adults more strongly because they are the primary population of interest. A more convincing case could be made if the split-brain patients did not show a similar hemispheric difference for arrow stimuli, as long as alternative interpretations for the different results could be ruled out.

Most studies of gaze cuing have examined only covert attention shifts in response to uninformative stimuli. However, in most situations in everyday life, people make overt attention shifts with eye and/or head movements. Ricciardelli et al. (2002) conducted an experiment in which participants made a signaled saccadic eye movement from a central fixation point to a left or right target location. The target was indicated by the central fixation point changing to a blue or orange color. At different time intervals after the onset of the instruction signal, a distractor stimulus of a woman's face with her eye gaze turned to the left or right was displayed briefly. Results showed that more antisaccades (i.e., eye movements to the wrong target location) were made when the face's eye-gaze direction was incongruent with the signaled saccade direction than when it was congruent. This difference was evident at the shortest onset interval of 50 ms but not at longer ones. Reaction times for the saccades also showed an 11-ms congruity effect, which did not vary as a function of onset interval. Kuhn and Kingstone (2009) obtained similar results with gaze-direction cues but also for arrows pointing to the left or right. These findings suggest that the "automatic" tendency to orient to the left or right is not restricted to gaze direction, even when it is counter to the intended eye-movement direction.

If orientation to gaze direction is automatic, one would expect a Simon-type congruity effect based on gaze direction to be obtained when people are to make a left or right key press to gaze stimuli based on stimulus color. This result was reported by Zorzi et al. (2003) and Ansorge (2003). Both studies found Simon-type effects of about 20 to 30 ms as a function of whether the eye-gaze direction was congruent with the response signaled by the color or not. Zorzi et al. did not get a significant Simon-type effect when the stimuli were two large outline squares with smaller filled squares inside, consistent with the hypothesis that eye-gaze direction is special. However, Ansorge noted that analyses of reaction-time distributions showed that the eye-gaze congruity effect was mainly evident for the longer reaction times, whereas it would be expected to be obtained mainly for the short reaction times if it were due to rapid, automatic activation. Moreover, Ricciardelli et al. (2005) found Simon-type effects of similar size for gaze-direction stimuli, square-"direction" stimuli of the type used by Zorzi et al., and arrow-direction stimuli located within an outline square. The Simon-type effect data are not in complete agreement, but on the whole, the results are counter to the idea that eye-gaze stimuli have a privileged status.

The strongest assessment of the issue of automaticity of activation for eye-gaze stimuli is that of Besner et al. (2021). They contrasted the relative automaticity of eye-gaze and arrow-direction stimuli in 10 experiments by presenting displays that contained both types of stimuli within a circular "face" (see Figure 12.3). The core stimuli used in most of their experiments were those in Quadrant 1 that included both eyes and arrows, with the arrow located in the position of a nose. In different experiments, participants were instructed to respond to the direction of eye gaze or the direction in which the arrow pointed. When the arrow direction was irrelevant, this produced a congruity effect regardless of whether the arrow appeared below or above the eyes, averaging about 45 ms. A congruity effect was also evident when gaze direction was irrelevant, but the effect was much smaller, averaging less than 10 ms. Thus, by relative interference as a metric, these data imply that the eye-gaze cues are less automatic than the arrow-direction cues. In other words, at least with schematic faces of the type used by Besner et al., arrows seem more privileged than eye-gaze stimuli to signal left or right direction.

Social Factors and Shared Attention

The third-order processes in Stephenson et al.'s (2021) shared attention model relate to determining and processing the social outcomes that one's actions have had. These processes include the creation of gaze coordination and the various social outcomes that may result from the shared attention episode, such as emotional evaluation, a sense of self and agency, and social bonding and affiliation (see Figure 12.1). Stephenson et al. noted that the most novel

FIGURE 12.3. Eyes and Arrow Stimuli Used by Besner et al. (2021)

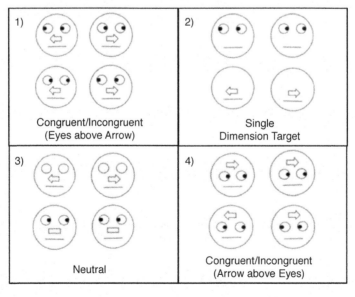

Note. From "On the Determination of Eye Gaze and Arrow Direction: Automaticity Reconsidered," by D. Besner, D. McLean, and T. Young, 2021, *Canadian Journal of Experimental Psychology*, *75*(3), p. 263 (https://doi.org/10.1037/cep0000261). Copyright 2021 by the Canadian Psychological Association. Adapted with permission.

aspect of their model is the third-order social cognition, which considers the dynamic nature of social interactions, the mechanisms that need to be coordinated between the initiator and responder, and more of the social outcomes than have typically been considered.

Even though the social factors are most closely linked to the shared attention concept, Dalmaso et al. (2020) pointed out that most research attempting to study the role of social factors in moderating the effects of eye-gaze stimuli on attention have been conducted using the gaze-cuing paradigm. In accord with the results we have described, Dalmaso et al. acknowledged that when schematic faces without any social features are used in a cuing task, the behavioral results are like those observed in response to arrow stimuli. Hence, they argued that gaze-cuing studies should use realistic face images and look at social variables (for the faces used and of the people performing the task). They indicated that recent research has focused on the modulatory effects of several social variables. For the most part, the results they reviewed for individual differences among participants showed little consistent effect. Exceptions concerned properties of the face used for the gaze-cuing task, for which results suggested that gaze-direction stimuli higher in dominance and social status may elicit a larger orienting response than those of lower dominance and status. Also, perhaps not too surprisingly, results of some studies suggest that attentional affects are larger when the face is familiar to the performer than when it is not.

We describe one example from each of the three research categories. For dominance, Jones et al. (2010) found that masculinized versions of male and female prototype faces yielded correspondence effects of 17 and 6 ms, respectively, when viewing time was brief (200 ms). With regard to social status, Dalmaso et al. (2012) found that after reading fictitious curricula vitae (CVs; résumés) associated with the faces of 16 individuals, the gaze-cuing effect was 15 ms for faces associated with high-status CVs compared with 5 ms for those associated with low-status CVs. Deaner et al. (2007) found that females who worked in a department from which the faces were selected and who were thus familiar with them showed a larger gaze-cuing effect than did females who unfamiliar with the people. However, this effect was not obtained for male participants, which requires an ad hoc explanation.

Dalmaso et al. (2020) reasoned that research on gaze-direction cuing should continue even though there is little evidence that gaze-direction cues for schematic faces are any stronger than arrow-direction cues. This is a strategy that proceeds with research into more complex situations looking at social variables in which the results are interpreted as if they have a social basis. It should be clear that nonsocial factors could be responsible for results like those described in the prior paragraph. The social interpretations depend on the assumption that gaze-direction cues are uniquely social, which has not been validated unambiguously in more controlled settings with schematic face and eye-gaze stimuli.

In their shared attention model, Stephenson et al. (2021) emphasized a need to consider initiators as well as responders. This was done in a study by

Kim and Mundy (2012) that used a virtual-reality setup to obtain evidence of a possible difference between initiators and responders. The participant faced a head and shoulders display of an avatar (see Figure 12.4). For a responder joint-attention condition (bottom panel), the avatar made an eye movement to the left or right, for which the participant's gaze was to follow. Then, two pictures appeared, one to the gaze-cued side of the avatar and one to the opposite side. For an initiator joint-attention condition (top panel), the procedure was similar except that the participant freely chose to move their eyes to fixate on the left or right location, after which the avatar moved their eyes to that location. Participants performed the tasks separately for several trials, with instructions to remember as many pictures as possible, and after each task condition, they were given a memory test.

The memory test included target pictures that had been at the gaze-cued location in the block, nontarget pictures that were at the uncued location, and novel pictures that had not been seen. Participants were to indicate whether they had seen each picture in the prior task. Of most interest, they were better at discriminating target gaze-cued pictures from novel ones on the memory test in the initiator condition ($d' = 1.77$) than in the responder condition ($d' = 1.11$). Kim and Mundy (2012) concluded that the picture stimuli to which attention was shifted were processed at a deeper level when initiating shared attention than responding to the avatar's cued direction. They proposed several possible explanations in terms of social attention but acknowledged that they could not rule out that the effects were due to free versus forced choice

FIGURE 12.4. Virtual Reality Joint Attention Task of Initiator Joint Attention and Responder Joint Attention

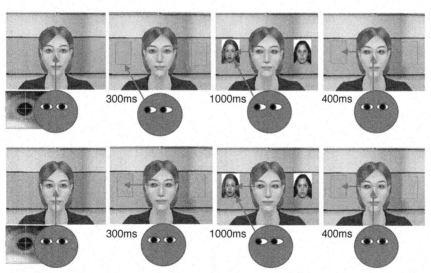

Note. From "Joint Attention, Social-Cognition, and Recognition Memory in Adults," by K. Kim and P. Mundy, 2012, *Frontiers in Human Neuroscience*, *6*, Article 172, p. 3 (https://doi.org/10.3389/fnhum.2012.00172). CC BY-NC 3.0.

more generally or some other aspect of their method besides coordination of joint attention.

Shteynberg's Shared Attention State

Shteynberg (2015, 2018), as mentioned earlier, focused mainly on the social aspects in broader contexts. He emphasized that shared attention can be experienced in public and private contexts and with other persons who are physically present (e.g., a rally) or imagined (e.g., on social media). He argued that shared attention not only establishes a common knowledge base among group members but also results in deeper level cognitive processing and, thus, better learning and memory. In his 2015 article, Shteynberg adopted a social cognition stance, stating, "If awareness of shared attention changes cognitive, affective, and behavioral responses to targets of attention, it would suggest that the psychological process of attention is, in part, socially grounded" (p. 580). He also conveyed a similar view in his 2018 article but allowed that the mechanisms might not be strictly social.

Several studies have found better performance on memory tests in shared attention conditions, but we focus on only two. Eskenazi et al. (2013) had two participants seated beside each other perform a word classification task. Words from three categories (fruit or vegetable, animal, or household object) were shown one at a time, and each participant was to make a key press response when a word from an assigned category appeared. The third category was not assigned to either participant, and neither participant was to respond to it. This condition of joint task performance was compared with a control condition of individual task performance in which a person had to discriminate the two relevant categories with a left or right key press and not respond to words in the third category. The main finding was that on a subsequent unexpected memory test in which the participants were to recall as many words as possible, more words were remembered when that category had been assigned to the partner than when it was one of the response categories in individual task performance (the control condition). No significant difference was found in the joint task for the category to which the participant responded or to the one that required no response for either person. The benefit seemed to be due to attending to the stimuli relevant to the partner, which the authors credited to task corepresentation.

U. Wagner et al. (2017) noted that many perceptual factors differed between the joint and individual conditions that could have accounted for Eskenazi et al.'s (2013) results. Thus, they controlled for these in an experiment like that of Eskenazi et al. One joint condition was equivalent to Eskenazi et al.'s in that the participants were seated next to each other at the same computer. For a second condition, each participant performed on a different computer in the same room but was separated by a partition and wearing headphones so that they could not see or hear the other person responding. For the third condition, the participants were in separate rooms. The results for the memory test replicated those of Eskenazi et al. for the identical situation. There was a smaller but significant effect when the participants were in the same room but separated by a partition but no effect when they were in different rooms. The authors attributed the joint-action effect on memory to the social meaning attached to the stimuli to which the partner is to respond in the joint task context and not due to attention-related perceptual cues. They also took the results as suggesting that physical distance is a critical variable. As this experiment and the others show, it is difficult to obtain evidence that uniquely requires a social explanation.

In summary, directing another person's attention to a specific object or event, either by looking at the target object or using some other cue, is key to communication between humans. There is no doubt that there is a social component in that a person often intends to direct someone else's attention to an object for the purpose of coattention. However, much of the relevant research has been conducted under controlled conditions in laboratory experiments in which many nonsocial factors are known to influence performance. Consequently, it is difficult to attribute the results uniquely to social explanations. This difficulty is evident in studies of the joint Simon and flanker effects, discussed next.

JOINT REPRESENTATION AND SOCIAL PRIMING

The joint performance procedure of Eskenazi et al. (2013) was adopted from widely studied topics called joint Simon and flanker effects. These studies used procedures in which the effect of another participant on a person's performance in Simon and flanker tasks is examined. *Social priming* is a closely related type of experiment aimed at studying the unconscious influence of social cues on people's judgments and actions.

Joint Simon Task

In a go/no-go version of a Simon task, participants respond to only one of the two alternatives on the relevant stimulus dimension instead of making a unique response to each. For example, a person is to respond to a red stimulus with a right key press and not respond if the stimulus is green in one trial block and then, in another block, respond only if the stimulus is green. In this case, the Simon effect is not evident, with little difference in performance for congruent and incongruent stimulus and response locations (Hommel, 1996; Sebanz et al., 2003).

Sebanz et al. (2003) found, however, that a Simon effect was obtained for a Simon task performed by two people if the person on the left responded to one stimulus value (green color, in this example) and the person on the right responded to the other (red color). In their study, participants performed both a joint go/no-go task and an individual go/no-go task. For the former, they were seated side by side in front of a computer display screen, with one response button for each person mounted on the tabletop. In the individual go/no-go task, only one of the participants was at the table, and that person responded in the same manner as in the joint task. The stimuli were rather unusual in that they were photographs of a right hand with the index finger pointing to the left or right or straight (see Figure 12.5). The finger contained a red or green ring, and the instructions were to respond to one of the two colors.

The critical finding in Sebanz et al.'s (2003) experiment was that the joint task showed a Simon effect of 11 ms, whereas the individual task showed a nonsignificant effect of only 3 ms. Although 8 ms may seem like a small difference, it was statistically significant because responses in go/no-go tasks are fast and show little variability. Note that for an individual participant, their task was the same in the joint and individual conditions because the participant responded to the same color, which occurred equally often in both conditions. Sebanz et al. emphasized social factors differentiating the joint task from the individual one, which led to the phenomenon initially being called the social Simon effect. However, because many nonsocial factors differentiated the conditions as well, a more neutral label of *joint Simon effect* has come to be more widely used.

The initial account provided for the joint Simon effect was *corepresentation of action*; each person in the joint task represents the actions of the coactor much like they were performing the task themselves (Sebanz et al., 2003, 2005). Thus, rather than representing the task in terms of the individual as go/no-go, the shared task is represented as a choice reaction in which the corepresented participants must decide whether the left or right response is signaled by the stimulus. This notion of a shared representation is like that for shared attention, discussed earlier in the chapter, and similar issues arise as to whether the representations are indeed shared or even social.

FIGURE 12.5. Setting in the Joint Go/No-Go Task of Sebanz et al. (2003)

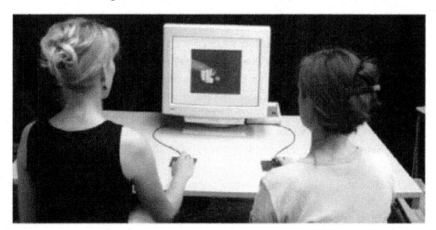

Note. From "Representing Others' Actions: Just Like One's Own?," by N. Sebanz, G. Knoblich, and W. Prinz, 2003, *Cognition, 88*(3), p. B14 (https://doi.org/10.1016/S0010-0277(03)00043-X). Copyright 2003 by Elsevier. Reprinted with permission.

An alternative explanation favored by many researchers is *referential coding*. According to the referential coding account, nothing is unique about a person being located next to a performer or anything social in the situation. Instead, the effect is attributed to representational and attentional processes that operate in a variety of settings. Dolk et al. (2013) provided evidence favoring the referential coding account in a study that used research designs like that for the joint Simon task but for which the other "participant" was a Japanese waving cat. Participants sat in the position normally occupied by the right-side person in the joint Simon task—to the right side of the display screen—and pressed a single response key with the right index finger. They responded to one of two distinct tone stimuli, which were presented from the location of a left or right loudspeaker. The main manipulation was whether the waving cat was placed in the location corresponding to where the other person would be responding in a joint task setup. Results showed a 19-ms Simon effect in the cat-present condition compared with a 7-ms nonsignificant effect in the cat-absent condition. Dolk et al. replicated this pattern of results with a clock or beating metronome in place of the cat, but not when the metronome was present without making a sound (or doing anything else). Their conclusion, based in large part on this last result, was that they did not find any evidence of a joint Simon effect in the absence of an attention-attracting event, suggesting that it is the dynamic event component rather than the social one that is responsible for producing the joint Simon effect.

Because the movement of Dolk et al.'s (2013) waving cat was accompanied by a sound produced by the waving, Puffe et al. (2017) conducted a study dissociating the visual and auditory components. They replicated the result obtained by Dolk et al., obtaining a Simon effect of 10 ms for the condition with both components. The effect was a numerically smaller 4 ms—which was still statistically significant—when the waving cat was not visible but the sound was present and only a nonsignificant 3 ms when only the visual waving cat alone was present. A similar experiment that required categorization of visual stimuli occurring in left and right locations as red or green did not show any joint Simon effect, even with the visual plus auditory waving cat. Overall, the results indicate that the waving cat does yield a joint Simon effect with an auditory stimulus version of the task, and the essential components of the waving event are unclear. Puffe et al. interpreted their results as consistent with a referential coding account for the auditory modality, indicating that the nonsocial object contains cues that must be ignored due to their spatial correspondence, which increases the salience of the spatial alignment.

Additional evidence consistent with referential coding was obtained by Xiong and Proctor (2015) in a simulated driving environment. Their participants performed a go/no-go Simon task in which they responded with their hands holding the steering wheel and the thumbs located on buttons that could be pressed. They responded to one of two tone frequencies presented from a left or right speaker, using a left button press in one trial block and a right button press in another. Because both hands were on the response buttons, a Simon effect based on left and right location on the wheel was obtained for the go/no-go task. The critical manipulation was the presence of an irrelevant simulated dynamic display located to the right or left. Results showed that the Simon effect was smaller for the response that was on the same side as the display than for the response on the opposite side. In other words, the results suggest the push-button responses were coded as left and right not only with respect to the wheel-based reference frame but also relative to the visually salient dynamic display. Although they are slightly different from Puffe et al.'s (2017) results, these findings suggest that a dynamic visual event itself can be sufficiently salient to influence the relative location coding of stimuli in the auditory modality.

Liepelt et al. (2019) examined whether saccadic eye-movement responses showed a joint Simon effect. A square or diamond stimulus could appear to the left or right of a fixation point. Two additional dots were placed on the left or right side as targets for the eye movements. In the individual condition, the participant sat to the left side of the screen and was to make a saccade to the left as soon as a square appeared to turn on a left light and not to respond when a diamond appeared. For the joint task, a confederate of the experimenters sat to the right side of the participant and responded to the diamond stimulus with a saccade to the right target location. The results showed an 11-ms Simon effect overall, which did not differ as a function of whether the task was individual or joint. That the effect did not increase in the joint condition provides evidence that neither the saccadic responses of the other person nor the corresponding action effects produced by their responses (light onsets) had any influence on the Simon effect.

Yamaguchi, Wall, and Hommel (2018) had participants perform individual and joint Simon tasks (with red and green stimuli) and obtained a 7-ms Simon effect in the joint task compared with a 1-ms nonsignificant effect in the individual task. This pattern replicates prior results. Of most interest was the second session, in which for some sets of trials, 90% of the trials for Participant A were spatially congruent and 10% spatially incongruent or vice versa. The performance of Participant B, for whom the percentages of congruent and incongruent trials remained 50%, was examined. The trial-proportion manipulation had a significant effect on the performance of Participant A, who received the 90/10 condition, but little effect on the performance of Participant B, who received the 50/50 condition. These results imply that Participant B did not represent the bias of trial types in Participant A's task but just the stimulus–response mapping.

Joint Flanker Task

The *flanker* task, in which a target stimulus is flanked by instances of an alternative stimulus that can be congruent or incongruent with the target, is also a two-choice task in which one or more stimuli are assigned to left and right key press responses. Atmaca et al. (2011) obtained evidence that a joint version of the flanker task yields a flanker congruity effect, which they attributed to shared representations, as in Sebanz et al.'s (2003) study with the joint Simon task. For the joint task, one person makes one response, and the other makes the other response. Atmaca et al. assigned two letters to each response and had participants perform a standard two-choice task, a joint task, and an individual task that was the same as the joint task but without a partner performing the other response. The flanker effect was largest in the typical two-choice task (57 ms), and it was evident even in the individual go/no-go task (30 ms), but it was larger in the joint task (45 ms). The authors interpreted this latter difference as consistent with the corepresentation hypothesis. They provided further evidence in support of the corepresentation hypothesis in another experiment, in which the joint flanker effect was larger when the partner intentionally responded to the target than when the partner's response was executed unintentionally through the activation of a magnet that "pulled down" the finger because of a metal ring on it. The implication was that the partner must be responding intentionally.

Dolk et al. (2014) conducted a study with the flanker task in which they compared joint flanker task performance with that for a condition in which the joint "performer" was the Japanese waving cat. Their reaction time data showed an 8-ms larger flanker effect in the joint condition than when no performer or cat accompanied the performer, and this did not interact with whether a person or the waving cat was located next to the performer. The authors interpreted this result as showing that another salient event (the waving cat) is sufficient to increase the response competition caused by incompatible flanking stimuli. This conclusion must be qualified somewhat in that the error data showed a larger increase in flanker effect in the joint condition than the waving cat did.

Dittrich et al. (2017) compared the joint Simon and joint flanker effects in experiments in which they manipulated whether the participant could see the coactor. This was accomplished by placing a partition between the two performers. The joint Simon effect was of similar size regardless of whether the coactor was visible, but the joint flanker effect was larger when participants saw their coactors than when they did not. Dittrich et al. attributed the joint Simon effect to spatial referential coding but concluded that the joint flanker effect is due to an impaired ability to focus spatial attention on the target stimulus in the presence of a visible coactor. Like gaze-cuing studies, researchers can give social interpretations to effects of variables such as social exclusion (J. Walter et al., 2021), but the evidence indicates that the basic joint Simon effect has its basis in nonsocial mechanisms, although the joint flanker effect may not.

Social Priming

One of the most widely known areas of social cognition research related to attention is *social priming*. As discussed in Chapter 1, semantic priming was established in the 1970s, with studies showing that a prime word facilitated processing of associated words or members of the prime category (Meyer et al., 1975; Neely, 1977). In subsequent years, several studies were reported that supposedly showed priming effects on the behavior of subtle social cues of which the participants were unaware. Bargh et al. (1996) showed that participants primed with words relating to the concept of rudeness interrupted the experimenter more often and more quickly than those who received a neutral list. Also, participants primed with an elderly stereotype walked more slowly down a hallway when leaving the experiment. Doyen et al. (2012) were unable to replicate this latter result unless the experimenters were aware of the expected outcome, and there have been numerous failed replications of related social priming results.

Carter et al. (2011) went so far as to argue that exposure to the American flag could affect citizens' attitudes and behaviors. Specifically, they reported that brief exposure to the flag led to a shift toward Republican beliefs, attitudes, and voting behavior among both Republican and Democratic participants and that some of these effects were evident 8 months later. Consequently, Carter et al. (2011) concluded that their results provided evidence that nonconscious priming effects from seeing the flag can bias citizens toward a particular political party for some time afterward. These conclusions seem suspect, and Carter et al. (2020) have indicated that their earlier results are, in fact, not replicable. They stated, on the basis of a meta-analysis of their studies, "Our analyses suggest that . . . American flag primes did create politically conservative shifts in attitudes and beliefs during the initial time period when data were collected . . ., but this effect has since declined over time to be roughly zero" (Carter et al., 2020, p. 489). They interpreted this "decline effect" as indicating the changing historical context of symbols such as the flag, but it more likely indicates that the first report of the phenomenon was due to chance error or another factor.

In a pithy assessment of the difficulty of replicating social priming effects, Meyer (2014) emphasized the distinction between semantic priming and social priming. He noted that "the "psychological phenomenon, called 'semantic priming,' has been demonstrated many times during the past decades" (p. 523). In contrast, though, the "recent failed replication attempts concern much more exotic types of putative behavior priming" (p. 523). In short, the basic information-processing phenomena are well-established and replicable, whereas the social priming phenomena are not.

ATTENTION WITH AVATARS

Because avatars are used in many electronic games and are easy to implement on computers, much research concerning social attention and perspective taking has been conducted with them. Two such lines of research are perspective taking in the Simon task and attentional orienting in the dot perception task.

Perspective Taking of Avatars in the Simon Task

Research on perspective taking with avatars in the Simon task is closely related to that on the joint Simon effect, except that the participant usually performs a two-choice task. The relation between the participant and the avatar's positioning is varied. Böffel and Müsseler (2018) conducted experiments in which the spatial relations were varied. In their first experiment, an avatar was displayed on the screen, as in Figure 12.6. Each participant performed two trial blocks, each with a right (–90°) or a left (90°) avatar position. They responded to the color of a circle (light or dark blue) with an assigned left or right key press. Half the participants were told to ignore the avatar, but half were told to control the avatar's hand. The main result was that a Simon effect of 15 ms was obtained relative to the avatar: Left responses were faster when the stimulus occurred near the avatar's left hand, and right responses were faster when it occurred near the right hand, regardless of the avatar orientation. The ignore or control instructions had no significant effect, indicating that an explicit intent to adopt the avatar's perspective was unnecessary. Böffel and Müsseler (2019) showed that this avatar-based Simon effect occurs when the left or right avatar orientation changes randomly from trial to trial and when the avatar appears at the same time as the color circle (although the effect is smaller).

Müsseler et al. (2019) examined stimulus–response compatibility proper, in which the participant responds to stimulus location as the relevant dimension to determine contradictory response tendencies with an avatar. In this case, the avatar was rotated 180° relative to the participant, making the avatar's left hand correspond with the participant's right hand and vice versa. Performance with this arrangement was compared with one in which the avatar was oriented

FIGURE 12.6. Examples of the Conditions in Böffel and Müsseler's (2019) Experiment

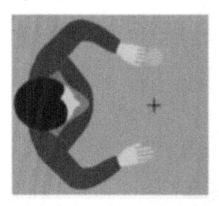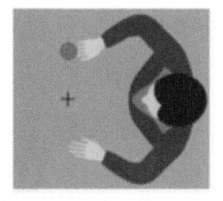

Note. From "Visual Perspective Taking for Avatars in a Simon Task," by C. Böffel and J. Müsseler, 2019, *Attention, Perception, & Psychophysics*, *81*(1), p. 162 (https://doi.org/10.3758/s13414-018-1573-0). Copyright 2019 by Springer Nature. Reprinted with permission.

at 0° rotation, aligned with the orientation of the participant. Participants responded from the perspective of the avatar, and stimulus color (light or dark blue) designated whether the corresponding or noncorresponding response was to be made. With the 0° rotation, a typical compatibility effect of 34 ms was evident, but with the 180° rotation, the effect reversed to be 29 ms faster for the participant's noncorresponding response than for the corresponding response. That is, the faster response was the one compatible with the avatar's hand rather than the participant's hand. Müsseler et al. established that this effect depended on the instructions: With avatars rotated plus and minus 135°, they found that the compatibility effect followed the avatar's hand locations when instructed to adopt the avatar's view but was relative to the self when instructed to ignore the avatar.

Von Salm-Hoogstraeten et al. (2020) evaluated whether perspective taking or referential coding accounted for the avatar effects found in the prior experiments. They used the displays shown in Figure 12.7. The critical aspect of these displays is that they allowed the left- and right-hand distinction to be dissociated from the avatar's perspective. If hand position is crucial, the two displays on the left of the figure (Panels A and C) should yield similar results because

FIGURE 12.7. The Four Avatars Used by Von Salm-Hoogstraeten et al. (2020)

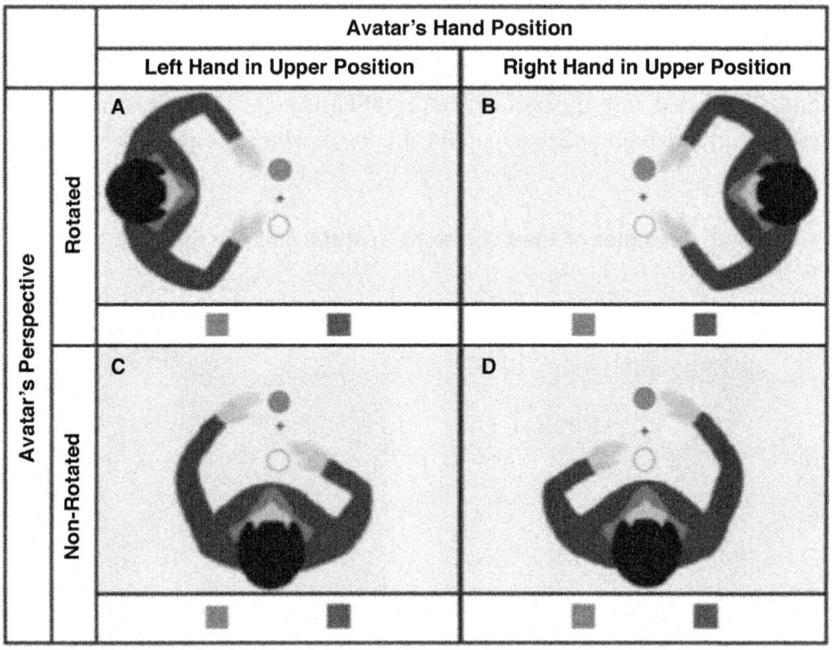

Note. From "Seeing the World Through the Eyes of an Avatar? Comparing Perspective Taking and Referential Coding," by S. von Salm-Hoogstraeten, K. Bolzius, and J. Müsseler, 2020, *Journal of Experimental Psychology: Human Perception and Performance, 46*(3), p. 266 (https://doi.org/10.1037/xhp0000711). Copyright 2020 by the American Psychological Association.

the left and right hands are assigned to the same locations, and the same holds for the two displays on the right (Panels B and D). The avatar's perspective gives a clear left–right coding distinction for the top displays (A and B) but not the bottom ones (C and D).

Participants performed the Simon task with the different avatars in distinct trial blocks and were instructed to adopt the avatar's perspective. The results replicated the prior findings that the Simon effect was determined by the avatar orientation when it was rotated 90° relative to the participant. The nonrotated avatars not only showed the same congruity effects relative to the avatars' hands, but the effects were also even larger than those shown by the rotated avatars. Given that only in the latter case is the perspective different between the avatar and the performer, this result pattern provides evidence against the perspective-taking account and is consistent with a referential coding account.

Attentional Orienting in the Dot Perception Task

The dot perception task was introduced by Samson et al. (2010). Their stimuli comprised a room with three visible walls and a human avatar oriented toward the left or right wall (see Figure 12.8, a and b). The gender of the avatar was matched to that of the participant, with the idea that this would encourage the adoption of the avatar's perspective. Two red discs were positioned on one or two walls, and on half of the trials, the avatar could not "see" some of the discs that the person could see. On each trial, the participant was cued

FIGURE 12.8. Examples of Stimuli Used in the Dot Perspective Task

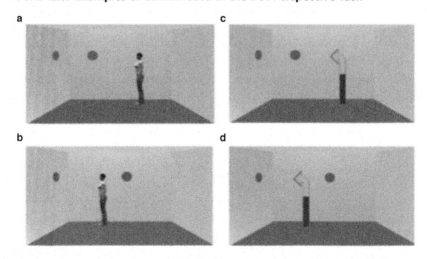

Note. From "Avatars and Arrows: Implicit Mentalizing or Domain-General Processing?," by I. Santiesteban, C. Catmur, S. C. Hopkins, G. Bird, and C. Heyes, 2014, *Journal of Experimental Psychology: Human Perception and Performance, 40*(3), p. 930 (https://doi.org/10.1037/a0035175). Copyright 2014 by the American Psychological Association.

to take their own perspective (YOU) or that of the avatar (HE or SHE). A short while later, a number from 0 to 3 appeared, followed soon thereafter by the depiction of the room. The participant responded "yes" if the number presented matched what could be seen from the designated perspective and "no" otherwise.

Of most interest were trials in which the response would be the same from both perspectives (congruent trials; Panel a) compared with ones for which they were not (incongruent trials; Panel b). On the basis of what we have covered in this book, you can probably predict that reaction time would be longer on incongruent trials than on congruent trials, which indeed was the case. This congruity effect averaged about 75 ms, regardless of whether the cued perspective was the participant's or the avatar's. Note that the results obtained with the avatar might have nothing to do with taking its perspective because the avatar is an object in the display relative to which the locations of other stimuli can be coded.

Samson et al. (2010) reported another experiment in which participants made only judgments from the self-perspective but with the avatar or a rectangle of about the same height and width placed in the middle of the room. Again, there was a congruity effect, but of only 21 ms for the avatar, with no similar effect for the rectangle. The authors took the absence of the congruity effect with the rectangle as indicating that the effect with the avatar was not due to the specific spatial disc layout but to what the avatar could "see." Statements such as these strongly imply a social basis to the avatar results, but near the end of the article, Samson et al. conceded that the mechanisms producing their results need not be specific to the social domain.

The social, implicit mentalizing account of the self–avatar congruity effect depends on two assumptions (Heyes, 2014; Santiesteban et al., 2014). The first is that the results are due to an automatic process, which several other studies have confirmed (McCleery et al., 2011; Qureshi et al., 2010). The second assumption is that the process represents what the avatar can see, but this assumption has been questioned. Santiesteban et al. (2014) had participants perform two versions of the dot perspective task, with the avatar presented on some trials and an arrow with similar visual features on other trials (see Figure 12.8, panels c and d). Self–avatar congruity effects of similar size were obtained in both conditions, suggesting that there is nothing special to the human properties of the avatar. This result was evident not only when the perspective changed randomly from trial to trial but also when participants responded from the self-perspective on all trials. That the same results were obtained with the arrows provides evidence that the self–avatar congruity effects are due to domain-general processes involved in spatial coding and attentional orienting.

Similar results to the dot perception experiments were reported by Kovács et al. (2010), whose participants watched one of four films. In each, an avatar agent entered the scene and placed a ball on a table. The ball then rolled behind an object that occluded the ball (occluder) and, with the avatar still present, either remained behind the occluder or rolled out from it and left the scene. The avatar then left the scene, thinking that the ball was still behind the occluder or not. Then, in the avatar's absence, if the ball was behind the occluder, it either left or did not, and if the ball had previously left the scene, it either returned behind the occluder or did not. Thus, the participant's belief about whether the ball was behind the occluder could be congruent or incongruent with the belief of the avatar. As a final step, the avatar reentered the scene, and the occluder was removed to reveal the presence or absence of the ball, and the participant responded as quickly as possible if they detected the ball. Responses were influenced by both the participant's belief and the avatar's belief, with reaction times approximately 50 ms shorter when the expectancies for both were that the ball would be behind the occluder than when the expectancies of one or the other were that it would not be there. Note that the avatar's beliefs were irrelevant to the task, which Kovács et al. interpreted as showing that the participants automatically tracked the avatar's beliefs.

Phillips et al. (2015) replicated the main findings supporting automaticity of belief representation when they conducted their experiments much like Kovács et al. (2010). But by varying whether participants responded to the ball's presence or absence and eliminating the avatar agent's perceptual access to the ball, they obtained results inconsistent with the automatic belief hypothesis. Phillips et al. also provided evidence that the effects in the original paradigm were due to a subtle methodological issue associated with an attention check. The effect was present when the attention-check timing (but not the avatar's beliefs) varied across conditions but not when the avatar's beliefs (but not the attention-check timing) varied across conditions. Again, the evidence runs counter to a social, mentalizing account.

As Dalmaso et al. (2020) did with the gaze-cuing task, Capozzi and Ristic (2020) acknowledged that much of the data in the dot perspective task can be explained by general attentional processes but said, "Showing an involvement of domain-general attentional processes in social orienting does not necessarily rule out a contribution of mentalizing processes" (p. 98) and proposed a synthesis of the two accounts. Given that many results do not require a social, mentalizing explanation, the responsibility should be on the researchers who favor social, mentalizing accounts to demonstrate unequivocally that their findings cannot be explained by nonsocial attentional accounts to satisfy the skeptics (see Box 12.1).

AFFECT AND EMOTION

In a chapter on attention and emotion, Matthews and Wells (1999) began by stating, "Emotion and attention are intimately linked" (p. 172). Emotion can increase the cognitive resources and effort one has to devote to a task. Emotional stimuli can attract attention and, depending on whether they are task relevant or not, benefit or detract from task performance. Perhaps most

BOX 12.1 | **LIMITATIONS OF LABORATORY RESEARCH FOR STUDYING SOCIAL PROCESSES**

It is not too surprising that it is difficult to get solid evidence for social processes in laboratory tasks with two people or one person and a pictorial image of another person or an avatar. Responding to stimuli presented on a screen with key press responses as quickly as possible in many cases is the domain of cognitive psychologists. They have a thorough knowledge of the many basic factors in perception, cognition, and action that can influence the performance of such laboratory tasks that have little to do with the social level of processing. The manipulations of having an unknown person sit next to you, presenting eyes on a screen that gaze to the left and right, or presenting circles relative to an avatar are not strong forms of social interaction. But does that mean that social attention and cognition do not occur in other contexts?

The obvious answer to that question is "no," and there are reasons to think that unique aspects of attention and cognition emerge when two people work together closely. Anyone who has watched *Star Trek* knows that Spock and other Vulcans engaged in what is known as the "Vulcan mind meld." It was typically initiated by touching the responder's head, but the main point is that it enabled "the participants to become one mind, sharing consciousness in a kind of gestalt" (Memory Alpha, 2021, para. 1). This "one mind" seems to be what advocates of social attention think occurs, but it would seem to require much more than performing identification or detection tasks together with an unfamiliar person or acquaintance.

Moving from the realm of science fiction, real-life examples come from famous duos. In cognitive psychology, the joint work of Amos Tversky and Daniel Kahneman revolutionized thinking about reasoning and decision making, leading them to be awarded the 2002 Nobel Prize in Economic Sciences (which was awarded only to Kahneman because Tversky was already deceased at the time). Although both are prominent psychologists who individually made many contributions (e.g., Kahneman's resource theory of attention, described in Chapter 6, this volume), there is no doubt that their joint work could not have emerged from either of them alone. The basis for this work was their close relationship, as explained in their biography by M. L. Lewis (2016): "They connected with each other more deeply than either had connected with anyone else. Their wives noticed it. 'Their relationship was more intense than a marriage'" (p. 238), said Barbara Tversky, Amos Tversky's wife (and herself a noted cognitive psychologist). Another indication of this is in a description about deciding who should be lead author on an article: "And yet the collaboration was so complete that neither of them felt comfortable taking credit as the lead author; to decide whose name would appear first, they flipped a coin" (pp. 158–159).

Another famous pair of researchers is David Hubel and Torsten Wiesel. They also won a Nobel Prize for Physiology and Medicine in 1981 for their research on information processing in the visual system. They also worked closely for approximately 20 years, and Wiesel noted, "Our special bond and private

BOX 12.1 | **LIMITATIONS OF LABORATORY RESEARCH FOR STUDYING SOCIAL PROCESSES *(Continued)***

dialogues, took place while we carried out our experiments" (Hubel & Wiesel, 2004, p. 32). As a final research example, Frances Crick and James Watson were winners of the 1962 Nobel Prize for Physiology and Medicine for their discoveries of DNA (along with Maurice Wilkins; like Tversky, Rosalind Franklin, who worked with Wilkins, was not among the recipients because she was already deceased). Crick (1988) noted that one advantage he and Watson had was that they were doing the research for their own interest, not because of outside pressure. He went on to say, "Our other advantage was that we had evolved unstated but fruitful methods of collaboration" (p. 70).

Corepresentation is evident as well in the arts. Stan Laurel and Oliver Hardy, famous comedians in silent movies and early movies with sound, worked together for 30 years. Drop (2014) noted that the two were complete opposites from their on-screen personas, but "there was one thing that the movies and real life had in common. Stan and Oliver were the best of friends who truly cared for each other" (para. 5). Shortly after Oliver Hardy died in 1957, Laurel wrote, "I feel lost without him after 30 odd years of close friendship & happy association" (para. 6). In music, such corepresentation is illustrated by brothers Ron and Russell Mael, featured in the documentary film *The Sparks Brothers* (Wright, 2021), who have been making pop music for 50 years as the band Sparks. As with Laurel and Hardy, their talents complement each other, and in line with the description of a mind meld, the whole is greater than the sum of the parts.

important, when interacting with people, expressions and perceptions of affective state and emotion are often crucial. If a partner is unhappy with something you have done, you need to be able to detect that. Conversely, if the partner is in a happy mood, it is important to perceive that as well. People rely on cues to convey and process emotions, and sometimes the communication is ambiguous. The close link between emotion and attention makes it difficult to interpret any findings that are obtained.

The influence of emotion on attention and performance has been studied using various laboratory tasks, including the Stroop and Simon tasks. Emotional stimuli yield congruity effects similar to those found in the basic tasks. As reviewed by J. M. G. Williams et al. (1996), in the 1960s and 1970s, several researchers began using the *emotional Stroop task* to measure "automatic" processing of negative affect words. In that task, colored words are presented, and participants are to say the ink color as quickly as possible, as in the standard Stroop color-naming task. Half of the words have a negative meaning, and the other half are of neutral affect. Even though there is no dimensional overlap of this irrelevant affective dimension with color, the color-identification responses to the negative words are slower and less accurate than those to

neutral words. The basic idea is that this longer time to name the color of negative words was due to the automatic allocation of attention to that irrelevant
stimulus dimension.

Song et al. (2017) performed a meta-analysis of neuroimaging studies
that used an emotional Stroop task, comparing brain activation patterns on
incongruent trials with that on congruent trials. Incongruity produced more
activation in the lateral prefrontal cortex (including the dorsolateral prefrontal
cortex, which plays a role in cognitive control), inferior frontal gyrus (the
functions of which include language processing), medial prefrontal cortex (which
is more specifically involved in processing emotional information in working
memory), and dorsal anterior cingulate cortex (the ACC, which plays a role
in cognition and action, possibly in inhibiting responses that are incorrect for
the task).

Evidence that the dorsal ACC is involved both in processing emotions and
monitoring and inhibiting conflict has led some researchers to propose that
the trial-to-trial sequential effects in congruity tasks, which can be modeled
by conflict adaptation, are due to negative affect produced by the conflict and
reflect affective regulation (Dreisbach & Fischer, 2015). Dignath et al. (2020)
evaluated the literature on this affective-signaling hypothesis and concluded
that the evidence indicates that conflict does induce negative affect. But the
evidence is ambiguous as to whether this negative affect is monitored and is
a basis for cognitive control.

A limitation of the emotional Stroop task is that it deviates from the Stroop
task in its structure because the irrelevant affective dimension has no obvious
overlap with the relevant stimulus–response dimension of color. Thus, the
possibility exists that the effect of the negative words is due to a mechanism
other than the competition that produces the typical Stroop effect. Algom et al.
(2004) obtained results consistent with this possibility in experiments showing
that reading and lexical decisions, as well as color naming, were slower with
emotional words. They concluded that the effect was not due to selective
attention mechanisms but to a threat-driven slowdown in processing. Frings
et al. (2010) conducted experiments in which they separated emotional valence
on the prior and current trials and concluded that there was evidence not only
for threat-driven slowing of the type described by Algom et al. but also for a
component that was due to automatic allocation of attention to high arousal
stimuli, as initially proposed.

The Simon task seems to offer a more straightforward way to evaluate
activation produced by emotional stimuli. De Houwer and Eelen (1998) first
reported what is called the *affective Simon effect* for a task in which participants
classified words as nouns or adjectives by saying the word "positive" or "negative." An irrelevant dimension of the words that varied randomly from trial
to trial was whether the word had a positive or negative connotation. A congruity effect like that in spatial tasks was obtained for faster responses when
the word affect was congruent with the response affect than when it was
incongruent. Similar results are obtained when responding "good" or "bad" to

the red or green color of schematic faces that have positive or negative expressions (Y. Zhang & Proctor, 2008). Emotional stimuli also may affect the processing of stimulus location. When schematic face stimuli for which left or right stimulus location is irrelevant are classified as happy or sad with a left or right key press, the spatial Simon effect is larger for the happy face (Lien et al., 2020; Schlaghecken et al., 2017). This outcome suggests a bias of attention toward the positive stimuli, although it is also possible that some visual feature of the stimuli is crucial.

Shared experiences, both positive and negative, are essential to people, as emphasized by the shared attention model discussed at the beginning of the chapter. Part of the enjoyment of attending movies, stage plays, and musical concerts comes from the positive shared experience. Likewise, funerals and associated events involve sharing grief among many persons. Shteynberg et al. (2014) performed a systematic study of the influence of group attention on emotional experience. They compared the reported experience of simultaneous coattention with one's group members with that when attending alone, coattending with strangers, or attending nonsimultaneously with one's group members. In one study, scary advertisements were judged as scarier under group attention, and in another, group attention increased reported feelings of sadness to negative images and happiness to positive images. In an experiment, group attention to a video depicting homelessness led not only to greater reported sadness but also larger donations to charities for the homeless. Finally, group attention increased the cognitive resources devoted to processing sad and amusing videos (as indexed by the percentage of thoughts referencing video content), which was correlated with more sadness and happiness, respectively.

The hypothesis supported by Shteynberg et al.'s (2014) study was that group attention "increases the intensity of valenced events and, hence, the likelihood of emotion-based action" (p. 1102). Note the latter point on "emotion-based action," which is especially critical. Such intensified emotion could explain the actions of many attendees at the rally in Washington, DC, on the morning of January 6, 2021, that led to the storming of the U.S. Capitol Building. Many of the individuals would likely never have engaged in such an action if not for the strong emotions developed by the group as a consequence of attending to the heated rhetoric of the speakers. This is reflected by one participant who Billeaud and Tarm (2021) reported as saying that he "was seized by the 'passion of the moment'" and by other participants who apologized for their actions.

TEAM MENTAL MODELS AND SITUATION AWARENESS

One of the points of the joint Simon and joint flanker tasks is that each participant is nominally performing their respective task individually. Each person responds when a stimulus assigned to them occurs and not otherwise. However, for many tasks, two or more individuals must work together to accomplish a common goal. The examples just described are of two-person teams for which the members work in a coordinated fashion. Other two-person team examples include doubles tennis partners and pairings of an airline pilot and copilot. Larger teams can be found in the numerous team sports, surgical teams, businesses, and research teams of many scientific laboratories. For teams, coordinated performance is crucial, which becomes more difficult when teams extend to three or more people. As such, teams need to have shared mental models representing the team knowledge (Gardner et al., 2017), which support team situation awareness (Demir et al., 2017).

The concept of individual mental models refers to understanding a particular event on the basis of the activation of relevant schemas from long-term memory and, sometimes, simulation of possible scenarios (see also Chapter 10). Bower and Morrow (1990) pointed out that a crucial role in mental models is to shift and focus attention. Although their main concern was narrative comprehension, the implications are broader and include significant aspects of the social world. In social and team environments, one needs to attend to relevant cues related to achieving team goals.

Shared mental models refer to a collective understanding among team members of the task to be performed and how it can be accomplished. This understanding includes the responsibilities of the individual team members and dependencies between teammates on other members' progress. The term *team mental models* is sometimes used when the context is teamwork that needs to be coordinated and executed (Jonker et al., 2010). The idea is that teams will perform better if they share mental models. Some evidence for this comes from surgical teams (Gardner et al., 2017). Surgery interns were randomly assigned to different teams, and they performed one unique medical simulation for 5 days. Each day, the team members filled out a concept similarity tool, for which greater similarity across members implies more comparable mental models. Similarity scores and performance on the simulated surgical task increased across the 5 days. On Day 1, there was no correlation of team mental models with performance, but on Days 2 to 5, better team mental models were correlated with better team performance.

The surgery intern study illustrates that shared mental models are learned, leading to the question of how this learning can be facilitated. Van den Bossche et al. (2011) evaluated team learning behavior, mental model acquisition, and performance of three-person teams who performed a business simulation game. Team learning behavior was measured through subjective ratings provided to closed-ended questions, whereas team members' mental models were obtained by analyzing answers to two open-ended questions in relation to the importance of game variables and their relations. Results showed that *constructive conflict*—expressions of differences of opinions, asking other team members critical questions, and directly addressing differences in opinion—was associated with the development of shared mental models, which in turn predicted team performance. Behaviors the authors classified as coconstruction, those involving agreement with or elaboration of other team members' ideas, were negatively correlated with the development of shared mental models. This study seems to show that constructive discussion of disagreements is most beneficial, likely due to its directing other team members' attention to critical issues that need to be resolved.

Team leadership can be effective at getting members to be engaged in activities that will promote shared mental models. Boies and Fiset (2018) found evidence that leaders can facilitate the development of shared mental models by involving team members in the consideration of the to-be-accomplished task and their roles in its accomplishment. This involvement, again, likely directs members' attention to information relevant for achieving team goals and enables more domain-specific group discussion, which then furthers the emergence of a shared mental model.

Although it has been customary to think of mental models, shared or otherwise, as involving humans, developments in artificial intelligence (AI) and robotics have led to the view that for many activities, it is best to think of the human and automation as a team (Demir et al., 2020). An implication of this is that the AI needs to be able to communicate with humans and, as a team member, possess a mental model that coincides with that of the human team members. A core assumption of explainable AI (XAI) is that the algorithms used by the AI system and why the system is recommending or doing what it does should be comprehensible to the user (i.e., transparent) and contribute to the user developing a more accurate and appropriate mental model for the system (Gunning & Aha, 2019). A related idea is that the AI system needs to be able to develop a model of the human from which it can predict the human's behavior. It has been argued that appropriately capturing and accounting for the user's mental model is key to successful XAI (Rutjes et al., 2019).

Gervits et al. (2020) applied this notion to teams of robots. They had human participants perform a task in virtual reality that involved marking the location of three types of rocks and a radiation zone on a map based on coordinates verbally announced by a planetary rover. The participants were accompanied by two virtual robots who could assist in the task. For half the participants, the robots were programmed with shared mental models, whereas, for the other half, the robots were independent. Time and accuracy of task performance were better with the robots that had shared mental models than with those that did not. At least—in this case—the performance of human–robot teams was improved when the robots had shared mental models.

Situation awareness is a broader concept than mental models, focusing on an explicit understanding of events and contexts. *Shared situation awareness* differs from individual situation awareness, discussed in Chapter 9, in the information required for operators to have effective coordination (Chiappe et al., 2016). For example, paramedics delivering a patient to an emergency room need to coordinate with the hospital and its staff members to ensure that the hospital has the capacity and that the doctors receiving the patient have the vital information they need to treat the patient. Once the patient is in the emergency room, nurses, doctors, and technicians need to coordinate with each other to make sure that the patient is being properly cared for. Endsley et al. (2003)

indicated that team members have unique tasks they can perform independently and some tasks that are shared with other team members. Thus, team situation awareness is based on a shared understanding of a common "picture" relevant to all members of the team. This picture or model of the team and its members is not static but constantly updated with new information relevant to the team performance, again implying a key role for attention.

In contrast to the shared view of team situation awareness, Stanton et al. (2017) took a distributed situation awareness view, according to which information can be transferred among individuals in the team system without members having a shared model of the overall situation. This idea of distributed situation awareness assumes that effective coordination among team members results from two kinds of situation awareness, compatible and transactive. *Compatible situation awareness* refers to the unique goals and tasks that each team member in a system holds that are consistent with their roles. This awareness is an individual one that will be different for each team member. Other team members do not need to be aware of a specific team member's role and goals, and the system achieves its goals by having each team member fulfill their role. When team members need to share information, *transactive situation awareness* comes into play, for which the transacting members communicate the information relevant to the transaction. Note that for transactive awareness, attention only needs to be paid to information relevant to the communicating parties.

Chiappe et al. (2012) proposed a situated view of team situation awareness, which is intermediate to those of Endsley et al. (2003) and Stanton et al. (2017). In it, team members need to create a partial shared representation of the team's situation to support their task goals. The shared representation does not have to be an internal picture or model, but operators can use displays in their environment to offload information and retrieve it when needed. The situated view differs from Endsley et al.'s shared awareness in that it does not require team members to share the complete internal representation but only enough to communicate essential information based on their mutual understanding. Unlike Stanton et al.'s claim that no shared awareness is needed, the situated approach does assume some shared elements for effective coordination, but the team can take advantage of the two types of awareness (compatible and transactive) distinguished by Stanton et al. to communicate relevant information among team members. According to the situated view, displays for complex systems should be designed to direct members' attention to information that will help them develop mutual knowledge of the situation.

The development of a shared mental model can occur by way of *cross-training*, in which team members receive information and training in the tasks performed by other team members. In addition to providing the team with mutual knowledge should a team member be absent, this strategy can contribute to the development of more efficient communication strategies and enhanced task performance (Volpe et al., 1996). Teams that must function in high-workload environments may also benefit from special training to recognize high-stress conditions and adapt their behavior accordingly. One of the most important adaptive strategies seems to be learning to anticipate the information needs of other team members (Entin & Serfaty, 1999).

In summary, more than individual task demands, workload and situation awareness are essential to team performance. Team members must be able to function as an entire system, increasingly incorporating nonhuman, automated technologies as well. There is a debate about how much team members must "be on the same page"—that is, to have a complete shared awareness that is updated as new information becomes available and events transpire. Regardless, team members need to establish a representation of the dynamically evolving situation that allows them to know the status of relevant aspects of their task and communicate with others.

VALUATION OF CONSUMER PRODUCTS

Consumer psychology refers to how buyers perceive and react to products and their marketing (Proctor et al., 2022). Attention has increasingly attracted interest in this area because of the advent of the *attention economy*. This term refers to the fact people are constantly and increasingly bombarded with demands on their attention by the social and physical world and all of the devices by which content can be delivered electronically. It is not too surprising that the concept is based loosely on resource models of attention because they were derived largely from analogy to economic resources. The basic idea is that the demands on people's attentional resources far exceed the supply, so many different sources of information compete for these resources.

Romaniuk and Nguyen (2017) identified three levels of competition for attention with regard to consumer behavior and marketing: (a) Marketing stimuli must compete for attention with other stimuli in the consumers' internal and external environment. For example, during an advertisement on a television show, a viewer's attention may be directed toward a conversation with a friend, preventing attention from being allocated to the advertisement. (b) Marketing stimuli for one brand often must compete with those for related products. This is the case for supermarkets, where there may be multiple options for a product such as potato chips, and for multiplex theaters that may be showing many movies. The concern is how to get consumers to attend to the company's product and choose it if a comparison is made with rival products. (c) The third level of attention competition involves the components of the marketing stimuli, including the brand name, advertising message, and claims on the packaging.

Throughout the book, evidence has been presented that irrelevant, salient stimuli can capture attention. Peschel et al. (2019) varied the large or small size and salience (low or high contrast) of a Danish organic food label across three food product categories and used an eye tracker to determine how much overt attention was captured by the label. Results showed much greater attention capture for the larger, more visually salient labels. Participants were required to choose between alternatives with or without the label, and the effects of size and salience were evident in these choices as well.

Studies have also shown that stimuli that are highly valued due to being associated with a monetary reward can attract attention. B. A. Anderson et al. (2011) had participants discriminate the orientation of a bar inside a red or green stimulus, and a reward given at the end of each trial depended on the color, with the probability being .8 for a high reward (5 cents) for one color and .2 for a low reward (1 cent) for the other color. After completing over 1,000 trials of this training phase, participants then performed a task of searching for a unique shape among six differently colored shapes (e.g., a diamond among circles), with color being irrelevant to the task. The visual display contained a high-value distractor color, a low-value distractor color, or neither. Reaction times across the three conditions were 681 ms, 673 ms, and 665 ms, respectively, indicating that the stimuli of a prior irrelevant color slowed responses. More important, this effect was larger for the color with a high trained reward value than for the color with a lower value reward. B. A. Anderson et al. obtained a similar, though weaker, result pattern after only 240 training trials and, even more remarkably, when participants were invited back 4 to 21 days later. The persistence of these valuation effects across time conforms with studies of practice with an incompatible spatial mapping (Tagliabue et al., 2000; Vu et al., 2003) and occurred despite the fact that the distractors were not physically salient or goal relevant.

Janiszewski et al. (2013) conducted a study in which they provided evidence suggesting that repeatedly selectively attending to a product and not to others influences later choices between those products and alternative ones. Participants first performed a task in which they were to identify a product at a designated location in a display and ignore an alternative product at the undesignated location. In a second task, half the participants indicated a preference between the designated alternative and a "neutral" option, whereas the other half were to do the same for the neglected alternative and a neutral option. The main finding was that the previously attended to "designated" product was chosen more than half the time, and the previously unattended to "neglected" product was chosen less than half the time. Another experiment showed that these effects were larger when the products were closer together than farther apart, which, along with other findings, the authors interpreted as evidence that both excitatory and inhibitory processes contributed to the subsequent preference decisions.

Makarina et al. (2019) noted that because Janiszewski et al.'s (2013) stimuli were initially neutral, their results did not speak to the issue of whether effects of selective attention occur when people have preexisting attitudes toward products. Makarina et al. were able to replicate the attentional-selection effect on choice with known products. Items that served as targets in an initial search task were preferred to ones that previously served as distractors. Also, ratings of value were higher for former targets than for former distractors. Thus, attentional selection can affect not only preference choices but also the perceived value of the attended to and selected items.

CHAPTER SUMMARY

Sharing attention with others when interacting in pairs or large groups is essential in life. Sharing attention relies on cues and communication about the objects or events to which one should attend. Whether social influences on shared attention and cognitive representation are mainly a consequence of social implicit mentalizing due to adopting other people's mental states or sub-mentalizing based on fundamental perceptual and attentional operations is a matter of dispute. Many results in gaze-cuing studies and the joint Simon and joint flanker tasks can be interpreted in terms of social variables, but in almost all cases, accounts in terms of more basic cognitive mechanisms cannot be ruled out.

The same can be said about findings obtained with avatar perspectives and the dot perspective task. In each case, results counter to a perspective-taking view have been found. A limitation of the laboratory experiments for investigating social factors is that many factors other than social ones influence performance on any given task, and explanations in terms of those factors must be ruled out if more skeptical researchers are to find the social explanations compelling.

The concepts of mental models and situation awareness have been extended to teams in shared mental models and team situation awareness. Although there are disagreements about how much shared awareness is required for team performance, there is agreement that more than the accuracy of an individual's mental model is needed for teams to function well. Finally, businesses and other organizations are concerned with attracting people's attention to their products and messages. Many of the principles covered in the text can be used to enable one's goods and creations to stand out from those of competitors.

KEY POINTS

- **Fact:** People can attend to the same information, which is called *shared attention*.

- **Theory:** The shared-attention system theory specifies three levels at which shared attention is accomplished: gaze perception, joint perception, and shared perception.

- **Fact:** The direction of eye gaze from a schematic or photographed face can cue a left or right location, but this may be due to general properties of attention.

- **Phenomenon:** Joint Simon and flanker effects are obtained when each participant makes a single response to one or more of the stimuli.

- **Theory:** Although many favor a social, shared representation view of joint Simon and flanker effects, a general referential coding account can explain most, if not all, the results.

- **Phenomenon:** In avatar orientation tasks, participants' performance is influenced by the direction of the avatar's gaze.

- **Theory:** There is considerable evidence that the gaze-cuing results are due to domain-general attentional processes, although there may also be a contribution of mentalizing processes.

- **Phenomenon:** Stroop-like and Simon-like effects based on negative and positive affect occur and are called *emotional Stroop effects* and *affective Simon effects*, respectively.

- **Phenomenon:** Simultaneous coattention with other group members may increase the intensity of emotionally valenced events and the likelihood of emotion-based action.

- **Theory:** Team mental models and situation awareness are essential for effective team performance.

- **Fact:** Selectively attending to a product can result in its being chosen more often than those of competitors.

Afterword

After reading this book, you should have an awareness of the breadth of topics included in the study of attention. You should realize that attention is not a unidimensional construct and that multiple processes and regions of the brain underlie the various components of attention. Many of the experimental phenomena (e.g., the Stroop and Simon effects) identified in the Key Points sections of each chapter are robust, and the factors known to modulate them are well established. In many cases, there is also agreement on the general aspect of human information processing that gives rise to the phenomena. For example, essentially all researchers agree that bottom-up (stimulus-driven) and top-down (goal-driven) processes are involved in all attentional phenomena, but they differ as to how much of a role each process plays. Likewise, some tasks do not require much attention, whereas others do, and a significant bottleneck limits performance when multiple responses must be selected.

The disagreements are mainly in the exact natures of the underlying processes for respective phenomena, including the role of attention. Because theories require assumptions to interpret results, it is often possible to interpret results within theoretical frameworks that differ in detail. Consequently, even though the research findings are established, they may not uniquely favor one particular theory. Over time, though, many theoretical issues get resolved or refined, although there are limits to the constraints that data can provide.

https://doi.org/10.1037/0000317-013
Attention: Selection and Control in Human Information Processing, by R. W. Proctor and K.-P. L. Vu

We end by emphasizing that in any experimental science, the interplay between theory and data is crucial. Theoretical proposals based on existing empirical facts generate research questions to which new studies can be directed. The body of knowledge developed about attentional processes and phenomena can be applied to the design of systems and products that are compatible with human capabilities, even when this knowledge is incomplete.

REFERENCES

Ach, N. S. (1964). Über die willenstätigkeit und das denken [About volition and thinking]. In J. M. Mandler & G. Mandler (Eds.), *Thinking: From association to Gestalt* (pp. 201–207). Wiley. (Original work published 1905)

Afergan, D., Peck, E. M., Solovey, E. T., Jenkins, A., Hincks, S. W., Brown, E. T., Chang, R., & Jacob, R. J. (2014, April 26–May 1). Dynamic difficulty using brain metrics of workload. In M. Jones & P. Palanque (Chairs), *Proceedings of the SIGCHI Conference on Human Factors in Computing Systems*. CHI Conference on Human Factors in Computing Systems, Toronto, Canada.

Akyeampong, J., Udoka, S., Caruso, G., & Bordegoni, M. (2014). Evaluation of hydraulic excavator human–machine interface concepts using NASA TLX. *International Journal of Industrial Ergonomics, 44*(3), 374–382. https://doi.org/10.1016/j.ergon.2013.12.002

Algom, D., & Chajut, E. (2019). Reclaiming the Stroop effect back from control to input-driven attention and perception. *Frontiers in Psychology, 10,* Article 1683. https://doi.org/10.3389/fpsyg.2019.01683

Algom, D., Chajut, E., & Lev, S. (2004). A rational look at the emotional Stroop phenomenon: A generic slowdown, not a Stroop effect. *Journal of Experimental Psychology: General, 133*(3), 323–338. https://doi.org/10.1037/0096-3445.133.3.323

Allport, A. (1987). Selection for action: Some behavioral and neurophysiological considerations of attention and action. In H. Heuer & A. F. Sanders (Eds.), *Perspectives on perception and action* (pp. 395–419). Erlbaum.

Allport, A., & Wylie, G. (2000). Task switching, stimulus-response bindings, and negative priming. In S. Monsell & J. Driver (Eds.), *Control of cognitive processes: Attention and performance XVIII* (pp. 35–70). MIT Press.

Allport, D. A., Antonis, B., & Reynolds, P. (1972). On the division of attention: A disproof of the single channel hypothesis. *Quarterly Journal of Experimental Psychology, 24*(2), 225–235. https://doi.org/10.1080/00335557243000102

Al-Shargie, F., Tariq, U., Mir, H., Alawar, H., Babiloni, F., & Al-Nashash, H. (2019). Vigilance decrement and enhancement techniques: A review. *Brain Sciences*, *9*(8), 178. https://doi.org/10.3390/brainsci9080178

Alsius, A., Paré, M., & Munhall, K. G. (2018). Forty years after hearing lips and seeing voices: The McGurk effect revisited. *Multisensory Research*, *31*(1-2), 111–144. https://doi.org/10.1163/22134808-00002565

Altmann, E. M., & Trafton, J. G. (2007). Timecourse of recovery from task interruption: Data and a model. *Psychonomic Bulletin & Review*, *14*(6), 1079–1084. https://doi.org/10.3758/BF03193094

American Psychiatric Association. (2013). *Diagnostic and statistical manual of mental disorders* (5th ed.). https://doi.org/10.1176/appi.books.9780890425596

Andersen, S. K., Müller, M. M., & Hillyard, S. A. (2009). Color-selective attention need not be mediated by spatial attention. *Journal of Vision*, *9*(6), 2–7. https://doi.org/10.1167/9.6.2

Anderson, B. A. (2019). Neurobiology of value-driven attention. *Current Opinion in Psychology*, *29*, 27–33. https://doi.org/10.1016/j.copsyc.2018.11.004

Anderson, B. A., Laurent, P. A., & Yantis, S. (2011). Value-driven attentional capture. *PNAS*, *108*(25), 10367–10371. https://doi.org/10.1073/pnas.1104047108

Anderson, J. R. (1982). Acquisition of cognitive skill. *Psychological Review*, *89*(4), 369–406. https://doi.org/10.1037/0033-295X.89.4.369

Anderson, J. R., Bothell, D., Byrne, M. D., Douglass, S., Lebiere, C., & Qin, Y. (2004). An integrated theory of the mind. *Psychological Review*, *111*(4), 1036–1060. https://doi.org/10.1037/0033-295X.111.4.1036

Anderson, J. R., Matessa, M., & Lebiere, C. (1997). ACT-R: A theory of higher level cognition and its relation to visual attention. *Human–Computer Interaction*, *12*(4), 439–462. https://doi.org/10.1207/s15327051hci1204_5

Andre, A. D., & Wickens, C. D. (1990). *Display-control compatibility in the cockpit: Guidelines for display layout analysis*. NASA Ames Research Center.

Ansorge, U. (2003). Spatial Simon effects and compatibility effects induced by observed gaze direction. *Visual Cognition*, *10*(3), 363–383. https://doi.org/10.1080/13506280244000122

Ansorge, U., & Wühr, P. (2004). A response-discrimination account of the Simon effect. *Journal of Experimental Psychology: Human Perception and Performance*, *30*(2), 365–377. https://doi.org/10.1037/0096-1523.30.2.365

Arbuthnott, K., & Frank, J. (2000). Executive control in set switching: Residual switch cost and task-set inhibition. *Canadian Journal of Experimental Psychology*, *54*(1), 33–41. https://doi.org/10.1037/h0087328

Aru, J., & Bachmann, T. (2017). Expectation creates something out of nothing: The role of attention in iconic memory reconsidered. *Consciousness and Cognition*, *53*, 203–210. https://doi.org/10.1016/j.concog.2017.06.017

Atienza, M., Cantero, J. L., & Gómez, C. M. (2001). The initial orienting response during human REM sleep as revealed by the N1 component of auditory event-related potentials. *International Journal of Psychophysiology*, *41*(2), 131–141. https://doi.org/10.1016/S0167-8760(00)00196-3

Atkinson, R. C., & Shiffrin, R. M. (1968). Human memory: A proposed system and its control processes. In K. W. Spence (Ed.), *The psychology of learning and motivation: Advances in research and theory* (Vol. 2, pp. 89–195). Academic Press/Elsevier.

Atmaca, S., Sebanz, N., & Knoblich, G. (2011). The joint flanker effect: Sharing tasks with real and imagined co-actors. *Experimental Brain Research*, *211*(3-4), 371–385. https://doi.org/10.1007/s00221-011-2709-9

Attwood, J. E., Kennard, C., Harris, J., Humphreys, G., & Antoniades, C. A. (2018). A comparison of change blindness in real-world and on-screen viewing of museum artefacts. *Frontiers in Psychology, 9,* Article 151. https://doi.org/10.3389/fpsyg.2018.00151

Awh, E., Anllo-Vento, L., & Hillyard, S. A. (2000). The role of spatial selective attention in working memory for locations: Evidence from event-related potentials. *Journal of Cognitive Neuroscience, 12*(5), 840–847. https://doi.org/10.1162/089892900562444

Awh, E., & Jonides, J. (1998). Spatial working memory and spatial selective attention. In R. Parasuraman (Ed.), *The attentive brain* (pp. 353–380). MIT Press.

Awh, E., Jonides, J., & Reuter-Lorenz, P. A. (1998). Rehearsal in spatial working memory. *Journal of Experimental Psychology: Human Perception and Performance, 24*(3), 780–790. https://doi.org/10.1037/0096-1523.24.3.780

Awh, E., Smith, E. E., & Jonides, J. (1995). Human rehearsal processes and the frontal lobes: PET evidence. In J. Grafman, K. Holyoak, & F. Boller (Eds.), *Structure and function of the prefrontal cortex* (pp. 97–118). New York Academy of Sciences. https://doi.org/10.1111/j.1749-6632.1995.tb38134.x

Baber, C., Morar, N. S., & McCabe, F. (2019). Ecological interface design, the proximity compatibility principle, and automation reliability in road traffic management. *IEEE Transactions on Human-Machine Systems, 49*(3), 241–249. https://doi.org/10.1109/THMS.2019.2896838

Babiloni, F., & Astolfi, L. (2014). Social neuroscience and hyperscanning techniques: Past, present and future. *Neuroscience and Biobehavioral Reviews, 44,* 76–93. https://doi.org/10.1016/j.neubiorev.2012.07.006

Badart, P., McDowall, J., & Prime, S. L. (2018). Multimodal sustained attention superiority in concentrative meditators compared to nonmeditators. *Mindfulness, 9*(3), 824–835. https://doi.org/10.1007/s12671-017-0822-y

Baddeley, A. (1998a). *Human memory: Theory and practice.* Allyn & Bacon.

Baddeley, A. (1998b). Recent developments in working memory. *Current Opinion in Neurobiology, 8*(2), 234–238. https://doi.org/10.1016/S0959-4388(98)80145-1

Baddeley, A. (2000). The episodic buffer: A new component of working memory? *Trends in Cognitive Sciences, 4*(11), 417–423. https://doi.org/10.1016/S1364-6613(00)01538-2

Baddeley, A. (2012). Working memory: Theories, models, and controversies. *Annual Review of Psychology, 63*(1), 1–29. https://doi.org/10.1146/annurev-psych-120710-100422

Baddeley, A. D., & Hitch, G. (1974). Working memory. In G. A. Bower (Ed.), *Recent advances in learning and motivation* (Vol. 8, pp. 47–89). Academic Press.

Baddeley, A. D., & Hitch, G. J. (2019). The phonological loop as a buffer store: An update. *Cortex, 112,* 91–106. https://doi.org/10.1016/j.cortex.2018.05.015

Baddeley, A. D., Hitch, G. J., & Allen, R. J. (2019). From short-term store to multicomponent working memory: The role of the modal model. *Memory & Cognition, 47*(4), 575–588. https://doi.org/10.3758/s13421-018-0878-5

Baethge, A., Müller, A., & Rigotti, T. (2016). Nursing performance under high workload: A diary study on the moderating role of selection, optimization and compensation strategies. *Journal of Advanced Nursing, 72*(3), 545–557. https://doi.org/10.1111/jan.12847

Baier, D., Goller, F., & Ansorge, U. (2020). Awareness and stimulus-driven spatial attention as independent processes. *Frontiers in Human Neuroscience, 14,* Article 352. https://doi.org/10.3389/fnhum.2020.00352

Baldwin, C. L., & Lewis, B. A. (2014). Perceived urgency mapping across modalities within a driving context. *Applied Ergonomics, 45*(5), 1270–1277. https://doi.org/10.1016/j.apergo.2013.05.002

Baldwin, C. L., Roberts, D. M., Barragan, D., Lee, J. D., Lerner, N., & Higgins, J. S. (2017). Detecting and quantifying mind wandering during simulated driving. *Frontiers in Human Neuroscience, 11*, Article 406. https://doi.org/10.3389/fnhum.2017.00406

Bálint, R. (1909). Seelenlähmung des "schauens," optische ataxie, räumliche störung der aufmerksamkeit [Mental paralysis of "looking," optical ataxia, spatial disturbance of attention]. *Monatsschrift für Psychiatrie und Neurologie, 25*(1), 51–66. https://doi.org/10.1159/000210464

Ball, F., Bernasconi, F., & Busch, N. A. (2015). Semantic relations between visual objects can be unconsciously processed but not reported under change blindness. *Journal of Cognitive Neuroscience, 27*(11), 2253–2268. https://doi.org/10.1162/jocn_a_00860

Ballard, J. C. (1996). Computerized assessment of sustained attention: A review of factors affecting vigilance performance. *Journal of Clinical and Experimental Neuropsychology, 18*(6), 843–863. https://doi.org/10.1080/01688639608408307

Banich, M. T. (2019). The Stroop effect occurs at multiple points along a cascade of control: Evidence from cognitive neuroscience approaches. *Frontiers in Psychology, 10*, Article 2164. https://doi.org/10.3389/fpsyg.2019.02164

Banks, W. P., & Prinzmetal, W. (1976). Configurational effects in visual information processing. *Perception & Psychophysics, 19*(4), 361–367. https://doi.org/10.3758/BF03204244

Bargh, J. A., Chen, M., & Burrows, L. (1996). Automaticity of social behavior: Direct effects of trait construct and stereotype-activation on action. *Journal of Personality and Social Psychology, 71*(2), 230–244. https://doi.org/10.1037/0022-3514.71.2.230

Barker, L. M., & Weaver, C. A., III. (1983). Rapid, permanent, loss of memory for absolute intensity of taste and smell. *Bulletin of the Psychonomic Society, 21*(4), 281–284. https://doi.org/10.3758/BF03334710

Barnas, A. J., & Greenberg, A. S. (2016). Visual field meridians modulate the reallocation of object-based attention. *Attention, Perception, & Psychophysics, 78*(7), 1985–1997. https://doi.org/10.3758/s13414-016-1116-5

Barnas, A. J., & Greenberg, A. S. (2019). Object-based attention shifts are driven by target location, not object placement. *Visual Cognition, 27*(9-10), 768–791. https://doi.org/10.1080/13506285.2019.1680587

Bartolomeo, P. (2021). Visual and motor neglect: Clinical and neurocognitive aspects. *Revue Neurologique, 177*(6), 619–626. https://doi.org/10.1016/j.neurol.2020.09.003

Bartz, W. H., Satz, P., & Fennell, E. (1967). Grouping strategies in dichotic listening: The effects of instructions, rate, and ear asymmetry. *Journal of Experimental Psychology, 74*(1), 132–136. https://doi.org/10.1037/h0024487

Bavelier, D., Achtman, R. L., Mani, M., & Föcker, J. (2012). Neural bases of selective attention in action video game players. *Vision Research, 61*, 132–143. https://doi.org/10.1016/j.visres.2011.08.007

Bayer, M., Rubens, M. T., & Johnstone, T. (2018). Simultaneous EEG-fMRI reveals attention-dependent coupling of early face processing with a distributed cortical network. *Biological Psychology, 132*, 133–142. https://doi.org/10.1016/j.biopsycho.2017.12.002

Baylis, G. C., & Driver, J. (1992). Visual parsing and response competition: The effect of grouping factors. *Perception & Psychophysics, 51*(2), 145–162. https://doi.org/10.3758/BF03212239

Beatty, J. (1982). Phasic not tonic pupillary responses vary with auditory vigilance performance. *Psychophysiology, 19*(2), 167–172. https://doi.org/10.1111/j.1469-8986.1982.tb02540.x

Bediou, B., Adams, D. M., Mayer, R. E., Tipton, E., Green, C. S., & Bavelier, D. (2018). Meta-analysis of action video game impact on perceptual, attentional, and cognitive skills. *Psychological Bulletin, 144*(1), 77–110. https://doi.org/10.1037/bul0000130

Beim, J. A., Oxenham, A. J., & Wojtczak, M. (2019). No effects of attention or visual perceptual load on cochlear function, as measured with stimulus-frequency otoacoustic emissions. *The Journal of the Acoustical Society of America, 146*(2), 1475–1491. https://doi.org/10.1121/1.5123391

Benda, N. C., & Fairbanks, R. J. (2017). Are you paying attention? Related guidance on how concepts of attention may inform effective time sharing of tasks in emergency medicine. *Annals of Emergency Medicine, 69*(5), 669–670. https://doi.org/10.1016/j.annemergmed.2017.01.027

Bennett, K. B., Bryant, A., & Sushereba, C. (2018). Ecological interface design for computer network defense. *Human Factors, 60*(5), 610–625. https://doi.org/10.1177/0018720818769233

Bennett, K. B., & Flach, J. M. (1992). Graphical displays: Implications for divided attention, focused attention, and problem solving. *Human Factors, 34*(5), 513–533. https://doi.org/10.1177/001872089203400502

Benoni, H. (2018). Can automaticity be verified utilizing a perceptual load manipulation? *Psychonomic Bulletin & Review, 25*(6), 2037–2046. https://doi.org/10.3758/s13423-018-1444-7

Bentin, S., Moscovitch, M., & Nirhod, O. (1998). Levels of processing and selective attention effects on encoding in memory. *Acta Psychologica, 98*(2-3), 311–341. https://doi.org/10.1016/S0001-6918(97)00048-6

Berlucchi, G. (2006). Inhibition of return: A phenomenon in search of a mechanism and a better name. *Cognitive Neuropsychology, 23*(7), 1065–1074. https://doi.org/10.1080/02643290600588426

Berlyne, D. E. (1974). Attention. In E. C. Carterette & M. P. Friedman (Eds.), *Handbook of perception: Vol. 1. Historical and philosophical roots of perception* (pp. 123–147). Academic Press.

Bertelson, P., & Aschersleben, G. (1998). Automatic visual bias of perceived auditory location. *Psychonomic Bulletin & Review, 5*(3), 482–489. https://doi.org/10.3758/BF03208826

Besner, D., Davies, J., & Daniels, S. (1981). Reading for meaning: The effects of concurrent articulation. *Quarterly Journal of Experimental Psychology, 33*(4), 415–437. https://doi.org/10.1080/14640748108400801

Besner, D., McLean, D., & Young, T. (2021). On the determination of eye gaze and arrow direction: Automaticity reconsidered. *Canadian Journal of Experimental Psychology, 75*(3), 261–278. https://doi.org/10.1037/cep0000261

Best, V., Jennings, T. R., & Kidd, G., Jr. (2020). An effect of eye position in cocktail party listening. *Proceedings of Meetings on Acoustics, 42*(1), Article 050001.

Bialystok, E., Craik, F. I. M., Klein, R., & Viswanathan, M. (2004). Bilingualism, aging, and cognitive control: Evidence from the Simon task. *Psychology and Aging, 19*(2), 290–303. https://doi.org/10.1037/0882-7974.19.2.290

Bialystok, E., Craik, F., & Luk, G. (2008). Cognitive control and lexical access in younger and older bilinguals. *Journal of Experimental Psychology: Learning, Memory, and Cognition, 34*(4), 859–873. https://doi.org/10.1037/0278-7393.34.4.859

Billeaud, J., & Tarm, M. (2021, March 31). Some U.S. Capitol riot participants apologize for actions in court. *CP24.* https://www.cp24.com/world/some-u-s-capitol-riot-participants-apologize-for-actions-in-court-1.5369289?cache=yes%3FclipId%3D89750%3FclipId%3D373266

Bills, A. G. (1931). Blocking: A new principle of mental fatigue. *The American Journal of Psychology, 43*(2), 230–245. https://doi.org/10.2307/1414771

Binet, A. (1890). La concurrence des états psychologiques [The competition of psychological states]. *Revue Philosophique de la France et de l'Etranger, 24,* 138–155.

Bischoff, M., Walter, B., Blecker, C. R., Morgen, K., Vaitl, D., & Sammer, G. (2007). Utilizing the ventriloquism-effect to investigate audio-visual binding. *Neuropsychologia, 45*(3), 578–586. https://doi.org/10.1016/j.neuropsychologia.2006.03.008

Bishop, D. V. M. (1992). The underlying nature of specific language impairment. *Journal of Child Psychology and Psychiatry, 33*(1), 3–66. https://doi.org/10.1111/j.1469-7610.1992.tb00858.x

Bisley, J. W., & Mirpour, K. (2019). The neural instantiation of a priority map. *Current Opinion in Psychology, 29,* 108–112. https://doi.org/10.1016/j.copsyc.2019.01.002

Bissonnette, J. N., Francis, A. M., Hull, K. M., Leckey, J., Pimer, L., Berrigan, L. I., & Fisher, D. J. (2020). MMN-indexed auditory change detection in major depressive disorder. *Clinical EEG and Neuroscience, 51*(6), 365–372. https://doi.org/10.1177/1550059420914200

Blais, C., & Besner, D. (2006). Reverse Stroop effects with untranslated responses. *Journal of Experimental Psychology: Human Perception and Performance, 32*(6), 1345–1353. https://doi.org/10.1037/0096-1523.32.6.1345

Bliss, J. C., Crane, H. D., Mansfield, P. K., & Townsend, J. T. (1966). Information available in brief tactile presentations. *Perception & Psychophysics, 1*(4), 273–283. https://doi.org/10.3758/BF03207391

Blumenthal, A. L. (1980). Wilhelm Wundt and early American psychology. In R. W. Rieber (Ed.), *Wilhelm Wundt and the making of scientific psychology* (pp. 117–135). Plenum. https://doi.org/10.1007/978-1-4684-8340-6_4

Blundon, E. G., Rumak, S. P., & Ward, L. M. (2017). Sequential search asymmetry: Behavioral and psychophysiological evidence from a dual oddball task. *PLOS ONE, 12*(3), Article e0173237. https://doi.org/10.1371/journal.pone.0173237

Boag, R. J., Strickland, L., Loft, S., & Heathcote, A. (2019). Strategic attention and decision control support prospective memory in a complex dual-task environment. *Cognition, 191,* 103974. https://doi.org/10.1016/j.cognition.2019.05.011

Böffel, C., & Müsseler, J. (2018). Perceived ownership of avatars influences visual perspective taking. *Frontiers in Psychology, 9,* Article 743. https://doi.org/10.3389/fpsyg.2018.00743

Böffel, C., & Müsseler, J. (2019). Visual perspective taking for avatars in a Simon task. *Attention, Perception, & Psychophysics, 81*(1), 158–172. https://doi.org/10.3758/s13414-018-1573-0

Boies, K., & Fiset, J. (2018). Leadership and communication as antecedents of shared mental models emergence. *Performance Improvement Quarterly, 31*(3), 293–316. https://doi.org/10.1002/piq.21267

Boot, W. R., Kramer, A. F., Simons, D. J., Fabiani, M., & Gratton, G. (2008). The effects of video game playing on attention, memory, and executive control. *Acta Psychologica, 129*(3), 387–398. https://doi.org/10.1016/j.actpsy.2008.09.005

Boronat, C. B., & Logan, G. D. (1997). The role of attention in automatization: Does attention operate at encoding, or retrieval, or both? *Memory & Cognition, 25*, 36–46. https://doi.org/10.3758/BF03197283

BotoxZombie. (2008, December 29). *Penn and Teller explain sleight of hand* [Video]. YouTube. https://www.youtube.com/watch?v=oXGr76CfoCs&feature=emb_title

Botvinick, M. M., Braver, T. S., Barch, D. M., Carter, C. S., & Cohen, J. D. (2001). Conflict monitoring and cognitive control. *Psychological Review, 108*(3), 624–652. https://doi.org/10.1037/0033-295X.108.3.624

Botvinick, M., & Cohen, J. (1998, February 19). Rubber hands 'feel' touch that eyes see. *Nature, 391*(6669), 756. https://doi.org/10.1038/35784

Boudewijnse, G. J., Murray, D. J., & Bandomir, C. A. (1999). Herbart's mathematical psychology. *History of Psychology, 2*(3), 163–193. https://doi.org/10.1037/1093-4510.2.3.163

Bower, G. H., & Morrow, D. G. (1990, January 5). Mental models in narrative comprehension. *Science, 247*(4938), 44–48. https://doi.org/10.1126/science.2403694

Boxhoorn, S., Lopez, E., Schmidt, C., Schulze, D., Hänig, S., & Freitag, C. M. (2018). Attention profiles in autism spectrum disorder and subtypes of attention-deficit/hyperactivity disorder. *European Child & Adolescent Psychiatry, 27*(11), 1433–1447. https://doi.org/10.1007/s00787-018-1138-8

Breitmeyer, B. G., & Ganz, L. (1976). Implications of sustained and transient channels for theories of visual pattern masking, saccadic suppression, and information processing. *Psychological Review, 83*(1), 1–36. https://doi.org/10.1037/0033-295X.83.1.1

Briand, K. A., & Klein, R. M. (1987). Is Posner's "beam" the same as Treisman's "glue"? On the relation between visual orienting and feature integration theory. *Journal of Experimental Psychology: Human Perception and Performance, 13*(2), 228–241. https://doi.org/10.1037/0096-1523.13.2.228

Brickner, M., & Gopher, D. (1981). *Improving time-sharing performance by enhancing voluntary control on processing resources.* Technion-Israel Institute of Technology Haifa Center of Human Engineering and Industrial Safety Research.

Broadbent, D. E. (1954). The role of auditory localization in attention and memory span. *Journal of Experimental Psychology, 47*(3), 191–196. https://doi.org/10.1037/h0054182

Broadbent, D. E. (1957). A mechanical model for human attention and immediate memory. *Psychological Review, 64*(3), 205–215. https://doi.org/10.1037/h0047313

Broadbent, D. E. (1958). *Perception and communication.* Pergamon Press. https://doi.org/10.1037/10037-000

Broadbent, D. E. (1982). Task combination and selective intake of information. *Acta Psychologica, 50*(3), 253–290. https://doi.org/10.1016/0001-6918(82)90043-9

Broadbent, D. E., & Broadbent, M. H. (1987). From detection to identification: Response to multiple targets in rapid serial visual presentation. *Perception & Psychophysics, 42*(2), 105–113. https://doi.org/10.3758/BF03210498

Broadbent, D. E., Cooper, P. F., FitzGerald, P., & Parkes, K. R. (1982). The Cognitive Failures Questionnaire (CFQ) and its correlates. *British Journal of Clinical Psychology, 21*(1), 1–16. https://doi.org/10.1111/j.2044-8260.1982.tb01421.x

Brockmole, J. R., & Henderson, J. M. (2006). Using real-world scenes as contextual cues for search. *Visual Cognition, 13*(1), 99–108. https://doi.org/10.1080/13506280500165188

Bronkhorst, A. W. (2015). The cocktail-party problem revisited: Early processing and selection of multi-talker speech. *Attention, Perception, & Psychophysics, 77*(5), 1465–1487. https://doi.org/10.3758/s13414-015-0882-9

Brooks, L. R. (1968). Spatial and verbal components of the act of recall. *Canadian Journal of Psychology, 22*(5), 349–368. https://doi.org/10.1037/h0082775

Buetti, S., Lleras, A., & Moore, C. M. (2014). The flanker effect does not reflect the processing of "task-irrelevant" stimuli: Evidence from inattentional blindness. *Psychonomic Bulletin & Review, 21*(5), 1231–1237. https://doi.org/10.3758/s13423-014-0602-9

Bugg, J. M., & Hutchison, K. A. (2013). Converging evidence for control of color–word Stroop interference at the item level. *Journal of Experimental Psychology: Human Perception and Performance, 39*(2), 433–449. https://doi.org/10.1037/a0029145

Bundesen, C. (1990). A theory of visual attention. *Psychological Review, 97*(4), 523–547. https://doi.org/10.1037/0033-295X.97.4.523

Bundesen, C., Pedersen, L. F., & Larsen, A. (1984). Measuring efficiency of selection from briefly exposed visual displays: A model for partial report. *Journal of Experimental Psychology: Human Perception and Performance, 10*(3), 329–339. https://doi.org/10.1037/0096-1523.10.3.329

Burack, J. A., Russo, N., Kovshoff, H., Palma Fernandes, T., Ringo, J., Landry, O., & Iarocci, G. (2016). How I attend—Not how well do I attend: Rethinking developmental frameworks of attention and cognition in autism spectrum disorder and typical development. *Journal of Cognition and Development, 17*(4), 553–567. https://doi.org/10.1080/15248372.2016.1197226

Burgess, P. W., & Stuss, D. T. (2017). Fifty years of prefrontal cortex research: Impact on assessment. *Journal of the International Neuropsychological Society, 23*(9-10), 755–767. https://doi.org/10.1017/S1355617717000704

Cakir, J., Frye, R. E., & Walker, S. J. (2020). The lifetime social cost of autism: 1990–2029. *Research in Autism Spectrum Disorders, 72*, Article 101502. https://doi.org/10.1016/j.rasd.2019.101502

Calder, A. J., Jenkins, R., Cassel, A., & Clifford, C. W. G. (2008). Visual representation of eye gaze is coded by a nonopponent multichannel system. *Journal of Experimental Psychology: General, 137*(2), 244–261. https://doi.org/10.1037/0096-3445.137.2.244

Calderwood, C., Ackerman, P. L., & Conklin, E. M. (2014). What else do college students "do" while studying? An investigation of multitasking. *Computers & Education, 75*, 19–29. https://doi.org/10.1016/j.compedu.2014.02.004

Camos, V., Lagner, P., & Barrouillet, P. (2009). Two maintenance mechanisms of verbal information in working memory. *Journal of Memory and Language, 61*(3), 457–469. https://doi.org/10.1016/j.jml.2009.06.002

Camus, T., Hommel, B., Brunel, L., & Brouillet, T. (2018). From anticipation to integration: The role of integrated action-effects in building sensorimotor contingencies. *Psychonomic Bulletin & Review, 25*(3), 1059–1065. https://doi.org/10.3758/s13423-017-1308-6

Capozzi, F., & Ristic, J. (2020). Attention AND mentalizing? Reframing a debate on social orienting of attention. *Visual Cognition, 28*(2), 97–105. https://doi.org/10.1080/13506285.2020.1725206

Cardoso-Leite, P., Kludt, R., Vignola, G., Ma, W. J., Green, C., & Bavelier, D. (2016). Technology consumption and cognitive control: Contrasting action video game experience with media multitasking. *Attention, Perception, & Psychophysics*, *78*(1), 218–241. https://doi.org/10.3758/s13414-015-0988-0

Carlson, R. A., & Sohn, M.-H. (2000). Cognitive control of multistep routines: Information processing and conscious intentions. In S. Monsell & J. Driver (Eds.), *Control of cognitive processes: Attention and performance XVIII* (pp. 443–464). MIT Press.

Carpenter, W. B. (1852). On the influence of suggestion in modifying and directing muscular movement, independently of volition. *Proceedings of the Royal Institution of Great Britain*, *1*, 147–153.

Carral, V., Corral, M. J., & Escera, C. (2005). Auditory event-related potentials as a function of abstract change magnitude. *Neuroreport*, *16*(3), 301–305. https://doi.org/10.1097/00001756-200502280-00020

Carrasco, M. (2011). Visual attention: The past 25 years. *Vision Research*, *51*(13), 1484–1525. https://doi.org/10.1016/j.visres.2011.04.012

Carrasco, M. (2018). How visual spatial attention alters perception. *Cognitive Processing*, *19*(S1), 77–88. https://doi.org/10.1007/s10339-018-0883-4

Carrasco, M., & Barbot, A. (2019). Spatial attention alters visual appearance. *Current Opinion in Psychology*, *29*, 56–64. https://doi.org/10.1016/j.copsyc.2018.10.010

Carter, T. J., Ferguson, M. J., & Hassin, R. R. (2011). A single exposure to the American flag shifts support toward Republicanism up to 8 months later. *Psychological Science*, *22*(8), 1011–1018. https://doi.org/10.1177/0956797611414726

Carter, T. J., Pandey, G., Bolger, N., Hassin, R. R., & Ferguson, M. J. (2020). Has the effect of the American flag on political attitudes declined over time? A case study of the historical context of American flag priming. *Social Cognition*, *38*(6), 489–520. https://doi.org/10.1521/soco.2020.38.6.489

Casey, B. J. (2005). Frontostriatal and frontocerebellar circuitry underlying cognitive control. In U. Mayr, E. Awh, & S. W. Keele (Eds.), *Developing individuality in the human brain: A tribute to Michael I. Posner* (pp. 141–166). American Psychological Association. https://doi.org/10.1037/11108-008

Casteau, S., & Smith, D. T. (2020). Covert attention beyond the range of eye-movements: Evidence for a dissociation between exogenous and endogenous orienting. *Cortex*, *122*, 170–186. https://doi.org/10.1016/j.cortex.2018.11.007

Castillo, R., Alvarado, J., Moreno, P., Billeke, P., Martínez, C., Varas, J., & Jarufe, N. (2018). Validation of a visual-spatial secondary task to assess automaticity in laparoscopic skills. *Journal of Surgical Education*, *75*(4), 1001–1005. https://doi.org/10.1016/j.jsurg.2017.11.007

Cavanagh, J. F., & Frank, M. J. (2014). Frontal theta as a mechanism for cognitive control. *Trends in Cognitive Sciences*, *18*(8), 414–421. https://doi.org/10.1016/j.tics.2014.04.012

Cavanagh, J. F., & Shackman, A. J. (2015). Frontal midline theta reflects anxiety and cognitive control: Meta-analytic evidence. *Journal of Physiology, Paris*, *109*(1-3), 3–15. https://doi.org/10.1016/j.jphysparis.2014.04.003

Cave, K. R., & Pashler, H. (1995). Visual selection mediated by location: Selecting successive visual objects. *Perception & Psychophysics*, *57*(4), 421–432. https://doi.org/10.3758/BF03213068

Centers for Disease Control and Prevention. (n.d.). *Attention-deficit/hyperactivity disorder (ADHD)*. https://www.cdc.gov/ncbddd/adhd/data.html

Centers for Disease Control and Prevention. (2021, February 18). *Learn the signs: Act early.* https://www.cdc.gov/ncbddd/actearly/index.html?CDC_AA_refVal= https%3A%2F%2Fwww.cdc.gov%2Factearly%2Findex.html

Cepeda, N. J., Cave, K. R., Bichot, N. P., & Kim, M.-S. (1998). Spatial selection via feature-driven inhibition of distractor locations. *Perception & Psychophysics, 60*(5), 727–746. https://doi.org/10.3758/BF03206059

Chakrabarty, M., Badgio, D., Ptacek, J., Biswas, A., Ghosal, M., & Chatterjee, G. (2017). Hemispheric asymmetry in attention and its impact on our consciousness: A review with reference to altered consciousness in right hemisphere damaged subjects. *Journal of Consciousness Studies, 24*(7-8), 51–78.

Chapanis, A., & Lindenbaum, L. E. (1959). A reaction time study of four control-display linkages. *Human Factors, 1*(4), 1–7. https://doi.org/10.1177/001872085900100401

Charles, R. L., & Nixon, J. (2019). Measuring mental workload using physiological measures: A systematic review. *Applied Ergonomics, 74*, 221–232. https://doi.org/10.1016/j.apergo.2018.08.028

Chen, A., Wang, A., Wang, T., Tang, X., & Zhang, M. (2017). Behavioral oscillations in visual attention modulated by task difficulty. *Frontiers in Psychology, 8*, Article 1630. https://doi.org/10.3389/fpsyg.2017.01630

Chen, J., & Proctor, R. W. (2013). Response-effect compatibility defines the natural scrolling direction. *Human Factors, 55*(6), 1112–1129. https://doi.org/10.1177/0018720813482329

Chen, Z. (2012). Object-based attention: A tutorial review. *Attention, Perception, & Psychophysics, 74*(5), 784–802. https://doi.org/10.3758/s13414-012-0322-z

Chen, Z., & Cave, K. R. (2019). When is object-based attention not based on objects? *Journal of Experimental Psychology: Human Perception and Performance, 45*(8), 1062–1082. https://doi.org/10.1037/xhp0000657

Chen, Z., Cave, K. R., Basu, D., Suresh, S., & Wiltshire, J. (2020). A region complexity effect masquerading as object-based attention. *Journal of Vision, 20*(7), Article 24. https://doi.org/10.1167/jov.20.7.24

Cheng, P. W. (1985). Restructuring versus automaticity: Alternative accounts of skill acquisition. *Psychological Review, 92*(3), 414–423. https://doi.org/10.1037/0033-295X.92.3.414

Cherry, E. C. (1953). Some experiments on the recognition of speech, with one and with two ears. *The Journal of the Acoustical Society of America, 25*(5), 975–979. https://doi.org/10.1121/1.1907229

Chetverikov, A., Kuvaldina, M., MacInnes, W. J., Jóhannesson, Ó. I., & Kristjánsson, Á. (2018). Implicit processing during change blindness revealed with mouse-contingent and gaze-contingent displays. *Attention, Perception, & Psychophysics, 80*(4), 844–859. https://doi.org/10.3758/s13414-017-1468-5

Chiappe, D., Conger, M., Liao, J., Caldwell, J. L., & Vu, K. P. L. (2013). Improving multi-tasking ability through action videogames. *Applied Ergonomics, 44*(2), 278–284. https://doi.org/10.1016/j.apergo.2012.08.002

Chiappe, D., Morgan, C. A., Kraut, J., Ziccardi, J., Sturre, L., Strybel, T. Z., & Vu, K. L. (2016). Evaluating probe techniques and a situated theory of situation awareness. *Journal of Experimental Psychology: Applied, 22*(4), 436–454. https://doi.org/10.1037/xap0000097

Chiappe, D. L., Strybel, T. Z., & Vu, K. P. L. (2012). Mechanisms for the acquisition of situation awareness in situated agents. *Theoretical Issues in Ergonomics Science, 13*(6), 625–647. https://doi.org/10.1080/1463922X.2011.611267

Chong, S. C., & Treisman, A. (2005). Attentional spread in the statistical processing of visual displays. *Perception & Psychophysics, 67*(1), 1–13. https://doi.org/10.3758/BF03195009

Christie, J., & Klein, R. M. (2001). Negative priming for spatial location? *Canadian Journal of Experimental Psychology, 55*(1), 24–38. https://doi.org/10.1037/h0087350

Chun, M. M., & Potter, M. C. (1995). A two-stage model for multiple target detection in rapid serial visual presentation. *Journal of Experimental Psychology: Human Perception and Performance, 21*(1), 109–127. https://doi.org/10.1037/0096-1523.21.1.109

Clark, S. V., King, T. Z., & Turner, J. A. (2020). Cerebellar contributions to proactive and reactive control in the stop signal task: A systematic review and meta-analysis of functional magnetic resonance imaging studies. *Neuropsychology Review, 30*(3), 362–385. https://doi.org/10.1007/s11065-020-09432-w

Clark, V. P., & Hillyard, S. A. (1996). Spatial selective attention affects early extrastriate but not striate components of the visual evoked potential. *Journal of Cognitive Neuroscience, 8*(5), 387–402. https://doi.org/10.1162/jocn.1996.8.5.387

Cohen, A., & Ivry, R. (1989). Illusory conjunctions inside and outside the focus of attention. *Journal of Experimental Psychology: Human Perception and Performance, 15*(4), 650–663. https://doi.org/10.1037/0096-1523.15.4.650

Cohen, A., Ivry, R. I., & Keele, S. W. (1990). Attention and structure in sequence learning. *Journal of Experimental Psychology: Learning, Memory, and Cognition, 16*(1), 17–30. https://doi.org/10.1037/0278-7393.16.1.17

Cohen, J. D., Dunbar, K., & McClelland, J. L. (1990). On the control of automatic processes: A parallel distributed processing account of the Stroop effect. *Psychological Review, 97*(3), 332–361. https://doi.org/10.1037/0033-295X.97.3.332

Colavita, F. B. (1974). Human sensory dominance. *Perception & Psychophysics, 16*(2), 409–412. https://doi.org/10.3758/BF03203962

Coles, M. G., Gratton, G., Bashore, T. R., Eriksen, C. W., & Donchin, E. (1985). A psychophysiological investigation of the continuous flow model of human information processing. *Journal of Experimental Psychology: Human Perception and Performance, 11*(5), 529–553. https://doi.org/10.1037/0096-1523.11.5.529

Colflesh, G. J., & Conway, A. R. (2007). Individual differences in working memory capacity and divided attention in dichotic listening. *Psychonomic Bulletin & Review, 14*(4), 699–703. https://doi.org/10.3758/BF03196824

Colle, H. A., & Reid, G. B. (1999). Double trade-off curves with different cognitive processing combinations: Testing the cancellation axiom of mental workload measurement theory. *Human Factors, 41*(1), 35–50. https://doi.org/10.1518/001872099779577327

Collet, C., Salvia, E., & Petit-Boulanger, C. (2014). Measuring workload with electrodermal activity during common braking actions. *Ergonomics, 57*(6), 886–896. https://doi.org/10.1080/00140139.2014.899627

Colombo, J. (2001). The development of visual attention in infancy. *Annual Review of Psychology, 52*(1), 337–367. https://doi.org/10.1146/annurev.psych.52.1.337

Connelly, S. L., & Hasher, L. (1993). Aging and the inhibition of spatial location. *Journal of Experimental Psychology: Human Perception and Performance, 19*(6), 1238–1250. https://doi.org/10.1037/0096-1523.19.6.1238

Conrad, R., & Hull, A. J. (1964). Information, acoustic confusion and memory span. *British Journal of Psychology, 55*(4), 429–432. https://doi.org/10.1111/j.2044-8295.1964.tb00928.x

Corbetta, M. (1998). Functional anatomy of visual attention in the human brain: Studies with positron emission tomography. In R. Parasuraman (Ed.), *The attentive brain* (pp. 95–122). MIT Press.

Corteen, R. S., & Wood, B. (1972). Autonomic responses to shock-associated words in an unattended channel. *Journal of Experimental Psychology, 94*(3), 308–313. https://doi.org/10.1037/h0032759

Cowan, N. (1984). On short and long auditory stores. *Psychological Bulletin, 96*(2), 341–370. https://doi.org/10.1037/0033-2909.96.2.341

Cowan, N. (1988). Evolving conceptions of memory storage, selective attention, and their mutual constraints within the human information-processing system. *Psychological Bulletin, 104*(2), 163–191. https://doi.org/10.1037/0033-2909.104.2.163

Cowan, N. (1997). *Attention and memory: An integrated framework.* Oxford University Press.

Cowan, N. (2001). The magical number 4 in short-term memory: A reconsideration of mental storage capacity. *Behavioral and Brain Sciences, 24*(1), 87–114. https://doi.org/10.1017/S0140525X01003922

Cowan, N. (2017). The many faces of working memory and short-term storage. *Psychonomic Bulletin & Review, 24*(4), 1158–1170. https://doi.org/10.3758/s13423-016-1191-6

Cowan, N. (2019). Short-term memory based on activated long-term memory: A review in response to Norris (2017). *Psychological Bulletin, 145*(8), 822–847. https://doi.org/10.1037/bul0000199

Cowan, N., & Rachev, N. R. (2018). Merging with the path not taken: Wilhelm Wundt's work as a precursor to the embedded-processes approach to memory, attention, and consciousness. *Consciousness and Cognition, 63*, 228–238. https://doi.org/10.1016/j.concog.2018.06.001

Craig, F., Margari, F., Legrottaglie, A. R., Palumbi, R., de Giambattista, C., & Margari, L. (2016). A review of executive function deficits in autism spectrum disorder and attention-deficit/hyperactivity disorder. *Neuropsychiatric Disease and Treatment, 12*, 1191–1202.

Craik, F. I. M. (1977). Age differences in human memory. In J. Birren & K. Schaie (Eds.), *Handbook of the psychology of aging* (pp. 384–420). Van Nostrand Reinhold.

Craik, F. I. M., & Grady, C. L. (2002). Aging, memory, and frontal lobe functioning. In D. T. Stuss & R. T. Knight (Eds.), *Principles of frontal lobe function* (pp. 528–540). Oxford University Press. https://doi.org/10.1093/acprof:oso/9780195134971.003.0031

Craik, F. I. M., & Lockhart, R. S. (1972). Levels of processing: A framework for memory research. *Journal of Verbal Learning and Verbal Behavior, 11*(6), 671–684. https://doi.org/10.1016/S0022-5371(72)80001-X

Craik, K. J. W. (1948). Theory of the human operator in control systems; man as an element in a control system. *British Journal of Psychology, 38*(3), 142–148.

Crick, F. (1988). *What mad pursuit: A personal view of scientific discovery.* Basic Books.

Crossley, M., & Hiscock, M. (1992). Age-related differences in concurrent-task performance of normal adults: Evidence for a decline in processing resources. *Psychology and Aging, 7*(4), 499–506. https://doi.org/10.1037/0882-7974.7.4.499

Dahl, M., Granér, S., Fransson, P. A., Bertilsson, J., & Fredriksson, P. (2018). Analysis of eyewitness testimony in a police shooting with fatal outcome–Manifestations of spatial and temporal distortions. *Cogent Psychology, 5*(1), Article 1487271. https://doi.org/10.1080/23311908.2018.1487271

Dalmaso, M., Castelli, L., & Galfano, G. (2020). Social modulators of gaze-mediated orienting of attention: A review. *Psychonomic Bulletin & Review, 27*(5), 833–855. https://doi.org/10.3758/s13423-020-01730-x

Dalmaso, M., Pavan, G., Castelli, L., & Galfano, G. (2012). Social status gates social attention in humans. *Biology Letters, 8*(3), 450–452. https://doi.org/10.1098/rsbl.2011.0881

D'Angelo, M. C., Thomson, D. R., Tipper, S. P., & Milliken, B. (2016). Negative priming 1985 to 2015: A measure of inhibition, the emergence of alternative accounts, and the multiple process challenge. *Quarterly Journal of Experimental Psychology, 69*(10), 1890–1909. https://doi.org/10.1080/17470218.2016.1173077

Darwin, C. J., Turvey, M. T., & Crowder, R. G. (1972). An auditory analogue of the Sperling partial report procedure: Evidence for brief auditory storage. *Cognitive Psychology, 3*(2), 255–267. https://doi.org/10.1016/0010-0285(72)90007-2

Davis, R. (1957). The human operator as a single channel information system. *Quarterly Journal of Experimental Psychology, 9*(3), 119–129. https://doi.org/10.1080/17470215708416232

Dawson, M. E., & Schell, A. M. (1982). Electrodermal responses to attended and nonattended significant stimuli during dichotic listening. *Journal of Experimental Psychology: Human Perception and Performance, 8*(2), 315–324. https://doi.org/10.1037/0096-1523.8.2.315

Deaner, R. O., Shepherd, S. V., & Platt, M. L. (2007). Familiarity accentuates gaze cuing in women but not men. *Biology Letters, 3*(1), 65–68. https://doi.org/10.1098/rsbl.2006.0564

Deatherage, B. H., & Evans, T. R. (1969). Binaural masking: Backward, forward, and simultaneous effects. *The Journal of the Acoustical Society of America, 46*(2B), 362–371. https://doi.org/10.1121/1.1911698

de Bruin, A., Treccani, B., & Della Sala, S. (2015). Cognitive advantage in bilingualism: An example of publication bias? *Psychological Science, 26*(1), 99–107. https://doi.org/10.1177/0956797614557866

De Houwer, J., & Eelen, P. (1998). An affective variant of the Simon paradigm. *Cognition and Emotion, 12*(1), 45–62. https://doi.org/10.1080/026999398379772

De Jagger, J. J. (1970). *Reaction time and mental processes* (J. Brozek & M. S. Sibinga, Trans.). B. De Graf. (Original work published 1865)

de Jong, R. (1993). Multiple bottlenecks in overlapping task performance. *Journal of Experimental Psychology: Human Perception and Performance, 19*(5), 965–980. https://doi.org/10.1037/0096-1523.19.5.965

de Jong, R. (2000). An intention-activation account of residual switch costs. In S. Monsell & J. Driver (Eds.), *Control of cognitive processes: Attention and performance XVIII* (pp. 357–376). MIT Press.

de Jong, R., Coles, M. G. H., Logan, G. D., & Gratton, G. (1990). In search of the point of no return: The control of response processes. *Journal of Experimental Psychology: Human Perception and Performance, 16*(1), 164–182. https://doi.org/10.1037/0096-1523.16.1.164

de Jong, R., Liang, C.-C., & Lauber, E. (1994). Conditional and unconditional automaticity: A dual-process model of effects of spatial stimulus-response correspondence. *Journal of Experimental Psychology: Human Perception and Performance, 20*(4), 731–750. https://doi.org/10.1037/0096-1523.20.4.731

Delgado, P., & Salmerón, L. (2021). The inattentive on-screen reading: Reading medium affects attention and reading comprehension under time pressure.

Learning and Instruction, 71, 101396. https://doi.org/10.1016/j.learninstruc. 2020.101396

Delorme, A., Westerfield, M., & Makeig, S. (2007). Medial prefrontal theta bursts precede rapid motor responses during visual selective attention. *The Journal of Neuroscience, 27*(44), 11949–11959. https://doi.org/10.1523/JNEUROSCI. 3477-07.2007

Demir, M., McNeese, N. J., & Cooke, N. J. (2017). Team situation awareness within the context of human-autonomy teaming. *Cognitive Systems Research, 46,* 3–12. https://doi.org/10.1016/j.cogsys.2016.11.003

Demir, M., McNeese, N. J., & Cooke, N. J. (2020). Understanding human-robot teams in light of all-human teams: Aspects of team interaction and shared cognition. *International Journal of Human–Computer Studies, 140,* Article 102436. https://doi.org/10.1016/j.ijhcs.2020.102436

Desimone, R., & Duncan, J. (1995). Neural mechanisms of selective visual attention. *Annual Review of Neuroscience, 18*(1), 193–222. https://doi.org/10.1146/ annurev.ne.18.030195.001205

Desjardins, J. L., & Fernandez, F. (2018). Performance on auditory and visual tasks of inhibition in English monolingual and Spanish–English bilingual adults: Do bilinguals have a cognitive advantage? *Journal of Speech, Language, and Hearing Research, 61*(2), 410–419. https://doi.org/10.1044/2017_JSLHR-H-17-0160

D'Esposito, M., Zarahn, E., & Aguirre, G. K. (1999). Event-related functional MRI: Implications for cognitive psychology. *Psychological Bulletin, 125*(1), 155–164. https://doi.org/10.1037/0033-2909.125.1.155

Deutsch, J. A., & Deutsch, D. (1963). Some theoretical considerations. *Psychological Review, 70*(1), 80–90. https://doi.org/10.1037/h0039515

Deveau, J., Ozer, D. J., & Seitz, A. R. (2014). Improved vision and on-field performance in baseball through perceptual learning. *Current Biology, 24*(4), R146–R147. https://doi.org/10.1016/j.cub.2014.01.004

Dignath, D., Eder, A. B., Steinhauser, M., & Kiesel, A. (2020). Conflict monitoring and the affective-signaling hypothesis-An integrative review. *Psychonomic Bulletin & Review, 27*(2), 193–216. https://doi.org/10.3758/s13423-019-01668-9

Dillard, M. B., Warm, J. S., Funke, G. J., Nelson, W. T., Finomore, V. S., McClernon, C. K., Eggemeier, F. T., Tripp, L. D., & Funke, M. E. (2019). Vigilance tasks: Unpleasant, mentally demanding, and stressful even when time flies. *Human Factors, 61*(2), 225–242. https://doi.org/10.1177/0018720818796015

D'Imperio, D., Scandola, M., Gobbetto, V., Bulgarelli, C., Salgarello, M., Avesani, R., & Moro, V. (2017). Visual and cross-modal cues increase the identification of overlapping visual stimuli in Balint's syndrome. *Journal of Clinical and Experimental Neuropsychology, 39*(8), 786–802. https://doi.org/10.1080/13803395.2016. 1266307

Dittrich, K., Bossert, M.-L., Rothe-Wulf, A., & Klauer, K. C. (2017). The joint flanker effect and the joint Simon effect: On the comparability of processes underlying joint compatibility effects. *Quarterly Journal of Experimental Psychology, 70*(9), 1808–1823. https://doi.org/10.1080/17470218.2016.1207690

Doallo, S., Lorenzo-López, L., Vizoso, C., Rodríguez Holguín, S., Amenedo, E., Bará, S., & Cadaveira, F. (2004). The time course of the effects of central and peripheral cues on visual processing: An event-related potentials study. *Clinical Neurophysiology, 115*(1), 199–210. https://doi.org/10.1016/S1388-2457(03)00317-1

Dolk, T., Hommel, B., Prinz, W., & Liepelt, R. (2013). The (not so) social Simon effect: A referential coding account. *Journal of Experimental Psychology:*

Human Perception and Performance, 39(5), 1248–1260. https://doi.org/10.1037/a0031031

Dolk, T., Hommel, B., Prinz, W., & Liepelt, R. (2014). The joint flanker effect: Less social than previously thought. *Psychonomic Bulletin & Review, 21*(5), 1224–1230. https://doi.org/10.3758/s13423-014-0583-8

Donchin, E., & Coles, M. G. H. (1988). Is the P300 component a manifestation of context updating? *Behavioral and Brain Sciences, 11*(03), 357–427. https://doi.org/10.1017/S0140525X00058027

Donchin, E., Ritter, W., & McCallum, W. C. (1978). Cognitive psychophysiology: The endogenous components of the ERP. In E. Callaway, P. Tueting, & S. H. Koslow (Eds.), *Event-related brain potentials in man* (pp. 349–411). Academic Press. https://doi.org/10.1016/B978-0-12-155150-6.50019-5

Donders, F. C. (1969). On the speed of mental processes. In W. G. Koster (Ed.), *Acta Psychologica, 30, Attention and Performance II* (pp. 412–431). North-Holland. (Original work published 1868)

Donk, M., & Theeuwes, J. (2003). Prioritizing selection of new elements: Bottom-up versus top-down control. *Perception & Psychophysics, 65*(8), 1231–1242. https://doi.org/10.3758/BF03194848

Donkin, C., & Brown, S. D. (2018). Response times and decision-making. In E.-J. Wagenmakers & J. T. Wixted (Eds.), *Stevens' handbook of experimental psychology and cognitive neuroscience: Vol. 5. Methodology* (4th ed., pp. 349–382). Wiley. https://doi.org/10.1002/9781119170174.epcn509

Donkin, C., Tran, S. C., & Nosofsky, R. (2014). Landscaping analyses of the ROC predictions of discrete-slots and signal-detection models of visual working memory. *Attention, Perception, & Psychophysics, 76*(7), 2103–2116. https://doi.org/10.3758/s13414-013-0561-7

Donovan, I., Zhou, Y. J., & Carrasco, M. (2020). In search of exogenous feature-based attention. *Attention, Perception, & Psychophysics, 82*(1), 312–329. https://doi.org/10.3758/s13414-019-01815-3

Downing, C. J., & Pinker, S. (1985). The spatial structure of visual attention. In M. I. Posner & O. S. M. Marin (Eds.), *Attention and performance XI* (pp. 171–187). Erlbaum.

Downing, P., Liu, J., & Kanwisher, N. (2001). Testing cognitive models of visual attention with fMRI and MEG. *Neuropsychologia, 39*(12), 1329–1342. https://doi.org/10.1016/S0028-3932(01)00121-X

Doyen, S., Klein, O., Pichon, C. L., & Cleeremans, A. (2012). Behavioral priming: It's all in the mind, but whose mind? *PLoS One, 7*(1), Article e29081. https://doi.org/10.1371/journal.pone.0029081

Dreisbach, G., & Fischer, R. (2015). Conflicts as aversive signals for control adaptation. *Current Directions in Psychological Science, 24*(4), 255–260. https://doi.org/10.1177/0963721415569569

Drewing, K., & Lezkan, A. (2021). Masking interferes with haptic texture perception from sequential exploratory movements. *Attention, Perception, & Psychophysics, 83*(4), 1766–1776. https://doi.org/10.3758/s13414-021-02253-w

Driver, J. (1996, May 2). Enhancement of selective listening by illusory mislocation of speech sounds due to lip-reading. *Nature, 381*(6577), 66–68. https://doi.org/10.1038/381066a0

Driver, J., Baylis, G. C., Goodrich, S. J., & Rafal, R. D. (1994). Axis-based neglect of visual shapes. *Neuropsychologia, 32*(11), 1353–1356. https://doi.org/10.1016/0028-3932(94)00068-9

Driver, J., IV, Davis, G., Ricciardelli, P., Kidd, P., Maxwell, E., & Baron-Cohen, S. (1999). Gaze perception triggers reflexive visuospatial orienting. *Visual Cognition*, *6*(5), 509–540. https://doi.org/10.1080/135062899394920

Driver, J., & Pouget, A. (2000). Object-centered visual neglect, or relative egocentric neglect? *Journal of Cognitive Neuroscience*, *12*(3), 542–545. https://doi.org/10.1162/089892900562192

Driver, J., & Spence, C. J. (1994). Spatial synergies between auditory and visual attention. In C. Umiltà & M. Moscovitch (Eds.), *Attention and performance XV: Conscious and nonconscious information processing* (pp. 311–331). MIT Press.

Driver, J., & Spence, C. (1998). Attention and the crossmodal construction of space. *Trends in Cognitive Sciences*, *2*(7), 254–262. https://doi.org/10.1016/S1364-6613(98)01188-7

Driver, J., & Spence, C. (2004). Crossmodal spatial attention: Evidence from human performance. In J. Driver & C. Spence (Eds.), *Crossmodal space and crossmodal attention* (pp. 178–220). Oxford University Press. https://doi.org/10.1093/acprof:oso/9780198524861.003.0008

Drop, L. (2014, November 25). Laurel and Hardy: Best friends for life. *GERM Magazine*. https://germmagazine.com/laurel-and-hardy-best-friends-for-life/

Dugué, L., Merriam, E. P., Heeger, D. J., & Carrasco, M. (2020). Differential impact of endogenous and exogenous attention on activity in human visual cortex. *Scientific Reports*, *10*, Article 21274. https://doi.org/10.1038/s41598-020-78172-x

Dukewich, K. R., & Klein, R. M. (2015). Inhibition of return: A phenomenon in search of a definition and a theoretical framework. *Attention, Perception, & Psychophysics*, *77*(5), 1647–1658. https://doi.org/10.3758/s13414-015-0835-3

Duncan, J. (1980). The locus of interference in the perception of simultaneous stimuli. *Psychological Review*, *87*(3), 272–300. https://doi.org/10.1037/0033-295X.87.3.272

Duncan, J. (1983). Perceptual selection based on alphanumeric class: Evidence from partial reports. *Perception & Psychophysics*, *33*(6), 533–547. https://doi.org/10.3758/BF03202935

Duncan, J. (1984). Selective attention and the organization of visual information. *Journal of Experimental Psychology: General*, *113*(4), 501–517. https://doi.org/10.1037/0096-3445.113.4.501

Duncan, J., Emslie, H., Williams, P., Johnson, R., & Freer, C. (1996). Intelligence and the frontal lobe: The organization of goal-directed behavior. *Cognitive Psychology*, *30*(3), 257–303. https://doi.org/10.1006/cogp.1996.0008

Duncan, J., & Humphreys, G. W. (1989). Visual search and stimulus similarity. *Psychological Review*, *96*(3), 433–458. https://doi.org/10.1037/0033-295X.96.3.433

Duncan, J., Martens, S., & Ward, R. (1997, June 19). Restricted attentional capacity within but not between sensory modalities. *Nature*, *387*(6635), 808–810. https://doi.org/10.1038/42947

Duncan, J., Ward, R., & Shapiro, K. (1994, May 26). Direct measurement of attentional dwell time in human vision. *Nature*, *369*(6478), 313–315. https://doi.org/10.1038/369313a0

Durgin, F. H. (2000). The reverse Stroop effect. *Psychonomic Bulletin & Review*, *7*(1), 121–125. https://doi.org/10.3758/BF03210730

Durso, F. T., Bleckley, M. K., & Dattel, A. R. (2006). Does situation awareness add to the validity of cognitive tests? *Human Factors*, *48*(4), 721–733. https://doi.org/10.1518/001872006779166316

Durso, F. T., & Dattel, A. R. (2004). SPAM: The real-time assessment of SA. In S. Banbury & S. Tremblay (Eds.), *A cognitive approach to situation awareness: Theory and application* (pp. 137–154). Ashgate.

Dux, P. E., & Marois, R. (2009). The attentional blink: A review of data and theory. *Attention, Perception, & Psychophysics, 71*(8), 1683–1700. https://doi.org/10.3758/APP.71.8.1683

Dvorsky, M. R., & Langberg, J. M. (2016). A review of factors that promote resilience in youth with ADHD and ADHD symptoms. *Clinical Child and Family Psychology Review, 19*(4), 368–391. https://doi.org/10.1007/s10567-016-0216-z

Eben, C., Koch, I., Jolicoeur, P., & Nolden, S. (2020). The persisting influence of unattended auditory information: Negative priming in intentional auditory attention switching. *Attention, Perception, & Psychophysics, 82*(4), 1835–1846. https://doi.org/10.3758/s13414-019-01909-y

Edgar, G. K., Edgar, H. E., & Curry, M. B. (2003, October). Using signal detection theory to measure situation awareness in command and control. *Proceedings of the Human Factors and Ergonomics Society Annual Meeting, 47*(18), 2019–2023. https://doi.org/10.1177/154193120304701815

Egan, J., Carterette, E., & Thwing, E. (1954). Some factors affecting multichannel listening. *The Journal of the Acoustical Society of America, 26*(5), 774–782. https://doi.org/10.1121/1.1907416

Eggemeier, F. T., & Wilson, G. F. (1991). Performance-based and subjective assessment of workload in multi-task environments. In D. L. Damos (Ed.), *Multiple-task performance* (pp. 217–278). Taylor & Francis.

Eggemeier, F. T., Wilson, G. F., Kramer, A. F., & Damos, D. L. (1991). Workload assessment in multi-task environments. In D. L. Damos (Ed.), *Multiple-task performance* (pp. 207–216). Taylor & Francis.

Egly, R., Driver, J., & Rafal, R. D. (1994). Shifting visual attention between objects and locations: Evidence from normal and parietal lesion subjects. *Journal of Experimental Psychology: General, 123*(2), 161–177. https://doi.org/10.1037/0096-3445.123.2.161

Eimer, M., Cockburn, D., Smedley, B., & Driver, J. (2001). Cross-modal links in endogenous spatial attention are mediated by common external locations: Evidence from event-related brain potentials. *Experimental Brain Research, 139*(4), 398–411. https://doi.org/10.1007/s002210100773

Eimer, M., & Schröger, E. (1998). ERP effects of intermodal attention and cross-modal links in spatial attention. *Psychophysiology, 35*(3), 313–327. https://doi.org/10.1017/S004857729897086X

Elander, J., West, R., & French, D. (1993). Behavioral correlates of individual differences in road-traffic crash risk: An examination method and findings. *Psychological Bulletin, 113*(2), 279–294. https://doi.org/10.1037/0033-2909.113.2.279

Elio, R. (1986). Representation of similar well-learned cognitive procedures. *Cognitive Science, 10*(1), 41–73. https://doi.org/10.1207/s15516709cog1001_2

Endsley, M. R. (1995a). Measurement of situation awareness in dynamic systems. *Human Factors, 37*(1), 65–84. https://doi.org/10.1518/001872095779049499

Endsley, M. R. (1995b). Toward a theory of situation awareness in dynamic systems. *Human Factors, 37*(1), 32–64. https://doi.org/10.1518/001872095779049543

Endsley, M. R. (2017). From here to autonomy: Lessons learned from human–automation research. *Human Factors, 59*(1), 5–27. https://doi.org/10.1177/0018720816681350

Endsley, M. R. (2020). The divergence of objective and subjective situation awareness: A meta-analysis. *Journal of Cognitive Engineering and Decision Making, 14*(1), 34–53. https://doi.org/10.1177/1555343419874248

Endsley, M. R., Bolstad, C. A., Jones, D. G., & Riley, J. M. (2003, October). Situation awareness oriented design: From user's cognitive requirements to creating effective supporting technologies. *Proceedings of the Human Factors and Ergonomics Society Annual Meeting, 47*(3), 268–272. https://doi.org/10.1177/154193120304700304

Endsley, M. R., & Kiris, E. O. (1995). The out-of-the-loop performance problem and level of control in automation. *Human Factors, 37*(2), 381–394. https://doi.org/10.1518/001872095779064555

Engle, R. W. (2002). Working memory capacity as executive attention. *Current Directions in Psychological Science, 11*(1), 19–23. https://doi.org/10.1111/1467-8721.00160

Engle, R. W. (2018). Working memory and executive attention: A revisit. *Perspectives on Psychological Science, 13*(2), 190–193. https://doi.org/10.1177/1745691617720478

Enns, J. T., & Girgus, J. S. (1985). Developmental changes in selective and integrative visual attention. *Journal of Experimental Child Psychology, 40*(2), 319–337. https://doi.org/10.1016/0022-0965(85)90093-1

Enns, J. T., & Rensink, R. A. (1990, February 9). Influence of scene-based properties on visual search. *Science, 247*(4943), 721–723. https://doi.org/10.1126/science.2300824

Entin, E. E., & Serfaty, D. (1999). Adaptive team coordination. *Human Factors, 41*(2), 312–325. https://doi.org/10.1518/001872099779591196

Eramudugolla, R., Irvine, D. R., McAnally, K. I., Martin, R. L., & Mattingley, J. B. (2005). Directed attention eliminates 'change deafness' in complex auditory scenes. *Current Biology, 15*(12), 1108–1113. https://doi.org/10.1016/j.cub.2005.05.051

Erel, H., & Levy, D. A. (2016). Orienting of visual attention in aging. *Neuroscience and Biobehavioral Reviews, 69*, 357–380. https://doi.org/10.1016/j.neubiorev.2016.08.010

Erev, I., & Gopher, D. (1999). A cognitive game-theoretic analysis of attention strategies, ability, and incentives. In D. Gopher & A. Koriat (Eds.), *Attention and performance XVII: Cognitive regulation of performance: Interaction of theory and application* (pp. 343–371). MIT Press.

Eriksen, B. A., & Eriksen, C. W. (1974). Effects of noise letters upon the identification of a target letter in a nonsearch task. *Perception & Psychophysics, 16*(1), 143–149. https://doi.org/10.3758/BF03203267

Eriksen, C. W. (1995). The flankers task and response competition: A useful tool for investigating a variety of cognitive problems. *Visual Cognition, 2*(2-3), 101–118. https://doi.org/10.1080/13506289508401726

Eriksen, C. W., & Hoffman, J. E. (1973). The extent of processing of noise elements during selective encoding from visual displays. *Perception & Psychophysics, 14*(1), 155–160. https://doi.org/10.3758/BF03198630

Eriksen, C. W., & Murphy, T. D. (1987). Movement of attentional focus across the visual field: A critical look at the evidence. *Perception & Psychophysics, 42*(3), 299–305. https://doi.org/10.3758/BF03203082

Eriksen, C. W., & St. James, J. D. (1986). Visual attention within and around the field of focal attention: A zoom lens model. *Perception & Psychophysics, 40*(4), 225–240. https://doi.org/10.3758/BF03211502

Eriksen, C. W., & Webb, J. M. (1989). Shifting of attentional focus within and about a visual display. *Perception & Psychophysics, 45*(2), 175–183. https://doi.org/10.3758/BF03208052

Eriksen, C. W., & Yeh, Y. Y. (1985). Allocation of attention in the visual field. *Journal of Experimental Psychology: Human Perception and Performance, 11*(5), 583–597. https://doi.org/10.1037/0096-1523.11.5.583

Ermutlu, M. N., Demiralp, T., & Karamürsel, S. (2007). The effects of interstimulus interval on sensory gating and on preattentive auditory memory in the oddball paradigm: Can magnitude of the sensory gating affect preattentive auditory comparison process? *Neuroscience Letters, 412*(1), 1–5. https://doi.org/10.1016/j.neulet.2006.09.006

Eskenazi, T., Doerrfeld, A., Logan, G. D., Knoblich, G., & Sebanz, N. (2013). Your words are my words: Effects of acting together on encoding. *Quarterly Journal of Experimental Psychology, 66*(5), 1026–1034. https://doi.org/10.1080/17470218.2012.725058

Exner, S. (1882). Zur kenntniss von der wechselwirkung der erregungen im central-nervensystem [To the knowledge of the interaction of the excitations in the central nervous system]. *Archiv für die gesamte Physiologie des Menschen und der Tiere, 28*, 487–506.

Fadden, D. M., Morton, P. M., Taylor, R. W., & Lindberg, T. (2015). *First-hand evolution of the 2-person crew jet transport flight deck.* https://ethw.org/First-Hand:Evolution_of_the_2-Person_Crew_Jet_Transport_Flight_Deck

Fairclough, S. H., & Venables, L. (2006). Prediction of subjective states from psycho-physiology: A multivariate approach. *Biological Psychology, 71*(1), 100–110. https://doi.org/10.1016/j.biopsycho.2005.03.007

Fan, J., McCandliss, B. D., Sommer, T., Raz, A., & Posner, M. I. (2002). Testing the efficiency and independence of attentional networks. *Journal of Cognitive Neuroscience, 14*(3), 340–347. https://doi.org/10.1162/089892902317361886

Fan, J., & Posner, M. (2004). Human attentional networks. *Psychiatrische Praxis, 31*(S2), 210–214.

Fan, J., & Smith, A. P. (2020). Effects of occupational fatigue on cognitive performance of staff from a train operating company: A field study. *Frontiers in Psychology, 11*, Article 558520. https://doi.org/10.3389/fpsyg.2020.558520

Farah, M. J., Wong, A. B., Monheit, M. A., & Morrow, L. A. (1989). Parietal lobe mechanisms of spatial attention: Modality-specific or supramodal? *Neuropsychologia, 27*(4), 461–470. https://doi.org/10.1016/0028-3932(89)90051-1

Fawcett, J. M., Russell, E. J., Peace, K. A., & Christie, J. (2013). Of guns and geese: A meta-analytic review of the 'weapon focus' literature. *Psychology, Crime & Law, 19*(1), 35–66. https://doi.org/10.1080/1068316X.2011.599325

Fechner, G. T. (1966). *Elements of psychophysics* (H. E. Adler, Trans.). Holt, Rinehart & Winston.

Fels, J., Oberem, J., & Koch, I. (2016). Examining auditory selective attention in realistic, natural environments with an optimized paradigm. *Proceedings of Meetings on Acoustics, 28*(1), Article 050001.

Ferber, S., & Karnath, H. O. (2001). How to assess spatial neglect—Line bisection or cancellation tasks? *Journal of Clinical and Experimental Neuropsychology, 23*(5), 599–607. https://doi.org/10.1076/jcen.23.5.599.1243

Fernández, A., & Carrasco, M. (2020). Extinguishing exogenous attention via transcranial magnetic stimulation. *Current Biology, 30*(20), 4078–4084. https://doi.org/10.1016/j.cub.2020.07.068

Ferrari, M., & Quaresima, V. (2012). A brief review on the history of human functional near-infrared spectroscopy (fNIRS) development and fields of application. *NeuroImage, 63*(2), 921–935. https://doi.org/10.1016/j.neuroimage.2012.03.049

Fischer, B. (1986). The role of attention in the preparation of visually guided eye movements in monkey and man. *Psychological Research, 48*(4), 251–257. https://doi.org/10.1007/BF00309089

Fischer, B., Biscaldi, M., & Gezeck, S. (1997). On the development of voluntary and reflexive components in human saccade generation. *Brain Research, 754*(1-2), 285–297. https://doi.org/10.1016/S0006-8993(97)00094-2

Fischer, G. (1991). The importance of models and making complex systems comprehensible. In M. J. Talber & D. Ackermann (Eds.), *Mental models and human-computer interaction 2* (pp. 3–36). North-Holland. https://doi.org/10.1016/B978-0-444-88602-6.50005-0

Fischer, R., & Plessow, F. (2015). Efficient multitasking: Parallel versus serial processing of multiple tasks. *Frontiers in Psychology, 6*, Article 1366. https://doi.org/10.3389/fpsyg.2015.01366

Fisher, R. A. (1937). *The design of experiments* (2nd ed.). Oliver and Boyd.

Fitts, P. M. (1964). Perceptual-motor skill learning. In A. W. Melton (Ed.), *Categories of human learning* (pp. 243–285). Academic Press. https://doi.org/10.1016/B978-1-4832-3145-7.50016-9

Fitts, P. M., & Deininger, R. L. (1954). S-R compatibility: Correspondence among paired elements within stimulus and response codes. *Journal of Experimental Psychology, 48*(6), 483–492. https://doi.org/10.1037/h0054967

Fitts, P. M., Jones, R. E., & Milton, J. L. (1950). Eye movements of aircraft pilots during instrument-landing approaches. *Aeronautical Engineering Review, 9*(2), 1–6.

Fitts, P. M., & Posner, M. I. (1967). *Human performance.* Brooks/Cole.

Fitts, P. M., & Seeger, C. M. (1953). S-R compatibility: Spatial characteristics of stimulus and response codes. *Journal of Experimental Psychology, 46*(3), 199–210. https://doi.org/10.1037/h0062827

Flach, J. M. (2001). A meaning processing approach to analysis and design. In M. J. Smith, G. Salvendy, D. Harris, & R. J. Koubek (Eds.), *Usability evaluation and interface design: Cognitive engineering, intelligent agents, and virtual reality* (Vol. 1, pp. 1405–1409). Erlbaum.

Floden, D., Vallesi, A., & Stuss, D. T. (2011). Task context and frontal lobe activation in the Stroop task. *Journal of Cognitive Neuroscience, 23*(4), 867–879. https://doi.org/10.1162/jocn.2010.21492

Folk, C. L., Remington, R. W., & Johnston, J. C. (1992). Involuntary covert orienting is contingent on attentional control settings. *Journal of Experimental Psychology: Human Perception and Performance, 18*(4), 1030–1044. https://doi.org/10.1037/0096-1523.18.4.1030

Foroughi, C. K., Werner, N. E., Barragán, D., & Boehm-Davis, D. A. (2015). Interruptions disrupt reading comprehension. *Journal of Experimental Psychology: General, 144*(3), 704–709. https://doi.org/10.1037/xge0000074

Forster, B., & Eimer, M. (2005). Covert attention in touch: Behavioral and ERP evidence for costs and benefits. *Psychophysiology, 42*(2), 171–179. https://doi.org/10.1111/j.1469-8986.2005.00268.x

Fosco, W. D., Kofler, M. J., Alderson, R. M., Tarle, S. J., Raiker, J. S., & Sarver, D. E. (2019). Inhibitory control and information processing in ADHD: Comparing the dual task and performance adjustment hypotheses. *Journal of Abnormal Child Psychology, 47*(6), 961–974. https://doi.org/10.1007/s10802-018-0504-9

Foundas, A. L., Corey, D. M., Hurley, M. M., & Heilman, K. M. (2006). Verbal dichotic listening in right and left-handed adults: Laterality effects of directed attention. *Cortex, 42*(1), 79–86. https://doi.org/10.1016/S0010-9452(08)70324-1

Fox, E., & De Fockert, J. W. (1998). Negative priming depends on prime-probe similarity: Evidence for episodic retrieval. *Psychonomic Bulletin & Review, 5*(1), 107–113. https://doi.org/10.3758/BF03209464

Foyle, D. C., Dowell, S. R., & Hooey, B. L. (2001). Cognitive tunneling in head-up display (HUD) superimposed symbology: Effects of information location. In R. S. Jensen (Ed.), *Proceedings of the Eleventh Symposium on Aviation Psychology* (pp. 143:1–143:6). Ohio State University.

Franceschini, S., Gori, S., Ruffino, M., Viola, S., Molteni, M., & Facoetti, A. (2013). Action video games make dyslexic children read better. *Current Biology, 23*(6), 462–466. https://doi.org/10.1016/j.cub.2013.01.044

Francis, G. (2000). Designing multifunction displays: An optimization approach. *International Journal of Cognitive Ergonomics, 4*(2), 107–124. https://doi.org/10.1207/S15327566IJCE0402_2

Frankmann, J. P., & Adams, J. A. (1962). Theories of vigilance. *Psychological Bulletin, 59*(4), 257–272. https://doi.org/10.1037/h0046142

Friesen, C. K., & Kingstone, A. (1998). The eyes have it! Reflexive orienting is triggered by nonpredictive gaze. *Psychonomic Bulletin & Review, 5*(3), 490–495. https://doi.org/10.3758/BF03208827

Frings, C., Englert, J., Wentura, D., & Bermeitinger, C. (2010). Decomposing the emotional Stroop effect. *Quarterly Journal of Experimental Psychology, 63*(1), 42–49. https://doi.org/10.1080/17470210903156594

Frings, C., Schneider, K. K., & Fox, E. (2015). The negative priming paradigm: An update and implications for selective attention. *Psychonomic Bulletin & Review, 22*(6), 1577–1597. https://doi.org/10.3758/s13423-015-0841-4

Frischen, A., Bayliss, A. P., & Tipper, S. P. (2007). Gaze cueing of attention: Visual attention, social cognition, and individual differences. *Psychological Bulletin, 133*(4), 694–724. https://doi.org/10.1037/0033-2909.133.4.694

Frith, C., & Frith, U. (2005). Theory of mind. *Current Biology, 15*(17), R644–R645. https://doi.org/10.1016/j.cub.2005.08.041

Fu, S., Fedota, J. R., Greenwood, P. M., & Parasuraman, R. (2010). Dissociation of visual C1 and P1 components as a function of attentional load: An event-related potential study. *Biological Psychology, 85*(1), 171–178. https://doi.org/10.1016/j.biopsycho.2010.06.008

Gabbay, C., Zivony, A., & Lamy, D. (2019). Splitting the attentional spotlight? Evidence from attentional capture by successive events. *Visual Cognition, 27*(5-8), 518–536. https://doi.org/10.1080/13506285.2019.1617377

Gage, N. M., & Baars, B. J. (2018). *Fundamentals of cognitive neuroscience: A beginner's guide* (2nd ed.). Academic Press.

Gallace, A., Tan, H. Z., & Spence, C. (2006). The failure to detect tactile change: A tactile analogue of visual change blindness. *Psychonomic Bulletin & Review, 13*(2), 300–303. https://doi.org/10.3758/BF03193847

Garavan, H. (1998). Serial attention within working memory. *Memory & Cognition, 26*(2), 263–276. https://doi.org/10.3758/BF03201138

Gardner, A. K., Scott, D. J., & AbdelFattah, K. R. (2017). Do great teams think alike? An examination of team mental models and their impact on team performance. *Surgery, 161*(5), 1203–1208. https://doi.org/10.1016/j.surg.2016.11.010

Garner, W. R. (1976). Interaction of stimulus dimensions in concept and choice processes. *Cognitive Psychology, 8*(1), 98–123. https://doi.org/10.1016/0010-0285(76)90006-2

Gartenberg, D., Gunzelmann, G., Hassanzadeh-Behbaha, S., & Trafton, J. G. (2018). Examining the role of task requirements in the magnitude of the vigilance decrement. *Frontiers in Psychology, 9,* Article 1504. https://doi.org/10.3389/fpsyg.2018.01504

Gaspelin, N., Leonard, C. J., & Luck, S. J. (2015). Direct evidence for active suppression of salient-but-irrelevant sensory inputs. *Psychological Science, 26*(11), 1740–1750. https://doi.org/10.1177/0956797615597913

Gaspelin, N., Leonard, C. J., & Luck, S. J. (2017). Suppression of overt attentional capture by salient-but-irrelevant color singletons. *Attention, Perception, & Psychophysics, 79*(1), 45–62. https://doi.org/10.3758/s13414-016-1209-1

Gaspelin, N., & Luck, S. J. (2019). Inhibition as a potential resolution to the attentional capture debate. *Current Opinion in Psychology, 29,* 12–18. https://doi.org/10.1016/j.copsyc.2018.10.013

Gaymard, B., Lynch, J., Ploner, C. J., Condy, C., & Rivaud-Péchoux, S. (2003). The parieto-collicular pathway: Anatomical location and contribution to saccade generation. *The European Journal of Neuroscience, 17*(7), 1518–1526. https://doi.org/10.1046/j.1460-9568.2003.02570.x

Geffen, G., & Sexton, M. A. (1978). The development of auditory strategies of attention. *Developmental Psychology, 14*(1), 11–17. https://doi.org/10.1037/0012-1649.14.1.11

Geissler, L. R. (1912). Analysis of consciousness under negative instruction. *The American Journal of Psychology, 23*(2), 183–213. https://doi.org/10.2307/1412840

Gervits, F., Thurston, D., Thielstrom, R., Fong, T., Pham, Q., & Scheutz, M. (2020, May 9–13). Toward genuine robot teammates: Improving human–robot team performance using robot shared mental models. In A. El Fallah Seghrouchni, G. Sukthankar, B. An, & N. Yorke Smith (Chairs), *Proceedings of the 19th International Conference on Autonomous Agents and Multiagent Systems* (pp. 429–437). International Conference on Autonomous Agents and Multiagent Systems, Auckland, New Zealand.

Gibson, J. J. (1941). A critical review of the concept of set in contemporary experimental psychology. *Psychological Bulletin, 38*(9), 781–817. https://doi.org/10.1037/h0055307

Gill, N. F., & Dallenbach, K. M. (1926). A preliminary study of the range of attention. *The American Journal of Psychology, 37*(2), 247–256. https://doi.org/10.2307/1413693

Glucksberg, S., & Cowan, G. N., Jr. (1970). Memory for nonattended auditory material. *Cognitive Psychology, 1*(2), 149–156. https://doi.org/10.1016/0010-0285(70)90010-1

Gola, M., Magnuski, M., Szumska, I., & Wróbel, A. (2013). EEG beta band activity is related to attention and attentional deficits in the visual performance of elderly subjects. *International Journal of Psychophysiology, 89*(3), 334–341. https://doi.org/10.1016/j.ijpsycho.2013.05.007

Goldsmith, M. (1998). What's in a location? Comparing object-based and space-based models of feature integration in visual search. *Journal of Experimental Psychology: General, 127*(2), 189–219. https://doi.org/10.1037/0096-3445.127.2.189

Gollwitzer, P. M. (1999). Implementation intentions: Strong effects of simple plans. *American Psychologist, 54*(7), 493–503. https://doi.org/10.1037/0003-066X.54.7.493

Goodhew, S. C., Shen, E., & Edwards, M. (2016). Selective spatial enhancement: Attentional spotlight size impacts spatial but not temporal perception. *Psychonomic Bulletin & Review*, *23*(4), 1144–1149. https://doi.org/10.3758/s13423-015-0904-6

Gopher, D. (1993). The skill of attention control: Acquisition and execution of attention strategies. In D. E. Meyer & S. Kornblum (Eds.), *Attention and performance XIV* (pp. 299–322). MIT Press.

Gopher, D. (1994). Analysis and measurement of mental load. In G. d'Ydewalle, P. Edlen, & P. Bertelson (Eds.), *International perspectives on psychological science: Vol. 2. The state of the art* (pp. 265–291). Erlbaum.

Gopher, D., & Barzilai, O. (1993). The effect of knowledge levels on operators' response to malfunctions and technical problems in the system. *Proceedings of IEEE Systems Man and Cybernetics Conference*, *1*, 185–190.

Gopher, D., Brickner, M., & Navon, D. (1982). Different difficulty manipulations interact differently with task emphasis: Evidence for multiple resources. *Journal of Experimental Psychology: Human Perception and Performance*, *8*(1), 146–157. https://doi.org/10.1037/0096-1523.8.1.146

Gopher, D., & Donchin, E. (1986). Workload: An examination of the concept. In K. R. Boff, L. Kaufman, & J. P. Thomas (Eds.), *Handbook of perception and human performance: Vol. 2. Cognitive processes and performance* (pp. 1–49). Wiley.

Gottsdanker, R., & Stelmach, G. E. (1971). The persistence of psychological refractoriness. *Journal of Motor Behavior*, *3*(4), 301–312. https://doi.org/10.1080/00222895.1971.10734910

Grassi, M., Crotti, C., Giofrè, D., Boedker, I., & Toffalini, E. (2021). Two replications of Raymond, Shapiro, and Arnell (1992), the attentional blink. *Behavior Research Methods*, *53*(2), 656–668. https://doi.org/10.3758/s13428-020-01457-6

Gratton, G., Coles, M. G., & Donchin, E. (1992). Optimizing the use of information: Strategic control of activation of responses. *Journal of Experimental Psychology: General*, *121*(4), 480–506. https://doi.org/10.1037/0096-3445.121.4.480

Gratton, G., Coles, M. G., Sirevaag, E. J., Eriksen, C. W., & Donchin, E. (1988). Pre- and poststimulus activation of response channels: A psychophysiological analysis. *Journal of Experimental Psychology: Human Perception and Performance*, *14*(3), 331–344. https://doi.org/10.1037/0096-1523.14.3.331

Gray, J. A., & Wedderburn, A. A. I. (1960). Grouping strategies with simultaneous stimuli. *Quarterly Journal of Experimental Psychology*, *12*(3), 180–184. https://doi.org/10.1080/17470216008416722

Green, C. S., & Bavelier, D. (2003, May 29). Action video game modifies visual selective attention. *Nature*, *423*(6939), 534–537. https://doi.org/10.1038/nature01647

Green, D. M., & Swets, J. A. (1966). *Signal detection theory and psychophysics*. Wiley.

Greenlee, M. W., & Kimmig, H. (2019). Visual perception and eye movements. In C. Klein & U. Ettinger (Eds.), *Eye movement research: An introduction to its scientific foundations and applications* (pp. 165–196). Springer. https://doi.org/10.1007/978-3-030-20085-5_5

Greenwald, A. G. (1970). Sensory feedback mechanisms in performance control: With special reference to the ideo-motor mechanism. *Psychological Review*, *77*(2), 73–99. https://doi.org/10.1037/h0028689

Greenwald, A. G., & Shulman, H. G. (1973). On doing two things at once: II. Elimination of the psychological refractory period effect. *Journal of Experimental Psychology*, *101*(1), 70–76. https://doi.org/10.1037/h0035451

Gregg, M. K., Irsik, V. C., & Snyder, J. S. (2017). Effects of capacity limits, memory loss, and sound type in change deafness. *Attention, Perception, & Psychophysics*, *79*(8), 2564–2575. https://doi.org/10.3758/s13414-017-1416-4

Grier, R. A. (2015). How high is high? A meta-analysis of NASA-TLX global workload scores. *Proceedings of the Human Factors and Ergonomics Society Annual Meeting*, *59*(1), 1727–1731. https://doi.org/10.1177/1541931215591373

Gunning, D., & Aha, D. (2019). DARPA's explainable artificial intelligence (XAI) program. *AI Magazine*, *40*(2), 44–58. https://doi.org/10.1609/aimag.v40i2.2850

Güntekin, B., Saatçi, E., & Yener, G. (2008). Decrease of evoked delta, theta and alpha coherences in Alzheimer patients during a visual oddball paradigm. *Brain Research*, *1235*, 109–116. https://doi.org/10.1016/j.brainres.2008.06.028

Hadlow, S. M., Panchuk, D., Mann, D. L., Portus, M. R., & Abernethy, B. (2018). Modified perceptual training in sport: A new classification framework. *Journal of Science and Medicine in Sport*, *21*(9), 950–958. https://doi.org/10.1016/j.jsams.2018.01.011

Haider, H., Esser, S., & Eberhardt, K. (2020). Feature codes in implicit sequence learning: Perceived stimulus locations transfer to motor response locations. *Psychological Research*, *84*(1), 192–203. https://doi.org/10.1007/s00426-018-0980-0

Haigh, S. M., Coffman, B. A., & Salisbury, D. F. (2017). Mismatch negativity in first-episode schizophrenia: A meta-analysis. *Clinical EEG and Neuroscience*, *48*(1), 3–10. https://doi.org/10.1177/1550059416645980

Hallett, P. E. (1978). Primary and secondary saccades to goals defined by instructions. *Vision Research*, *18*(10), 1279–1296. https://doi.org/10.1016/0042-6989(78)90218-3

Hamilton, W. (1859). *Lectures on metaphysics and logic: Vol. 1. Metaphysics.* Gould and Lincoln.

Han, B., & Leite, F. (2021). Measuring the impact of immersive virtual reality on construction design review applications: Head-mounted display versus desktop monitor. *Journal of Construction Engineering and Management*, *147*(6), Article 04021042. https://doi.org/10.1061/(ASCE)CO.1943-7862.0002056

Hancock, P. A., Oron-Gilad, T., & Szalma, J. L. (2007). Elaborations of the multiple-resource theory of attention. In A. F. Kramer, D. A. Wiegmann, & A. Kirlik (Eds.), *Attention: From theory to practice* (pp. 45–56). Oxford University Press.

Handy, T. C., & Mangun, G. R. (2000). Attention and spatial selection: Electrophysiological evidence for modulation by perceptual load. *Perception & Psychophysics*, *62*(1), 175–186. https://doi.org/10.3758/BF03212070

Hanslmayr, S., Gross, J., Klimesch, W., & Shapiro, K. L. (2011). The role of α oscillations in temporal attention. *Brain Research Reviews*, *67*(1-2), 331–343. https://doi.org/10.1016/j.brainresrev.2011.04.002

Happé, F., Cook, J. L., & Bird, G. (2017). The structure of social cognition: In(ter) dependence of sociocognitive processes. *Annual Review of Psychology*, *68*(1), 243–267. https://doi.org/10.1146/annurev-psych-010416-044046

Harding, B., & Cousineau, D. (2022). Is the fast–same phenomenon that fast? An investigation of identity priming in the same–different task. *Journal of Experimental Psychology: Learning, Memory, and Cognition*, *48*(4), 520–546. https://doi.org/10.1037/xlm0001076

Harjunen, V. J., Ahmed, I., Jacucci, G., Ravaja, N., & Spapé, M. M. (2017). Manipulating bodily presence affects cross-modal spatial attention: A virtual-reality-based ERP study. *Frontiers in Human Neuroscience*, *11*, Article 79. https://doi.org/10.3389/fnhum.2017.00079

Harleß, E. (1861). Der apparat des willens [The apparatus of will] (R. Pfister & M. Janczyk, Trans.). *Zeitschrift für Philosophie und philosophische Kritik, 38*, 50–73.

Harmony, T. (2013). The functional significance of delta oscillations in cognitive processing. *Frontiers in Integrative Neuroscience, 7*, Article 83. https://doi.org/10.3389/fnint.2013.00083

Harrison, J., İzzetoğlu, K., Ayaz, H., Willems, B., Hah, S., Ahlstrom, U., Woo, H., Shewokis, P. A., Bunce, S. C., & Onaral, B. (2014). Cognitive workload and learning assessment during the implementation of a next-generation air traffic control technology using functional near-infrared spectroscopy. *IEEE Transactions on Human-Machine Systems, 44*(4), 429–440. https://doi.org/10.1109/THMS.2014.2319822

Hart, S. G. (2006, October). NASA-task load index (NASA-TLX): 20 years later. *Proceedings of the Human Factors and Ergonomics Society Annual Meeting, 50*(9), 904–908. https://doi.org/10.1177/154193120605000909

Hart, S. G., & Staveland, L. E. (1988). Development of NASA-TLX (Task Load Index): Results of empirical and theoretical research. In P. A. Hancock & N. Meshkati (Eds.), *Advances in Psychology: Vol. 52. Human mental workload* (pp. 139–183). North-Holland. https://doi.org/10.1016/S0166-4115(08)62386-9

Hasbroucq, T., & Guiard, Y. (1992). The effects of intensity and irrelevant location of a tactile stimulation in a choice reaction time task. *Neuropsychologia, 30*(1), 91–94. https://doi.org/10.1016/0028-3932(92)90017-G

Hasher, L., Lustig, C., & Zacks, R. T. (2007). Inhibitory mechanisms and the control of attention. In A. R. A. Conway, C. Jarrold, M. J. Kane, A. Miyake, & J. N. Towse (Eds.), *Variation in working memory* (pp. 227–249). Oxford University Press.

Hatfield, G. (1998). Attention in early scientific psychology. In R. D. Wright (Ed.), *Visual attention* (pp. 3–25). Oxford University Press.

Haxby, J. V., Courtney, S. M., & Clark, V. P. (1998). Functional magnetic resonance imaging and the study of attention. In R. Parasuraman (Ed.), *The attentive brain* (pp. 123–142). MIT press.

Healy, A. F., & Bourne, L. E., Jr. (Eds.). (2012). *Training cognition: Optimizing efficiency, durability, and generalizability*. Psychology Press. https://doi.org/10.4324/9780203816783

Healy, A. F., Kole, J. A., & Bourne, L. E., Jr. (2014). Training principles to advance expertise. *Frontiers in Psychology, 5*, Article 131. https://doi.org/10.3389/fpsyg.2014.00131

Heathcote, A., Brown, S., & Mewhort, D. J. (2000). The power law repealed: The case for an exponential law of practice. *Psychonomic Bulletin & Review, 7*(2), 185–207. https://doi.org/10.3758/BF03212979

Heaton, R. K., Grant, I., & Mathews, C. G. (1991). *Comprehensive norms for expanded Halstead-Reitan battery*. Psychological Assessment Resources.

Hebb, D. O. (1949). *The organization of behavior*. Wiley-Interscience.

Heidlmayr, K., Kihlstedt, M., & Isel, F. (2020). A review on the electroencephalography markers of Stroop executive control processes. *Brain and Cognition, 146*, 105637. https://doi.org/10.1016/j.bandc.2020.105637

Heilman, K. M., Bowers, D., Coslett, H. B., Whelan, H., & Watson, R. T. (1985). Directional hypokinesia: Prolonged reaction times for leftward movements in patients with right hemisphere lesions and neglect. *Neurology, 35*(6), 855–859. https://doi.org/10.1212/WNL.35.6.855

Heilman, K. M., & Valenstein, E. (1979). Mechanisms underlying hemispatial neglect. *Annals of Neurology, 5*(2), 166–170. https://doi.org/10.1002/ana.410050210

Heilman, K. M., Watson, R. T., & Valenstein, E. (1985). Neglect and related disorders. In K. M. Heilman & E. Valenstein (Eds.), *Clinical neuropsychology* (2nd ed., pp. 243–293). Oxford University Press.

Hein, E., Rolke, B., & Ulrich, R. (2006). Visual attention and temporal discrimination: Differential effects of automatic and voluntary cueing. *Visual Cognition*, *13*(1), 29–50. https://doi.org/10.1080/13506280500143524

Heinke, W., Kenntner, R., Gunter, T. C., Sammler, D., Olthoff, D., & Koelsch, S. (2004). Sequential effects of increasing propofol sedation on frontal and temporal cortices as indexed by auditory event-related potentials. *Anesthesiology*, *100*(3), 617–625. https://doi.org/10.1097/00000542-200403000-00023

Heinze, H. J., Luck, S. J., Mangun, G. R., & Hillyard, S. A. (1990). Visual event-related potentials index focused attention within bilateral stimulus arrays: I. Evidence for early selection. *Electroencephalography and Clinical Neurophysiology*, *75*(6), 511–527. https://doi.org/10.1016/0013-4694(90)90138-A

Heister, G., Schroeder-Heister, P., & Ehrenstein, W. H. (1990). Spatial coding and spatio-anatomical mapping: Evidence for a hierarchical model of spatial stimulus-response compatibility. In R. W. Proctor & T. G. Reeve (Eds.), *Stimulus-response compatibility: An integrated perspective* (pp. 117–143). North-Holland. https://doi.org/10.1016/S0166-4115(08)61220-0

Heitz, R. P. (2014). The speed-accuracy tradeoff: History, physiology, methodology, and behavior. *Frontiers in Neuroscience*, *8*, Article 150. https://doi.org/10.3389/fnins.2014.00150

Heller, M. A. (1992). Haptic dominance in form perception: Vision versus proprioception. *Perception*, *21*(5), 655–660. https://doi.org/10.1068/p210655

Hendy, K. C., Hamilton, K. M., & Landry, L. N. (1993). Measuring subjective workload: When is one scale better than many? *Human Factors*, *35*(4), 579–601. https://doi.org/10.1177/001872089303500401

Herbart, J. F. (1824–1825). *Psychologie als wissenschaft neu gegründet auf erfahrung, metaphysik und mathematik* [Psychology as a science newly founded on experience, metaphysics and mathematics]. Unzer.

Herff, C., Heger, D., Fortmann, O., Hennrich, J., Putze, F., & Schultz, T. (2014). Mental workload during n-back task-quantified in the prefrontal cortex using fNIRS. *Frontiers in Human Neuroscience*, *7*, Article 935. https://doi.org/10.3389/fnhum.2013.00935

Hering, A., Kliegel, M., Rendell, P. G., Craik, F. I. M., & Rose, N. S. (2018). Prospective memory is a key predictor of functional independence in older adults. *Journal of the International Neuropsychological Society*, *24*(6), 640–645. https://doi.org/10.1017/S1355617718000152

Heyes, C. (2014). Submentalizing: I am not really reading your mind. *Perspectives on Psychological Science*, *9*(2), 131–143. https://doi.org/10.1177/1745691613518076

Hick, W. E. (1952). On the rate of gain of information. *Quarterly Journal of Experimental Psychology*, *4*(1), 11–26. https://doi.org/10.1080/17470215208416600

Hidalgo-Muñoz, A. R., Béquet, A. J., Astier-Juvenon, M., Pépin, G., Fort, A., Jallais, C., Tattegrain, H., & Gabaude, C. (2019). Respiration and heart rate modulation due to competing cognitive tasks while driving. *Frontiers in Human Neuroscience*, *12*, Article 525. https://doi.org/10.3389/fnhum.2018.00525

Hilchey, M. D., & Klein, R. M. (2011). Are there bilingual advantages on non-linguistic interference tasks? Implications for the plasticity of executive control processes. *Psychonomic Bulletin & Review, 18*(4), 625–658. https://doi.org/10.3758/s13423-011-0116-7

Hillyard, S. A., Hink, R. F., Schwent, V. L., & Picton, T. W. (1973, October 12). Electrical signs of selective attention in the human brain. *Science, 182*(4108), 177–180. https://doi.org/10.1126/science.182.4108.177

Hillyard, S. A., & Kutas, M. (1983). Electrophysiology of cognitive processing. *Annual Review of Psychology, 34*(1), 33–61. https://doi.org/10.1146/annurev.ps.34.020183.000341

Hintzman, D. L., Carre, F. A., Eskridge, V. L., Owens, A. M., Shaff, S. S., & Sparks, M. E. (1972). "Stroop" effect: Input or output phenomenon? *Journal of Experimental Psychology, 95*(2), 458–459. https://doi.org/10.1037/h0033644

Hirnstein, M., Hugdahl, K., & Hausmann, M. (2019). Cognitive sex differences and hemispheric asymmetry: A critical review of 40 years of research. *Laterality: Asymmetries of Body, Brain, and Cognition, 24*(2), 204–252. https://doi.org/10.1080/1357650X.2018.1497044

Hirsch, P., Nolden, S., Declerck, M., & Koch, I. (2018). Common cognitive control processes underlying performance in task-switching and dual-task contexts. *Advances in Cognitive Psychology, 14*(3), 62–74. https://doi.org/10.5709/acp-0239-y

Hirst, W., Spelke, E. S., Reaves, C. C., Caharack, G., & Neisser, U. (1980). Dividing attention without alternation or automaticity. *Journal of Experimental Psychology: General, 109*(1), 98–117. https://doi.org/10.1037/0096-3445.109.1.98

Hockey, G. R. J. (1993). Cognitive energetical control mechanisms in the management of work demands and psychological health. In A. D. Baddeley & L. Weiskrantz (Eds.), *Attention: Selection, awareness, and control: A tribute to Donald Broadbent* (pp. 328–345). Oxford University Press.

Hockey, G. R. J. (2003). Operator functional state as a framework for the assessment of performance degradation. In G. R. J. Hockey, A. W. Gaillard, & O. Burov (Eds.), *Operator functional state: The assessment and prediction of human performance degradation in complex tasks* (pp. 8–23). IOS Press.

Hodgetts, H. M., & Jones, D. M. (2006). Interruption of the Tower of London task: Support for a goal-activation approach. *Journal of Experimental Psychology: General, 135*(1), 103–115. https://doi.org/10.1037/0096-3445.135.1.103

Hoffman, J. E., Nelson, B., & Houck, M. R. (1983). The role of attentional resources in automatic detection. *Cognitive Psychology, 15*(3), 379–410. https://doi.org/10.1016/0010-0285(83)90013-0

Hoffmann, C. (2007). Constant differences: Friedrich Wilhelm Bessel, the concept of the observer in early nineteenth-century practical astronomy and the history of the personal equation. *British Journal for the History of Science, 40*(3), 333–365. https://doi.org/10.1017/S0007087407009478

Hommel, B. (1993). The role of attention for the Simon effect. *Psychological Research, 55*(3), 208–222. https://doi.org/10.1007/BF00419608

Hommel, B. (1994). Spontaneous decay of response-code activation. *Psychological Research, 56*(4), 261–268. https://doi.org/10.1007/BF00419656

Hommel, B. (1996). The cognitive representation of action: Automatic integration of perceived action effects. *Psychological Research, 59*(3), 176–186. https://doi.org/10.1007/BF00425832

Hommel, B. (1998). Automatic stimulus-response translation in dual-task performance. *Journal of Experimental Psychology: Human Perception and Performance, 24*(5), 1368–1384. https://doi.org/10.1037/0096-1523.24.5.1368

Hommel, B. (2004). Event files: Feature binding in and across perception and action. *Trends in Cognitive Sciences*, *8*(11), 494–500. https://doi.org/10.1016/j.tics.2004.08.007

Hommel, B. (2010). Grounding attention in action control: The intentional control of selection. In B. Bruya (Ed.), *Effortless attention: A new perspective in the cognitive science of attention and action* (pp. 121–140). MIT Press. https://doi.org/10.7551/mitpress/9780262013840.003.0006

Hommel, B. (2011a). Attention and spatial stimulus coding in the Simon task: A rejoinder to van der Lubbe and Abrahamse (2010). *Acta Psychologica*, *136*(2), 265–268. https://doi.org/10.1016/j.actpsy.2010.10.002

Hommel, B. (2011b). The Simon effect as tool and heuristic. *Acta Psychologica*, *136*(2), 189–202. https://doi.org/10.1016/j.actpsy.2010.04.011

Hommel, B. (2019). Theory of Event Coding (TEC) V2.0: Representing and controlling perception and action. *Attention, Perception, & Psychophysics*, *81*(7), 2139–2154. https://doi.org/10.3758/s13414-019-01779-4

Hommel, B., Chapman, C. S., Cisek, P., Neyedli, H. F., Song, J. H., & Welsh, T. N. (2019). No one knows what attention is. *Attention, Perception, & Psychophysics*, *81*(7), 2288–2303. https://doi.org/10.3758/s13414-019-01846-w

Hommel, B., & Frings, C. (2020). The disintegration of event files over time: Decay or interference? *Psychonomic Bulletin & Review*, *27*(4), 751–757. https://doi.org/10.3758/s13423-020-01738-3

Hommel, B., Müsseler, J., Aschersleben, G., & Prinz, W. (2001). The Theory of Event Coding (TEC): A framework for perception and action planning. *Behavioral and Brain Sciences*, *24*(5), 849–878. https://doi.org/10.1017/S0140525X01000103

Hommel, B., Proctor, R. W., & Vu, K. P. L. (2004). A feature-integration account of sequential effects in the Simon task. *Psychological Research*, *68*(1), 1–17. https://doi.org/10.1007/s00426-003-0132-y

Hooge, I. T. C., Over, E. A., van Wezel, R. J., & Frens, M. A. (2005). Inhibition of return is not a foraging facilitator in saccadic search and free viewing. *Vision Research*, *45*(14), 1901–1908. https://doi.org/10.1016/j.visres.2005.01.030

Hoonakker, P., Carayon, P., Gurses, A., Brown, R., McGuire, K., Khunlertkit, A., & Walker, J. M. (2011). Measuring workload of ICU nurses with a questionnaire survey: The NASA Task Load Index (TLX). *IIE Transactions on Healthcare Systems Engineering*, *1*(2), 131–143. https://doi.org/10.1080/19488300.2011.609524

Hopfinger, J. B., & Mangun, G. R. (1998). Reflexive attention modulates processing of visual stimuli in human extrastriate cortex. *Psychological Science*, *9*(6), 441–447. https://doi.org/10.1111/1467-9280.00083

Hout, M. C., Walenchok, S. C., Goldinger, S. D., & Wolfe, J. M. (2015). Failures of perception in the low-prevalence effect: Evidence from active and passive visual search. *Journal of Experimental Psychology: Human Perception and Performance*, *41*(4), 977–994. https://doi.org/10.1037/xhp0000053

Hovland, C. I. (1960). Computer simulation of thinking. *American Psychologist*, *15*(11), 687–693. https://doi.org/10.1037/h0044165

Howard, C. J., Pole, R., Montgomery, P., Woodward, A., Guest, D., Standen, B., Kent, C., & Crowe, E. M. (2020). Visual spatial attention and spatial working memory do not draw on shared capacity-limited core processes. *Quarterly Journal of Experimental Psychology*, *73*(5), 799–818. https://doi.org/10.1177/1747021819897882

Hubel, D. H., & Wiesel, T. N. (2004). *Brain and visual perception: The story of a 25-year collaboration*. Oxford University Press. https://doi.org/10.1093/acprof:oso/9780195176186.001.0001

Huestegge, L., Pieczykolan, A., & Koch, I. (2014). Talking while looking: On the encapsulation of output system representations. *Cognitive Psychology, 73*, 72–91. https://doi.org/10.1016/j.cogpsych.2014.06.001

Huey, E. B. (1908). *The psychology and pedagogy of reading*. Macmillan.

Hughes, C. (2011). Changes and challenges in 20 years of research into the development of executive functions. *Infant and Child Development, 20*(3), 251–271. https://doi.org/10.1002/icd.736

Human Performance Research Group. (n.d.). *NASA task load index (TLX)* (Version 1.0). NASA Ames Research Center, Moffett Field, CA. https://humansystems.arc.nasa.gov/groups/tlx/downloads/TLX_pappen_manual.pdf

Humphreys, G. W., Ford, E. M. E., & Francis, D. (2000). The organization of sequential actions. In S. Monsell & J. Driver (Eds.), *Control of cognitive processes: Attention and performance XVIII* (pp. 427–442). MIT Press.

Humphreys, G. W., & Müller, H. (1993). Search via recursive rejection (SERR): A connectionist model of visual search. *Cognitive Psychology, 25*(1), 43–110. https://doi.org/10.1006/cogp.1993.1002

Humphreys, M. S., & Revelle, W. (1984). Personality, motivation, and performance: A theory of the relationship between individual differences and information processing. *Psychological Review, 91*(2), 153–184. https://doi.org/10.1037/0033-295X.91.2.153

Hunt, A. R., Reuther, J., Hilchey, M. D., & Klein, R. M. (2019). The relationship between spatial attention and eye movements. In H. Hodgson (Ed.), *Processes of visuospatial attention and working memory* (pp. 255–278). Springer. https://doi.org/10.1007/7854_2019_95

Hurtienne, J. (2017). How cognitive linguistics inspires HCI: Image schemas and image-schematic metaphors. *International Journal of Human–Computer Interaction, 33*(1), 1–20. https://doi.org/10.1080/10447318.2016.1232227

Hüttermann, S., Memmert, D., & Liesner, F. (2014). Finding the happy medium: An analysis of gaze behavior strategies in a representative task design of soccer penalties. *Journal of Applied Sport Psychology, 26*(2), 172–181. https://doi.org/10.1080/10413200.2013.816892

Hyman, R. (1953). Stimulus information as a determinant of reaction time. *Journal of Experimental Psychology, 45*(3), 188–196. https://doi.org/10.1037/h0056940

Ignashchenkova, A., Dicke, P. W., Haarmeier, T., & Thier, P. (2004). Neuron-specific contribution of the superior colliculus to overt and covert shifts of attention. *Nature Neuroscience, 7*(1), 56–64. https://doi.org/10.1038/nn1169

International Ergonomics Association. (n.d.). *What is ergonomics?* https://iea.cc/what-is-ergonomics/

Inui, K., Urakawa, T., Yamashiro, K., Otsuru, N., Takeshima, Y., Nishihara, M., Motomura, E., Kida, T., & Kakigi, R. (2010). Echoic memory of a single pure tone indexed by change-related brain activity. *BMC Neuroscience, 11*(1), 135. https://doi.org/10.1186/1471-2202-11-135

Irwin-Chase, H., & Burns, B. (2000). Developmental changes in children's abilities to share and allocate attention in a dual task. *Journal of Experimental Child Psychology, 77*(1), 61–85. https://doi.org/10.1006/jecp.1999.2557

Itti, L., & Koch, C. (2001). Computational modelling of visual attention. *Nature Reviews Neuroscience, 2*(3), 194–203. https://doi.org/10.1038/35058500

Jacoby, L. L., Lindsay, D. S., & Hessels, S. (2003). Item-specific control of automatic processes: Stroop process dissociations. *Psychonomic Bulletin & Review, 10*(3), 638–644. https://doi.org/10.3758/BF03196526

James, W. (1950). *The principles of psychology* (Vol. 1). Dover Press. (Original work published 1890)

Janczyk, M., Renas, S., & Durst, M. (2018). Identifying the locus of compatibility-based backward crosstalk: Evidence from an extended PRP paradigm. *Journal of Experimental Psychology: Human Perception and Performance*, *44*(2), 261–276. https://doi.org/10.1037/xhp0000445

Janczyk, M., Xiong, A., & Proctor, R. W. (2019). Stimulus-response and response-effect compatibility with touchless gestures and moving action effects. *Human Factors*, *61*(8), 1297–1314. https://doi.org/10.1177/0018720819831814

Janiszewski, C., Kuo, A., & Tavassoli, N. T. (2013). The influence of selective attention and inattention to products on subsequent choice. *The Journal of Consumer Research*, *39*(6), 1258–1274. https://doi.org/10.1086/668234

Janssen, T. W. P., Heslenfeld, D. J., van Mourik, R., Geladé, K., Maras, A., & Oosterlaan, J. (2018). Alterations in the ventral attention network during the stop-signal task in children with ADHD: An event-related potential source imaging study. *Journal of Attention Disorders*, *22*(7), 639–650. https://doi.org/10.1177/1087054715580847

Jastrow, J. (1890). *The time-relations of mental phenomena*. N. D. C. Hodges.

Jefferies, L. N., Enns, J. T., & Di Lollo, V. (2019). The exogenous and endogenous control of attentional focusing. *Psychological Research*, *83*(5), 989–1006. https://doi.org/10.1007/s00426-017-0918-y

Jensen, M. S., Yao, R., Street, W. N., & Simons, D. J. (2011). Change blindness and inattentional blindness. *Wiley Interdisciplinary Reviews: Cognitive Science*, *2*(5), 529–546. https://doi.org/10.1002/wcs.130

Jersild, A. T. (1927). Mental set and shift. *Archives of Psychology* [Special issue], *89*.

Jeunet, C., Tonin, L., Albert, L., Chavarriaga, R., Bideau, B., Argelaguet, F., Millán, J. D. R., Lécuyer, A., & Kulpa, R. (2020). Uncovering EEG correlates of covert attention in soccer goalkeepers: Towards innovative sport training procedures. *Scientific Reports*, *10*(1), 1705. https://doi.org/10.1038/s41598-020-58533-2

Jevons, W. S. (1871, February 9). The power of numerical discrimination. *Nature*, *3*(67), 281–282. https://doi.org/10.1038/003281a0

Johnson, A., & Proctor, R. W. (2004). *Attention: Theory and practice*. SAGE. https://doi.org/10.4135/9781483328768

Johnson, A., & Proctor, R. W. (2017). *Skill acquisition and training: Achieving expertise in simple and complex tasks*. Routledge.

Johnson, M. H. (1990). Cortical maturation and the development of visual attention in early infancy. *Journal of Cognitive Neuroscience*, *2*(2), 81–95. https://doi.org/10.1162/jocn.1990.2.2.81

Johnson, R., Jr. (1993). On the neural generators of the P300 component of the event-related potential. *Psychophysiology*, *30*(1), 90–97. https://doi.org/10.1111/j.1469-8986.1993.tb03208.x

Jolicoeur, P. (1999). Concurrent response-selection demands modulate the attentional blink. *Journal of Experimental Psychology: Human Perception and Performance*, *25*(4), 1097–1113. https://doi.org/10.1037/0096-1523.25.4.1097

Jolicoeur, P., & Dell'Acqua, R. (1999). Attentional and structural constraints on visual encoding. *Psychological Research*, *62*(2-3), 154–164. https://doi.org/10.1007/s004260050048

Jolicoeur, P., Dell'Acqua, R., & Crebolder, J. (2000). Multitasking performance deficits: Forging links between the attentional blink and the psychological refractory period. In S. Monsell & J. Driver (Eds.), *Control of cognitive processes: Attention and performance XVIII* (pp. 309–330). MIT Press.

Jones, B. C., DeBruine, L. M., Main, J. C., Little, A. C., Welling, L. L., Feinberg, D. R., & Tiddeman, B. P. (2010). Facial cues of dominance modulate the short-term gaze-cuing effect in human observers. *Proceedings of the Royal Society B: Biological Sciences, 277*(1681), 617–624.

Jonides, J., & Mack, R. (1984). On the cost and benefit of cost and benefit. *Psychological Bulletin, 96*(1), 29–44. https://doi.org/10.1037/0033-2909.96.1.29

Jonker, C. M., Van Riemsdijk, M. B., & Vermeulen, B. (2010). Shared mental models. In M. De Vos, N. Fornara, & J. V. Pitt (Eds.), *Coordination, organizations, institutions, and norms in agent systems* (pp. 132–151). Springer.

Jónsdóttir, M. K., Adólfsdóttir, S., Cortez, R. D., Gunnarsdóttir, M., & Gústafsdóttir, Á. H. (2007). A diary study of action slips in healthy individuals. *The Clinical Neuropsychologist, 21*(6), 875–883. https://doi.org/10.1080/13854040701220044

Joseph, J. S., Chun, M. M., & Nakayama, K. (1997, June 19). Attentional requirements in a 'preattentive' feature search task. *Nature, 387*(6635), 805–807. https://doi.org/10.1038/42940

Ju, Y. J., & Lien, Y. W. (2018). Who is prone to wander and when? Examining an integrative effect of working memory capacity and mindfulness trait on mind wandering under different task loads. *Consciousness and Cognition, 63*, 1–10. https://doi.org/10.1016/j.concog.2018.06.006

Kahneman, D. (1968). Method, findings, and theory in studies of visual masking. *Psychological Bulletin, 70*(6), 404–425. https://doi.org/10.1037/h0026731

Kahneman, D. (1973). *Attention and effort.* Prentice Hall.

Kalckert, A., Perera, A. T. M., Ganesan, Y., & Tan, E. (2019). Rubber hands in space: The role of distance and relative position in the rubber hand illusion. *Experimental Brain Research, 237*(7), 1821–1832. https://doi.org/10.1007/s00221-019-05539-6

Kalra, P. B., Gabrieli, J. D. E., & Finn, A. S. (2019). Evidence of stable individual differences in implicit learning. *Cognition, 190*, 199–211. https://doi.org/10.1016/j.cognition.2019.05.007

Kamiński, J., Brzezicka, A., Gola, M., & Wróbel, A. (2012). β band oscillations engagement in human alertness process. *International Journal of Psychophysiology, 85*(1), 125–128. https://doi.org/10.1016/j.ijpsycho.2011.11.006

Kane, M. J., Bleckley, M. K., Conway, A. R. A., & Engle, R. W. (2001). A controlled-attention view of working-memory capacity. *Journal of Experimental Psychology: General, 130*(2), 169–183. https://doi.org/10.1037/0096-3445.130.2.169

Kane, N. M., Curry, S. H., Butler, S. R., & Cummins, B. H. (1993). Electrophysiological indicator of awakening from coma. *The Lancet, 341*(8846), 688. https://doi.org/10.1016/0140-6736(93)90453-N

Karamacoska, D., Barry, R. J., Steiner, G. Z., Coleman, E. P., & Wilson, E. J. (2018). Intrinsic EEG and task-related changes in EEG affect Go/NoGo task performance. *International Journal of Psychophysiology, 125*(3), 17–28. https://doi.org/10.1016/j.ijpsycho.2018.01.015

Karayanidis, F., & McKewen, M. (2021). More than "just a test"—Task-switching paradigms offer an early warning system for cognitive decline. In K. D. Federmeier (Ed.), *The psychology of learning and motivation* (pp. 141–193). Academic Press. https://doi.org/10.1016/bs.plm.2021.02.006

Karimi, D., Mann, D. D., & Yan, J. (2011). A comparison of textual, symbolic, and pictorial presentation of information on an air-seeder display. *Australian Journal of Agricultural Engineering, 2*(4), 90–95.

Karlin, L., & Kestenbaum, R. (1968). Effects of number of alternatives on the psychological refractory period. *Quarterly Journal of Experimental Psychology*, *20*(2), 167–178. https://doi.org/10.1080/14640746808400145

Keele, S. W. (1972). Attention demands of memory retrieval. *Journal of Experimental Psychology*, *93*(2), 245–248. https://doi.org/10.1037/h0032460

Keele, S. W. (1973). *Attention and human performance*. Goodyear Press.

Kellen, D., & Klauer, K. C. (2018). Elementary signal detection and threshold theory. In E.-J. Wagenmakers & J. T. Wixted (Eds.), *Stevens' handbook of experimental psychology and cognitive neuroscience: Vol. 5. Methodology* (pp. 161–199). Wiley. https://doi.org/10.1002/9781119170174.epcn505

Kerns, J. G., Cohen, J. D., MacDonald, A. W., III, Cho, R. Y., Stenger, V. A., & Carter, C. S. (2004, February 13). Anterior cingulate conflict monitoring and adjustments in control. *Science*, *303*(5660), 1023–1026. https://doi.org/10.1126/science.1089910

Kieras, D. E. (2017). A summary of the EPIC cognitive architecture. In S. E. F. Chipman (Ed.), *The Oxford handbook of cognitive science* (pp. 27–48). Oxford University Press.

Kiesel, A., Steinhauser, M., Wendt, M., Falkenstein, M., Jost, K., Philipp, A. M., & Koch, I. (2010). Control and interference in task switching—A review. *Psychological Bulletin*, *136*(5), 849–874. https://doi.org/10.1037/a0019842

Kim, K., & Mundy, P. (2012). Joint attention, social-cognition, and recognition memory in adults. *Frontiers in Human Neuroscience*, *6*, Article 172. https://doi.org/10.3389/fnhum.2012.00172

Kimura, D. (1961). Cerebral dominance and the perception of verbal stimuli. *Canadian Journal of Psychology*, *15*(3), 166–171. https://doi.org/10.1037/h0083219

Kingstone, A. (1992). Combining expectancies. *Quarterly Journal of Experimental Psychology*, *44*(1), 69–104. https://doi.org/10.1080/14640749208401284

Kingstone, A., Friesen, C. K., & Gazzaniga, M. S. (2000). Reflexive joint attention depends on lateralized cortical connections. *Psychological Science*, *11*(2), 159–166. https://doi.org/10.1111/1467-9280.00232

Kinsbourne, M. (1993). Orientational bias model of unilateral neglect: Evidence from attentional gradients within hemispace. In I. H. Robertson & J. C. Marshall (Eds.), *Unilateral neglect: Clinical and experimental studies* (pp. 63–86). Erlbaum.

Kinukawa, T., Takeuchi, N., Sugiyama, S., Nishihara, M., Nishiwaki, K., & Inui, K. (2019). Properties of echoic memory revealed by auditory-evoked magnetic fields. *Scientific Reports*, *9*(1), 12260. https://doi.org/10.1038/s41598-019-48796-9

Kitroeff, N., Gelles, D., Nicas, J., Kaplan, T., & Haberman, M. (2019, March 16). After 2 crashes of Boeing jet, pilot training now a focus. *The New York Times*. https://www.nytimes.com/2019/03/16/business/boeing-max-flight-simulator-ethiopia-lion-air.html?

Klaffehn, A. L., Schwarz, K. A., Kunde, W., & Pfister, R. (2018). Similar task-switching performance of real-time strategy and first-person shooter players: Implications for cognitive training. *Journal of Cognitive Enhancement*, *2*(3), 240–258. https://doi.org/10.1007/s41465-018-0066-3

Klapp, S. T., Maslovat, D., & Jagacinski, R. J. (2019). The bottleneck of the psychological refractory period effect involves timing of response initiation rather than response selection. *Psychonomic Bulletin & Review*, *26*(1), 29–47. https://doi.org/10.3758/s13423-018-1498-6

Klapp, S. T., Nelson, J. M., & Jagacinski, R. J. (1998). Can people tap concurrent bimanual rhythms independently? *Journal of Motor Behavior, 30*(4), 301–322. https://doi.org/10.1080/00222899809601346

Klauer, K. C., & Zhao, Z. (2004). Double dissociations in visual and spatial short-term memory. *Journal of Experimental Psychology: General, 133*(3), 355–381. https://doi.org/10.1037/0096-3445.133.3.355

Klein, R. (1980). Does oculomotor readiness mediate cognitive control of visual attention? In R. S. Nickerson (Ed.), *Attention and performance VIII* (pp. 259–276). Erlbaum.

Klein, R. (1988, August 1). Inhibitory tagging system facilitates visual search. *Nature, 334*(6181), 430–431. https://doi.org/10.1038/334430a0

Klein, R. (2009). On the control of attention. *Canadian Journal of Experimental Psychology, 63*(3), 240–252. https://doi.org/10.1037/a0015807

Klein, R. M. (2000). Inhibition of return. *Trends in Cognitive Sciences, 4*(4), 138–147. https://doi.org/10.1016/S1364-6613(00)01452-2

Klein, R. M., & MacInnes, W. J. (1999). Inhibition of return is a foraging facilitator in visual search. *Psychological Science, 10*(4), 346–352. https://doi.org/10.1111/1467-9280.00166

Klein, R. M., & Redden, R. S. (2018). Two "inhibitions of return" bias orienting differently. In T. Hubbard (Ed.), *Spatial biases in perception and cognition* (pp. 295–306). Cambridge University Press. https://doi.org/10.1017/9781316651247.021

Klemen, J., & Chambers, C. D. (2012). Current perspectives and methods in studying neural mechanisms of multisensory interactions. *Neuroscience and Biobehavioral Reviews, 36*(1), 111–133. https://doi.org/10.1016/j.neubiorev.2011.04.015

Klempe, S. H. (2021). The importance of Leibniz for Wundt. *Human Arenas, 4*(1), 20–31. https://doi.org/10.1007/s42087-020-00169-9

Koch, I., Lawo, V., Fels, J., & Vorländer, M. (2011). Switching in the cocktail party: Exploring intentional control of auditory selective attention. *Journal of Experimental Psychology: Human Perception and Performance, 37*(4), 1140–1147. https://doi.org/10.1037/a0022189

Koch, I., Poljac, E., Müller, H., & Kiesel, A. (2018). Cognitive structure, flexibility, and plasticity in human multitasking—An integrative review of dual-task and task-switching research. *Psychological Bulletin, 144*(6), 557–583. https://doi.org/10.1037/bul0000144

Kompus, K., Specht, K., Ersland, L., Juvodden, H. T., van Wageningen, H., Hugdahl, K., & Westerhausen, R. (2012). A forced-attention dichotic listening fMRI study on 113 subjects. *Brain and Language, 121*(3), 240–247. https://doi.org/10.1016/j.bandl.2012.03.004

Konstantopoulos, P., Chapman, P., & Crundall, D. (2010). Driver's visual attention as a function of driving experience and visibility. Using a driving simulator to explore drivers' eye movements in day, night and rain driving. *Accident; Analysis and Prevention, 42*(3), 827–834. https://doi.org/10.1016/j.aap.2009.09.022

Kornblum, S. (1992). Dimensional overlap and dimensional relevance in stimulus-response and stimulus-stimulus compatibility. In G. E. Stelmach & J. Requin (Eds.), *Tutorials in motor behavior II* (pp. 743–777). North-Holland.

Korteling, J. E. (1991). Effects of skill integration and perceptual competition on age-related differences in dual-task performance. *Human Factors, 33*(1), 35–44. https://doi.org/10.1177/001872089103300103

Korteling, J. E. (1993). Effects of age and task similarity on dual-task performance. *Human Factors, 35*(1), 99–113. https://doi.org/10.1177/001872089303500106

Kovács, Á. M., Téglás, E., & Endress, A. D. (2010, December 24). The social sense: Susceptibility to others' beliefs in human infants and adults. *Science, 330*(6012), 1830–1834. https://doi.org/10.1126/science.1190792

Kowal, M., Toth, A. J., Exton, C., & Campbell, M. J. (2018). Different cognitive abilities displayed by action video gamers and non-gamers. *Computers in Human Behavior, 88*, 255–262. https://doi.org/10.1016/j.chb.2018.07.010

Krafka, K., Khosla, A., Kellnhofer, P., Kannan, H., Bhandarkar, S., Matusik, W., & Torralba, A. (2016). Eye tracking for everyone. In *Proceedings of the IEEE conference on computer vision and pattern recognition* (pp. 2176–2184). Institute of Electrical and Electronics Engineers.

Kramer, A. F., Hahn, S., & Gopher, D. (1999). Task coordination and aging: Explorations of executive control processes in the task switching paradigm. *Acta Psychologica, 101*(2-3), 339–378. https://doi.org/10.1016/S0001-6918(99)00011-6

Kramer, A. F., Humphrey, D. G., Larish, J. F., Logan, G. D., & Strayer, D. L. (1994). Aging and inhibition: Beyond a unitary view of inhibitory processing in attention. *Psychology and Aging, 9*(4), 491–512. https://doi.org/10.1037/0882-7974.9.4.491

Kristjánsson, Á., & Egeth, H. (2020). How feature integration theory integrated cognitive psychology, neurophysiology, and psychophysics. *Attention, Perception, & Psychophysics, 82*(1), 7–23. https://doi.org/10.3758/s13414-019-01803-7

Kuhn, G., & Kingstone, A. (2009). Look away! Eyes and arrows engage oculomotor responses automatically. *Attention, Perception, & Psychophysics, 71*(2), 314–327. https://doi.org/10.3758/APP.71.2.314

Külpe, O. (1904). Versuche über abstraktion [Experiments about abstraction]. *Bericht über den Kongress für Experimentele Psychologie, 1*, 56–68.

Külpe, O. (1964). Über die modern psychologie des denkens [The modern psychology of thinking]. In G. Mandler & J. M. Mandler (Eds.), *Thinking: From association to Gestalt* (pp. 208–216). Greenwood Press. (Original work published 1922)

Kunde, W. (2001). Response-effect compatibility in manual choice reaction tasks. *Journal of Experimental Psychology: Human Perception and Performance, 27*(2), 387–394. https://doi.org/10.1037/0096-1523.27.2.387

Kurniawan, V. (2012). *The neural basis of multisensory spatial and feature-based attention in vision and somatosensation* [Unpublished doctoral dissertation]. Cardiff University.

Kutas, M., McCarthy, G., & Donchin, E. (1977, August 19). Augmenting mental chronometry: The P300 as a measure of stimulus evaluation time. *Science, 197*(4305), 792–795. https://doi.org/10.1126/science.887923

LaBerge, D. (1983). Spatial extent of attention to letters and words. *Journal of Experimental Psychology: Human Perception and Performance, 9*(3), 371–379. https://doi.org/10.1037/0096-1523.9.3.371

Labossière, D. I., & Leboe-McGowan, J. P. (2018). Specific and non-specific match effects in negative priming. *Acta Psychologica, 182*, 138–153. https://doi.org/10.1016/j.actpsy.2017.10.009

Laeng, B., & Alnaes, D. (2019). Pupillometry. In C. Klein & U. Ettinger (Eds.), *Eye movement research: An introduction to its scientific foundations and applications* (pp. 449–502). Springer. https://doi.org/10.1007/978-3-030-20085-5_11

Lagroix, H. E. P., Di Lollo, V., & Spalek, T. M. (2019). The attentional blink: Why does Lag-1 sparing occur when the dependent measure is accuracy, but Lag-1 deficit when it is RT? *Psychological Research, 83*(8), 1778–1797. https://doi.org/10.1007/s00426-018-1026-3

Laird, J. E. (2012). *The Soar cognitive architecture.* MIT Press. https://doi.org/10.7551/mitpress/7688.001.0001

Lakatos, S., & Shepard, R. N. (1997). Time-distance relations in shifting attention between locations on one's body. *Perception & Psychophysics, 59*(4), 557–566. https://doi.org/10.3758/BF03211864

Lamberts, K., Tavernier, G., & d'Ydewalle, G. (1992). Effects of multiple reference points in spatial stimulus-response compatibility. *Acta Psychologica, 79*(2), 115–130. https://doi.org/10.1016/0001-6918(92)90028-C

Land, M. F. (2019). The evolution of gaze shifting eye movements. In H. Hodgson (Ed.), *Processes of visuospatial attention and working memory* (pp. 3–11). Springer.

Lane, D. M., & Pearson, D. A. (1982). The development of selective attention. *Merrill-Palmer Quarterly, 28*(3), 317–337.

Lange, L. (1888). Neue experimente über den vorgang der einfachen reaction auf sinneseindrücke [New experiments on the process of the simple reaction to sensory impressions]. *Philosophische Studien (Wundt), 4,* 479–510.

Lange, S., & Süß, H. M. (2014). Measuring slips and lapses when they occur—Ambulatory assessment in application to cognitive failures. *Consciousness and Cognition, 24,* 1–11. https://doi.org/10.1016/j.concog.2013.12.008

Langfeld, H. S. (1913). Voluntary movement under positive and negative instruction. *Psychological Review, 20*(6), 459–478. https://doi.org/10.1037/h0075222

Larson, G. E., & Perry, Z. A. (1999). Visual capture and human error. *Applied Cognitive Psychology, 13*(3), 227–236. https://doi.org/10.1002/(SICI)1099-0720(199906)13:3<227::AID-ACP563>3.0.CO;2-J

Lavie, N. (1995). Perceptual load as a necessary condition for selective attention. *Journal of Experimental Psychology: Human Perception and Performance, 21*(3), 451–468. https://doi.org/10.1037/0096-1523.21.3.451

Lavie, N., & Tsal, Y. (1994). Perceptual load as a major determinant of the locus of selection in visual attention. *Perception & Psychophysics, 56*(2), 183–197. https://doi.org/10.3758/BF03213897

Lawrence, R. K., Edwards, M., & Goodhew, S. C. (2020). The impact of scaling rather than shaping attention: Changes in the scale of attention using global motion inducers influence both spatial and temporal acuity. *Journal of Experimental Psychology: Human Perception and Performance, 46*(3), 313–323. https://doi.org/10.1037/xhp0000708

Lawson, R. P., Clifford, C. W., & Calder, A. J. (2011). A real head turner: Horizontal and vertical head directions are multichannel coded. *Journal of Vision, 11*(9), 17. https://doi.org/10.1167/11.9.17

Leary, D. E. (1980). The historical foundation of Herbart's mathematization of psychology. *Journal of the History of the Behavioral Sciences, 16*(2), 150–163. https://doi.org/10.1002/1520-6696(198004)16:2<150::AID-JHBS2300160206>3.0.CO;2-1

Lee, E., & MacGregor, J. (1985). Minimizing user search time in menu retrieval systems. *Human Factors, 27*(2), 157–162. https://doi.org/10.1177/001872088502700203

Lee, J., Jung, K., & Han, S. W. (2021). Serial, self-terminating search can be distinguished from others: Evidence from multi-target search data. *Cognition, 212,* 104736. https://doi.org/10.1016/j.cognition.2021.104736

Leibniz, G. W. (1765). Nouveaux essais sure l'entendement humain [New essays on human understanding]. In R. E. Raspe (Ed.), *Oeuvres philosophiques de feu M. Leibnitz* (pp. 1–496). Schreuder.

Leibniz, G. W. (1985). *Textes inédits d'après des manuscrits de la Bibliothèque Provinciale d'Hanovre* [Unpublished texts from manuscripts in the Provincial Library of Hanover] (G. Grua, Ed.). Garland. (Original work published 1948)

Lennie, P. (2003). The cost of cortical computation. *Current Biology, 13*(6), 493–497. https://doi.org/10.1016/S0960-9822(03)00135-0

Leonards, U., Sunaert, S., Van Hecke, P., & Orban, G. A. (2000). Attention mechanisms in visual search—An fMRI study. *Journal of Cognitive Neuroscience, 12*(Suppl. 2), 61–75. https://doi.org/10.1162/089892900564073

Levin, A., & Suhartono, H. (2019, March 20). Pilot who hitched a ride saved Lion Air 737 day before deadly crash. *Bloomberg.* https://www.bloomberg.com/news/articles/2019-03-19/how-an-extra-man-in-cockpit-saved-a-737-max-that-later-crashed

Levin, D. T., & Simons, D. J. (1997). Failure to detect changes to attended objects in motion pictures. *Psychonomic Bulletin & Review, 4*(4), 501–506. https://doi.org/10.3758/BF03214339

Levy, F. (1980). The development of sustained attention (vigilance) and inhibition in children: Some normative data. *Journal of Child Psychology and Psychiatry, 21*(1), 77–84. https://doi.org/10.1111/j.1469-7610.1980.tb00018.x

Lewis, J. L. (1970). Semantic processing of unattended messages using dichotic listening. *Journal of Experimental Psychology, 85*(2), 225–228. https://doi.org/10.1037/h0029518

Lewis, M. L. (2016). *The undoing project: A friendship that changed our minds.* Norton.

Lewthwaite, R., & Wulf, G. (2017). Optimizing motivation and attention for motor performance and learning. *Current Opinion in Psychology, 16,* 38–42. https://doi.org/10.1016/j.copsyc.2017.04.005

Li, X., & Logan, G. D. (2008). Object-based attention in Chinese readers of Chinese words: Beyond Gestalt principles. *Psychonomic Bulletin & Review, 15*(5), 945–949. https://doi.org/10.3758/PBR.15.5.945

Lien, M.-C., McCann, R. S., Ruthruff, E., & Proctor, R. W. (2005). Dual-task performance with ideomotor-compatible tasks: Is the central processing bottleneck intact, bypassed, or shifted in locus? *Journal of Experimental Psychology: Human Perception and Performance, 31*(1), 122–144. https://doi.org/10.1037/0096-1523.31.1.122

Lien, M.-C., & Proctor, R. W. (2000). Multiple spatial correspondence effects on dual-task performance. *Journal of Experimental Psychology: Human Perception and Performance, 26*(4), 1260–1280. https://doi.org/10.1037/0096-1523.26.4.1260

Lien, M.-C., & Proctor, R. W. (2002). Stimulus-response compatibility and psychological refractory period effects: Implications for response selection. *Psychonomic Bulletin & Review, 9*(2), 212–238. https://doi.org/10.3758/BF03196277

Lien, M.-C., Proctor, R. W., & Allen, P. A. (2002). Ideomotor compatibility in the psychological refractory period effect: 29 years of oversimplification. *Journal of Experimental Psychology: Human Perception and Performance, 28*(2), 396–409. https://doi.org/10.1037/0096-1523.28.2.396

Lien, M.-C., Proctor, R. W., & Hinkson, J. (2020). Emotion-induced attentional bias: Does it modulate the spatial Simon effect? *Cognition and Emotion, 34*(8), 1591–1607. https://doi.org/10.1080/02699931.2020.1785847

Lien, M.-C., Ruthruff, E., Remington, R. W., & Johnston, J. C. (2005). On the limits of advance preparation for a task switch: Do people prepare all the task some of the time or some of the task all the time? *Journal of Experimental Psychology: Human Perception and Performance, 31*(2), 299–315. https://doi.org/10.1037/0096-1523.31.2.299

Liepelt, R., Porcu, E., Stenzel, A., & Lappe, M. (2019). Saccadic eye movements do not trigger a joint Simon effect. *Psychonomic Bulletin & Review, 26*(6), 1896–1904. https://doi.org/10.3758/s13423-019-01639-0

Light, G. A., & Swerdlow, N. R. (2015). Future clinical uses of neurophysiological biomarkers to predict and monitor treatment response for schizophrenia. *Annals of the New York Academy of Sciences, 1344*(1), 105–119. https://doi.org/10.1111/nyas.12730

Lindsen, J. P., & de Jong, R. (2010). Distinguishing between the partial-mapping preparation hypothesis and the failure-to-engage hypothesis of residual switch costs. *Journal of Experimental Psychology: Human Perception and Performance, 36*(5), 1207–1226. https://doi.org/10.1037/a0020362

Liu, W., Oulasvirta, A., Rioul, O., Beaudouin-Lafon, M., & Guiard, Y. (2019, May 4–9). *Information theory: An analysis and design tool for HCI* [Workshop]. ACM CHI Conference on Human Factors in Computing Systems, Glasgow, United Kingdom.

Lloyd, D. M., Merat, N., McGlone, F., & Spence, C. (2003). Crossmodal links between audition and touch in covert endogenous spatial attention. *Perception & Psychophysics, 65*(6), 901–924. https://doi.org/10.3758/BF03194823

Loft, S., Bowden, V., Braithwaite, J., Morrell, D. B., Huf, S., & Durso, F. T. (2015). Situation awareness measures for simulated submarine track management. *Human Factors, 57*(2), 298–310. https://doi.org/10.1177/0018720814545515

Logan, G. D. (1981). Attention, automaticity, and the ability to stop a speeded choice response. In J. Long & A. D. Baddeley (Eds.), *Attention and performance IX* (pp. 205–222). Erlbaum.

Logan, G. D. (1988). Toward an instance theory of automatization. *Psychological Review, 95*(4), 492–527. https://doi.org/10.1037/0033-295X.95.4.492

Logan, G. D. (1994). On the ability to inhibit thought and action: A user's guide to the stop signal paradigm. In D. Dagenbach & T. H. Carr (Eds.), *Inhibitory processes in attention, memory, and language* (pp. 189–239). Academic Press.

Logan, G. D., & Cowan, W. B. (1984). On the ability to inhibit thought and action: A theory of an act of control. *Psychological Review, 91*(3), 295–327. https://doi.org/10.1037/0033-295X.91.3.295

Logan, G. D., Cox, G. E., Annis, J., & Lindsey, D. R. B. (2021). The episodic flanker effect: Memory retrieval as attention turned inward. *Psychological Review, 128*(3), 397–445. https://doi.org/10.1037/rev0000272

Logan, G. D., & Etherton, J. L. (1994). What is learned during automatization? The role of attention in constructing an instance. *Journal of Experimental Psychology: Learning, Memory, and Cognition, 20*(5), 1022–1050. https://doi.org/10.1037/0278-7393.20.5.1022

Logan, G. D., & Irwin, D. E. (2000). Don't look! Don't touch! Inhibitory control of eye and hand movements. *Psychonomic Bulletin & Review, 7*(1), 107–112. https://doi.org/10.3758/BF03210728

Logan, G. D., Schachar, R. J., & Tannock, R. (1997). Impulsivity and inhibitory control. *Psychological Science, 8*(1), 60–64. https://doi.org/10.1111/j.1467-9280.1997.tb00545.x

Logan, G. D., & Schulkind, M. D. (2000). Parallel memory retrieval in dual-task situations: I. Semantic memory. *Journal of Experimental Psychology: Human Perception and Performance, 26*(3), 1072–1090. https://doi.org/10.1037/0096-1523.26.3.1072

Logan, G. D., & Zbrodoff, N. J. (1979). When it helps to be misled: Facilitative effects of increasing the frequency of conflicting stimuli in a Stroop-like task. *Memory & Cognition, 7*(3), 166–174. https://doi.org/10.3758/BF03197535

Lohse, K. R., Sherwood, D. E., & Healy, A. F. (2010). How changing the focus of attention affects performance, kinematics, and electromyography in dart throwing. *Human Movement Science, 29*(4), 542–555. https://doi.org/10.1016/j.humov.2010.05.001

Longo, L. (2015). A defeasible reasoning framework for human mental workload representation and assessment. *Behaviour & Information Technology, 34*(8), 758–786. https://doi.org/10.1080/0144929X.2015.1015166

Lotze, R. H. (1852). *Medicinische psychologie oder physiologie der seele* [Medical psychology or physiology of the soul]. Weidmann.

Lovie, A. D. (1983). Attention and behaviourism. *British Journal of Psychology, 74*(3), 301–310. https://doi.org/10.1111/j.2044-8295.1983.tb01864.x

Lowe, D. G. (1979). Strategies, context, and the mechanism of response inhibition. *Memory & Cognition, 7*(5), 382–389. https://doi.org/10.3758/BF03196943

Lu, C.-H., & Proctor, R. W. (1995). The influence of irrelevant location information on performance: A review of the Simon and spatial Stroop effects. *Psychonomic Bulletin & Review, 2*(2), 174–207. https://doi.org/10.3758/BF03210959

Lu, S. A., Wickens, C. D., Sarter, N. B., & Sebok, A. (2011). Informing the design of multimodal displays: A meta-analysis of empirical studies comparing auditory and tactile interruptions. *Proceedings of the Human Factors and Ergonomics Society Annual Meeting, 55*(1), 1170–1174. https://doi.org/10.1177/1071181311551244

Luck, S. J. (2014). *An introduction to the event-related potential technique* (2nd ed.). MIT Press.

Luck, S. J., Fan, S., & Hillyard, S. A. (1993). Attention-related modulation of sensory-evoked brain activity in a visual search task. *Journal of Cognitive Neuroscience, 5*(2), 188–195. https://doi.org/10.1162/jocn.1993.5.2.188

Luck, S. J., Gaspelin, N., Folk, C. L., Remington, R. W., & Theeuwes, J. (2021). Progress toward resolving the attentional capture debate. *Visual Cognition, 29*(1), 1–21. https://doi.org/10.1080/13506285.2020.1848949

Luck, S. J., & Girelli, M. (1998). Electrophysiological approaches to the study of selective attention in the human brain. In R. Parasuraman (Ed.), *The attentive brain* (pp. 71–94). MIT Press.

Luck, S. J., Woodman, G. F., & Vogel, E. K. (2000). Event-related potential studies of attention. *Trends in Cognitive Sciences, 4*(11), 432–440. https://doi.org/10.1016/S1364-6613(00)01545-X

Lukas, S., Philipp, A. M., & Koch, I. (2010). Switching attention between modalities: Further evidence for visual dominance. *Psychological Research, 74*(3), 255–267. https://doi.org/10.1007/s00426-009-0246-y

Lukas, S., Philipp, A. M., & Koch, I. (2014). Crossmodal attention switching: Auditory dominance in temporal discrimination tasks. *Acta Psychologica, 153*, 139–146. https://doi.org/10.1016/j.actpsy.2014.10.003

Lundberg, U., & Frankenhaeuser, M. (1978). Psychophysiological reactions to noise as modified by personal control over noise intensity. *Biological Psychology, 6*(1), 51–59. https://doi.org/10.1016/0301-0511(78)90006-6

Luo, C., & Proctor, R. W. (2018). The location-, word-, and arrow-based Simon effects: An ex-Gaussian analysis. *Memory & Cognition, 46*(3), 497–506. https://doi.org/10.3758/s13421-017-0767-3

Luo, C., & Proctor, R. W. (2020). Shared mechanisms underlying the location-, word- and arrow-based Simon effects. *Psychological Research, 84*(6), 1655–1667. https://doi.org/10.1007/s00426-019-01175-5

Lynn, S. K., & Barrett, L. F. (2014). "Utilizing" signal detection theory. *Psychological Science, 25*(9), 1663–1673. https://doi.org/10.1177/0956797614541991

Macaluso, E. (2010). Orienting of spatial attention and the interplay between the senses. *Cortex, 46*(3), 282–297. https://doi.org/10.1016/j.cortex.2009.05.010

MacDonald, P. A., Joordens, S., & Seergobin, K. N. (1999). Negative priming effects that are bigger than a breadbox: Attention to distractors does not eliminate negative priming, it enhances it. *Memory & Cognition, 27*(2), 197–207. https://doi.org/10.3758/BF03211405

Mack, A., Clarke, J., & Erol, M. (2018). Attention, expectation and iconic memory: A reply to Aru and Bachmann (2017). *Consciousness and Cognition, 59*, 60–63. https://doi.org/10.1016/j.concog.2017.10.001

Mack, A., Erol, M., & Clarke, J. (2015). Iconic memory is not a case of attention-free awareness. *Consciousness and Cognition, 33*, 291–299. https://doi.org/10.1016/j.concog.2014.12.016

Mack, A., Erol, M., Clarke, J., & Bert, J. (2016). No iconic memory without attention. *Consciousness and Cognition, 40*, 1–8. https://doi.org/10.1016/j.concog.2015.12.006

Macknik, S. L., King, M., Randi, J., Robbins, A., Teller, E., Thompson, J., & Martinez-Conde, S. (2008). Attention and awareness in stage magic: Turning tricks into research. *Nature Reviews Neuroscience, 9*(11), 871–879. https://doi.org/10.1038/nrn2473

Mackworth, N. H. (1948). The breakdown of vigilance during prolonged visual search. *Quarterly Journal of Experimental Psychology, 1*(1), 6–21. https://doi.org/10.1080/17470214808416738

Mackworth, N. H. (1961). Researches on the measurement of human performance. In H. W. Sinaiko (Ed.), *Selected papers on human factors in the design and use of control systems* (pp. 174–331). Dover. (Original work published 1950)

MacLeod, C. M. (1991). Half a century of research on the Stroop effect: An integrative review. *Psychological Bulletin, 109*(2), 163–203. https://doi.org/10.1037/0033-2909.109.2.163

MacLeod, C. M. (1992). The Stroop task: The "gold standard" of attentional measures. *Journal of Experimental Psychology: General, 121*(1), 12–14. https://doi.org/10.1037/0096-3445.121.1.12

Maier, A., & Tsuchiya, N. (2021). Growing evidence for separate neural mechanisms for attention and consciousness. *Attention, Perception, & Psychophysics, 83*(2), 558–576. https://doi.org/10.3758/s13414-020-02146-4

Makarina, N., Hübner, R., & Florack, A. (2019). Increased preference and value of consumer products by attentional selection. *Frontiers in Psychology, 10*, Article 2086. https://doi.org/10.3389/fpsyg.2019.02086

Maki, W. S., Frigen, K., & Paulson, K. (1997). Associative priming by targets and distractors during rapid serial visual presentation: Does word meaning survive the attentional blink? *Journal of Experimental Psychology: Human Perception and Performance, 23*(4), 1014–1034. https://doi.org/10.1037/0096-1523.23.4.1014

Mäkisalo, J. L., Gowases, T., & Pietinen, S. (2013). Using eye tracking to study the effect of badly synchronized subtitles on the gaze paths of television viewers. *New Voices in Translation Studies*, *10*, 72–86.

Malebranche, N. (1980). *De la recherché de la vérité/The search after truth*. Ohio University Press. (Original work published 1674)

Malienko, A., Harrar, V., & Khan, A. Z. (2018). Contrasting effects of exogenous cueing on saccades and reaches. *Journal of Vision*, *18*(9), Article 4. https://doi.org/10.1167/18.9.4

Maman, P., Gaurang, S., & Sandhu, J. S. (2011). The effect of vision training on performance in tennis players. *Serbian Journal of Sports Sciences*, *5*(1), 11–16.

Mandrick, K., Derosiere, G., Dray, G., Coulon, D., Micallef, J. P., & Perrey, S. (2013). Prefrontal cortex activity during motor tasks with additional mental load requiring attentional demand: A near-infrared spectroscopy study. *Neuroscience Research*, *76*(3), 156–162. https://doi.org/10.1016/j.neures.2013.04.006

Mangun, G. R., & Hillyard, S. A. (1991). Modulations of sensory-evoked brain potentials indicate changes in perceptual processing during visual-spatial priming. *Journal of Experimental Psychology: Human Perception and Performance*, *17*(4), 1057–1074. https://doi.org/10.1037/0096-1523.17.4.1057

Manly, T., Robertson, I. H., Galloway, M., & Hawkins, K. (1999). The absent mind: Further investigations of sustained attention to response. *Neuropsychologia*, *37*(6), 661–670. https://doi.org/10.1016/S0028-3932(98)00127-4

Marinescu, A. C., Sharples, S., Ritchie, A. C., Sánchez López, T., McDowell, M., & Morvan, H. P. (2018). Physiological parameter response to variation of mental workload. *Human Factors*, *60*(1), 31–56. https://doi.org/10.1177/0018720817733101

Markant, J., & Amso, D. (2014). Leveling the playing field: Attention mitigates the effects of intelligence on memory. *Cognition*, *131*(2), 195–204. https://doi.org/10.1016/j.cognition.2014.01.006

Marshall, D. C., Lee, J. D., & Austria, R. A. (2007). Alerts for in-vehicle information systems: Annoyance, urgency, and appropriateness. *Human Factors*, *49*(1), 145–157. https://doi.org/10.1518/001872007779598145

Martens, S., & Wyble, B. (2010). The attentional blink: Past, present, and future of a blind spot in perceptual awareness. *Neuroscience and Biobehavioral Reviews*, *34*(6), 947–957. https://doi.org/10.1016/j.neubiorev.2009.12.005

Marti, S., Sigman, M., & Dehaene, S. (2012). A shared cortical bottleneck underlying attentional blink and psychological refractory period. *NeuroImage*, *59*(3), 2883–2898. https://doi.org/10.1016/j.neuroimage.2011.09.063

Maslovat, D., Chua, R., Spencer, H. C., Forgaard, C. J., Carlsen, A. N., & Franks, I. M. (2013). Evidence for a response preparation bottleneck during dual-task performance: Effect of a startling acoustic stimulus on the psychological refractory period. *Acta Psychologica*, *144*(3), 481–487. https://doi.org/10.1016/j.actpsy.2013.08.005

Massaro, D. W. (1994). Introducing information processing: 25 years later [Review of the book *Memory and attention: An introduction to human information processing*, by D. A. Norman]. *The American Journal of Psychology*, *107*(4), 597–603. https://doi.org/10.2307/1423002

Mathewson, K. E., Lleras, A., Beck, D. M., Fabiani, M., Ro, T., & Gratton, G. (2011). Pulsed out of awareness: EEG alpha oscillations represent a pulsed-inhibition of ongoing cortical processing. *Frontiers in Psychology*, *2*, Article 99. https://doi.org/10.3389/fpsyg.2011.00099

Matthews, G. (2021). Stress states, personality and cognitive functioning: A review of research with the Dundee Stress State Questionnaire. *Personality and Individual Differences, 169,* 110083. https://doi.org/10.1016/j.paid.2020.110083

Matthews, G., & Davies, D. R. (2001). Individual differences in energetic arousal and sustained attention: A dual-task study. *Personality and Individual Differences, 31*(4), 575–589. https://doi.org/10.1016/S0191-8869(00)00162-8

Matthews, G., Davies, D. R., & Lees, J. L. (1990). Arousal, extraversion, and individual differences in resource availability. *Journal of Personality and Social Psychology, 59*(1), 150–168. https://doi.org/10.1037/0022-3514.59.1.150

Matthews, G., Jones, D. M., & Chamberlain, A. G. (1990). Refining the measurement of mood: The UWIST Mood Adjective Checklist. *British Journal of Psychology, 81*(1), 17–42. https://doi.org/10.1111/j.2044-8295.1990.tb02343.x

Matthews, G., Warm, J. S., Reinerman, L. E., Langheim, L. K., & Saxby, D. J. (2010). Task engagement, attention, and executive control. In A. Gruszka, G. Matthews, & B. Szymura (Eds.), *Handbook of individual differences in cognition* (pp. 205–230). Springer. https://doi.org/10.1007/978-1-4419-1210-7_13

Matthews, G., & Wells, A. (1999). The cognitive science of attention and emotion. In T. Dalgleish & M. J. Power (Eds.), *Handbook of cognition and emotion* (pp. 171–192). Wiley. https://doi.org/10.1002/0470013494.ch9

Mattingley, J. B., Phillips, J. G., & Bradshaw, J. L. (1994). Impairments of movement execution in unilateral neglect: A kinematic analysis of directional bradykinesia. *Neuropsychologia, 32*(9), 1111–1134. https://doi.org/10.1016/0028-3932(94)90157-0

Mattler, U. (2005). Flanker effects on motor output and the late-level response activation hypothesis. *Quarterly Journal of Experimental Psychology, 58*(4), 577–601. https://doi.org/10.1080/02724980443000089

Maunsell, J. H., & Treue, S. (2006). Feature-based attention in visual cortex. *Trends in Neurosciences, 29*(6), 317–322. https://doi.org/10.1016/j.tins.2006.04.001

May, C. P. (1999). Synchrony effects in cognition: The costs and a benefit. *Psychonomic Bulletin & Review, 6*(1), 142–147. https://doi.org/10.3758/BF03210822

May, C. P., & Hasher, L. (1998). Synchrony effects in inhibitory control over thought and action. *Journal of Experimental Psychology: Human Perception and Performance, 24*(2), 363–379. https://doi.org/10.1037/0096-1523.24.2.363

May, K. E., & Elder, A. D. (2018). Efficient, helpful, or distracting? A literature review of media multitasking in relation to academic performance. *International Journal of Educational Technology in Higher Education, 15*(1), 13–17. https://doi.org/10.1186/s41239-018-0096-z

Mayes, D. K., Sims, V. K., & Koonce, J. M. (2001). Comprehension and workload differences for VDT and paper-based reading. *International Journal of Industrial Ergonomics, 28*(6), 367–378. https://doi.org/10.1016/S0169-8141(01)00043-9

Mayr, U., Awh, E., & Laurey, P. (2003). Conflict adaptation effects in the absence of executive control. *Nature Neuroscience, 6*(5), 450–452. https://doi.org/10.1038/nn1051

Mayr, U., & Keele, S. W. (2000). Changing internal constraints on action: The role of backward inhibition. *Journal of Experimental Psychology: General, 129*(1), 4–26. https://doi.org/10.1037/0096-3445.129.1.4

McAvinue, L. P., Habekost, T., Johnson, K. A., Kyllingsbæk, S., Vangkilde, S., Bundesen, C., & Robertson, I. H. (2012). Sustained attention, attentional selectivity, and attentional capacity across the lifespan. *Attention, Perception, & Psychophysics, 74*(8), 1570–1582. https://doi.org/10.3758/s13414-012-0352-6

McCann, R. S., & Johnston, J. C. (1992). Locus of the single-channel bottleneck in dual-task interference. *Journal of Experimental Psychology: Human Perception and Performance, 18*(2), 471–484. https://doi.org/10.1037/0096-1523.18.2.471

McCarley, J. S., & Yamani, Y. (2021). Psychometric curves reveal three mechanisms of vigilance decrement. *Psychological Science, 32*(10), 1675–1683. https://doi.org/10.1177/09567976211007559

McCleery, J. P., Surtees, A. D., Graham, K. A., Richards, J. E., & Apperly, I. A. (2011). The neural and cognitive time course of theory of mind. *The Journal of Neuroscience, 31*(36), 12849–12854. https://doi.org/10.1523/JNEUROSCI.1392-11.2011

McClelland, J. L. (1979). On the time relations of mental processes: An examination of systems of processes in cascade. *Psychological Review, 86*(4), 287–330. https://doi.org/10.1037/0033-295X.86.4.287

McDonald, J. J., Green, J. J., Störmer, V. S., & Hillyard, S. A. (2012). Cross-modal spatial cueing of attention influences visual perception. In M. M. Murray & M. T. Wallace (Eds.), *The neural bases of multisensory processes* (pp. 509–528). CRC Press.

McDonald, J. J., Teder-Sälejärvi, W. A., Di Russo, F., & Hillyard, S. A. (2005). Neural basis of auditory-induced shifts in visual time-order perception. *Nature Neuroscience, 8*(9), 1197–1202. https://doi.org/10.1038/nn1512

McDonough, I. M., Wood, M. M., & Miller, W. S., Jr. (2019). Attention science: A review on the trajectory of attentional mechanisms in aging and the Alzheimer's disease continuum through the attention network test. *The Yale Journal of Biology and Medicine, 92*(1), 37–51.

McDowd, J. M. (1986). The effects of age and extended practice on divided attention performance. *Journal of Gerontology, 41*(6), 764–769. https://doi.org/10.1093/geronj/41.6.764

McGuinness, B., & Foy, L. (2000). A subjective measure of SA: The Crew Awareness Rating Scale (CARS). In *Proceedings of human performance, situation awareness, and automation: User-centered design for the new millennium* (Vol. 16, pp. 286–291). SA Technologies.

McGurk, H., & MacDonald, J. (1976, December 23). Hearing lips and seeing voices. *Nature, 264*(5588), 746–748. https://doi.org/10.1038/264746a0

McLaughlin, E. N., Shore, D. I., & Klein, R. M. (2001). The attentional blink is immune to masking-induced data limits. *Quarterly Journal of Experimental Psychology, 54A*(1), 169–196. https://doi.org/10.1080/02724980042000075

McNeese, N. J., & Cooke, N. J. (2020). Understanding human-robot teams in light of all-human teams: Aspects of team interaction and shared cognition. *International Journal of Human–Computer Studies, 140*, Article 102436. https://doi.org/10.1016/j.ijhcs.2020.102436

McRae, R. (1976). *Leibniz: Perception, apperception, and thought.* University of Toronto Press. https://doi.org/10.3138/9781487579777

Medin, D. L., Wattenmaker, W. D., & Hampson, S. E. (1987). Family resemblance, conceptual cohesiveness, and category construction. *Cognitive Psychology, 19*(2), 242–279. https://doi.org/10.1016/0010-0285(87)90012-0

Medina, J., McCloskey, M., Coslett, H. B., & Rapp, B. (2014). Somatotopic representation of location: Evidence from the Simon effect. *Journal of Experimental Psychology: Human Perception and Performance, 40*(6), 2131–2142. https://doi.org/10.1037/a0037975

Meiran, N. (1996). Reconfiguration of processing mode prior to task performance. *Journal of Experimental Psychology: Learning, Memory, and Cognition, 22*(6), 1423–1442. https://doi.org/10.1037/0278-7393.22.6.1423

Meiran, N. (2000). Reconfiguration of stimulus task sets and response task sets during task switching. In S. Monsell & J. Driver (Eds.), *Control of cognitive processes: Attention and performance XVIII* (pp. 377–399). MIT Press.

Melara, R. D., & Mounts, J. R. W. (1993). Selective attention to Stroop dimensions: Effects of baseline discriminability, response mode, and practice. *Memory & Cognition, 21*(5), 627–645. https://doi.org/10.3758/BF03197195

Melara, R. D., Wang, H., Vu, K. P. L., & Proctor, R. W. (2008). Attentional origins of the Simon effect: Behavioral and electrophysiological evidence. *Brain Research, 1215*, 147–159. https://doi.org/10.1016/j.brainres.2008.03.026

Memelink, J., & Hommel, B. (2013). Intentional weighting: A basic principle in cognitive control. *Psychological Research, 77*(3), 249–259. https://doi.org/10.1007/s00426-012-0435-y

Memory Alpha. (2021, June 30). Mind meld. *Fandom.* https://memory-alpha.fandom.com/wiki/Mind_meld

Merkel, J. (1885). Die zeitliche verhaltnisse de willenstatigkeit [The temporal relations of activities of the will]. *Philosophische Studien, 2*, 73–127.

Mesulam, M. M. (1990). Large-scale neurocognitive networks and distributed processing for attention, language, and memory. *Annals of Neurology, 28*(5), 597–613. https://doi.org/10.1002/ana.410280502

Meyer, D. E. (2014, August 1). Semantic priming well established. *Science, 345*(6196), 523. https://doi.org/10.1126/science.345.6196.523-b

Meyer, D. E., & Kieras, D. E. (1997a). A computational theory of executive cognitive processes and multiple-task performance: Part 1. Basic mechanisms. *Psychological Review, 104*(1), 3–65. https://doi.org/10.1037/0033-295X.104.1.3

Meyer, D. E., & Kieras, D. E. (1997b). A computational theory of executive cognitive processes and multiple-task performance: Part 2. Accounts of psychological refractory-period phenomena. *Psychological Review, 104*(4), 749–791. https://doi.org/10.1037/0033-295X.104.4.749

Meyer, D. E., Schvaneveldt, R. W., & Ruddy, M. G. (1975). Locus of contextual effects on visual word-recognition. In P. M. A. Rabbitt & S. Dornic (Eds.), *Attention and performance V* (pp. 98–118). Academic Press.

Miles, J. D., & Proctor, R. W. (2012). Correlations between spatial compatibility effects: Are arrows more like locations or words? *Psychological Research, 76*(6), 777–791. https://doi.org/10.1007/s00426-011-0378-8

Miller, G. A. (1956). The magical number seven plus or minus two: Some limits on our capacity for processing information. *Psychological Review, 63*(2), 81–97. https://doi.org/10.1037/h0043158

Miller, G. A. (2003). The cognitive revolution: A historical perspective. *Trends in Cognitive Sciences, 7*(3), 141–144. https://doi.org/10.1016/S1364-6613(03)00029-9

Miller, J. (1991). Channel interaction and the redundant-targets effect in bimodal divided attention. *Journal of Experimental Psychology: Human Perception and Performance, 17*(1), 160–169. https://doi.org/10.1037/0096-1523.17.1.160

Miller, J. (2006). Backward crosstalk effects in psychological refractory period paradigms: Effects of second-task response types on first-task response latencies. *Psychological Research, 70*(6), 484–493. https://doi.org/10.1007/s00426-005-0011-9

Miller, J., Atkins, S. G., & Van Nes, F. (2005). Compatibility effects based on stimulus and response numerosity. *Psychonomic Bulletin & Review, 12*(2), 265–270. https://doi.org/10.3758/BF03196370

Miller, J., & Durst, M. (2014). "Just do it when you get a chance": The effects of a background task on primary task performance. *Attention, Perception, & Psychophysics, 76*(8), 2560–2574. https://doi.org/10.3758/s13414-014-0730-3

Miller, J., & Hackley, S. A. (1992). Electrophysiological evidence for temporal overlap among contingent mental processes. *Journal of Experimental Psychology: General, 121*(2), 195–209. https://doi.org/10.1037/0096-3445.121.2.195

Miller, J., & Schwarz, W. (2018). Implications of individual differences in on-average null effects. *Journal of Experimental Psychology: General, 147*(3), 377–397. https://doi.org/10.1037/xge0000367

Miller, J., Ulrich, R., & Rolke, B. (2009). On the optimality of serial and parallel processing in the psychological refractory period paradigm: Effects of the distribution of stimulus onset asynchronies. *Cognitive Psychology, 58*(3), 273–310. https://doi.org/10.1016/j.cogpsych.2006.08.003

Miller, M. W., Rietschel, J. C., McDonald, C. G., & Hatfield, B. D. (2011). A novel approach to the physiological measurement of mental workload. *International Journal of Psychophysiology, 80*(1), 75–78. https://doi.org/10.1016/j.ijpsycho.2011.02.003

Miller, S. (2001). *Workload measures*. National Advanced Driving Simulator. https://www.nads-sc.uiowa.edu/publicationStorage/200501251347060.N01-006.pdf

Milliken, B., Joordens, S., Merikle, P. M., & Seiffert, A. E. (1998). Selective attention: A reevaluation of the implications of negative priming. *Psychological Review, 105*(2), 203–229. https://doi.org/10.1037/0033-295X.105.2.203

Milliken, B., Tipper, S. P., Houghton, G., & Lupiáñez, J. (2000). Attending, ignoring, and repetition: On the relation between negative priming and inhibition of return. *Perception & Psychophysics, 62*(6), 1280–1296. https://doi.org/10.3758/BF03212130

Milliken, B., Tipper, S. P., & Weaver, B. (1994). Negative priming in a spatial localization task: Feature mismatching and distractor inhibition. *Journal of Experimental Psychology: Human Perception and Performance, 20*(3), 624–646. https://doi.org/10.1037/0096-1523.20.3.624

Moncrieff, D. W. (2011). Dichotic listening in children: Age-related changes in direction and magnitude of ear advantage. *Brain and Cognition, 76*(2), 316–322. https://doi.org/10.1016/j.bandc.2011.03.013

Moncrieff, D., & Dubyne, L. (2017). Enhanced identification of long versus short voice onset time consonant–vowel syllables in a dichotic listening task. *American Journal of Audiology, 26*(4), 555–561. https://doi.org/10.1044/2017_AJA-17-0031

Mondy, S., & Coltheart, V. (2000). Detection and identification of change in naturalistic scenes. *Visual Cognition, 7*(1-3), 281–296. https://doi.org/10.1080/135062800394810

Monsell, S., & Driver, J. (Eds.). (2000). *Control of cognitive processes: Attention and performance XVIII*. MIT Press.

Moran, J., & Desimone, R. (1985, August 23). Selective attention gates visual processing in the extrastriate cortex. *Science, 229*(4715), 782–784. https://doi.org/10.1126/science.4023713

Moray, N. (1959). Attention in dichotic listening. *Quarterly Journal of Experimental Psychology, 11*(1), 56–60. https://doi.org/10.1080/17470215908416289

Moray, N. (1969). *Listening and attention*. Penguin.

Moray, N., Bates, A., & Barnett, T. (1965). Experiments on the four-eared man. *The Journal of the Acoustical Society of America, 38*(2), 196–201. https://doi.org/10.1121/1.1909631

Moroney, W. F., Biers, D. W., Eggemeier, F. T., & Mitchell, J. A. (1992). A comparison of two scoring procedures with the NASA task load index in a simulated flight task. In *Proceedings of the IEEE 1992 National Aerospace and Electronics Conference* (pp. 734–740). IEEE.

Morris, C. D., Bransford, J. D., & Franks, J. J. (1977). Levels of processing versus transfer appropriate processing. *Journal of Verbal Learning and Verbal Behavior*, *16*(5), 519–533. https://doi.org/10.1016/S0022-5371(77)80016-9

Moruzzi, G., & Magoun, H. W. (1949). Brain stem reticular formation and activation of the EEG. *Electroencephalography and Clinical Neurophysiology*, *1*(1-4), 455–473. https://doi.org/10.1016/0013-4694(49)90219-9

Moustafa, K., Luz, S., & Longo, L. (2017, June). Assessment of mental workload: A comparison of machine learning methods and subjective assessment techniques. In L. Longon & M. C. Leva (Eds.), *Human mental workload: Models and applications* (pp. 30–50). Springer.

Mowrer, O. H., Rayman, N. N., & Bliss, E. L. (1940). Preparatory set (expectancy)—An experimental demonstration of its 'central' locus. *Journal of Experimental Psychology*, *26*(4), 357–372. https://doi.org/10.1037/h0058172

Mudd, S. A., & McCormick, J. (1960). The use of auditory cues in a visual search task. *Journal of Applied Psychology*, *44*(3), 184–188. https://doi.org/10.1037/h0045878

Müller, H. J., & Rabbitt, P. M. A. (1989). Reflexive and voluntary orienting of visual attention: Time course of activation and resistance to interruption. *Journal of Experimental Psychology: Human Perception and Performance*, *15*(2), 315–330. https://doi.org/10.1037/0096-1523.15.2.315

Müller, M. M., Malinowski, P., Gruber, T., & Hillyard, S. A. (2003). Sustained division of the attentional spotlight. *Nature*, *424*(6946), 309–312. https://doi.org/10.1038/nature01812

Müller, N. G., Bartelt, O. A., Donner, T. H., Villringer, A., & Brandt, S. A. (2003). A physiological correlate of the "Zoom Lens" of visual attention. *The Journal of Neuroscience*, *23*(9), 3561–3565. https://doi.org/10.1523/JNEUROSCI.23-09-03561.2003

Mulligan, J. B., Stevenson, S. B., & Cormack, L. K. (2013). Reflexive and voluntary control of smooth eye movements. In B. E. Rogowitz, T. N. Pappas, & H. de Ridder (Eds.), *Human vision and electronic imaging XVIII* (Article 86510Z). International Society for Optics and Photonics. https://doi.org/10.1117/12.2010333

Mundy, P., Kim, K., McIntyre, N., Lerro, L., & Jarrold, W. (2016). Brief report: Joint attention and information processing in children with higher functioning autism spectrum disorders. *Journal of Autism and Developmental Disorders*, *46*(7), 2555–2560. https://doi.org/10.1007/s10803-016-2785-6

Murphy, G., & Greene, C. M. (2016). Perceptual load affects eyewitness accuracy and susceptibility to leading questions. *Frontiers in Psychology*, *7*, Article 1322. https://doi.org/10.3389/fpsyg.2016.01322

Murphy, G., & Greene, C. M. (2017). The elephant in the road: Auditory perceptual load affects driver perception and awareness. *Applied Cognitive Psychology*, *31*(2), 258–263. https://doi.org/10.1002/acp.3311

Murphy, G., Groeger, J. A., & Greene, C. M. (2016). Twenty years of load theory—Where are we now, and where should we go next? *Psychonomic Bulletin & Review*, *23*(5), 1316–1340. https://doi.org/10.3758/s13423-015-0982-5

Murphy, S., Spence, C., & Dalton, P. (2017). Auditory perceptual load: A review. *Hearing Research*, *352*, 40–48. https://doi.org/10.1016/j.heares.2017.02.005

Murray, D. J. (1968). Articulation and acoustic confusability in short-term memory. *Journal of Experimental Psychology*, *78*(4, Pt. 1), 679–684. https://doi.org/10.1037/h0026641

Murray, D. J., & Ross, H. E. (1982). Vives (1538) on memory and recall. *Canadian Psychology, 23*(1), 22–31. https://doi.org/10.1037/h0081226

Müsseler, J., & Hommel, B. (1997). Blindness to response-compatible stimuli. *Journal of Experimental Psychology: Human Perception and Performance, 23*(3), 861–872. https://doi.org/10.1037/0096-1523.23.3.861

Müsseler, J., Ruhland, L., & Böffel, C. (2019). Reversed effect of spatial compatibility when taking avatar's perspective. *Quarterly Journal of Experimental Psychology, 72*(6), 1539–1549. https://doi.org/10.1177/1747021818799240

Näätänen, R. (1992). *Attention and brain function.* Erlbaum.

Näätänen, R., Kujala, T., & Light, G. (2019). *Mismatch negativity: A window to the brain.* Oxford University Press. https://doi.org/10.1093/oso/9780198705079.001.0001

Näätänen, R., Paavilainen, P., Rinne, T., & Alho, K. (2007). The mismatch negativity (MMN) in basic research of central auditory processing: A review. *Clinical Neurophysiology, 118*(12), 2544–2590. https://doi.org/10.1016/j.clinph.2007.04.026

Nabavinik, M., Abaszadeh, A., Mehranmanesh, M., & Rosenbaum, D. A. (2018). Especial skills in experienced archers. *Journal of Motor Behavior, 50*(3), 249–253. https://doi.org/10.1080/00222895.2017.1327416

Naito, E., & Matsumura, M. (1996). Movement-related potentials associated with motor inhibition under different preparatory states during performance of two visual stop signal paradigms in humans. *Neuropsychologia, 34*(6), 565–573. https://doi.org/10.1016/0028-3932(95)00140-9

Nakayama, K., & Silverman, G. H. (1986, March 20). Serial and parallel processing of visual feature conjunctions. *Nature, 320*(6059), 264–265. https://doi.org/10.1038/320264a0

Narayana, S., Saboury, B., Newberg, A. B., Papanicolaou, A. C., & Alavi, A. (2017). Positron emission tomography: Blood flow and metabolic imaging. In A. C. Papanicolaou (Ed.), *The Oxford handbook of functional brain imaging in neuropsychology and cognitive neurosciences* (pp. 61–80). Oxford University Press.

Nash, E. B., Edwards, G. W., Thompson, J. A., & Barfield, W. (2000). A review of presence and performance in virtual environments. *International Journal of Human–Computer Interaction, 12*(1), 1–41. https://doi.org/10.1207/S15327590IJHC1201_1

Navon, D. (1984). Resources—A theoretical soup stone? *Psychological Review, 91*(2), 216–234. https://doi.org/10.1037/0033-295X.91.2.216

Navon, D., & Gopher, D. (1979). On the economy of the human-processing system. *Psychological Review, 86*(3), 214–255. https://doi.org/10.1037/0033-295X.86.3.214

Navon, D., & Miller, J. (1987). Role of outcome conflict in dual-task interference. *Journal of Experimental Psychology: Human Perception and Performance, 13*(3), 435–448. https://doi.org/10.1037/0096-1523.13.3.435

Navon, D., & Miller, J. (2002). Queuing or sharing? A critical evaluation of the single-bottleneck notion. *Cognitive Psychology, 44*(3), 193–251. https://doi.org/10.1006/cogp.2001.0767

Neely, J. H. (1977). Semantic priming and retrieval from lexical memory: Roles of inhibitionless spreading activation and limited-capacity attention. *Journal of Experimental Psychology: General, 106*(3), 226–254. https://doi.org/10.1037/0096-3445.106.3.226

Neigel, A. R., Claypoole, V. L., Smith, S. L., Waldfogle, G. E., Fraulini, N. W., Hancock, G. M., Helton, W. S., & Szalma, J. L. (2020). Engaging the human operator: A review of the theoretical support for the vigilance decrement and a discussion of practical applications. *Theoretical Issues in Ergonomics Science, 21*(2), 239–258. https://doi.org/10.1080/1463922X.2019.1682712

Neigel, A. R., Claypoole, V. L., & Szalma, J. L. (2019). Effects of state motivation in overload and underload vigilance task scenarios. *Acta Psychologica, 197*, 106–114. https://doi.org/10.1016/j.actpsy.2019.05.007

Neill, W. T. (1977). Inhibitory and facilitatory processes in selective attention. *Journal of Experimental Psychology: Human Perception and Performance, 3*(3), 444–450. https://doi.org/10.1037/0096-1523.3.3.444

Neill, W. T. (2007). Mechanisms of transfer-inappropriate processing. In D. S. Gorfein & C. M. MacLeod (Eds.), *Inhibition in cognition* (pp. 63–78). American Psychological Association. https://doi.org/10.1037/11587-004

Neill, W. T., & Kleinsmith, A. L. (2016). Spatial negative priming: Location or response? *Attention, Perception, & Psychophysics, 78*(8), 2411–2419. https://doi.org/10.3758/s13414-016-1176-6

Neill, W. T., Valdes, L. A., Terry, K. M., & Gorfein, D. S. (1992). Persistence of negative priming: II. Evidence for episodic trace retrieval. *Journal of Experimental Psychology: Learning, Memory, and Cognition, 18*(5), 993–1000. https://doi.org/10.1037/0278-7393.18.5.993

Neisser, U. (1967). *Cognitive psychology*. Appleton-Century-Crofts.

Neisser, U. (1969, July 27–August 2). *Selective reading: A method for the study of visual attention* [Paper presentation]. 19th International Congress of Psychology, London, United Kingdom.

Neisser, U. (1976). *Cognition and reality*. Freeman.

Neisser, U., & Becklen, R. (1975). Selective looking: Attending to visually specified events. *Cognitive Psychology, 7*(4), 480–494. https://doi.org/10.1016/0010-0285(75)90019-5

Neumann, O. (1987). Beyond capacity: A functional view of attention. In H. Heuer & A. F. Sanders (Eds.), *Perspectives on perception and action* (pp. 361–394). Erlbaum.

Newell, A., & Simon, H. A. (1972). *Human problem solving*. Prentice-Hall.

Newman, R. L. (2017). *Head-up displays: Designing the way ahead*. Routledge. https://doi.org/10.4324/9781315253596

Nicoletti, R., & Umiltà, C. (1985). Responding with hand and foot: The right/left prevalence in spatial compatibility is still present. *Perception & Psychophysics, 38*(3), 211–216. https://doi.org/10.3758/BF03207147

Nicoletti, R., & Umiltà, C. (1994). Attention shifts produce spatial stimulus codes. *Psychological Research, 56*(3), 144–150. https://doi.org/10.1007/BF00419701

Nieuwenhuis, S., De Geus, E. J., & Aston-Jones, G. (2011). The anatomical and functional relationship between the P3 and autonomic components of the orienting response. *Psychophysiology, 48*(2), 162–175. https://doi.org/10.1111/j.1469-8986.2010.01057.x

Nigg, J. T. (1999). The ADHD response-inhibition deficit as measured by the stop task: Replication with *DSM–IV* combined type, extension, and qualification. *Journal of Abnormal Child Psychology, 27*(5), 393–402. https://doi.org/10.1023/A:1021980002473

Nigg, J. T., Sibley, M. H., Thapar, A., & Karalunas, S. L. (2020). Development of ADHD: Etiology, heterogeneity, and early life course. *Annual Review of Developmental Psychology, 2*(1), 559–583. https://doi.org/10.1146/annurev-devpsych-060320-093413

Nijboer, M., Borst, J. P., van Rijn, H., & Taatgen, N. A. (2016). Driving and multitasking: The good, the bad, and the dangerous. *Frontiers in Psychology, 7*, Article 1718. https://doi.org/10.3389/fpsyg.2016.01718

Ninio, A., & Kahneman, D. (1974). Reaction time in focused and in divided attention. *Journal of Experimental Psychology, 103*(3), 394–399. https://doi.org/10.1037/h0037202

Nishimura, A., & Yokosawa, K. (2009). Effects of laterality and pitch height of an auditory accessory stimulus on horizontal response selection: The Simon effect and the SMARC effect. *Psychonomic Bulletin & Review, 16*(4), 666–670. https://doi.org/10.3758/PBR.16.4.666

Nishimura, A., & Yokosawa, K. (2010). Visual and auditory accessory stimulus offset and the Simon effect. *Attention, Perception, & Psychophysics, 72*(7), 1965–1974. https://doi.org/10.3758/APP.72.7.1965

Nissen, M. J., & Bullemer, P. (1987). Attentional requirements of learning: Evidence from performance measures. *Cognitive Psychology, 19*(1), 1–32. https://doi.org/10.1016/0010-0285(87)90002-8

Norman, D. (2013). *The design of everyday things* (Rev. ed.). Basic Books.

Norman, D. A. (1968). Toward a theory of memory and attention. *Psychological Review, 75*(6), 522–536. https://doi.org/10.1037/h0026699

Norman, D. A. (1969). *Memory and attention: An introduction to human information processing.* Wiley.

Norman, D. A. (1981). Categorization of action slips. *Psychological Review, 88*(1), 1–15. https://doi.org/10.1037/0033-295X.88.1.1

Norman, D. A., & Bobrow, D. G. (1975). On data-limited and resource-limited processes. *Cognitive Psychology, 7*(1), 44–64. https://doi.org/10.1016/0010-0285(75)90004-3

Norman, D. A., & Shallice, T. (1986). Attention to action: Willed and automatic control of behavior. In R. J. Davidson, G. E. Schwartz, & D. Shapiro (Eds.), *Consciousness and self-regulation* (Vol. 4, pp. 1–18). Plenum Press. https://doi.org/10.1007/978-1-4757-0629-1_1

Norris, D. (2017). Short-term memory and long-term memory are still different. *Psychological Bulletin, 143*(9), 992–1009. https://doi.org/10.1037/bul0000108

Norris, D., Butterfield, S., Hall, J., & Page, M. P. A. (2018). Phonological recoding under articulatory suppression. *Memory & Cognition, 46*(2), 173–180. https://doi.org/10.3758/s13421-017-0754-8

O'Regan, J. K., Deubel, H., Clark, J. J., & Rensink, R. A. (2000). Picture changes during blinks: Looking without seeing and seeing without looking. *Visual Cognition, 7*(1-3), 191–211. https://doi.org/10.1080/135062800394766

O'Riordan, M. A. (2004). Superior visual search in adults with autism. *Autism, 8*(3), 229–248. https://doi.org/10.1177/1362361304045219

O'Riordan, M. A., Plaisted, K. C., Driver, J., & Baron-Cohen, S. (2001). Superior visual search in autism. *Journal of Experimental Psychology: Human Perception and Performance, 27*(3), 719–730. https://doi.org/10.1037/0096-1523.27.3.719

Oberauer, K. (2002). Access to information in working memory: Exploring the focus of attention. *Journal of Experimental Psychology: Learning, Memory, and Cognition, 28*(3), 411–421. https://doi.org/10.1037/0278-7393.28.3.411

Oberauer, K. (2009). Design for a working memory. In B. H. Ross (Ed.), *The psychology of learning and motivation* (Vol. 51, pp. 45–100). Academic Press. https://doi.org/10.1016/S0079-7421(09)51002-X

Oberauer, K., & Hein, L. (2012). Attention to information in working memory. *Current Directions in Psychological Science, 21*(3), 164–169. https://doi.org/10.1177/0963721412444727

Oberauer, K., Lewandowsky, S., Awh, E., Brown, G. D. A., Conway, A., Cowan, N., Donkin, C., Farrell, S., Hitch, G. J., Hurlstone, M. J., Ma, W. J., Morey, C. C., Nee, D. E., Schweppe, J., Vergauwe, E., & Ward, G. (2018). Benchmarks for models of short-term and working memory. *Psychological Bulletin, 144*(9), 885–958. https://doi.org/10.1037/bul0000153

Oberem, J., Koch, I., & Fels, J. (2017). Intentional switching in auditory selective attention: Exploring age-related effects in a spatial setup requiring speech perception. *Acta Psychologica, 177*, 36–43. https://doi.org/10.1016/j.actpsy.2017.04.008

Øie, M. G., Sundet, K., Haug, E., Zeiner, P., Klungsøyr, O., & Rund, B. R. (2021). Cognitive performance in early-onset schizophrenia and attention-deficit/hyperactivity disorder: A 25-year follow-up study. *Frontiers in Psychology, 11*, Article 606365. https://doi.org/10.3389/fpsyg.2020.606365

Olivers, C. N. L., Humphreys, G. W., & Braithwaite, J. J. (2006). The preview search task: Evidence for visual marking. *Visual Cognition, 14*(4-8), 716–735. https://doi.org/10.1080/13506280500194188

Olivers, C. N. L., & Roelfsema, P. R. (2020). Attention for action in visual working memory. *Cortex, 131*, 179–194. https://doi.org/10.1016/j.cortex.2020.07.011

Opitz, B., Rinne, T., Mecklinger, A., von Cramon, D. Y., & Schröger, E. (2002). Differential contribution of frontal and temporal cortices to auditory change detection: fMRI and ERP results. *NeuroImage, 15*(1), 167–174. https://doi.org/10.1006/nimg.2001.0970

Opoku-Baah, C., Schoenhaut, A. M., Vassall, S. G., Tovar, D. A., Ramachandran, R., & Wallace, M. T. (2021). Visual influences on auditory behavioral, neural, and perceptual processes: A review. *Journal of the Association for Research in Otolaryngology, 22*(4), 365–386. https://doi.org/10.1007/s10162-021-00789-0

Osaka, N., Minamoto, T., Yaoi, K., Azuma, M., Shimada, Y. M., & Osaka, M. (2015). How two brains make one synchronized mind in the inferior frontal cortex: fNIRS-based hyperscanning during cooperative singing. *Frontiers in Psychology, 6*, Article 1811. https://doi.org/10.3389/fpsyg.2015.01811

Osman, A., Kornblum, S., & Meyer, D. E. (1990). Does motor programming necessitate response execution? *Journal of Experimental Psychology: Human Perception and Performance, 16*(1), 183–198. https://doi.org/10.1037/0096-1523.16.1.183

Osman, A., Lou, L., Muller-Gethmann, H., Rinkenauer, G., Mattes, S., & Ulrich, R. (2000). Mechanisms of speed-accuracy tradeoff: Evidence from covert motor processes. *Biological Psychology, 51*(2-3), 173–199. https://doi.org/10.1016/S0301-0511(99)00045-9

Osman, A., & Moore, C. M. (1993). The locus of dual-task interference: Psychological refractory effects on movement-related brain potentials. *Journal of Experimental Psychology: Human Perception and Performance, 19*(6), 1292–1312. https://doi.org/10.1037/0096-1523.19.6.1292

Otermans, P. C. J., Parton, A., & Szameitat, A. J. (2021). The working memory costs of a central attentional bottleneck in multitasking. *Psychological Research.* https://doi.org/10.1007/s00426-021-01615-1

Paap, K. (2019). The bilingual advantage debate: Quantity and quality of the evidence. In J. W. Schwieter & M. Paradis (Eds.), *The handbook of the neuroscience of multilingualism* (pp. 701–735). Wiley. https://doi.org/10.1002/9781119387725.ch34

Paap, K. R., & Cooke, N. J. (1997). Design of menus. In M. Helander, T. K. Landauer, & P. Prabhu (Eds.), *Handbook of human-computer interaction* (2nd ed., pp. 533–572). North-Holland. https://doi.org/10.1016/B978-044481862-1.50090-X

Paap, K. R., Johnson, H. A., & Sawi, O. (2015). Bilingual advantages in executive functioning either do not exist or are restricted to very specific and undetermined circumstances. *Cortex, 69*, 265–278. https://doi.org/10.1016/j.cortex.2015.04.014

Pachella, R. G. (1974). The interpretation of reaction time in information processing research. In B. H. Kantowitz (Ed.), *Human information processing: Tutorials in performance and cognition* (pp. 41–82). Erlbaum.

Palmer, S. E. (2003). Visual perception of objects. In A. F. Healy & R. W. Proctor (Eds.), *Experimental psychology* (pp. 179–212). Wiley. https://doi.org/10.1002/0471264385.wei0407

Panis, S., Moran, R., Wolkersdorfer, M. P., & Schmidt, T. (2020). Studying the dynamics of visual search behavior using RT hazard and micro-level speed-accuracy tradeoff functions: A role for recurrent object recognition and cognitive control processes. *Attention, Perception, & Psychophysics, 82*(2), 689–714. https://doi.org/10.3758/s13414-019-01897-z

Paprocki, R., & Lenskiy, A. (2017). What does eye-blink rate variability dynamics tell us about cognitive performance? *Frontiers in Human Neuroscience, 11*, Article 620. https://doi.org/10.3389/fnhum.2017.00620

Parasuraman, R., & Davies, D. R. (1977). A taxonomic analysis of vigilance performance. In R. R. Mackie (Ed.), *Vigilance theory, operational performance, and physiological correlates* (pp. 559–574). Plenum Press. https://doi.org/10.1007/978-1-4684-2529-1_26

Parducci, A. (1965). Category judgment: A range-frequency model. *Psychological Review, 72*(6), 407–418. https://doi.org/10.1037/h0022602

Park, E., Han, J., Kim, K. J., Cho, Y., & del Pobil, A. P. (2018). Effects of screen size in mobile learning over time. In *Proceedings of the 12th International Conference on Ubiquitous Information Management and Communication* (pp. 1–5). Association for Computing Machinery.

Park, J., & Park, W. (2019). Functional requirements of automotive head-up displays: A systematic review of literature from 1994 to present. *Applied Ergonomics, 76*, 130–146. https://doi.org/10.1016/j.apergo.2018.12.017

Parr, T., & Friston, K. J. (2017). Working memory, attention, and salience in active inference. *Scientific Reports, 7*(1), Article 14678. https://doi.org/10.1038/s41598-017-15249-0

Parton, A., Malhotra, P., & Husain, M. (2004). Hemispatial neglect. *Journal of Neurology, Neurosurgery, and Psychiatry, 75*(1), 13–21.

Pashler, H. (1984). Evidence against late selection: Stimulus quality effects in previewed displays. *Journal of Experimental Psychology: Human Perception and Performance, 10*(3), 429–448. https://doi.org/10.1037/0096-1523.10.3.429

Pashler, H. (1998). *The psychology of attention*. MIT Press.

Pashler, H., & Johnston, J. C. (1989). Chronometric evidence for central postponement in temporally overlapping tasks. *Quarterly Journal of Experimental Psychology, 41*(1), 19–45. https://doi.org/10.1080/14640748908402351

Pavani, F., Spence, C., & Driver, J. (2000). Visual capture of touch: Out-of-the-body experiences with rubber gloves. *Psychological Science, 11*(5), 353–359. https://doi.org/10.1111/1467-9280.00270

Pavani, F., & Turatto, M. (2008). Change perception in complex auditory scenes. *Perception & Psychophysics, 70*(4), 619–629. https://doi.org/10.3758/PP.70.4.619

Pavlov, I. P. (1960). *Conditioned reflexes*. Dover.

Peltier, C., & Becker, M. W. (2017). Eye movement feedback fails to improve visual search performance. *Cognitive Research: Principles and Implications, 2*(1), Article 47. https://doi.org/10.1186/s41235-017-0083-2

Pereira, D. R. (2017). Revisiting the contributions of The New Phrenology to the brain–mind debate. *Journal of Theoretical and Philosophical Psychology, 37*(3), 152–163. https://doi.org/10.1037/teo0000062

Perrott, D. R., & Saberi, K. (1990). Minimum audible angle thresholds for sources varying in both elevation and azimuth. *The Journal of the Acoustical Society of America, 87*(4), 1728–1731. https://doi.org/10.1121/1.399421

Persuh, M., Genzer, B., & Melara, R. D. (2012). Iconic memory requires attention. *Frontiers in Human Neuroscience, 6,* Article 126. https://doi.org/10.3389/fnhum.2012.00126

Peschel, A. O., Orquin, J. L., & Mueller Loose, S. (2019). Increasing consumers' attention capture and food choice through bottom-up effects. *Appetite, 132,* 1–7. https://doi.org/10.1016/j.appet.2018.09.015

Peterson, W. W. T. G., Birdsall, T., & Fox, W. (1954). The theory of signal detectability. *Transactions of the IRE Professional Group on Information Theory, 4*(4), 171–212.

Pfister, R. (2019). Effect-based action control with body-related effects: Implications for empirical approaches to ideomotor action control. *Psychological Review, 126*(1), 153–161. https://doi.org/10.1037/rev0000140

Pfurtscheller, G., & Berghold, A. (1989). Patterns of cortical activation during planning of voluntary movement. *Electroencephalography and Clinical Neurophysiology, 72*(3), 250–258. https://doi.org/10.1016/0013-4694(89)90250-2

Phansalkar, S., Edworthy, J., Hellier, E., Seger, D. L., Schedlbauer, A., Avery, A. J., & Bates, D. W. (2010). A review of human factors principles for the design and implementation of medication safety alerts in clinical information systems. *Journal of the American Medical Informatics Association, 17*(5), 493–501. https://doi.org/10.1136/jamia.2010.005264

Phillips, J., Ong, D. C., Surtees, A. D., Xin, Y., Williams, S., Saxe, R., & Frank, M. C. (2015). A second look at automatic theory of mind: Reconsidering Kovács, Téglás, and Endress (2010). *Psychological Science, 26*(9), 1353–1367. https://doi.org/10.1177/0956797614558717

Pick, D. F., & Proctor, R. W. (1999). Age differences in the effects of irrelevant location information. In M. W. Scerbo & M. Mouloua (Eds.), *Automation technology and human performance: Current research and trends* (pp. 258–261). Erlbaum.

Picton, T. W., Hillyard, S. A., Galambos, R., & Schiff, M. (1971, July 23). Human auditory attention: A central or peripheral process? *Science, 173*(3994), 351–353. https://doi.org/10.1126/science.173.3994.351

Piefke, M., & Glienke, K. (2017). The effects of stress on prospective memory: A systematic review. *Psychology & Neuroscience, 10*(3), 345–362. https://doi.org/10.1037/pne0000102

Pierce, J. E., Clements, B. A., & McDowell, J. E. (2019). Saccades: Fundamentals and neural mechanisms. In C. Klein & U. Ettinger (Eds.), *Eye movement research: An introduction to its scientific foundations and applications* (pp. 11–71). Springer. https://doi.org/10.1007/978-3-030-20085-5_2

Pierrot-Deseilligny, C., Milea, D., & Müri, R. M. (2004). Eye movement control by the cerebral cortex. *Current Opinion in Neurology, 17*(1), 17–25. https://doi.org/10.1097/00019052-200402000-00005

Pillsbury, W. B. (1973). *Attention*. Arno Press. (Original work published 1908)

Pilz, K. S., Roggeveen, A. B., Creighton, S. E., Bennett, P. J., & Sekuler, A. B. (2012). How prevalent is object-based attention? *PLOS ONE*, *7*(2), Article e30693. https://doi.org/10.1371/journal.pone.0030693

Pinti, P., Tachtsidis, I., Hamilton, A., Hirsch, J., Aichelburg, C., Gilbert, S., & Burgess, P. W. (2020). The present and future use of functional near-infrared spectroscopy (fNIRS) for cognitive neuroscience. *Annals of the New York Academy of Sciences*, *1464*(1), 5–29. https://doi.org/10.1111/nyas.13948

Pisoni, D. B., & Tash, J. (1974). Reaction times to comparisons within and across phonetic categories. *Perception & Psychophysics*, *15*(2), 285–290. https://doi.org/10.3758/BF03213946

Plaisted, K., O'Riordan, M., & Baron-Cohen, S. (1998). Enhanced visual search for a conjunctive target in autism: A research note. *Journal of Child Psychology and Psychiatry*, *39*(5), 777–783. https://doi.org/10.1111/1469-7610.00376

Plancher, G., & Barrouillet, P. (2020). On some of the main criticisms of the modal model: Reappraisal from a TBRS perspective. *Memory & Cognition*, *48*(3), 455–468. https://doi.org/10.3758/s13421-019-00982-w

Ploetzner, R., Berney, S., & Bétrancourt, M. (2021). When learning from animations is more successful than learning from static pictures: Learning the specifics of change. *Instructional Science*, *49*(4), 497–514. https://doi.org/10.1007/s11251-021-09541-w

Pohlmann, L. D., & Sorkin, R. D. (1976). Simultaneous three-channel signal detection: Performance and criterion as a function of order of report. *Perception & Psychophysics*, *20*(3), 179–186. https://doi.org/10.3758/BF03198598

Port, N. L., Trimberger, J., Hitzeman, S., Redick, B., & Beckerman, S. (2016). Micro and regular saccades across the lifespan during a visual search of "Where's Waldo" puzzles. *Vision Research*, *118*, 144–157. https://doi.org/10.1016/j.visres.2015.05.013

Posner, M. I. (1978). *Chronometric explorations of mind*. Erlbaum.

Posner, M. I. (1980). Orienting of attention. *Quarterly Journal of Experimental Psychology*, *32*(1), 3–25. https://doi.org/10.1080/00335558008248231

Posner, M. I. (1982). Cumulative development of attentional theory. *American Psychologist*, *37*(2), 168–179. https://doi.org/10.1037/0003-066X.37.2.168

Posner, M. I. (1986). Overview. In K. R. Boff, L. I. Kaufman, & J. P. Thomas (Eds.), *Handbook of perception and human performance: Vol. II. Cognitive processes and performance* (pp. V.3–V.10). Wiley.

Posner, M. I. (2016). Orienting of attention: Then and now. *Quarterly Journal of Experimental Psychology*, *69*(10), 1864–1875. https://doi.org/10.1080/17470218.2014.937446

Posner, M. I. (Ed.). (2017). *The psychology of attention*. Routledge.

Posner, M. I., & Boies, S. J. (1971). Components of attention. *Psychological Review*, *78*(5), 391–408. https://doi.org/10.1037/h0031333

Posner, M. I., & Cohen, Y. P. C. (1984). Components of visual orienting. In H. Bouma & D. Bouwhuis (Eds.), *Attention and performance X* (pp. 531–566). Erlbaum.

Posner, M. I., & Klein, M. (1973). On the functions of consciousness. In S. Kornblum (Ed.), *Attention and performance IV* (pp. 21–35). Academic Press.

Posner, M. I., & Mitchell, R. F. (1967). Chronometric analysis of classification. *Psychological Review*, *74*(5), 392–409. https://doi.org/10.1037/h0024913

Posner, M. I., Nissen, M. J., & Klein, R. M. (1976). Visual dominance: An information-processing account of its origins and significance. *Psychological Review, 83*(2), 157–171. https://doi.org/10.1037/0033-295X.83.2.157

Posner, M. I., & Petersen, S. E. (1990). The attention system of the human brain. *Annual Review of Neuroscience, 13*(1), 25–42. https://doi.org/10.1146/annurev.ne.13.030190.000325

Posner, M. I., Petersen, S. E., Fox, P. T., & Raichle, M. E. (1988, June 17). Localization of cognitive operations in the human brain. *Science, 240*(4859), 1627–1631. https://doi.org/10.1126/science.3289116

Posner, M. I., Rafal, R. D., Choate, L. S., & Vaughan, J. (1985). Inhibition of return: Neural basis and function. *Cognitive Neuropsychology, 2*(3), 211–228. https://doi.org/10.1080/02643298508252866

Posner, M. I., & Snyder, C. R. R. (1975). Facilitation and inhibition in the processing of signals. In P. M. A. Rabbitt & S. Dornic (Eds.), *Attention and performance V* (pp. 669–682). Academic Press.

Posner, M. I., Snyder, C. R. R., & Davidson, B. J. (1980). Attention and the detection of signals. *Journal of Experimental Psychology: General, 109*(2), 160–174. https://doi.org/10.1037/0096-3445.109.2.160

Postle, B. R., & Oberauer, K. (in press). Working memory. In M. J. Kahana & A. D. Wagner (Eds.), *The Oxford handbook of human memory*. Oxford University Press.

Potter, M. C. (1993). Very short-term conceptual memory. *Memory & Cognition, 21*(2), 156–161. https://doi.org/10.3758/BF03202727

Potter, M. C. (1999). Understanding sentences and scenes: The role of conceptual short-term memory. In K. Coltheart (Ed.), *Fleeting memories: Cognition of brief visual stimuli* (pp. 13–46). MIT Press.

Potter, M. C. (2012). Conceptual short term memory in perception and thought. *Frontiers in Psychology, 3*, Article 113. https://doi.org/10.3389/fpsyg.2012.00113

Potter, M. C., Wyble, B., Hagmann, C. E., & McCourt, E. S. (2014). Detecting meaning in RSVP at 13 ms per picture. *Attention, Perception, & Psychophysics, 76*(2), 270–279. https://doi.org/10.3758/s13414-013-0605-z

Pratt, J., & Sekuler, A. B. (2001). The effects of occlusion and past experience on the allocation of object-based attention. *Psychonomic Bulletin & Review, 8*(4), 721–727. https://doi.org/10.3758/BF03196209

Price, C. N., & Moncrieff, D. (2021). Defining the role of attention in hierarchical auditory processing. *Audiology Research, 11*(1), 112–128. https://doi.org/10.3390/audiolres11010012

Prime, D. J., McDonald, J. J., Green, J., & Ward, L. M. (2008). When cross-modal spatial attention fails. *Canadian Journal of Experimental Psychology, 62*(3), 192–197. https://doi.org/10.1037/1196-1961.62.3.192

Prinzmetal, W. (1981). Principles of feature integration in visual perception. *Perception & Psychophysics, 30*(4), 330–340. https://doi.org/10.3758/BF03206147

Prinzmetal, W., Amiri, H., Allen, K., & Edwards, T. (1998). Phenomenology of attention: I. Color, location, orientation, and spatial frequency. *Journal of Experimental Psychology: Human Perception and Performance, 24*(1), 261–282. https://doi.org/10.1037/0096-1523.24.1.261

Prinzmetal, W., & Banks, W. P. (1977). Good continuation affects visual detection. *Perception & Psychophysics, 21*(5), 389–395. https://doi.org/10.3758/BF03199491

Prinzmetal, W., Nwachuku, I., Bodanski, L., Blumenfeld, L., & Shimizu, N. (1997). The phenomenology of attention. *Consciousness and Cognition, 6*(2-3), 372–412. https://doi.org/10.1006/ccog.1997.0313

Prior, A., & MacWhinney, B. (2010). A bilingual advantage in task switching. *Bilingualism: Language and Cognition, 13*(2), 253–262. https://doi.org/10.1017/S1366728909990526

Proctor, R. W. (1981). A unified theory for matching-task phenomena. *Psychological Review, 88*(4), 291–326. https://doi.org/10.1037/0033-295X.88.4.291

Proctor, R. W., & Capaldi, E. J. (2006). *Why science matters: Understanding the methods of psychological research.* Blackwell. https://doi.org/10.1002/9780470773994

Proctor, R. W., & Cho, Y. S. (2006). Polarity correspondence: A general principle for performance of speeded binary classification tasks. *Psychological Bulletin, 132*(3), 416–442. https://doi.org/10.1037/0033-2909.132.3.416

Proctor, R. W., & Healy, A. F. (2021). Visual selection and response selection without effector selection in tasks with circular arrays. *Attention, Perception, & Psychophysics, 83*(2), 637–657. https://doi.org/10.3758/s13414-020-02116-w

Proctor, R. W., Miles, J. D., & Baroni, G. (2011). Reaction time distribution analysis of spatial correspondence effects. *Psychonomic Bulletin & Review, 18*(2), 242–266. https://doi.org/10.3758/s13423-011-0053-5

Proctor, R. W., Pick, D. F., Vu, K. P. L., & Anderson, R. E. (2005). The enhanced Simon effect for older adults is reduced when the irrelevant location information is conveyed by an accessory stimulus. *Acta Psychologica, 119*(1), 21–40. https://doi.org/10.1016/j.actpsy.2004.10.014

Proctor, R. W., & Reeve, T. G. (Eds.). (1990). *Stimulus-response compatibility: An integrated perspective.* North-Holland.

Proctor, R. W., & Schneider, D. W. (2018). Hick's law for choice reaction time: A review. *Quarterly Journal of Experimental Psychology, 71*(6), 1281–1299. https://doi.org/10.1080/17470218.2017.1322622

Proctor, R. W., Tan, H. Z., Vu, K.-P. L., Gray, R., & Spence, C. (2005). Implications of compatibility and cuing effects for multimodal interfaces. In D. D. Schmorrow (Ed.), *Foundations of augmented cognition* (Vol. 11, pp. 3–12). Erlbaum.

Proctor, R. W., & Van Zandt, T. (2018). *Human factors in simple and complex systems* (3rd ed.). CRC Press.

Proctor, R. W., & Vu, K.-P. L. (2006a). The cognitive revolution at age 50: Has the promise of the human information-processing approach been fulfilled? *International Journal of Human–Computer Interaction, 21*(3), 253–284. https://doi.org/10.1207/s15327590ijhc2103_1

Proctor, R. W., & Vu, K.-P. L. (2006b). *Stimulus-response compatibility principles: Data, theory, and application.* CRC Press. https://doi.org/10.1201/9780203022795

Proctor, R. W., & Vu, K.-P. L. (2021). Selection and control of action. In G. Salvendy & W. Karwowski (Eds.), *Handbook of human factors and ergonomics* (Vol. 5, pp. 91–113). Wiley. https://doi.org/10.1002/9781119636113.ch4

Proctor, R. W., & Xiong, A. (2017). The method of negative instruction: Herbert S. Langfeld's and Ludwig R. Geissler's 1910–1913 insightful studies. *The American Journal of Psychology, 130*(1), 11–21. https://doi.org/10.5406/amerjpsyc.130.1.0011

Proctor, R. W., Zeng, L., & Vu, K. P. L. (2022). Human factors research and user-centered design. In L. Kahle, J. Huber, & T. M. Lowrey (Eds.), *APA handbook of consumer psychology* (pp. 725–738). American Psychological Association. https://doi.org/10.1037/0000262-033

Puel, J. L., Bonfils, P., & Pujol, R. (1988). Selective attention modifies the active micromechanical properties of the cochlea. *Brain Research, 447*(2), 380–383. https://doi.org/10.1016/0006-8993(88)91144-4

Puffe, L., Dittrich, K., & Klauer, K. C. (2017). The influence of the Japanese waving cat on the joint spatial compatibility effect: A replication and extension of Dolk, Hommel, Prinz, and Liepelt (2013). *PLoS One, 12*(9), Article e0184844. https://doi.org/10.1371/journal.pone.0184844

Pulvermüller, F., & Shtyrov, Y. (2006). Language outside the focus of attention: The mismatch negativity as a tool for studying higher cognitive processes. *Progress in Neurobiology, 79*(1), 49–71. https://doi.org/10.1016/j.pneurobio.2006.04.004

Pulvermüller, F., Shtyrov, Y., Hasting, A. S., & Carlyon, R. P. (2008). Syntax as a reflex: Neurophysiological evidence for early automaticity of grammatical processing. *Brain and Language, 104*(3), 244–253. https://doi.org/10.1016/j.bandl.2007.05.002

Pulvermüller, F., Shtyrov, Y., Kujala, T., & Näätänen, R. (2004). Word-specific cortical activity as revealed by the mismatch negativity. *Psychophysiology, 41*(1), 106–112. https://doi.org/10.1111/j.1469-8986.2003.00135.x

Quinlan, P. T., & Bailey, P. J. (1995). An examination of attentional control in the auditory modality: Further evidence for auditory orienting. *Perception & Psychophysics, 57*(5), 614–628. https://doi.org/10.3758/BF03213267

Quinlivan, B., Butler, J. S., Beiser, I., Williams, L., McGovern, E., O'Riordan, S., Hutchinson, M., & Reilly, R. B. (2016). Application of virtual reality head mounted display for investigation of movement: A novel effect of orientation of attention. *Journal of Neural Engineering, 13*(5), 056006. https://doi.org/10.1088/1741-2560/13/5/056006

Qureshi, A. W., Apperly, I. A., & Samson, D. (2010). Executive function is necessary for perspective selection, not Level-1 visual perspective calculation: Evidence from a dual-task study of adults. *Cognition, 117*(2), 230–236. https://doi.org/10.1016/j.cognition.2010.08.003

Ranchet, M., Morgan, J. C., Akinwuntan, A. E., & Devos, H. (2017). Cognitive workload across the spectrum of cognitive impairments: A systematic review of physiological measures. *Neuroscience and Biobehavioral Reviews, 80*, 516–537. https://doi.org/10.1016/j.neubiorev.2017.07.001

Rasmussen, J. (1986). *Information processing and human–machine interaction: An approach to cognitive engineering.* North-Holland.

Ratcliff, R. (1978). A theory of memory retrieval. *Psychological Review, 85*(2), 59–108. https://doi.org/10.1037/0033-295X.85.2.59

Rauschenberger, R., Lin, J. J.-W., Zheng, X. S., & Lafleur, C. (2009). Subset search for icons of different spatial frequencies. In *Proceedings of the Human Factors and Ergonomics Society Annual Meeting* (pp. 1101–1105). Human Factors and Ergonomics Society.

Raymond, J. E., Shapiro, K. L., & Arnell, K. M. (1992). Temporary suppression of visual processing in an RSVP task: An attentional blink? *Journal of Experimental Psychology: Human Perception and Performance, 18*(3), 849–860. https://doi.org/10.1037/0096-1523.18.3.849

Rayner, K. (1978). Eye movements in reading and information processing. *Psychological Bulletin, 85*(3), 618–660. https://doi.org/10.1037/0033-2909.85.3.618

Rayner, K. (1998). Eye movements in reading and information processing: 20 years of research. *Psychological Bulletin, 124*(3), 372–422. https://doi.org/10.1037/0033-2909.124.3.372

Reason, J. (1979). Actions not as planned: The price of automatization. In G. Underwood & R. Stevens (Eds.), *Aspects of consciousness* (Vol. 1, pp. 67–89). Academic Press.

Reason, J. (1990). *Human error.* Cambridge University Press. https://doi.org/10.1017/CBO9781139062367

Reason, J. (2017). *A life in error: From little slips to big disasters.* CRC Press. https://doi.org/10.1201/9781315263830

Redden, R. S., MacInnes, W. J., & Klein, R. M. (2021). Inhibition of return: An information processing theory of its natures and significance. *Cortex, 135*, 30–48. https://doi.org/10.1016/j.cortex.2020.11.009

Reed, C. L., & Hartley, A. A. (2021). Embodied attention: Integrating the body and senses to act in the world. In M. R. Robinson & L. E. Thomas (Eds.), *Embodied psychology: Thinking, feeling, and acting* (pp. 265–290). Springer. https://doi.org/10.1007/978-3-030-78471-3_12

Reeve, T. G., & Proctor, R. W. (1990). The salient features coding principle for spatial- and symbolic-compatibility effects. In R. W. Proctor & T. G. Reeve (Eds.), *Stimulus-response compatibility: An integrated perspective* (pp. 163–180). North-Holland. https://doi.org/10.1016/S0166-4115(08)61222-4

Reid, G. B., Shingledecker, C. A., & Eggemeier, F. T. (1981). Application of conjoint measurement to workload scale development. In *Proceedings of the Human Factors Society 25th Annual Meeting* (pp. 522–526). Human Factors Society.

Reimer, C. B., Strobach, T., Frensch, P. A., & Schubert, T. (2015). Are processing limitations of visual attention and response selection subject to the same bottleneck in dual-tasks? *Attention, Perception, & Psychophysics, 77*(4), 1052–1069. https://doi.org/10.3758/s13414-015-0874-9

Reimer, C. B., Strobach, T., & Schubert, T. (2017). Concurrent deployment of visual attention and response selection bottleneck in a dual-task: Electrophysiological and behavioural evidence. *Quarterly Journal of Experimental Psychology, 70*(12), 2460–2477. https://doi.org/10.1080/17470218.2016.1245348

Reisberg, D., Scheiber, R., & Potemken, L. (1981). Eye position and the control of auditory attention. *Journal of Experimental Psychology: Human Perception and Performance, 7*(2), 318–323. https://doi.org/10.1037/0096-1523.7.2.318

Remington, R., & Pierce, L. (1984). Moving attention: Evidence for time-invariant shifts of visual selective attention. *Perception & Psychophysics, 35*(4), 393–399. https://doi.org/10.3758/BF03206344

Renshaw, I., Davids, K., Araújo, D., Lucas, A., Roberts, W. M., Newcombe, D. J., & Franks, B. (2019). Evaluating weaknesses of "perceptual-cognitive training" and "brain training" methods in sport: An ecological dynamics critique. *Frontiers in Psychology, 9*, Article 2468. https://doi.org/10.3389/fpsyg.2018.02468

Rensink, R. A. (2002). Change detection. *Annual Review of Psychology, 53*(1), 245–277. https://doi.org/10.1146/annurev.psych.53.100901.135125

Rensink, R. A., O'Regan, J. K., & Clark, J. J. (1997). To see or not to see: The need for attention to perceive changes in scenes. *Psychological Science, 8*(5), 368–373. https://doi.org/10.1111/j.1467-9280.1997.tb00427.x

Reuter-Lorenz, P. A., & Cappell, K. A. (2008). Neurocognitive aging and the compensation hypothesis. *Current Directions in Psychological Science, 17*(3), 177–182. https://doi.org/10.1111/j.1467-8721.2008.00570.x

Rey-Mermet, A., & Gade, M. (2018). Inhibition in aging: What is preserved? What declines? A meta-analysis. *Psychonomic Bulletin & Review, 25*(5), 1695–1716. https://doi.org/10.3758/s13423-017-1384-7

Rhodes, S., Jaroslawska, A. J., Doherty, J. M., Belletier, C., Naveh-Benjamin, M., Cowan, N., Camos, V., Barrouillet, P., & Logie, R. H. (2019). Storage and processing in working memory: Assessing dual-task performance and task prioritization across the adult lifespan. *Journal of Experimental Psychology: General, 148*(7), 1204–1227. https://doi.org/10.1037/xge0000539

Ribot, T. (1890). *The psychology of attention.* Open Court Press.

Ricciardelli, P., Bonfigliolo, C., Iani, C., Nicoletti, R., & Rubichi, S. (2005). Is there any difference between the spatial response code elicited by bilateral symmetrical biological and non-biological stimuli? In *Proceedings of the Annual Meeting of the Cognitive Science Society* (Vol. 27, pp. 1845–1849). Cognitive Science Society.

Ricciardelli, P., Bricolo, E., Aglioti, S. M., & Chelazzi, L. (2002). My eyes want to look where your eyes are looking: Exploring the tendency to imitate another individual's gaze. *Neuroreport, 13*(17), 2259–2264. https://doi.org/10.1097/00001756-200212030-00018

Richards, R. J. (1980). Christian Wolff's prolegomena to empirical and rational psychology: Translation and commentary. *Proceedings of the American Philosophical Society, 124*(3), 227–239.

Ricker, T. J., Sandry, J., Vergauwe, E., & Cowan, N. (2020). Do familiar memory items decay? *Journal of Experimental Psychology: Learning, Memory, and Cognition, 46*(1), 60–76. https://doi.org/10.1037/xlm0000719

Ridderinkhof, K. R. (2002a). Activation and suppression in conflict tasks: Empirical clarification through distributional analyses. In W. Prinz & B. Hommel (Eds.), *Common mechanisms in perception and action: Attention and performance XIX* (pp. 494–519). Oxford University Press.

Ridderinkhof, K. R. (2002b). Micro- and macro-adjustments of task set: Activation and suppression in conflict tasks. *Psychological Research, 66*(4), 312–323. https://doi.org/10.1007/s00426-002-0104-7

Ridderinkhof, K. R., Band, G. P. H., & Logan, G. D. (1999). A study of adaptive behavior: Effects of age and irrelevant information on the ability to inhibit one's actions. *Acta Psychologica, 101,* 315–337. https://doi.org/10.1016/S0001-6918(99)00010-4

Rieger, D., Reinecke, L., & Bente, G. (2017). Media-induced recovery: The effects of positive versus negative media stimuli on recovery experience, cognitive performance, and energetic arousal. *Psychology of Popular Media Culture, 6*(2), 174–191. https://doi.org/10.1037/ppm0000075

Rieger, M., & Gauggel, S. (1999). Inhibitory after-effects in the stop signal paradigm. *British Journal of Psychology, 90*(4), 509–518. https://doi.org/10.1348/000712699161585

Riggs, S. L., & Sarter, N. (2019). Tactile, visual, and crossmodal visual-tactile change blindness: The effect of transient type and task demands. *Human Factors, 61*(1), 5–24. https://doi.org/10.1177/0018720818818028

Ristic, J., Friesen, C. K., & Kingstone, A. (2002). Are eyes special? It depends on how you look at it. *Psychonomic Bulletin & Review, 9*(3), 507–513. https://doi.org/10.3758/BF03196306

Ristic, J., & Kingstone, A. (2012). A new form of human spatial attention: Automated symbolic orienting. *Visual Cognition, 20*(3), 244–264. https://doi.org/10.1080/13506285.2012.658101

Rivenez, M., Darwin, C. J., & Guillaume, A. (2006). Processing unattended speech. *The Journal of the Acoustical Society of America, 119*(6), 4027–4040. https://doi.org/10.1121/1.2190162

Rizzolatti, G., Riggio, L., Dascola, I., & Umiltá, C. (1987). Reorienting attention across the horizontal and vertical meridians: Evidence in favor of a premotor theory of attention. *Neuropsychologia, 25*(1, Pt. 1), 31–40. https://doi.org/10.1016/0028-3932(87)90041-8

Roberts, S., & Sternberg, S. (1993). The meaning of additive reaction-time effects: Tests of three alternatives. In D. E. Meyer & S. Kornblum (Eds.), *Attention and performance XIV: Synergies in experimental psychology, artificial intelligence, and cognitive neuroscience* (pp. 611–653). MIT Press.

Robertson, I. H., & Marshall, J. C. (Eds.). (1993). *Unilateral neglect: Clinical and experimental studies.* Psychology Press.

Robinson, D. K. (2001). Reaction-time experiments in Wundt's Institute and beyond. In R. W. Rieber & D. K. Robinson (Eds.), *Wilhelm Wundt in history: The making of a scientific psychology* (pp. 161–204). Kluwer/Plenum. https://doi.org/10.1007/978-1-4615-0665-2_6

Robinson, M. R., & Thomas, L. E. (Eds.). (2021). *Embodied psychology: Thinking, feeling, and acting.* Springer. https://doi.org/10.1007/978-3-030-78471-3

Roediger, H. L., III. (1990). Implicit memory. Retention without remembering. *American Psychologist, 45*(9), 1043–1056. https://doi.org/10.1037/0003-066X.45.9.1043

Röer, J. P., & Cowan, N. (2021). A preregistered replication and extension of the cocktail party phenomenon: One's name captures attention, unexpected words do not. *Journal of Experimental Psychology: Learning, Memory, and Cognition, 47*(2), 234–242. https://doi.org/10.1037/xlm0000874

Rogers, R. D., & Monsell, S. (1995). Costs of a predictable switch between simple cognitive tasks. *Journal of Experimental Psychology: General, 124*(2), 207–231. https://doi.org/10.1037/0096-3445.124.2.207

Romaiguère, P., Hasbroucq, T., Possamaï, C. A., & Seal, J. (1993). Intensity to force translation: A new effect of stimulus-response compatibility revealed by analysis of response time and electromyographic activity of a prime mover. *Cognitive Brain Research, 1*(3), 197–201. https://doi.org/10.1016/0926-6410(93)90028-4

Romaniuk, J., & Nguyen, C. (2017). Is consumer psychology research ready for today's attention economy? *Journal of Marketing Management, 33*(11–12), 909–916. https://doi.org/10.1080/0267257X.2017.1305706

Roscoe, A. H. (1992). Assessing pilot workload. Why measure heart rate, HRV and respiration? *Biological Psychology, 34*(2-3), 259–287. https://doi.org/10.1016/0301-0511(92)90018-P

Rosenholtz, R. (2001). Search asymmetries? What search asymmetries? *Perception & Psychophysics, 63*(3), 476–489. https://doi.org/10.3758/BF03194414

Rosenstreich, E., & Ruderman, L. (2016). Not sensitive, yet less biased: A signal detection theory perspective on mindfulness, attention, and recognition memory. *Consciousness and Cognition, 43*, 48–56. https://doi.org/10.1016/j.concog.2016.05.007

Roswarski, T. E., & Proctor, R. W. (2000). Auditory stimulus-response compatibility: Is there a contribution of stimulus-hand correspondence? *Psychological Research, 63*(2), 148–158. https://doi.org/10.1007/PL00008173

Rothermund, K., Wentura, D., & De Houwer, J. (2005). Retrieval of incidental stimulus-response associations as a source of negative priming. *Journal of Experimental Psychology: Learning, Memory, and Cognition, 31*(3), 482–495. https://doi.org/10.1037/0278-7393.31.3.482

Röttger, E., & Haider, H. (2017). Investigating the characteristics of "not responding": Backward crosstalk in the PRP paradigm with forced vs. free no-go decisions. *Psychological Research*, *81*(3), 596–610. https://doi.org/10.1007/s00426-016-0772-3

Rubichi, S., Vu, K. P. L., Nicoletti, R., & Proctor, R. W. (2006). Spatial coding in two dimensions. *Psychonomic Bulletin & Review*, *13*(2), 201–216. https://doi.org/10.3758/BF03193832

Rubin, O., & Meiran, N. (2005). On the origins of the task mixing cost in the cuing task-switching paradigm. *Journal of Experimental Psychology: Learning, Memory, and Cognition*, *31*(6), 1477–1491. https://doi.org/10.1037/0278-7393.31.6.1477

Russo, N., Mottron, L., Burack, J. A., & Jemel, B. (2012). Parameters of semantic multisensory integration depend on timing and modality order among people on the autism spectrum: Evidence from event-related potentials. *Neuropsychologia*, *50*(9), 2131–2141. https://doi.org/10.1016/j.neuropsychologia.2012.05.003

Ruthruff, E., Johnston, J. C., & Van Selst, M. (2001). Why practice reduces dual-task interference. *Journal of Experimental Psychology: Human Perception and Performance*, *27*(1), 3–21. https://doi.org/10.1037/0096-1523.27.1.3

Ruthruff, E., Johnston, J. C., Van Selst, M., Whitsell, S., & Remington, R. (2003). Vanishing dual-task interference after practice: Has the bottleneck been eliminated or is it merely latent? *Journal of Experimental Psychology: Human Perception and Performance*, *29*(2), 280–289. https://doi.org/10.1037/0096-1523.29.2.280

Rutjes, H., Willemsen, M., & IJsselsteijn, W. (2019, May 4). Considerations on explainable AI and users' mental models. In *Where is the human? Bridging the gap between AI and HCI* [Workshop]. CHI 2019, Glasgow, Scotland.

Ruzzoli, M., & Soto-Faraco, S. (2017). Modality-switching in the Simon task: The clash of reference frames. *Journal of Experimental Psychology: General*, *146*(10), 1478–1497. https://doi.org/10.1037/xge0000342

Sabri, M., De Lugt, D. R., & Campbell, K. B. (2000). The mismatch negativity to frequency deviants during the transition from wakefulness to sleep. *Canadian Journal of Experimental Psychology*, *54*(4), 230–242. https://doi.org/10.1037/h0087343

Salamé, P., & Baddeley, A. (1987). Noise, unattended speech and short-term memory. *Ergonomics*, *30*(8), 1185–1194. https://doi.org/10.1080/00140138708966007

Salmela, V., Salo, E., Salmi, J., & Alho, K. (2018). Spatiotemporal dynamics of attention networks revealed by representational similarity analysis of EEG and fMRI. *Cerebral Cortex*, *28*(2), 549–560.

Salmon, P. M., Stanton, N. A., Walker, G. H., Jenkins, D., Ladva, D., Rafferty, L., & Young, M. (2009). Measuring situation awareness in complex systems: Comparison of measures study. *International Journal of Industrial Ergonomics*, *39*(3), 490–500. https://doi.org/10.1016/j.ergon.2008.10.010

Salthouse, T. A., & Ellis, C. L. (1980). Determinants of eye-fixation duration. *The American Journal of Psychology*, *93*(2), 207–234. https://doi.org/10.2307/1422228

Salthouse, T. A., & Miles, J. D. (2002). Aging and time-sharing aspects of executive control. *Memory & Cognition*, *30*(4), 572–582. https://doi.org/10.3758/BF03194958

Saltzman, I. J., & Garner, W. R. (1948). Reaction time as a measure of span of attention. *The Journal of Psychology*, *25*(2), 227–241. https://doi.org/10.1080/00223980.1948.9917373

Salvucci, D. D. (2017). ACT-R and beyond. In S. E. F. Chipman (Ed.), *The Oxford handbook of cognitive science* (pp. 15–26). Oxford University Press.

Salvucci, D. D., & Taatgen, N. A. (2011). *The multitasking mind*. Oxford University Press.

Sams, M., Paavilainen, P., Alho, K., & Näätänen, R. (1985). Auditory frequency discrimination and event-related potentials. *Electroencephalography & Clinical Neurophysiology: Evoked Potentials, 62*(6), 437–448. https://doi.org/10.1016/0168-5597(85)90054-1

Samson, D., Apperly, I. A., Braithwaite, J. J., Andrews, B. J., & Bodley Scott, S. E. (2010). Seeing it their way: Evidence for rapid and involuntary computation of what other people see. *Journal of Experimental Psychology: Human Perception and Performance, 36*(5), 1255–1266. https://doi.org/10.1037/a0018729

Sanders, A. F. (1990). Issues and trends in the debate on discrete vs. continuous processing of information. *Acta Psychologica, 74*(2-3), 123–167. https://doi.org/10.1016/0001-6918(90)90004-Y

Santiesteban, I., Catmur, C., Hopkins, S. C., Bird, G., & Heyes, C. (2014). Avatars and arrows: Implicit mentalizing or domain-general processing? *Journal of Experimental Psychology: Human Perception and Performance, 40*(3), 929–937. https://doi.org/10.1037/a0035175

Sarter, N. (2008). Investigating mode errors on automated flight decks: Illustrating the problem-driven, cumulative, and interdisciplinary nature of human factors research. *Human Factors, 50*(3), 506–510. https://doi.org/10.1518/001872008X312233

Sarter, N. B. (2000). The need for multisensory interfaces in support of effective attention allocation and highly dynamic event-driven domains: The case of cockpit automation. *International Journal of Aviation Psychology, 10*, 231–245. https://doi.org/10.1207/S15327108IJAP1003_02

Sarter, N. B., & Woods, D. D. (1992). Pilot interaction with cockpit automation: Operational experiences with the flight management system. *The International Journal of Aviation Psychology, 2*(4), 303–321. https://doi.org/10.1207/s15327108ijap0204_5

Sarter, N. B., & Woods, D. D. (1995). "How in the world did we ever get into that mode?" Mode error and awareness in supervisory control. *Human Factors, 37*(1), 5–19. https://doi.org/10.1518/001872095779049516

Sasin, E., & Fougnie, D. (2021). The road to long-term memory: Top-down attention is more effective than bottom-up attention for forming long-term memories. *Psychonomic Bulletin & Review, 28*(3), 937–945. https://doi.org/10.3758/s13423-020-01856-y

Satel, J., Wilson, N. R., & Klein, R. M. (2019). What neuroscientific studies tell us about inhibition of return. *Vision, 3*(4), 58. https://doi.org/10.3390/vision3040058

Schachar, R. J., & Logan, G. D. (1990). Impulsivity and inhibitory control in normal development and childhood psychopathology. *Developmental Psychology, 26*(5), 710–720. https://doi.org/10.1037/0012-1649.26.5.710

Scharf, B., & Buus, S. (1986). Audition I: Stimulus, physiology, thresholds. In K. Boff, L. Kaufman, & J. Thomas (Eds.), *Handbook of perception and performance* (Vol. I, pp. 14.1–14.71). Wiley.

Schlaghecken, F., Blagrove, E., Mantantzis, K., Maylor, E. A., & Watson, D. G. (2017). Look on the bright side: Positivity bias modulates interference effects in the Simon task. *Journal of Experimental Psychology: General, 146*(6), 763–770. https://doi.org/10.1037/xge0000316

Schmidgen, H. (2002). Of frogs and men: The origins of psychophysiological time experiments, 1850–1865. *Endeavour, 26*(4), 142–148. https://doi.org/10.1016/S0160-9327(02)01466-7

Schmidt, J. R. (2013). Questioning conflict adaptation: Proportion congruent and Gratton effects reconsidered. *Psychonomic Bulletin & Review, 20*(4), 615–630. https://doi.org/10.3758/s13423-012-0373-0

Schmidt, J. R. (2019). Evidence against conflict monitoring and adaptation: An updated review. *Psychonomic Bulletin & Review, 26*(3), 753–771. https://doi.org/10.3758/s13423-018-1520-z

Schneider, D. W. (2017). Phasic alertness and residual switch costs in task switching. *Journal of Experimental Psychology: Human Perception and Performance, 43*(2), 317–327. https://doi.org/10.1037/xhp0000318

Schneider, D. W. (2019). Alertness and cognitive control: Is there a spatial attention constraint? *Attention, Perception, & Psychophysics, 81*(1), 119–136. https://doi.org/10.3758/s13414-018-1613-9

Schneider, D. W., & Dixon, P. (2009). Visuospatial cues for reinstating mental models in working memory during interrupted reading. *Canadian Journal of Experimental Psychology, 63*(3), 161–172. https://doi.org/10.1037/a0014867

Schneider, W., & Fisk, A. D. (1982). Concurrent automatic and controlled visual search: Can processing occur without resource cost? *Journal of Experimental Psychology: Learning, Memory, and Cognition, 8*(4), 261–278. https://doi.org/10.1037/0278-7393.8.4.261

Schneider, W., & Shiffrin, R. M. (1977). Controlled and automatic human information processing: I. Detection, search, and attention. *Psychological Review, 84*(1), 1–66. https://doi.org/10.1037/0033-295X.84.1.1

Scholkmann, F., Holper, L., Wolf, U., & Wolf, M. (2013). A new methodical approach in neuroscience: Assessing inter-personal brain coupling using functional near-infrared imaging (fNIRI) hyperscanning. *Frontiers in Human Neuroscience, 7,* Article 813. https://doi.org/10.3389/fnhum.2013.00813

Schröger, E. (1996). A neural mechanism for involuntary attention shifts to changes in auditory stimulation. *Journal of Cognitive Neuroscience, 8*(6), 527–539. https://doi.org/10.1162/jocn.1996.8.6.527

Schumacher, N., Reer, R., & Braumann, K. M. (2020). On-field perceptual-cognitive training improves peripheral reaction in soccer: A controlled trial. *Frontiers in Psychology, 11,* Article 1948. https://doi.org/10.3389/fpsyg.2020.01948

Schweickert, R. (1978). A critical path generalization of the additive factor method: Analysis of a Stroop task. *Journal of Mathematical Psychology, 18*(2), 105–139. https://doi.org/10.1016/0022-2496(78)90059-7

Schweickert, R., & Boruff, B. (1986). Short-term memory capacity: Magic number or magic spell? *Journal of Experimental Psychology: Learning, Memory, and Cognition, 12*(3), 419–425. https://doi.org/10.1037/0278-7393.12.3.419

Sciberras, E., Streatfeild, J., Ceccato, T., Pezzullo, L., Scott, J. G., Middeldorp, C. M., Hutchins, P., Paterson, R., Bellgrove, M. A., & Coghill, D. (2022). Social and economic costs of attention-deficit/hyperactivity disorder across the lifespan. *Journal of Attention Disorders, 26*(1), 72–87. https://doi.org/10.1177/1087054720961828

Sebanz, N., Knoblich, G., & Prinz, W. (2003). Representing others' actions: Just like one's own? *Cognition, 88*(3), B11–B21. https://doi.org/10.1016/S0010-0277(03)00043-X

Sebanz, N., Knoblich, G., & Prinz, W. (2005). How two share a task: Corepresenting stimulus-response mappings. *Journal of Experimental Psychology: Human Perception and Performance, 31*(6), 1234–1246. https://doi.org/10.1037/0096-1523.31.6.1234

See, J. E., Howe, S. R., Warm, J. S., & Dember, W. N. (1995). Meta-analysis of the sensitivity decrement in vigilance. *Psychological Bulletin, 117*(2), 230–249. https://doi.org/10.1037/0033-2909.117.2.230

Selcon, S. J., & Taylor, R. M. (1990). *Evaluation of the situational awareness rating technique (SART) as a tool for aircrew systems design.* https://ext.eurocontrol.int/ehp/?q=node/1608

Senderecka, M., Grabowska, A., Szewczyk, J., Gerc, K., & Chmylak, R. (2012). Response inhibition of children with ADHD in the stop-signal task: An event-related potential study. *International Journal of Psychophysiology, 85*(1), 93–105. https://doi.org/10.1016/j.ijpsycho.2011.05.007

Servant, M., Cassey, P., Woodman, G. F., & Logan, G. D. (2018). Neural bases of automaticity. *Journal of Experimental Psychology: Learning, Memory, and Cognition, 44*(3), 440–464. https://doi.org/10.1037/xlm0000454

Shaffer, L. H. (1965). Choice reaction with variable S–R mapping. *Journal of Experimental Psychology, 70*(3), 284–288. https://doi.org/10.1037/h0022207

Shaffer, L. H. (1975). Multiple attention in continuous verbal tasks. In P. M. A. Rabbitt & S. Dorn (Eds.), *Attention and performance V* (pp. 157–167). Academic Press.

Shannon, C. E., & Weaver, W. (1949). *The mathematical theory of communication.* University of Illinois Press.

Shapiro, K. L., Hanslmayr, S., Enns, J. T., & Lleras, A. (2017). Alpha, beta: The rhythm of the attentional blink. *Psychonomic Bulletin & Review, 24*(6), 1862–1869. https://doi.org/10.3758/s13423-017-1257-0

Sheehan, W. (2013). From the transits of Venus to the birth of experimental psychology. *Physics in Perspective, 15*(2), 130–159. https://doi.org/10.1007/s00016-012-0101-1

Shell, D. F., & Flowerday, T. (2019). Affordances and attention: Learning and culture. In K. A. Renninger & S. E. Hidi (Eds.), *The Cambridge handbook of motivation and learning* (pp. 759–782). Cambridge University Press. https://doi.org/10.1017/9781316823279.032

Shen, J., & Reingold, E. M. (2001). Visual search asymmetry: The influence of stimulus familiarity and low-level features. *Perception & Psychophysics, 63*(3), 464–475. https://doi.org/10.3758/BF03194413

Shiffrin, R. M., Diller, D., & Cohen, A. (1996). Processing visual information in an unattended location. In A. F. Kramer & M. G. H. Coles (Eds.), *Converging operations in the study of visual selective attention* (pp. 225–245). American Psychological Association. https://doi.org/10.1037/10187-007

Shiffrin, R. M., & Schneider, W. (1977). Controlled and automatic human information processing: II. Perceptual learning, automatic attending, and a general theory. *Psychological Review, 84*(2), 127–190. https://doi.org/10.1037/0033-295X.84.2.127

Shirama, A., Kato, N., & Kashino, M. (2017). When do individuals with autism spectrum disorder show superiority in visual search? *Autism, 21*(8), 942–951. https://doi.org/10.1177/1362361316656943

Shmueli, Y., Degani, A., Zelman, I., Asherov, R., Zande, D., Weiss, J., & Bernard, A. (2013, September). Toward a formal approach to information integration evaluation of an automotive instrument display. *Proceedings of the Human Factors and*

Ergonomics Society Annual Meeting, 57(1), 1658–1662. https://doi.org/10.1177/1541931213571368

Shomstein, S. (2012). Cognitive functions of the posterior parietal cortex: Top-down and bottom-up attentional control. *Frontiers in Integrative Neuroscience, 6,* Article 38. https://doi.org/10.3389/fnint.2012.00038

Shortliffe, E. H. (1976). *MYCIN: Computer-based medical consultation.* Elsevier.

Shteynberg, G. (2015). Shared attention. *Perspectives on Psychological Science, 10*(5), 579–590. https://doi.org/10.1177/1745691615589104

Shteynberg, G. (2018). A collective perspective: Shared attention and the mind. *Current Opinion in Psychology, 23,* 93–97. https://doi.org/10.1016/j.copsyc.2017.12.007

Shteynberg, G., Hirsh, J. B., Apfelbaum, E. P., Larsen, J. T., Galinsky, A. D., & Roese, N. J. (2014). Feeling more together: Group attention intensifies emotion. *Emotion, 14*(6), 1102–1114. https://doi.org/10.1037/a0037697

Shtyrov, Y., & Pulvermüller, F. (2002). Neurophysiological evidence of memory traces for words in the human brain. *Neuroreport, 13*(4), 521–525. https://doi.org/10.1097/00001756-200203250-00033

Simione, L., Di Pace, E., Chiarella, S. G., & Raffone, A. (2019). Visual attention modulates phenomenal consciousness: Evidence from a change detection study. *Frontiers in Psychology, 10,* Article 2150. https://doi.org/10.3389/fpsyg.2019.02150

Simon, H. A. (1979). Information processing models of cognition. *Annual Review of Psychology, 30*(1), 363–396. https://doi.org/10.1146/annurev.ps.30.020179.002051

Simon, J. R. (1969). Reactions toward the source of stimulation. *Journal of Experimental Psychology, 81*(1), 174–176. https://doi.org/10.1037/h0027448

Simon, J. R. (1990). The effects of an irrelevant directional cue on human information processing. In R. W. Proctor & T. G. Reeve (Eds.), *Stimulus-response compatibility: An integrated perspective* (pp. 31–86). North-Holland. https://doi.org/10.1016/S0166-4115(08)61218-2

Simon, J. R., & Pouraghabagher, A. R. (1978). The effect of aging on the stages of processing in a choice reaction time task. *Journal of Gerontology, 33*(4), 553–561. https://doi.org/10.1093/geronj/33.4.553

Simon, J. R., & Rudell, A. P. (1967). Auditory S-R compatibility: The effect of an irrelevant cue on information processing. *Journal of Applied Psychology, 51*(3), 300–304. https://doi.org/10.1037/h0020586

Simon, J. R., & Small, A. M., Jr. (1969). Processing auditory information: Interference from an irrelevant cue. *Journal of Applied Psychology, 53*(5), 433–435. https://doi.org/10.1037/h0028034

Simons, D. J. (1996). In sight, out of mind: When object representations fail. *Psychological Science, 7*(5), 301–305. https://doi.org/10.1111/j.1467-9280.1996.tb00378.x

Simons, D. J., & Chabris, C. F. (1999). Gorillas in our midst: Sustained inattentional blindness for dynamic events. *Perception, 28*(9), 1059–1074. https://doi.org/10.1068/p281059

Simons, D. J., & Levin, D. T. (1998). Failure to detect changes to people in a real-world interaction. *Psychonomic Bulletin & Review, 5*(4), 644–649. https://doi.org/10.3758/BF03208840

Singh, I. L., Molloy, R., & Parasuraman, R. (1993). Individual differences in monitoring failures of automation. *The Journal of General Psychology, 120*(3), 357–373. https://doi.org/10.1080/00221309.1993.9711153

Slagter, H. A., Prinssen, S., Reteig, L. C., & Mazaheri, A. (2016). Facilitation and inhibition in attention: Functional dissociation of pre-stimulus alpha activity, P1, and N1 components. *NeuroImage, 125,* 25–35. https://doi.org/10.1016/j.neuroimage.2015.09.058

Slotnick, S. D. (2005). Source localization of ERP generators. In T. C. Handy (Ed.), *Event-related potentials: A methods handbook* (pp. 149–166). MIT Press.

Smallman, H. S., & St. John, M. (2005). Naive realism: Misplaced faith in realistic displays. *Ergonomics in Design, 13*(3), 6–13. https://doi.org/10.1177/106480460501300303

Smirl, J. D., Wright, A. D., Bryk, K., & van Donkelaar, P. (2016). Where's Waldo? The utility of a complicated visual search paradigm for transcranial Doppler-based assessments of neurovascular coupling. *Journal of Neuroscience Methods, 270,* 92–101. https://doi.org/10.1016/j.jneumeth.2016.06.007

Smith, D. T., & Casteau, S. (2019). The effect of offset cues on saccade programming and covert attention. *Quarterly Journal of Experimental Psychology, 72*(3), 481–490. https://doi.org/10.1177/1747021818759468

Smith, M. C. (1967). Theories of the psychological refractory period. *Psychological Bulletin, 67*(3), 202–213. https://doi.org/10.1037/h0020419

Smulders, F. T., Miller, J. O., & Luck, S. J. (2012). The lateralized readiness potential. In S. J. Luck & E. S. Kappenman (Eds.), *The Oxford handbook of event-related potential components* (pp. 209–229). Oxford University Press.

Sobel, K. V., Puri, A. M., & York, A. K. (2020). Visual search inverts the classic Stroop asymmetry. *Acta Psychologica, 205,* Article 103054. https://doi.org/10.1016/j.actpsy.2020.103054

Soetens, E. (1998). Localizing sequential effects in serial choice reaction time with the information reduction procedure. *Journal of Experimental Psychology: Human Perception and Performance, 24*(2), 547–568. https://doi.org/10.1037/0096-1523.24.2.547

Sokolov, E. N. (1963). *Perception and the conditioned reflex.* Macmillan.

Solís-Marcos, I., & Kircher, K. (2019). Event-related potentials as indices of mental workload while using an in-vehicle information system. *Cognition Technology and Work, 21*(1), 55–67. https://doi.org/10.1007/s10111-018-0485-z

Song, S., Zilverstand, A., Song, H., Uquillas, F. D., Wang, Y., Xie, C., Cheng, L., & Zou, Z. (2017). The influence of emotional interference on cognitive control: A meta-analysis of neuroimaging studies using the emotional Stroop task. *Scientific Reports, 7*(1), Article 2088.

Sorkin, R. D., Pohlmann, L. D., & Gilliom, J. D. (1973). Simultaneous two-channel signal detection. III. 630- and 1400-Hz signals. *The Journal of the Acoustical Society of America, 53*(4), 1045–1050. https://doi.org/10.1121/1.1913422

Soroker, N., Calamaro, N., Glicksohn, J., & Myslobodsky, M. S. (1997). Auditory inattention in right-hemisphere-damaged patients with and without visual neglect. *Neuropsychologia, 35*(3), 249–256. https://doi.org/10.1016/S0028-3932(96)00038-3

Soto-Faraco, S., Morein-Zamir, S., & Kingstone, A. (2005). On audiovisual spatial synergy: The fragility of the phenomenon. *Perception & Psychophysics, 67*(3), 444–457. https://doi.org/10.3758/BF03193323

Spector, A., & Biederman, I. (1976). Mental set and mental shift revisited. *The American Journal of Psychology, 89*(4), 669–679. https://doi.org/10.2307/1421465

Spelke, E., Hirst, W., & Neisser, U. (1976). Skills of divided attention. *Cognition, 4*(3), 215–230. https://doi.org/10.1016/0010-0277(76)90018-4

Spence, C. (2010). Crossmodal spatial attention. *Annals of the New York Academy of Sciences, 1191*(1), 182–200. https://doi.org/10.1111/j.1749-6632.2010.05440.x

Spence, C., & Driver, J. (1996). Audiovisual links in endogenous covert spatial attention. *Journal of Experimental Psychology: Human Perception and Performance, 22*(4), 1005–1030. https://doi.org/10.1037/0096-1523.22.4.1005

Spence, C., & Driver, J. (1997). Audiovisual links in exogenous covert spatial orienting. *Perception & Psychophysics, 59*(1), 1–22. https://doi.org/10.3758/BF03206843

Spence, C., & Driver, J. (2000). Attracting attention to the illusory location of a sound: Reflexive crossmodal orienting and ventriloquism. *Neuroreport, 11*(9), 2057–2061. https://doi.org/10.1097/00001756-200006260-00049

Spence, C., & Gallace, A. (2007). Recent developments in the study of tactile attention. *Canadian Journal of Experimental Psychology, 61*(3), 196–207. https://doi.org/10.1037/cjep2007021

Spence, C., Lloyd, D., McGlone, F., Nicholls, M. E., & Driver, J. (2000). Inhibition of return is supramodal: A demonstration between all possible pairings of vision, touch, and audition. *Experimental Brain Research, 134*(1), 42–48. https://doi.org/10.1007/s002210000442

Spence, C., & McGlone, F. P. (2001). Reflexive spatial orienting of tactile attention. *Experimental Brain Research, 141*(3), 324–330. https://doi.org/10.1007/s002210100883

Spence, C., Parise, C., & Chen, Y. C. (2012). The Colavita visual dominance effect. In M. M. Murray & M. T. Wallace (Eds.), *The neural bases of multisensory processes* (pp. 529–556). CRC Press.

Spence, C., Pavani, F., & Driver, J. (2000). Crossmodal links between vision and touch in covert endogenous spatial attention. *Journal of Experimental Psychology: Human Perception and Performance, 26*(4), 1298–1319. https://doi.org/10.1037/0096-1523.26.4.1298

Spence, C., Shore, D. I., & Klein, R. M. (2001). Multisensory prior entry. *Journal of Experimental Psychology: General, 130*(4), 799–832. https://doi.org/10.1037/0096-3445.130.4.799

Spence, C., & Soto-Foraco, S. (2020). *Crossmodal attention applied: Lessons for driving.* Cambridge University Press. https://doi.org/10.1017/9781108919951

Sperling, G. (1960). The information available in brief visual presentations. *Psychological Monographs, 74*(11), 1–29. https://doi.org/10.1037/h0093759

Sperling, G., & Melchner, M. J. (1978, October 20). The attention operating characteristic: Examples from visual search. *Science, 202*(4365), 315–318. https://doi.org/10.1126/science.694536

Spitz, G. (1988). Flexibility in resource allocation and the performance of time-sharing tasks. In *Proceedings of the Human Factors Society 32nd Annual Meeting* (pp. 1466–1470). Human Factors Society.

Squire, L. R. (2009). The legacy of patient H.M. for neuroscience. *Neuron, 61*(1), 6–9. https://doi.org/10.1016/j.neuron.2008.12.023

Stamatakis, E. A., Orfanidou, E., & Papanicolaou, A. C. (2017). Functional magnetic resonance imaging. In A. C. Papanicolaou (Ed.), *The Oxford handbook of functional brain imaging in neuropsychology and cognitive neurosciences* (pp. 41–59). Oxford University Press.

Stanton, N. A., Stewart, R., Harris, D., Houghton, R. J., Baber, C., McMaster, R., & Green, D. (2017). Distributed situation awareness in dynamic systems: Theoretical development and application of an ergonomics methodology. In E. Salas

& A. S. Dietz (Eds.), *Situational awareness* (pp. 419–442). Routledge. https://doi.org/10.4324/9781315087924-25

Stapel, J., Mullakkal-Babu, F. A., & Happee, R. (2019). Automated driving reduces perceived workload, but monitoring causes higher cognitive load than manual driving. *Transportation Research Part F: Traffic Psychology and Behaviour, 60*, 590–605. https://doi.org/10.1016/j.trf.2018.11.006

Stein, B. E., London, N., Wilkinson, L. K., & Price, D. D. (1996). Enhancement of perceived visual intensity by auditory stimuli: A psychophysical analysis. *Journal of Cognitive Neuroscience, 8*(6), 497–506. https://doi.org/10.1162/jocn.1996.8.6.497

Stein, B. E., & Meredith, M. A. (1993). *The merging of the senses.* MIT Press.

Stein, E. (1985). *Controller workload: An examination of workload probe* (DOT/FAA/CT-TN84/24). Federal Aviation Administration Technical Center.

Stephenson, L. J., Edwards, S. G., & Bayliss, A. P. (2021). From gaze perception to social cognition: The shared-attention system. *Perspectives on Psychological Science, 16*(3), 553–576. https://doi.org/10.1177/1745691620953773

Sternberg, S. (1969). The discovery of processing stages: Extensions of Donders' method. *Acta Psychologica, 30*, 276–315. https://doi.org/10.1016/0001-6918(69)90055-9

Stewart, L., Ellison, A., Walsh, V., & Cowey, A. (2001). The role of transcranial magnetic stimulation (TMS) in studies of vision, attention and cognition. *Acta Psychologica, 107*(1-3), 275–291. https://doi.org/10.1016/S0001-6918(01)00035-X

Stoffer, T. H. (1991). Attentional focussing and spatial stimulus-response compatibility. *Psychological Research, 53*(2), 127–135. https://doi.org/10.1007/BF01371820

Störmer, V. S. (2019). Orienting spatial attention to sounds enhances visual processing. *Current Opinion in Psychology, 29*, 193–198. https://doi.org/10.1016/j.copsyc.2019.03.010

Störmer, V. S., Feng, W., Martinez, A., McDonald, J. J., & Hillyard, S. A. (2016). Salient, irrelevant sounds reflexively induce alpha rhythm desynchronization in parallel with slow potential shifts in visual cortex. *Journal of Cognitive Neuroscience, 28*(3), 433–445. https://doi.org/10.1162/jocn_a_00915

Störmer, V. S., McDonald, J. J., & Hillyard, S. A. (2009). Cross-modal cueing of attention alters appearance and early cortical processing of visual stimuli. *PNAS, 106*(52), 22456–22461. https://doi.org/10.1073/pnas.0907573106

Störmer, V. S., McDonald, J. J., & Hillyard, S. A. (2019). Involuntary orienting of attention to sight or sound relies on similar neural biasing mechanisms in early visual processing. *Neuropsychologia, 132*, 107122. https://doi.org/10.1016/j.neuropsychologia.2019.107122

Strater, L. D., Endsley, M. R., Pleban, R. J., & Matthews, M. D. (2001). *Measures of platoon leader situation awareness in virtual decision-making exercises* (Research Report 1770). U.S. Army Institute for the Behavioral and Social Sciences. https://apps.dtic.mil/sti/pdfs/ADA390238.pdf

Strayer, D. L., & Kramer, A. F. (1990). Attentional requirements of automatic and controlled processing. *Journal of Experimental Psychology: Learning, Memory, and Cognition, 16*(1), 67–82. https://doi.org/10.1037/0278-7393.16.1.67

Strayer, D. L., Wickens, C. D., & Braune, R. (1987). Adult age differences in the speed and capacity of information processing: 2. An electrophysiological approach. *Psychology and Aging, 2*(2), 99–110. https://doi.org/10.1037/0882-7974.2.2.99

Strevens, M. (2020). *The knowledge machine: How irrationality created modern science.* Liveright.

Strobach, T., & Schubert, T. (2021). Video game training and effects on executive functions. In T. Srobach & J. Karbach (Eds.), *Cognitive training* (pp. 229–241). Springer. https://doi.org/10.1007/978-3-030-39292-5_16

Stroop, J. R. (1992). Studies of interference in serial verbal reactions. *Journal of Experimental Psychology: General, 121,* 15–23. https://doi.org/10.1037/0096-3445.121.1.15 (Original work published 1935)

Strybel, T. Z., Boucher, J. M., Fujawa, G. E., & Volp, C. S. (1995). Auditory spatial cueing in visual search tasks: Effects of amplitude, contrast and duration. In *Proceedings of the Human Factors and Ergonomics Society 39th Annual Meeting* (pp. 109–113). Human Factors and Ergonomics Society.

Stuiver, A., Brookhuis, K. A., de Waard, D., & Mulder, B. (2014). Short-term cardiovascular measures for driver support: Increasing sensitivity for detecting changes in mental workload. *International Journal of Psychophysiology, 92*(1), 35–41. https://doi.org/10.1016/j.ijpsycho.2014.01.010

Stürmer, B., Leuthold, H., Soetens, E., Schröter, H., & Sommer, W. (2002). Control over location-based response activation in the Simon task: Behavioral and electrophysiological evidence. *Journal of Experimental Psychology: Human Perception and Performance, 28*(6), 1345–1363. https://doi.org/10.1037/0096-1523.28.6.1345

Stuss, D. T., & Alexander, M. P. (2007). Is there a dysexecutive syndrome? *Philosophical Transactions of the Royal Society of London: Series B. Biological Sciences, 362*(1481), 901–915. https://doi.org/10.1098/rstb.2007.2096

Stuss, D. T., Shallice, T., Alexander, M. P., & Picton, T. W. (1995). A multidisciplinary approach to anterior attentional functions. *Annals of the New York Academy of Sciences, 769*(1), 191–212. https://doi.org/10.1111/j.1749-6632.1995.tb38140.x

Suedfeld, P., & Landon, P. B. (1970). Motivational arousal and task complexity. *Journal of Experimental Psychology, 83*(2, Pt. 1), 329–330. https://doi.org/10.1037/h0028523

Sushereba, C. E. L., Bennett, K. B., & Bryant, A. (2020). Visual displays for cyber network defense. *Ergonomics, 63*(2), 191–209. https://doi.org/10.1080/00140139.2019.1694181

Suzuki, S., & Cavanagh, P. (1997). Focused attention distorts visual space: An attentional repulsion effect. *Journal of Experimental Psychology: Human Perception and Performance, 23*(2), 443–463. https://doi.org/10.1037/0096-1523.23.2.443

Swick, D., Ashley, V., & Turken, A. U. (2008). Left inferior frontal gyrus is critical for response inhibition. *BMC Neuroscience, 9*(1), 102. https://doi.org/10.1186/1471-2202-9-102

Sykes, D. H., Douglas, V. I., & Morgenstern, G. (1973). Sustained attention in hyperactive children. *Journal of Child Psychology and Psychiatry, 14*(3), 213–220. https://doi.org/10.1111/j.1469-7610.1973.tb01189.x

Tada, M., Kirihara, K., Mizutani, S., Uka, T., Kunii, N., Koshiyama, D., Fujioka, M., Usui, K., Nagai, T., Araki, T., & Kasai, K. (2019). Mismatch negativity (MMN) as a tool for translational investigations into early psychosis: A review. *International Journal of Psychophysiology, 145,* 5–14. https://doi.org/10.1016/j.ijpsycho.2019.02.009

Tagliabue, M., Zorzi, M., Umiltà, C., & Bassignani, F. (2000). The role of long-term-memory and short-term-memory links in the Simon effect. *Journal of Experimental Psychology: Human Perception and Performance, 26*(2), 648–670. https://doi.org/10.1037/0096-1523.26.2.648

Takio, F., Koivisto, M., Jokiranta, L., Rashid, F., Kallio, J., Tuominen, T., Laukka, S. J., & Hämäläinen, H. (2009). The effect of age on attentional modulation in Dichotic listening. *Developmental Neuropsychology, 34*(3), 225–239. https://doi.org/10.1080/87565640902805669

Tanji, J., & Evarts, E. V. (1976). Anticipatory activity of motor cortex neurons in relation to direction of an intended movement. *Journal of Neurophysiology, 39*(5), 1062–1068. https://doi.org/10.1152/jn.1976.39.5.1062

Tao, J., Yafeng, N., & Lei, Z. (2017). Are the warning icons more attentional? *Applied Ergonomics, 65*, 51–60. https://doi.org/10.1016/j.apergo.2017.05.012

Taylor, T. L., & Klein, R. M. (2000). Visual and motor effects in inhibition of return. *Journal of Experimental Psychology: Human Perception and Performance, 26*(5), 1639–1656. https://doi.org/10.1037/0096-1523.26.5.1639

Teder-Sälejärvi, W. A., McDonald, J. J., Di Russo, F., & Hillyard, S. A. (2002). An analysis of audio-visual crossmodal integration by means of event-related potential (ERP) recordings. *Cognitive Brain Research, 14*(1), 106–114. https://doi.org/10.1016/S0926-6410(02)00065-4

Telford, C. W. (1931). Refractory phase of voluntary and associative responses. *Journal of Experimental Psychology, 14*(1), 1–36. https://doi.org/10.1037/h0073262

Tenison, C., Fincham, J. M., & Anderson, J. R. (2016). Phases of learning: How skill acquisition impacts cognitive processing. *Cognitive Psychology, 87*, 1–28. https://doi.org/10.1016/j.cogpsych.2016.03.001

Theeuwes, J. (1989). Effects of location and form cuing on the allocation of attention in the visual field. *Acta Psychologica, 72*(2), 177–192. https://doi.org/10.1016/0001-6918(89)90043-7

Theeuwes, J. (1991). Exogenous and endogenous control of attention: The effect of visual onsets and offsets. *Perception & Psychophysics, 49*(1), 83–90. https://doi.org/10.3758/BF03211619

Theeuwes, J. (1993). Visual selective attention: A theoretical analysis. *Acta Psychologica, 83*(2), 93–154. https://doi.org/10.1016/0001-6918(93)90042-P

Theeuwes, J. (1995). Abrupt luminance change pops out; abrupt color change does not. *Perception & Psychophysics, 57*(5), 637–644. https://doi.org/10.3758/BF03213269

Theeuwes, J., & Van der Burg, E. (2007). The role of spatial and nonspatial information in visual selection. *Journal of Experimental Psychology: Human Perception and Performance, 33*(6), 1335–1351. https://doi.org/10.1037/0096-1523.33.6.1335

Thompson, K. G., Biscoe, K. L., & Sato, T. R. (2005). Neuronal basis of covert spatial attention in the frontal eye field. *The Journal of Neuroscience, 25*(41), 9479–9487. https://doi.org/10.1523/JNEUROSCI.0741-05.2005

Thomson, D. R., Besner, D., & Smilek, D. (2015). A resource-control account of sustained attention: Evidence from mind-wandering and vigilance paradigms. *Perspectives on Psychological Science, 10*(1), 82–96. https://doi.org/10.1177/1745691614556681

Thomson, S. J., Danis, L. K., & Watter, S. (2015). PRP training shows Task1 response selection is the locus of the backward response compatibility effect. *Psychonomic Bulletin & Review, 22*(1), 212–218. https://doi.org/10.3758/s13423-014-0660-z

Thropp, J. E., Szalma, J. L., & Hancock, P. A. (2004). Performance operating characteristics for spatial and temporal discriminations: Common or separate capacities? *Proceedings of the Human Factors and Ergonomics Society Annual Meeting, 48*(16), 1880–1884. https://doi.org/10.1177/154193120404801619

Timme, N. M., & Lapish, C. (2018). A tutorial for information theory in neuroscience. *eNeuro*, *5*(3), Article e0052-18.2018, 1–40. https://doi.org/10.1523/ENEURO.0052-18.2018

Tipper, S. P. (1985). The negative priming effect: Inhibitory priming by ignored objects. *Quarterly Journal of Experimental Psychology*, *37*(4), 571–590. https://doi.org/10.1080/14640748508400920

Tipper, S. P., Brehaut, J. C., & Driver, J. (1990). Selection of moving and static objects for the control of spatially directed action. *Journal of Experimental Psychology: Human Perception and Performance*, *16*(3), 492–504. https://doi.org/10.1037/0096-1523.16.3.492

Tipper, S. P., Howard, L. A., & Houghton, G. (1998). Action-based mechanisms of attention. *Philosophical Transactions of the Royal Society of London: Series B. Biological Sciences*, *353*(1373), 1385–1393. https://doi.org/10.1098/rstb.1998.0292

Tipper, S. P., Lortie, C., & Baylis, G. C. (1992). Selective reaching: Evidence for action-centered attention. *Journal of Experimental Psychology: Human Perception and Performance*, *18*(4), 891–905. https://doi.org/10.1037/0096-1523.18.4.891

Tipper, S. P., Meegan, D., & Howard, L. A. (2002). Action-centred negative priming: Evidence for reactive inhibition. *Visual Cognition*, *9*(4-5), 591–614. https://doi.org/10.1080/13506280143000593

Tipples, J. (2002). Eye gaze is not unique: Automatic orienting in response to uninformative arrows. *Psychonomic Bulletin & Review*, *9*(2), 314–318. https://doi.org/10.3758/BF03196287

Titchener, E. B. (1910). Attention as sensory clearness. *The Journal of Philosophy, Psychology, and Scientific Methods*, *7*(7), 180–182. https://doi.org/10.2307/2010783

Titchener, E. B. (1973). *Psychology of feeling and attention*. Arno Press. (Original work published 1908)

Todd, R. D., & Botteron, K. N. (2001). Is attention-deficit/hyperactivity disorder an energy deficiency syndrome? *Biological Psychiatry*, *50*(3), 151–158. https://doi.org/10.1016/S0006-3223(01)01173-8

Tombu, M., & Jolicoeur, P. (2002). All-or-none bottleneck versus capacity sharing accounts of the psychological refractory period phenomenon. *Psychological Research*, *66*(4), 274–286. https://doi.org/10.1007/s00426-002-0101-x

Tombu, M., & Jolicoeur, P. (2005). Testing the predictions of the central capacity sharing model. *Journal of Experimental Psychology: Human Perception and Performance*, *31*(4), 790–802. https://doi.org/10.1037/0096-1523.31.4.790

Tomko, L., & Proctor, R. W. (2017). Crossmodal spatial congruence effects: Visual dominance in conditions of increased and reduced selection difficulty. *Psychological Research*, *81*(5), 1035–1050. https://doi.org/10.1007/s00426-016-0801-2

Townsend, J. T. (1971). A note on the identifiability of parallel and serial processes. *Perception & Psychophysics*, *10*(3), 161–163. https://doi.org/10.3758/BF03205778

Townsend, J. T. (1972). Some results concerning the identifiability of parallel and serial processes. *British Journal of Mathematical & Statistical Psychology*, *25*(2), 168–199. https://doi.org/10.1111/j.2044-8317.1972.tb00490.x

Treat, J., Tumbas, N., McDonald, S., Shinar, D., Hume, R., Mayer, R., Stansifer, R., & Castellan, N. (1979). *Tri-level study of the causes of traffic accidents: Executive summary* (National Technical Information Services Technical Report No. DOT HS-805 099). University of Indiana.

Treccani, B., Argyri, E., Sorace, A., & Sala, S. D. (2009). Spatial negative priming in bilingualism. *Psychonomic Bulletin & Review*, *16*(2), 320–327. https://doi.org/10.3758/PBR.16.2.320

Treisman, A. (1991). Search, similarity, and integration of features between and within dimensions. *Journal of Experimental Psychology: Human Perception and Performance, 17*(3), 652–676. https://doi.org/10.1037/0096-1523.17.3.652

Treisman, A. (1998). The perception of features and objects. In R. D. Wright (Ed.), *Visual attention* (pp. 26–54). Oxford University Press.

Treisman, A., & Gormican, S. (1988). Feature analysis in early vision: Evidence from search asymmetries. *Psychological Review, 95*(1), 15–48. https://doi.org/10.1037/0033-295X.95.1.15

Treisman, A., Kahneman, D., & Burkell, J. (1983). Perceptual objects and the cost of filtering. *Perception & Psychophysics, 33*(6), 527–532. https://doi.org/10.3758/BF03202934

Treisman, A., & Sato, S. (1990). Conjunction search revisited. *Journal of Experimental Psychology: Human Perception and Performance, 16*(3), 459–478. https://doi.org/10.1037/0096-1523.16.3.459

Treisman, A., & Schmidt, H. (1982). Illusory conjunctions in the perception of objects. *Cognitive Psychology, 14*(1), 107–141. https://doi.org/10.1016/0010-0285(82)90006-8

Treisman, A., Squire, R., & Green, J. (1974). Semantic processing in dichotic listening? A replication. *Memory & Cognition, 2*(4), 641–646. https://doi.org/10.3758/BF03198133

Treisman, A. M. (1960). Contextual cues in selective listening. *Quarterly Journal of Experimental Psychology, 12*(4), 242–248. https://doi.org/10.1080/17470216008416732

Treisman, A. M. (1964a). The effect of irrelevant material on the efficiency of selective listening. *The American Journal of Psychology, 77*(4), 533–546. https://doi.org/10.2307/1420765

Treisman, A. M. (1964b). Monitoring and storage of irrelevant messages in selective attention. *Journal of Verbal Learning and Verbal Behavior, 3*(6), 449–459. https://doi.org/10.1016/S0022-5371(64)80015-3

Treisman, A. M. (1964c). Verbal cues, language, and meaning in attention. *The American Journal of Psychology, 77*(2), 206–219. https://doi.org/10.2307/1420127

Treisman, A. M. (1969). Strategies and models of selective attention. *Psychological Review, 76*(3), 282–299. https://doi.org/10.1037/h0027242

Treisman, A. M., & Gelade, G. (1980). A feature-integration theory of attention. *Cognitive Psychology, 12*(1), 97–136. https://doi.org/10.1016/0010-0285(80)90005-5

Treisman, A. M., & Riley, J. G. A. (1969). Is selective attention selective perception or selective response? A further test. *Journal of Experimental Psychology, 79*(1, Pt. 1), 27–34. https://doi.org/10.1037/h0026890

Tremper, K. K., Mace, J. J., Gombert, J. M., Tremper, T. T., Adams, J. F., & Bagian, J. P. (2018). Design of a novel multifunction decision support display for anesthesia care: AlertWatch® OR. *BMC Anesthesiology, 18*(1), 16. https://doi.org/10.1186/s12871-018-0478-8

Tsal, Y. (1983). Movements of attention across the visual field. *Journal of Experimental Psychology: Human Perception and Performance, 9*(4), 523–530. https://doi.org/10.1037/0096-1523.9.4.523

Tsal, Y., & Benoni, H. (2010). Diluting the burden of load: Perceptual load effects are simply dilution effects. *Journal of Experimental Psychology: Human Perception and Performance, 36*(6), 1645–1656. https://doi.org/10.1037/a0018172

Tsal, Y., & Lamy, D. (2000). Attending to an object's color entails attending to its location: Support for location-special views of visual attention. *Perception & Psychophysics, 62*(5), 960–968. https://doi.org/10.3758/BF03212081

Tsogli, V., Jentschke, S., Daikoku, T., & Koelsch, S. (2019). When the statistical MMN meets the physical MMN. *Scientific Reports, 9*(1), 5563. https://doi.org/10.1038/s41598-019-42066-4

Tufano, D. R. (1997). Automotive HUDs: The overlooked safety issues. *Human Factors, 39*(2), 303–311. https://doi.org/10.1518/001872097778543840

Tulving, E. (1985). How many memory systems are there? *American Psychologist, 40*(4), 385–398. https://doi.org/10.1037/0003-066X.40.4.385

Turatto, M., & Bridgeman, B. (2005). Change perception using visual transients: Object substitution and deletion. *Experimental Brain Research, 167*(4), 595–608. https://doi.org/10.1007/s00221-005-0056-4

Turvey, M. T. (1973). On peripheral and central processes in vision: Inferences from an information-processing analysis of masking with patterned stimuli. *Psychological Review, 80*(1), 1–52. https://doi.org/10.1037/h0033872

Ulrich, R., Mattes, S., & Miller, J. (1999). Donders's assumption of pure insertion: An evaluation on the basis of response dynamics. *Acta Psychologica, 102*(1), 43–76. https://doi.org/10.1016/S0001-6918(99)00019-0

Ulrich, R., Schröter, H., Leuthold, H., & Birngruber, T. (2015). Automatic and controlled stimulus processing in conflict tasks: Superimposed diffusion processes and delta functions. *Cognitive Psychology, 78*, 148–174. https://doi.org/10.1016/j.cogpsych.2015.02.005

Umiltà, C. (2022). The prefix neuro. In S. Della Sala (Ed.), *Encyclopedia of behavioral neuroscience* (2nd ed., pp. 569–572). Academic Press. https://doi.org/10.1016/B978-0-12-819641-0.00014-1

Umiltà, C., & Liotti, M. (1987). Egocentric and relative spatial codes in S-R compatibility. *Psychological Research, 49*(2-3), 81–90. https://doi.org/10.1007/BF00308672

Umiltà, C., & Nicoletti, R. (1990). Spatial stimulus-response compatibility. In R. W. Proctor & T. G. Reeve (Eds.), *Stimulus-response compatibility: An integrated perspective* (pp. 89–116). North-Holland.

Underwood, G. (1974). Moray vs. the rest: The effects of extended shadowing practice. *Quarterly Journal of Experimental Psychology, 26*(3), 368–372. https://doi.org/10.1080/14640747408400426

Unsworth, N., Robison, M. K., & Miller, A. L. (2021). Individual differences in lapses of attention: A latent variable analysis. *Journal of Experimental Psychology: General, 150*(7), 1303–1331. https://doi.org/10.1037/xge0000998

Utoomprurkporn, N., Hardy, C. J. D., Stott, J., Costafreda, S. G., Warren, J., & Bamiou, D. E. (2020). "The Dichotic Digit Test" as an index indicator for hearing problem in dementia: Systematic review and meta-analysis. *Journal of the American Academy of Audiology, 31*(9), 646–655. https://doi.org/10.1055/s-0040-1718700

Uttal, W. R. (2001). *The new phrenology: The limits of localizing cognitive processes in the brain.* MIT Press.

Valdez, P. (2019). Circadian rhythms in attention. *The Yale Journal of Biology and Medicine, 92*(1), 81–92.

Valian, V. (2015). Bilingualism and cognition. *Bilingualism: Language and Cognition, 18*(1), 3–24. https://doi.org/10.1017/S1366728914000522

Van den Bossche, P., Gijselaers, W., Segers, M., Woltjer, G., & Kirschner, P. (2011). Team learning: Building shared mental models. *Instructional Science, 39*(3), 283–301. https://doi.org/10.1007/s11251-010-9128-3

van den Brink, R. L., Murphy, P. R., & Nieuwenhuis, S. (2016). Pupil diameter tracks lapses of attention. *PLOS ONE, 11*(10), Article e0165274. https://doi.org/10.1371/journal.pone.0165274

van der Heijden, A. H. C. (1992). *Selective attention in vision*. Routledge.

van der Heijden, A. H. C. (1993). The role of position in object selection in vision. *Psychological Research, 56*(1), 44–58. https://doi.org/10.1007/BF00572132

van der Lubbe, R. H., & Abrahamse, E. L. (2011). The premotor theory of attention and the Simon effect. *Acta Psychologica, 136*(2), 259–264. https://doi.org/10.1016/j.actpsy.2010.09.007

van der Lubbe, R. H. J., Jaśkowski, P., Wauschkuhn, B., & Verleger, R. (2001). Influence of time pressure in a simple response task, a choice-by-location task, and the Simon task. *Journal of Psychophysiology, 15*(4), 241–255. https://doi.org/10.1027//0269-8803.15.4.241

van der Lubbe, R. H. J., Keuss, P. J. G., & Stoffels, E.-J. (1996). Threefold effect of peripheral precues: Alertness, orienting, and response tendencies. *Acta Psychologica, 94*(3), 319–337. https://doi.org/10.1016/S0001-6918(96)00005-4

van der Lubbe, R. H., & Verleger, R. (2002). Aging and the Simon task. *Psychophysiology, 39*(1), 100–110. https://doi.org/10.1111/1469-8986.3910100

Van Diepen, R. M., Foxe, J. J., & Mazaheri, A. (2019). The functional role of alpha-band activity in attentional processing: The current zeitgeist and future outlook. *Current Opinion in Psychology, 29*, 229–238. https://doi.org/10.1016/j.copsyc.2019.03.015

Van Doorn, L., & Zijlstra, F. R. H. (1988). Variation in response functions complicates the evaluation of scales. In W. E. Saris (Ed.), *Variation in response functions: A source of measurement error in attitude research* (pp. 87–97). Sociometric Research Foundation.

van Opstal, J. (2016). *The auditory system and human sound-localization behavior*. Academic Press.

Van Selst, M., Ruthruff, E., & Johnston, J. C. (1999). Can practice eliminate the psychological refractory period effect? *Journal of Experimental Psychology: Human Perception and Performance, 25*(5), 1268–1283. https://doi.org/10.1037/0096-1523.25.5.1268

Van Zandt, T. (2000). How to fit a response time distribution. *Psychonomic Bulletin & Review, 7*(3), 424–465. https://doi.org/10.3758/BF03214357

Vandierendonck, A., Liefooghe, B., & Verbruggen, F. (2010). Task switching: Interplay of reconfiguration and interference control. *Psychological Bulletin, 136*(4), 601–626. https://doi.org/10.1037/a0019791

Varghese, L., Bharadwaj, H. M., & Shinn-Cunningham, B. G. (2015). Evidence against attentional state modulating scalp-recorded auditory brainstem steady-state responses. *Brain Research, 1626*, 146–164. https://doi.org/10.1016/j.brainres.2015.06.038

Veltman, J. A., & Gaillard, A. W. K. (1993). Pilot workload evaluated with subjective and physiological measures. In K. Brookhuis, C. Weikert, J. Moraal, & D. de Waard (Eds.), *Aging and human factors* (pp. 107–128). University of Groningen Traffic Control Centre.

Veltman, J. A., & Gaillard, A. W. K. (1998). Physiological workload reactions to increasing levels of task difficulty. *Ergonomics, 41*(5), 656–669. https://doi.org/10.1080/001401398186829

Verbruggen, F., Aron, A. R., Band, G. P., Beste, C., Bissett, P. G., Brockett, A. T., Brown, J. W., Chamberlain, S. R., Chambers, C. D., Colonius, H., Colzato, L. S., Corneil, B. D., Coxon, J. P., Dupuis, A., Eagle, D. M., Garavan, H., Greenhouse, I., Heathcote, A., Huster, R. J., . . . Boehler, C. N. (2019). A consensus guide to capturing the ability to inhibit actions and impulsive behaviors in the stop-signal task. *eLife, 8*, Article e46323. https://doi.org/10.7554/eLife.46323

Verbruggen, F., & Logan, G. D. (2017). Control in response inhibition. In T. Egner (Ed.), *The Wiley handbook of cognitive control* (pp. 97–110). Wiley. https://doi.org/10.1002/9781118920497.ch6

Verhaeghen, P., & De Meersman, L. (1998). Aging and the Stroop effect: A meta-analysis. *Psychology and Aging, 13*(1), 120–126. https://doi.org/10.1037/0882-7974.13.1.120

Verleger, R. (1997). On the utility of P3 latency as an index of mental chronometry. *Psychophysiology, 34*(2), 131–156. https://doi.org/10.1111/j.1469-8986.1997.tb02125.x

Verwey, W. B., & Veltman, H. A. (1996). Detecting short periods of elevated workload: A comparison of nine workload assessment techniques. *Journal of Experimental Psychology: Applied, 2*(3), 270–285. https://doi.org/10.1037/1076-898X.2.3.270

Vicente, K. J., & Rasmussen, J. (1992). Ecological interface design: Theoretical foundations. *IEEE Transactions on Systems, Man, and Cybernetics, 22*(4), 589–606. https://doi.org/10.1109/21.156574

Vidulich, M. A. (2000). Testing the sensitivity of situation awareness metrics in interface evaluations. In M. R. Endsley & D. J. Garland (Eds.), *Situation awareness analysis and measurement* (pp. 227–246). Erlbaum.

Vidulich, M. A., & Tsang, P. S. (2012). Mental workload and situation awareness. In G. Salvendy (Ed.), *Handbook of human factors and ergonomics* (pp. 243–273). Wiley. https://doi.org/10.1002/9781118131350.ch8

Vince, M. A. (1948). The intermittency of control movements and the psychological refractory period. *British Journal of Psychology, 38*(Pt. 3), 149–157.

Virzi, R. A., & Egeth, H. E. (1985). Toward a translational model of Stroop interference. *Memory & Cognition, 13*(4), 304–319. https://doi.org/10.3758/BF03202499

Vitevitch, M. S. (2003). Change deafness: The inability to detect changes between two voices. *Journal of Experimental Psychology: Human Perception and Performance, 29*(2), 333–342. https://doi.org/10.1037/0096-1523.29.2.333

Vives, J. L. (1948). *Obras completas* [Complete works] (L. Riber, Trans.). M. Aguilar. (Original work published 1538)

Vogel, E. K., & Luck, S. J. (2000). The visual N1 component as an index of a discrimination process. *Psychophysiology, 37*(2), 190–203. https://doi.org/10.1111/1469-8986.3720190

Vogel, E. K., Luck, S. J., & Shapiro, K. L. (1998). Electrophysiological evidence for a postperceptual locus of suppression during the attentional blink. *Journal of Experimental Psychology: Human Perception and Performance, 24*(6), 1656–1674. https://doi.org/10.1037/0096-1523.24.6.1656

Volpe, C. E., Cannon-Bowers, J. A., Salas, E., & Spector, P. E. (1996). The impact of cross-training on team functioning: An empirical investigation. *Human Factors*, *38*(1), 87–100. https://doi.org/10.1518/001872096778940741

von Helmholtz, H. (1968). The origin of the correct interpretation of our sensory impressions. In R. M. Warren & R. P. Warren (Eds.), *Helmholtz on perception: Its physiology and development* (pp. 249–260). Wiley. (Original work published 1894)

von Salm-Hoogstraeten, S., Bolzius, K., & Müsseler, J. (2020). Seeing the world through the eyes of an avatar? Comparing perspective taking and referential coding. *Journal of Experimental Psychology: Human Perception and Performance*, *46*(3), 264–273. https://doi.org/10.1037/xhp0000711

Von Wright, J. M. (1968). Selection in visual immediate memory. *Quarterly Journal of Experimental Psychology*, *20*(1), 62–68. https://doi.org/10.1080/14640746808400128

Voyer, D. (2011). Sex differences in dichotic listening. *Brain and Cognition*, *76*(2), 245–255. https://doi.org/10.1016/j.bandc.2011.02.001

Vu, K.-P. L., & Chiappe, D. (2015). Situation awareness in human systems integration. In D. A. Boehm-Davis, F. T. Durso, & J. D. Lee (Eds.), *APA handbook of human systems integration* (pp. 293–308). American Psychological Association. https://doi.org/10.1037/14528-019

Vu, K.-P. L., Lachter, J., Battiste, V., & Strybel, T. Z. (2018). Single pilot operations in domestic commercial aviation. *Human Factors*, *60*(6), 755–762. https://doi.org/10.1177/0018720818791372

Vu, K.-P. L., & Proctor, R. W. (2001). Determinants of right-left and top-bottom prevalence for two-dimensional spatial compatibility. *Journal of Experimental Psychology: Human Perception and Performance*, *27*(4), 813–828. https://doi.org/10.1037/0096-1523.27.4.813

Vu, K.-P. L., & Proctor, R. W. (2002). The prevalence effect in two-dimensional stimulus-response compatibility is a function of the relative salience of the dimensions. *Perception & Psychophysics*, *64*(5), 815–828. https://doi.org/10.3758/BF03194748

Vu, K.-P. L., & Proctor, R. W. (2004). Mixing compatible and incompatible mappings: Elimination, reduction, and enhancement of spatial compatibility effects. *Quarterly Journal of Experimental Psychology*, *57*(3), 539–556. https://doi.org/10.1080/02724980343000387

Vu, K.-P. L., Proctor, R. W., & Hung, Y.-H. (2021). Website design and evaluation. In G. Salvendy & W. Karwowski (Eds.), *Handbook of human factors and ergonomics* (5th ed., pp. 1016–1036). Wiley. https://doi.org/10.1002/9781119636113.ch39

Vu, K.-P. L., Proctor, R. W., & Urcuioli, P. (2003). Transfer effects of incompatible location-relevant mappings on a subsequent visual or auditory Simon task. *Memory & Cognition*, *31*(7), 1146–1152. https://doi.org/10.3758/BF03196135

Vu, K.-P. L., Strybel, T. Z., & Proctor, R. W. (2006). Effects of displacement magnitude and direction of auditory cues on auditory spatial facilitation of visual search. *Human Factors*, *48*(3), 587–599. https://doi.org/10.1518/001872006778606796

Vu, K.-P. L., & Sun, Y. (2019). Population stereotypes for objects and representations: Response tendencies for interacting with everyday objects and interfaces. *Human Factors*, *61*(6), 953–975. https://doi.org/10.1177/0018720818823570

Wagenmakers, E. J., van der Maas, H. L., & Grasman, R. P. (2007). An EZ-diffusion model for response time and accuracy. *Psychonomic Bulletin & Review*, *14*(1), 3–22. https://doi.org/10.3758/BF03194023

Wagner, I., & Schnotz, W. (2017). Learning from static and dynamic visualizations: What kind of questions should we ask? In R. Lowe & R. Ploetzner (Eds.), *Learning from dynamic visualization* (pp. 69–91). Springer. https://doi.org/10.1007/978-3-319-56204-9_4

Wagner, U., Giesen, A., Knausenberger, J., & Echterhoff, G. (2017). The joint action effect on memory as a social phenomenon: The role of cued attention and psychological distance. *Frontiers in Psychology, 8*, Article 1697. https://doi.org/10.3389/fpsyg.2017.01697

Walker, B. N., & Ehrenstein, A. (2000). Pitch and pitch change interact in auditory displays. *Journal of Experimental Psychology: Applied, 6*(1), 15–30. https://doi.org/10.1037/1076-898X.6.1.15

Wallace, R. J. (1971). S-R compatibility and the idea of a response code. *Journal of Experimental Psychology, 88*(3), 354–360. https://doi.org/10.1037/h0030892

Walter, J., Buon, M., Glaviaux, B., & Brunel, L. (2021). Excluded but not alone. Does social exclusion prevent the occurrence of a Joint Simon Effect (JSE)? *Acta Psychologica, 218*, Article 103337. https://doi.org/10.1016/j.actpsy.2021.103337

Walter, S., & Meier, B. (2014). How important is importance for prospective memory? A review. *Frontiers in Psychology, 5*, Article 657. https://doi.org/10.3389/fpsyg.2014.00657

Wang, D.-Y. D., Proctor, R. W., & Pick, D. F. (2007). Acquisition and transfer of attention allocation strategies in a multiple-task work environment. *Human Factors, 49*(6), 995–1004. https://doi.org/10.1518/001872007X249866

Ward, L. M. (1994). Supramodal and modality-specific mechanisms for stimulus-driven shifts of auditory and visual attention. *Canadian Journal of Experimental Psychology, 48*(2), 242–259. https://doi.org/10.1037/1196-1961.48.2.242

Ward, L. M., McDonald, J. J., & Golestani, N. (1998). Crossmodal control of attention shifts. In R. D. Wright (Ed.), *Visual attention* (pp. 232–268). Oxford University Press.

Ward, L. M., McDonald, J. J., & Lin, D. (2000). On asymmetries in cross-modal spatial attention orienting. *Perception & Psychophysics, 62*(6), 1258–1264. https://doi.org/10.3758/BF03212127

Warm, J. S., Dember, W. N., & Hancock, P. A. (1996). Vigilance and workload in automated systems. In R. Parasuraman & M. Mouloua (Eds.), *Attention and human performance: Theories and applications* (pp. 183–200). Erlbaum.

Warm, J. S., Parasuraman, R., & Matthews, G. (2008). Vigilance requires hard mental work and is stressful. *Human Factors, 50*(3), 433–441. https://doi.org/10.1518/001872008X312152

Washburn, M. F. (1914). The function of incipient motor processes. *Psychological Review, 21*(5), 376–390. https://doi.org/10.1037/h0072419

Wassermann, E. M., & Lisanby, S. H. (2001). Therapeutic application of repetitive transcranial magnetic stimulation: A review. *Clinical Neurophysiology, 112*(8), 1367–1377. https://doi.org/10.1016/S1388-2457(01)00585-5

Watson, D. G., & Humphreys, G. W. (1997). Visual marking: Prioritizing selection for new objects by top-down attentional inhibition of old objects. *Psychological Review, 104*(1), 90–122. https://doi.org/10.1037/0033-295X.104.1.90

Watson, D. G., & Humphreys, G. W. (1998). Visual marking of moving objects: A role for top-down feature-based inhibition in selection. *Journal of Experimental Psychology: Human Perception and Performance, 24*(3), 946–962. https://doi.org/10.1037/0096-1523.24.3.946

Watson, D. G., & Humphreys, G. W. (2000). Visual marking: Evidence for inhibition using a probe-dot detection paradigm. *Perception & Psychophysics*, *62*(3), 471–481. https://doi.org/10.3758/BF03212099

Watson, D. G., Humphreys, G. W., & Olivers, C. N. (2003). Visual marking: Using time in visual selection. *Trends in Cognitive Sciences*, *7*(4), 180–186. https://doi.org/10.1016/S1364-6613(03)00033-0

Watson, P., van Wingen, G., & de Wit, S. (2018). Conflicted between goal-directed and habitual control, an fMRI investigation. *eNeuro*, *5*(4), Article 0240-18.2018. https://doi.org/10.1523/ENEURO.0240-18.2018

Watt, H. J. (1906). Experimental contribution to a theory of thinking. *Journal of Anatomy and Physiology*, *40*, 257–266. (Original work published 1904)

Weber, E. H. (1978). *The sense of touch* (D. J. Murray, Trans.). Academic Press. (Original work published 1846)

Webster, J. C., & Thompson, P. O. (1954). Responding to both of two overlapping messages. *The Journal of the Acoustical Society of America*, *26*(3), 396–402. https://doi.org/10.1121/1.1907348

Weintraub, D. J., & Ensing, M. (1992). *Human factors issues in head-up display: The book of HUD.* CSERIAC.

Weissman, D. H., Drake, B., Colella, K., & Samuel, D. (2018). Perceptual load is not always a crucial determinant of early versus late selection. *Acta Psychologica*, *185*, 125–135. https://doi.org/10.1016/j.actpsy.2018.02.004

Welch, J. C. (1898). On the measurement of mental activity through muscular activity and the determination of a constant of attention. *The American Journal of Physiology*, *1*(3), 283–306. https://doi.org/10.1152/ajplegacy.1898.1.3.283

Welford, A. T. (1952). The "psychological refractory period" and the timing of high-speed performance: A review and a theory. *British Journal of Psychology*, *43*, 2–19.

Welford, A. T. (1976). *Skilled performance: Perceptual and motor skills.* Scott & Foresman.

Welford, A. T. (1980). On the nature of higher-order skills. *Journal of Occupational Psychology*, *53*(2), 107–110. https://doi.org/10.1111/j.2044-8325.1980.tb00013.x

Weltman, G., Smith, J. E., & Egstrom, G. H. (1971). Perceptual narrowing during simulated pressure-chamber exposure. *Human Factors*, *13*(2), 99–107. https://doi.org/10.1177/001872087101300202

Wesslein, A. K., Spence, C., Mast, F., & Frings, C. (2016). Spatial negative priming: In touch, it's all about location. *Attention, Perception, & Psychophysics*, *78*(2), 464–473. https://doi.org/10.3758/s13414-015-1028-9

West, R., & Baylis, G. C. (1998). Effects of increased response dominance and con-textual disintegration on the Stroop interference effect in older adults. *Psychology and Aging*, *13*(2), 206–217. https://doi.org/10.1037/0882-7974.13.2.206

Westerhausen, R. (2019). A primer on dichotic listening as a paradigm for the assessment of hemispheric asymmetry. *Laterality*, *24*(6), 740–771. https://doi.org/10.1080/1357650X.2019.1598426

Weyers, B., Bowen, J., Dix, A., & Palanque, P. (Eds.). (2017). *The handbook of formal methods in human-computer interaction.* Springer. https://doi.org/10.1007/978-3-319-51838-1

Wheeler, M. E., & Treisman, A. M. (2002). Binding in short-term visual memory. *Journal of Experimental Psychology: General*, *131*(1), 48–64. https://doi.org/10.1037/0096-3445.131.1.48

Wickelgren, W. A. (1977). Speed-accuracy tradeoff and information processing dynamics. *Acta Psychologica, 41*(1), 67–85. https://doi.org/10.1016/0001-6918(77) 90012-9

Wickens, C. D. (1980). The structure of attentional resources. In R. Nickerson (Ed.), *Attention and performance VIII* (pp. 239–257). Erlbaum.

Wickens, C. D. (1984). Processing resources in attention. In R. Parasuraman & D. R. Davies (Eds.), *Varieties of attention* (pp. 63–102). Academic Press.

Wickens, C. D. (1999). Cognitive factors in aviation. In F. T. Durso (Ed.), *Handbook of applied cognition* (pp. 247–282). Wiley.

Wickens, C. D. (2008). Multiple resources and mental workload. *Human Factors, 50*(3), 449–455. https://doi.org/10.1518/001872008X288394

Wickens, C. D. (2021). Attention: Theory, principles, models and applications. *International Journal of Human–Computer Interaction, 37*(5), 403–417. https://doi.org/ 10.1080/10447318.2021.1874741

Wickens, C. D., & Andre, A. D. (1990). Proximity compatibility and information display: Effects of color, space, and object display on information integration. *Human Factors, 32*(1), 61–77. https://doi.org/10.1177/001872089003200105

Wickens, C. D., & Carswell, C. M. (1995). The proximity compatibility principle: Its psycho-logical foundation and relevance to display design. *Human Factors, 37*(3), 473–494. https://doi.org/10.1518/001872095779049408

Wickens, C. D., & Carswell, C. M. (2021). Information processing. In G. Salvendy & W. Karwowski (Eds.), *Handbook of human factors and ergonomics* (Vol. 5, pp. 114–158). Wiley. https://doi.org/10.1002/9781119636113.ch5

Wickens, C. D., Gordon Becker, S. E., Liu, Y., & Lee, J. D. (2004). *An introduction to human factors engineering* (2nd ed.). Pearson.

Wickens, C. D., Hollands, J. G., Banbury, S., & Parasuraman, R. (2016). *Engineering psychology and human performance* (5th ed.). Routledge.

Wickens, C. D., Hyman, F., Dellinger, J., Taylor, H., & Meador, M. (1986). The Sternberg memory search task as an index of pilot workload. *Ergonomics, 29*(11), 1371–1383. https://doi.org/10.1080/00140138608967252

Wickens, C. D., & Long, J. (1995). Object versus space-based models of visual attention: Implications for the design of head-up displays. *Journal of Experimental Psychology: Applied, 1*(3), 179–193. https://doi.org/10.1037/1076-898X. 1.3.179

Widyanti, A., Muslim, K., & Sutalaksana, I. Z. (2017). The sensitivity of Galvanic Skin Response for assessing mental workload in Indonesia. *Work, 56*(1), 111–117. https://doi.org/10.3233/WOR-162479

Wiener, N. (1950). Cybernetics. *Bulletin of the American Academy of Arts and Sciences, 3*(7), 2–4. https://doi.org/10.2307/3822945

Wiesman, A. I., Rezich, M. T., O'Neill, J., Morsey, B., Wang, T., Ideker, T., Swindells, S., Fox, H. S., & Wilson, T. W. (2020). Epigenetic markers of aging predict the neural oscillations serving selective attention. *Cerebral Cortex, 30*(3), 1234–1243. https://doi.org/10.1093/cercor/bhz162

Wijers, A. A., Lange, J. J., Mulder, G., & Mulder, L. J. (1997). An ERP study of visual spatial attention and letter target detection for isoluminant and non-isoluminant stimuli. *Psychophysiology, 34*(5), 553–565. https://doi.org/10.1111/ j.1469-8986.1997.tb01742.x

Wikman, A.-S., Nieminen, T., & Summala, N. (1998). Driving experience and time-sharing during in-car tasks on roads of different width. *Ergonomics, 41*(3), 358–372. https://doi.org/10.1080/001401398187080

Wilcocks, R. W. (1925). An examination of Külpe's experiments on abstraction. *The American Journal of Psychology*, *36*(3), 324–341. https://doi.org/10.2307/1414160

Wilkinson, R. T. (1962). Muscle tension during mental work under sleep deprivation. *Journal of Experimental Psychology*, *64*(6), 565–571. https://doi.org/10.1037/h0043570

Willcutt, E. G., Doyle, A. E., Nigg, J. T., Faraone, S. V., & Pennington, B. F. (2005). Validity of the executive function theory of attention-deficit/hyperactivity disorder: A meta-analytic review. *Biological Psychiatry*, *57*(11), 1336–1346. https://doi.org/10.1016/j.biopsych.2005.02.006

Williams, J. M. G., Mathews, A., & MacLeod, C. (1996). The emotional Stroop task and psychopathology. *Psychological Bulletin*, *120*(1), 3–24. https://doi.org/10.1037/0033-2909.120.1.3

Williams, P., & Simons, D. J. (2000). Detecting changes in novel, complex three-dimensional objects. *Visual Cognition*, *7*(1-3), 297–322. https://doi.org/10.1080/135062800394829

Wilson, G. F. (2002). An analysis of mental workload in pilots during flight using multiple psychophysiological measures. *The International Journal of Aviation Psychology*, *12*(1), 3–18. https://doi.org/10.1207/S15327108IJAP1201_2

Wittgenstein, L. (1953). *Philosophical investigations*. Blackwell.

Wixted, J. T. (2020). The forgotten history of signal detection theory. *Journal of Experimental Psychology: Learning, Memory, and Cognition*, *46*(2), 201–233. https://doi.org/10.1037/xlm0000732

Woldorff, M. G., Hillyard, S. A., Gallen, C. C., Hampson, S. R., & Bloom, F. E. (1998). Magnetoencephalographic recordings demonstrate attentional modulation of mismatch-related neural activity in human auditory cortex. *Psychophysiology*, *35*(3), 283–292. https://doi.org/10.1017/S0048577298961601

Wolfe, J. M. (1994). Guided Search 2.0 A revised model of visual search. *Psychonomic Bulletin & Review*, *1*(2), 202–238. https://doi.org/10.3758/BF03200774

Wolfe, J. M. (1998). What can 1 million trials tell us about visual search? *Psychological Science*, *9*(1), 33–39. https://doi.org/10.1111/1467-9280.00006

Wolfe, J. M. (2001). Asymmetries in visual search: An introduction. *Perception & Psychophysics*, *63*(3), 381–389. https://doi.org/10.3758/BF03194406

Wolfe, J. M. (2020). Forty years after feature integration theory: An introduction to the special issue in honor of the contributions of Anne Treisman. *Attention, Perception, & Psychophysics*, *82*(1), 1–6. https://doi.org/10.3758/s13414-019-01966-3

Wolfe, J. M. (2021). Guided Search 6.0: An updated model of visual search. *Psychonomic Bulletin & Review*, *28*(4), 1060–1092. https://doi.org/10.3758/s13423-020-01859-9

Wolfe, J. M., Butcher, S. J., Lee, C., & Hyle, M. (2003). Changing your mind: On the contributions of top-down and bottom-up guidance in visual search for feature singletons. *Journal of Experimental Psychology: Human Perception and Performance*, *29*(2), 483–502. https://doi.org/10.1037/0096-1523.29.2.483

Wolfe, J. M., Cave, K. R., & Franzel, S. L. (1989). Guided search: An alternative to the feature integration model for visual search. *Journal of Experimental Psychology: Human Perception and Performance*, *15*(3), 419–433. https://doi.org/10.1037/0096-1523.15.3.419

Wolfe, J. M., & Horowitz, T. S. (2017). Five factors that guide attention in visual search. *Nature Human Behaviour, 1,* Article 0058. https://doi.org/10.1038/s41562-017-0058

Wolfe, J. M., & Utochkin, I. S. (2019). What is a preattentive feature? *Current Opinion in Psychology, 29,* 19–26. https://doi.org/10.1016/j.copsyc.2018.11.005

Wolff, C. (1738). *Psychologia empirica* [Empirical psychology]. Officina Libraria Rengeriana.

Wolff, C. (1740). *Psychologia rationalis* [Rational psychology]. Officina Libraria Rengeriana.

Wolters, N. C. W., & Schiano, D. J. (1989). On listening where we look: The fragility of a phenomenon. *Perception & Psychophysics, 45*(2), 184–186. https://doi.org/10.3758/BF03208053

Wood, N. L., & Cowan, N. (1995). The cocktail party phenomenon revisited: Attention and memory in the classic selective listening procedure of Cherry (1953). *Journal of Experimental Psychology: General, 124*(3), 243–262. https://doi.org/10.1037/0096-3445.124.3.243

Woodman, G. F., & Luck, S. J. (2003). Serial deployment of attention during visual search. *Journal of Experimental Psychology: Human Perception and Performance, 29*(1), 121–138. https://doi.org/10.1037/0096-1523.29.1.121

Woodworth, R. S. (1899). The accuracy of voluntary movement. *The Psychological Review: Monograph Supplements, 3*(3), i–114. https://doi.org/10.1037/h0092992

Woodworth, R. S. (1938). *Experimental psychology.* Holt.

Wright, E. (Director). (2021). *The Sparks brothers* [Film]. Complete Fiction Pictures.

Wright, R. D., & Ward, L. M. (2008). *Orienting of Attention.* Oxford University Press.

Wundt, W. (1880). *Grundzüge der physiologischen* [Basic features of physiology] (2nd ed.). Wilhelm Engelman.

Wundt, W. (1907a). *Lectures on human and animal psychology* (J. B. Creighton & E. B. Titchener, Trans.). Macmillan.

Wundt, W. (1907b). *Outlines of psychology* (3rd rev., C. H. Judd, Trans.). Engelmann.

Wundt, W. (1912). *An introduction to psychology.* Allen & Unwin. https://doi.org/10.1037/13784-000

Wurtz, R. H., & Goldberg, M. E. (1972). The primate superior colliculus and the shift of visual attention. *Investigative Ophthalmology & Visual Science, 11*(6), 441–450.

Xiang, W. (2021). Implicit detection observation in different features, exposure duration, and delay during change blindness. *Frontiers in Psychology, 11,* Article 607863. https://doi.org/10.3389/fpsyg.2020.607863

Xiong, A., & Proctor, R. W. (2015). Referential coding of steering-wheel button presses in a simulated driving cockpit. *Journal of Experimental Psychology: Applied, 21*(4), 418–428. https://doi.org/10.1037/xap0000060

Xiong, A., & Proctor, R. W. (2018). Information processing: The language and analytical tools for cognitive psychology in the information age. *Frontiers in Psychology, 9,* Article 1270. https://doi.org/10.3389/fpsyg.2018.01270

Xu, J., Monterosso, J., Kober, H., Balodis, I. M., & Potenza, M. N. (2011). Perceptual load-dependent neural correlates of distractor interference inhibition. *PLOS ONE, 6*(1), Article e14552. https://doi.org/10.1371/journal.pone.0014552

Xu, J., Slagle, J. M., Banerjee, A., Bracken, B., & Weinger, M. B. (2019). Use of a portable functional near-infrared spectroscopy (fnirs) system to examine team experience during crisis event management in clinical simulations.

Frontiers in Human Neuroscience, 13, Article 85. https://doi.org/10.3389/fnhum. 2019.00085

Yamaguchi, M., Chen, J., Mishler, S., & Proctor, R. W. (2018). Flowers and spiders in spatial stimulus-response compatibility: Does affective valence influence selection of task-sets or selection of responses? *Cognition and Emotion, 32*(5), 1003–1017. https://doi.org/10.1080/02699931.2017.1381073

Yamaguchi, M., & Proctor, R. W. (2012). Multidimensional vector model of stimulus-response compatibility. *Psychological Review, 119*(2), 272–303. https://doi.org/10.1037/a0026620

Yamaguchi, M., Wall, H. J., & Hommel, B. (2018). Sharing tasks or sharing actions? Evidence from the joint Simon task. *Psychological Research, 82*(2), 385–394. https://doi.org/10.1007/s00426-016-0821-y

Yang, Q., Song, X., Dong, M., Li, J., & Proctor, R. W. (2021). The underlying neural mechanisms of interpersonal situations on collaborative ability: A hyperscanning study using functional near-infrared spectroscopy. *Social Neuroscience, 16*(5), 549–563. https://doi.org/10.1080/17470919.2021.1965017

Yantis, S. (1988). On analog movements of visual attention. *Perception & Psychophysics, 43*(2), 203–206. https://doi.org/10.3758/BF03214200

Yantis, S., & Hilstrom, A. P. (1994). Stimulus-driven attentional capture: Evidence from equiluminant visual objects. *Journal of Experimental Psychology: Human Perception and Performance, 20*, 95–107. https://doi.org/10.1037/0096-1523.20.1.95

Yantis, S., & Johnston, J. C. (1990). On the locus of visual selection: Evidence from focused attention tasks. *Journal of Experimental Psychology: Human Perception and Performance, 16*(1), 135–149. https://doi.org/10.1037/0096-1523.16.1.135

Yantis, S., & Jonides, J. (1984). Abrupt visual onsets and selective attention: Evidence from visual search. *Journal of Experimental Psychology: Human Perception and Performance, 10*(5), 601–621. https://doi.org/10.1037/0096-1523.10.5.601

Yaple, Z., & Arsalidou, M. (2017). Negative priming: A meta-analysis of fMRI studies. *Experimental Brain Research, 235*(11), 3367–3374. https://doi.org/10.1007/s00221-017-5065-6

Yarbus, A. L. (1967). *Eye movements and vision*. Springer. https://doi.org/10.1007/978-1-4899-5379-7

Yerkes, R. M., & Dodson, J. D. (1908). The relation of strength of stimulus to rapidity of habit formation. *Journal of Comparative Neurology & Psychology, 18*, 459–482. https://doi.org/10.1002/cne.920180503

Yi, W., Kang, M.-S., & Lee, K.-M. (2018). Visual attribute modulates the time course of iconic memory decay. *Visual Cognition, 26*(4), 223–230. https://doi.org/10.1080/13506285.2017.1416007

Yuan, P., & Raz, N. (2014). Prefrontal cortex and executive functions in healthy adults: A meta-analysis of structural neuroimaging studies. *Neuroscience and Biobehavioral Reviews, 42*, 180–192. https://doi.org/10.1016/j.neubiorev.2014.02.005

Zhang, Q., Walsh, M. M., & Anderson, J. R. (2018). The impact of inserting an additional mental process. *Computational Brain & Behavior, 1*(1), 22–35. https://doi.org/10.1007/s42113-018-0002-8

Zhang, Y., Chen, Y., Bressler, S. L., & Ding, M. (2008). Response preparation and inhibition: The role of the cortical sensorimotor beta rhythm. *Neuroscience, 156*(1), 238–246. https://doi.org/10.1016/j.neuroscience.2008.06.061

Zhang, Y., & Proctor, R. W. (2008). Influence of intermixed emotion-relevant trials on the affective Simon effect. *Experimental Psychology, 55*(6), 409–416. https://doi.org/10.1027/1618-3169.55.6.409

Zimmermann, K. M., Bischoff, M., Lorey, B., Stark, R., Munzert, J., & Zentgraf, K. (2012). Neural correlates of switching attentional focus during finger movements: An fMRI study. *Frontiers in Psychology, 3,* 1–11. https://doi.org/10.3389/fpsyg.2012.00555

Zorzi, M., Mapelli, D., Rusconi, E., & Umiltà, C. (2003). Automatic spatial coding of perceived gaze direction is revealed by the Simon effect. *Psychonomic Bulletin & Review, 10*(2), 423–429. https://doi.org/10.3758/BF03196501

Zwahlen, H. T., Adams, C. C., Jr., & DeBald, D. P. (1988). Safety aspects of CRT touch panel controls in automobiles. In A. G. Gale, M. H. Freeman, C. M. Haselgrave, P. Smith, & S. P. Taylor (Eds.), *Vision in vehicles II* (pp. 335–344). North-Holland.

INDEX

ABOUT THE AUTHORS

Robert W. Proctor, PhD, is a distinguished professor of psychological sciences at Purdue University. Dr. Proctor has published over 275 articles in basic and applied human performance and numerous books and chapters. His coauthored books include *Attention: Theory and Practice* (2004), *Human Factors in Simple and Complex Systems* (3rd ed., 2018), and *Skill Acquisition and Training* (2017). Dr. Proctor is the editor of the *American Journal of Psychology*, which was established in 1887. He is a fellow of the American Psychological Association (APA), the Psychonomic Society, the Association for Psychological Science, and the Human Factors and Ergonomics Society. Dr. Proctor received the 2013 Franklin V. Taylor Award for Outstanding Contributions in the Field of Applied Experimental/ Engineering Psychology from APA's Division 21 (Applied Experimental and Engineering Psychology) and the 2018 Paul M. Fitts Education Award for outstanding contributions to the education and training of human factors and ergonomics specialties from the Human Factors and Ergonomics Society.

Kim-Phuong L. Vu, PhD, is a professor of psychology at California State University, Long Beach. Dr. Vu has over 100 publications relating to human performance, human factors, and human–computer interaction. She coedited the *Handbook of Human Factors in Web Design* (2011) and has served as associate editor for *Behavior Research Methods* and *Human Factors*. Dr. Vu is a fellow of the American Psychological Association (APA), the Association for Psychological Science, and the Human Factors and Ergonomics Society and recipient of the 2021 Franklin V. Taylor Award for Outstanding Contributions in the Field of Applied Experimental/Engineering Psychology from APA's Division 21 (Applied Experimental and Engineering Psychology). She specializes in developing implications of basic research findings for applied design problems.

Drs. Proctor and Vu have coauthored many publications relating to attention and performance. They are coauthors of the book *Stimulus–Response Compatibility Principles: Data, Theory, and Application* (2006). Much of their recent work has been bringing together basic and applied knowledge of attention and performance in the context of multidisciplinary research. They coedited special issues of *American Psychologist* on "How Psychologists Help Solve Real-World Problems in Multidisciplinary Research Teams" and the *International Journal of Human–Computer Interaction* on "Foundations of Cognitive Science for the Design of Human–Computer Interactive Systems."